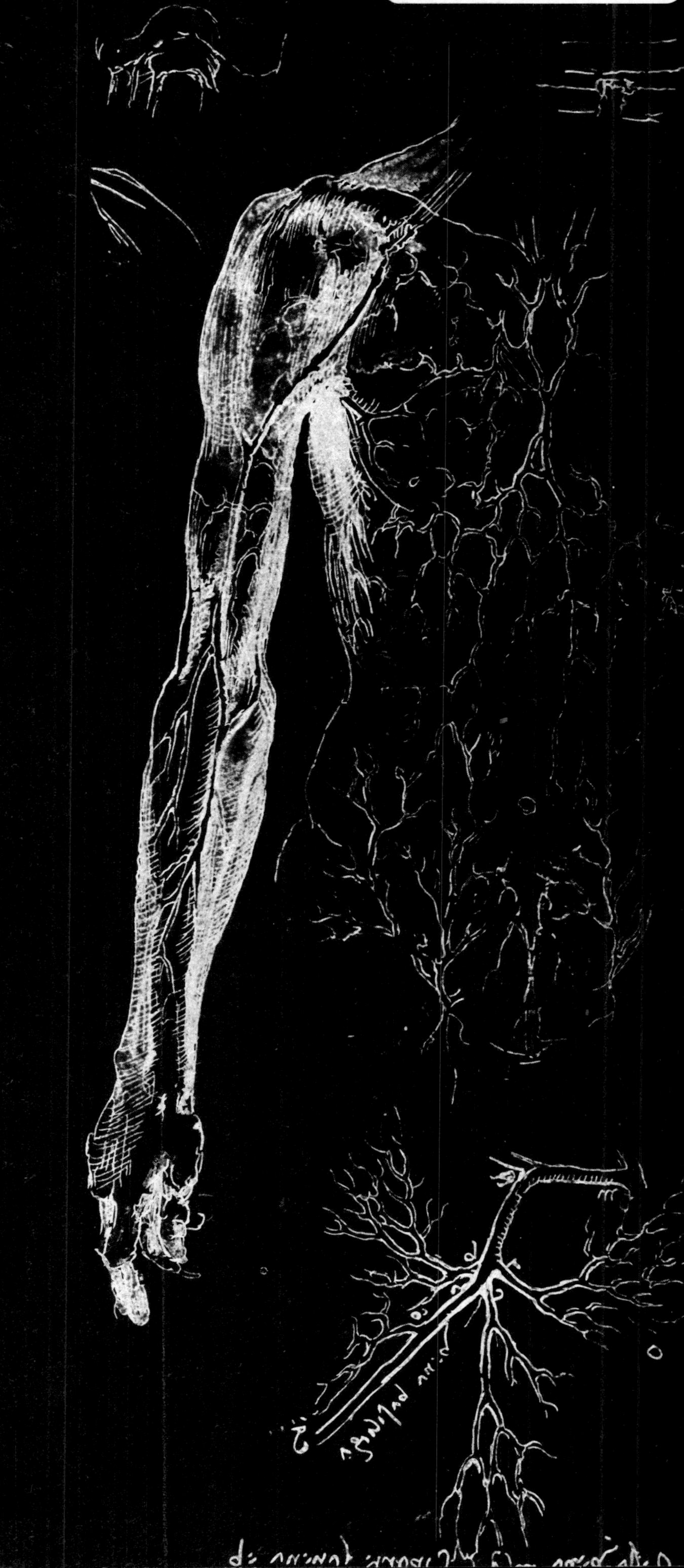

An Illustrated History of Medicine

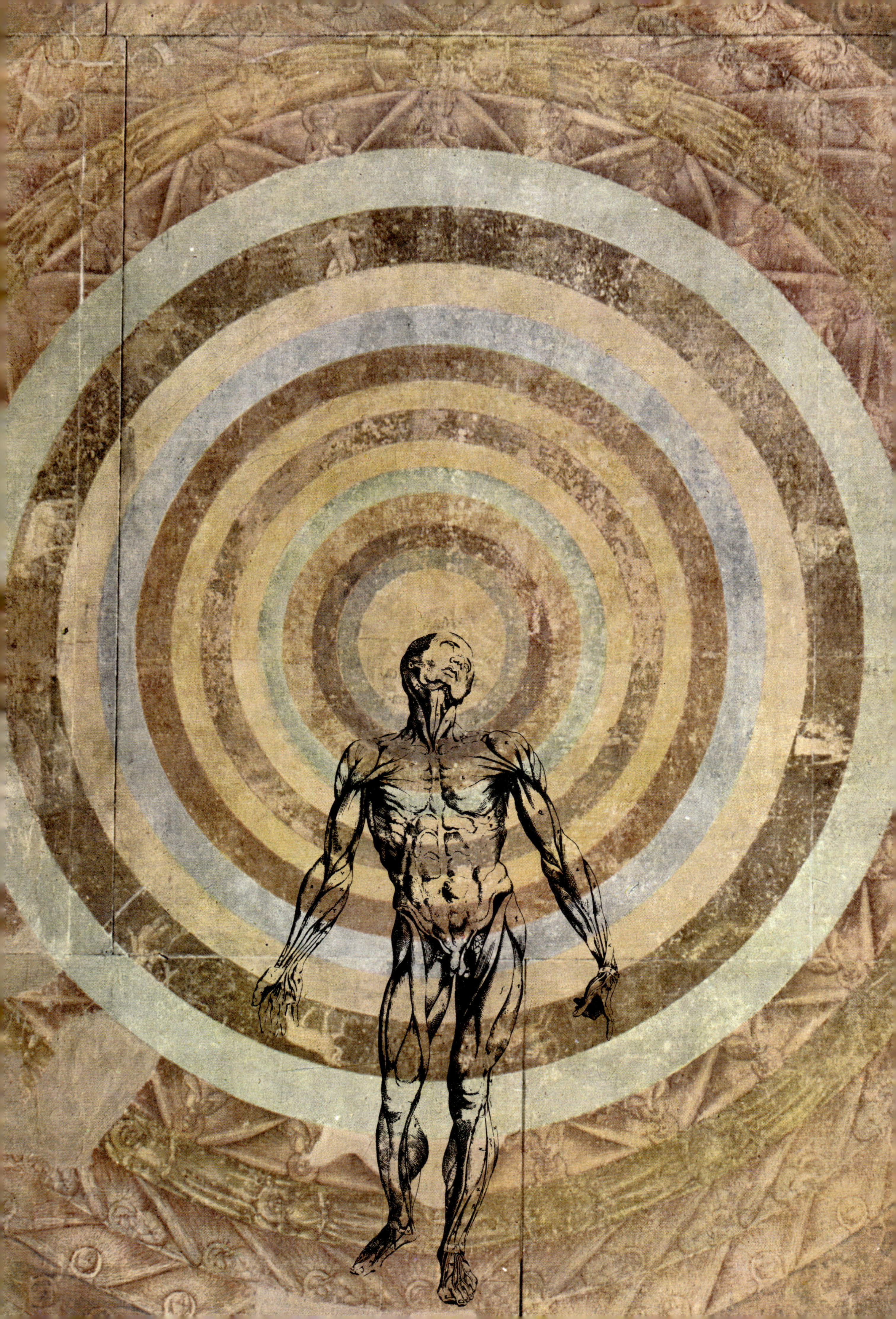

An Illustrated History of

MEDICINE

By Roberto Margotta

Edited by Paul Lewis
M.B., M.R.C.P., Institute of Neurology, London

Paul Hamlyn

Foreword

The purpose of this book is to present, in simple terms, a picture of the main stages of medicine in its evolution through the centuries. The story begins with the magic-imbued medicine of primitive man and concludes with a survey of modern achievements.

This book will have fulfilled its aim if the reader becomes aware of two themes in particular. One is the continuous nature of medical development, which must be regarded as still at an early stage. Thus present-day theory and practice incorporates knowledge acquired over hundreds of years, while indeed many ancient ideas and some ancient forms of medicine survive to this day, especially in societies resembling those that evolved them and remaining to a greater or lesser extent cut off from modern scientific thought. Despite the achievements of the last century, orthodox medical practice, unlike the scientific disciplines on which it is founded, remains by and large a matter of observation, opinion, and experience, and a knowledge of the wrong turnings of the past is essential if the doctor of today is not to be arrogant in his overestimation of his powers. This applies not only to the clinician but also sometimes to the research worker, who, forgetting the heritage of William Harvey, starts from an incomplete set of findings and attempts to construct an edifice of knowledge based on Aristotelian logic and the power of argument, ignoring outside evidence and putting forward shaky new concepts–thereby committing a fundamental error and turning the clock back two thousand years.

The other theme is the importance of the act of faith on the part of the patient in his relationship with the doctor, something which is no less a vital element of healing today, when rational and radical cures are available for many diseases, than it was when medicine was entirely magical and empirical. At this point it should be added that because the concern of this book is with the mainstream of medical development through the ages, such highly efficient and beneficial contemporary practices as osteopathy, whose rationale or system goes against the generally accepted concepts of anatomy, physiology and pathology, will not be considered.

Published by The Hamlyn Publishing Group, 42 The Centre, Feltham, Middlesex

Printed and bound in Italy–Officine Grafiche A. Mondadori–Verona

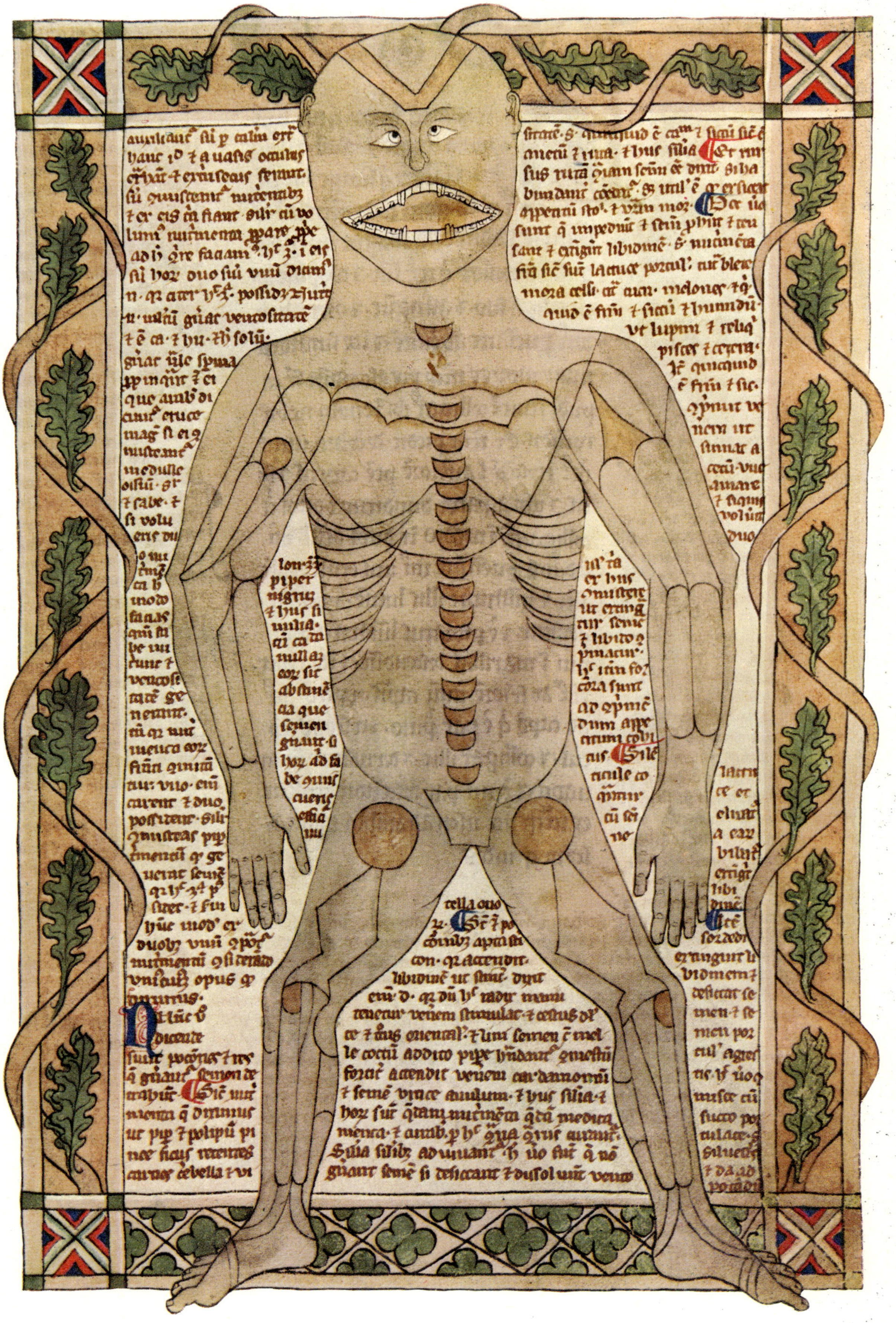

Contents

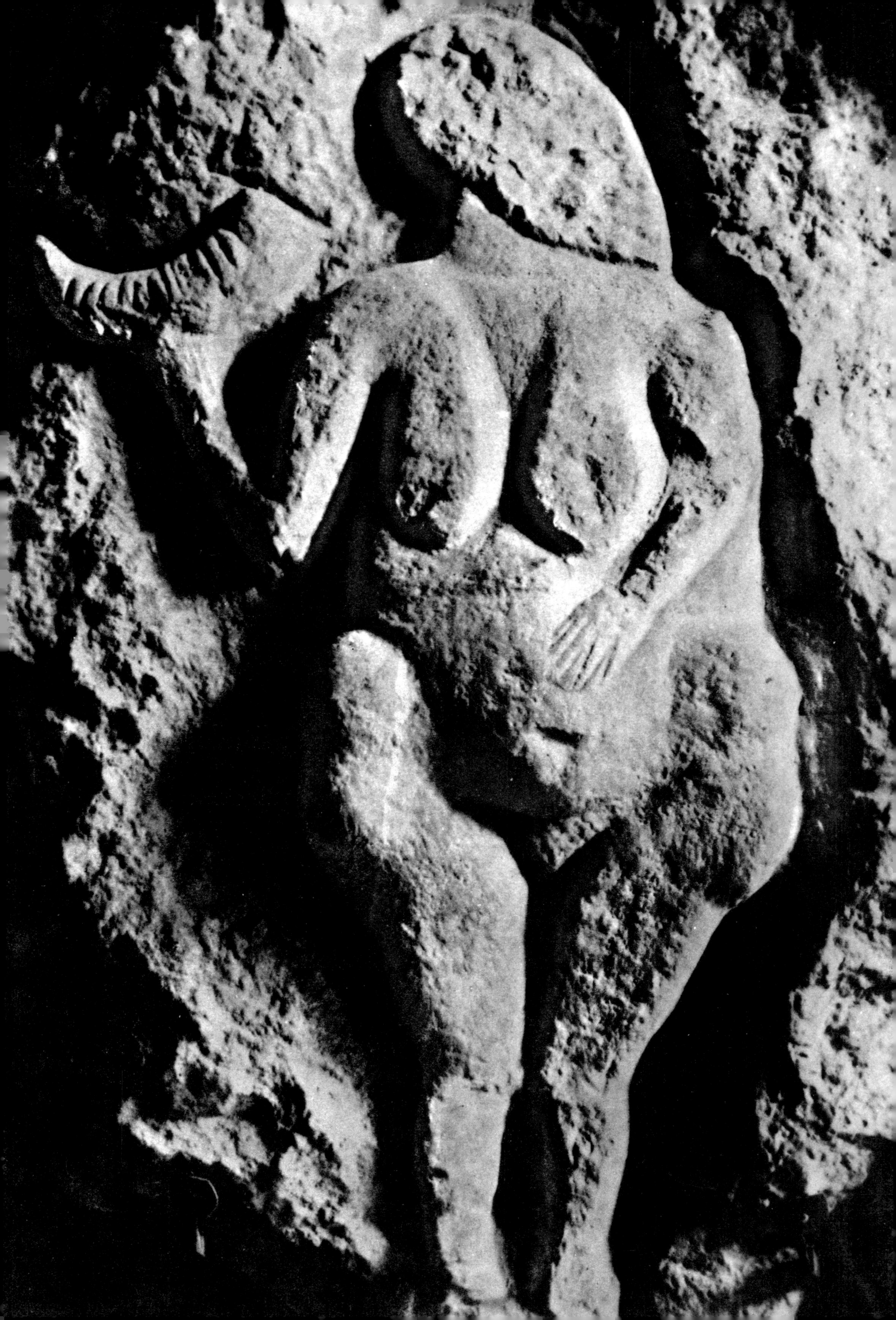

PRIMITIVE MAN
Magic and empirical medicine

If we understand medicine to be the conscious attempt by man to fight disease, then the art must surely be as old as human consciousness itself. Palaeontologists have revealed signs of pathological conditions in very ancient remains; injuries and diseases have always been hazards of living beings, and man is as vulnerable as any other. But what form the earliest medicine took must be entirely a matter for conjecture, in the absence of documentary evidence.

Medical historians have suggested many different origins, but until fairly recent times none of them come close to the truth. Many writers, like John Freind (1675–1728), the first Englishman in this field, did not acknowledge the existence of medicine before Galen and the Christian era, while subsequent historians saw fit to enumerate the achievements of individuals, presenting a mixture of freakish notions and quasi-modern concepts, without illuminating the continuously evolving nature of history.

An early attempt at a guess, perhaps the first, was that of Hippocrates of Cos, who in the fifth century BC wrote:

'In the first place the science of medicine would never have been discovered, nor, indeed, sought for, were there no need for it. If sick men fared just as well eating and drinking and living exactly as healthy men do, and no better on some different regimen, there would be little need for the science. But the reason why the art of medicine became necessary was because sick men did not get well on the same regimen as the healthy, any more than they do now. What is more, I am of the opinion that our present way of living and our present diet would not have come about if it had proved adequate for a man to eat and drink the same things as . . . all the other animals. . . . In primitive times, men often suffered terribly from their indigestible and animal-like diet, eating raw and uncooked food, difficult to digest. They suffered as men would suffer now from such a diet, being liable to violent pain and sickness and a speedy death.

'For this reason I believe these primitive men sought food suitable to their constitutions and discovered that which we now use. They boiled and baked and mixed and diluted the strong raw foods with the weaker ones and subjected them to many other processes always with a view to man's nature and his capabilities. They knew that if strong food

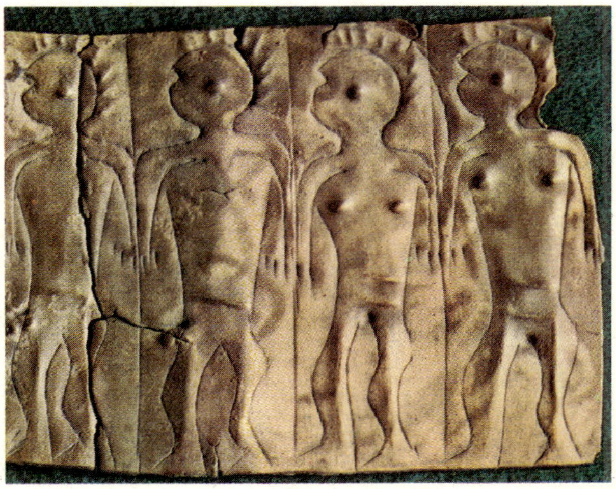

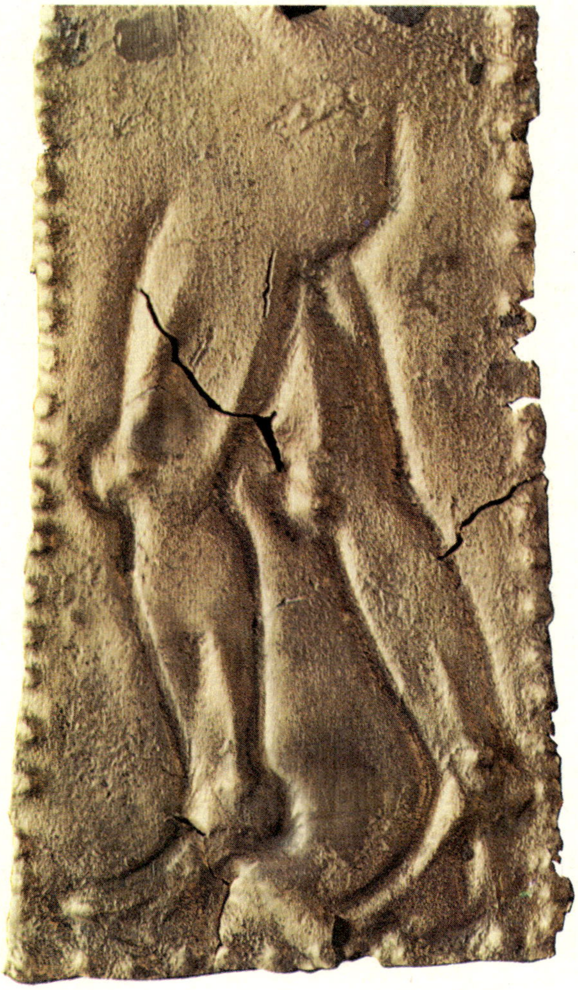

Previous pages :
Prehistoric Venus of Laussel. *Rock carving. Dordogne.*

Early representations of the human body. *Palaeo-venetic art. Civic Museum, Vicenza.*

These pages :
Prehistoric skull showing trephine holes. *Ethnological Museum, Berlin.*

Cult ceremony round a sick man. *Graffito on rock at Nacquane, Valcamonica.*

was eaten the body could not digest it and thus it would bring about pain, sickness and death, where-

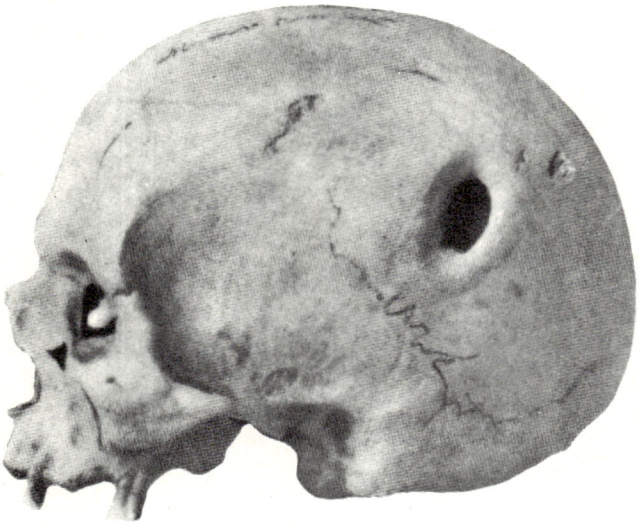

as the body draws nourishment and thus grows and is healthy from food it is able to digest. What fairer or more fitting name can be given to such research and discovery than that of medicine, which was founded for the health, preservation and nourishment of man?'

As far as it goes, much of Hippocrates' conjecture is probably true. But more explanation is required for the great step from the basic protective and remedial behaviour which the earliest men no doubt shared with animals—licking wounds and removing parasites and other foreign bodies—to the arrival of true medicine.

In the light of the researches and great medical histories of the nineteenth and present centuries, as well as the evidence of palaeontology and anthropology, it can now be affirmed that medicine, far from being akin to the rational process described by Hippocrates, originated in magic, and was from the beginning a priestly art.

Perhaps prehistoric man started by drawing a distinction between what could be seen and explained and what could not. Certainly fossil remains show evidence of such diseases as arthritis and tuberculosis as well as bone deformities caused by injury. On the one hand there were wounds incurred in fighting other men or animals or due to foreign bodies, and infestations with parasites, in all of which the cause was obvious and empirical

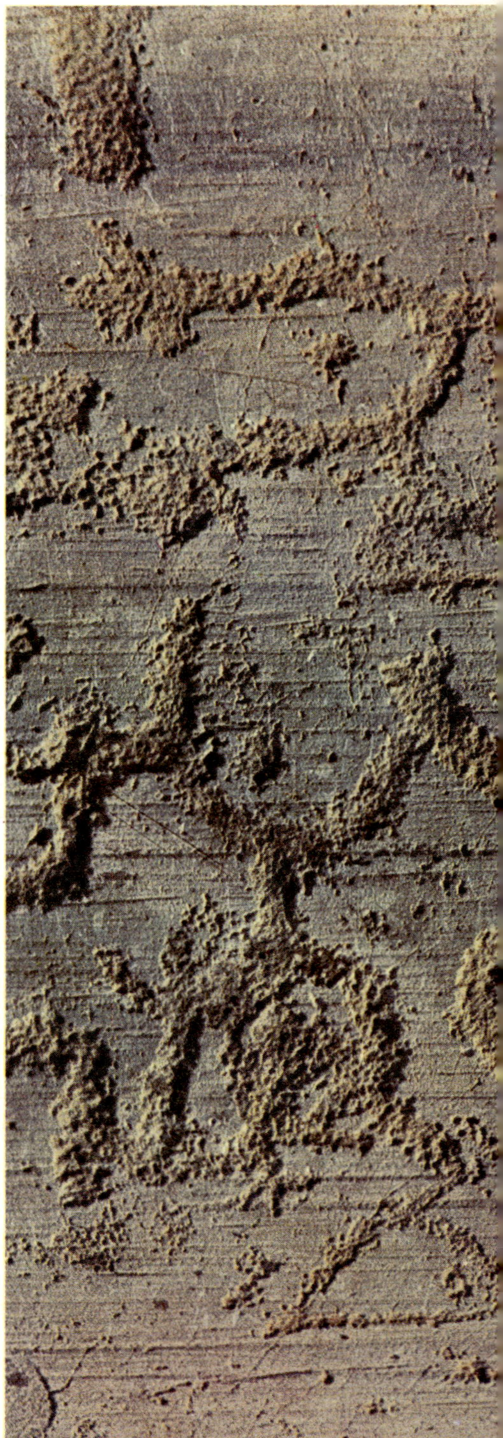

Medicine has its origins largely in magic and priestly practices. The dances of primitive peoples are often a part of complex rites in the course of which the aid of the supernatural forces is invoked: witch-doctors or sorcerers pray to the good demons and threaten the bad, while the dancers join hands to form a chain as a token of defence and protection.

From carvings on some cave walls and from other artifacts it appears that similar rites were performed also among prehistoric peoples. In addition, attempts to rid the sick of demons took other forms, including the practice of trephining or boring holes in the skull, in which evil demons were presumably thought to reside in some illnesses. The lore of the sorcerers also included empirical knowledge, for example of the effect of numerous plant and animal poisons.

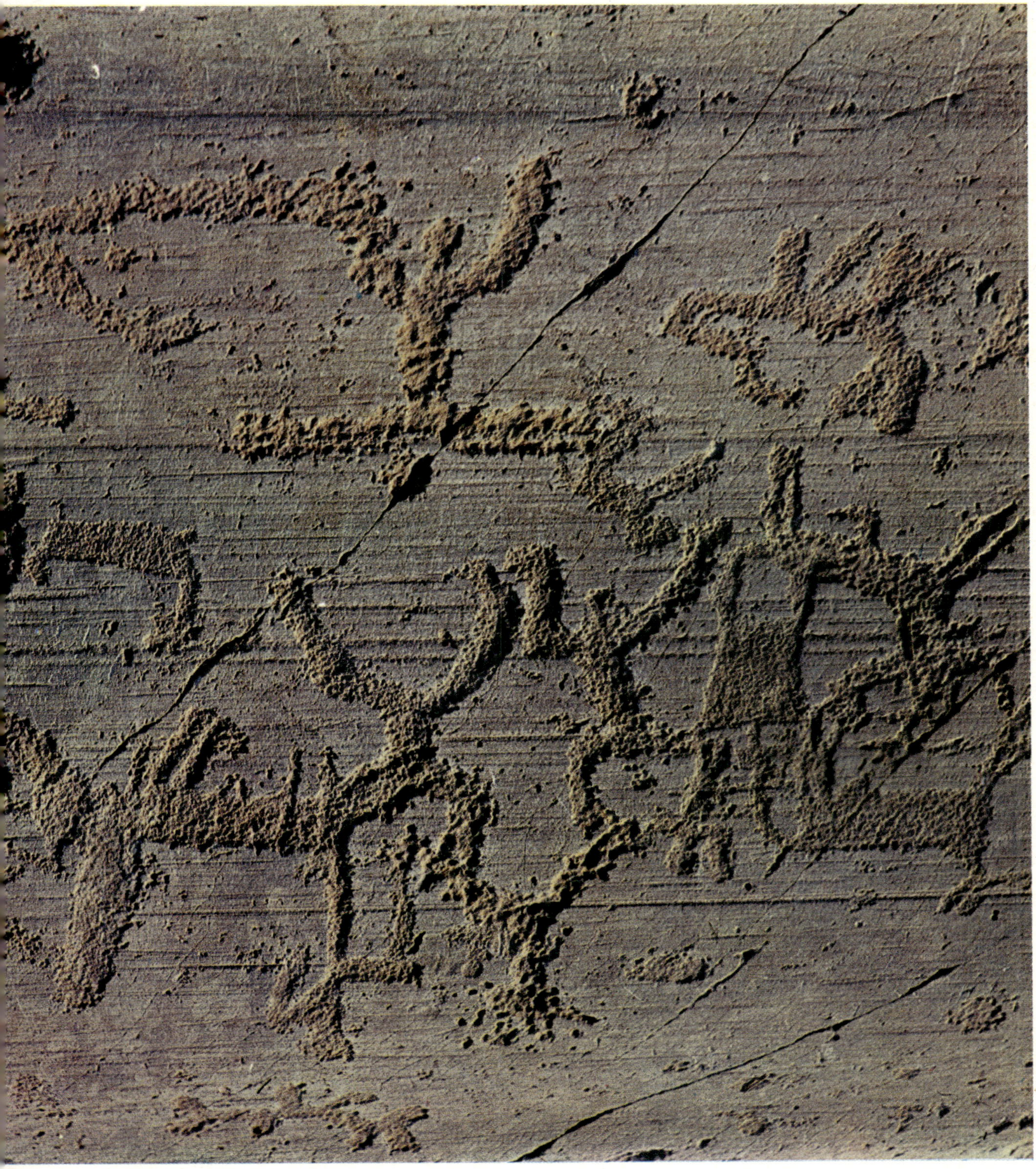

From the earliest times sorcerers formed a separate and exclusive caste in order to safeguard their secrets and heighten their authority, while animal-masks and other special clothing were also important in the attempt to impress and command the trust of their patients. Initiation into the caste often included cruel and bloodthirsty rites; blood was an essential ingredient, its importance to life already understood.

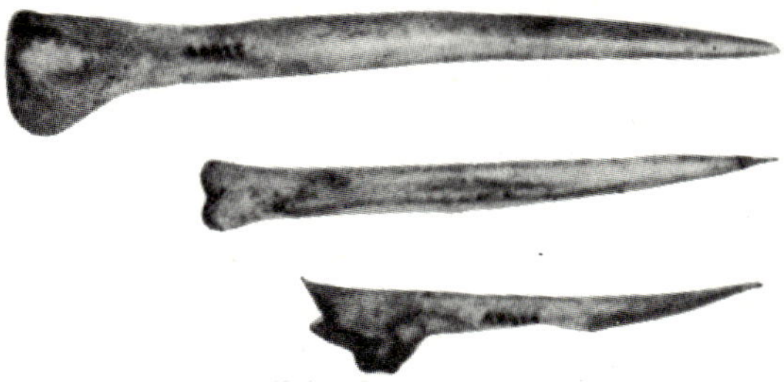

treatment relatively easy; on the other hand there were diseases for which there was no apparent cause, which came from nowhere to threaten health and life. Thus in fear of disease and death man began to investigate the nature of life itself.

Powerless, he had to stand by and see his fellow-beings stricken by unknown forces. The conviction grew in him that the painful mysteries–like illness and death–were the work of demons, while there were undoubtedly kindly divinities too, responsible for the good and pleasant things in life. Other frightening and inexplicable things occurred besides pain and death, like rain and storms, and the dark of moonless nights. Man associated these phenomena, too, with demons, supposing that they might be angry spirits of the dead or of animals killed in the hunt. It was as well, in any event, to propitiate the supernatural powers by worship and sacrifice. Sorcerers came into being, who claimed to have knowledge of the stars, of the herbs of healing and poisons, and of the means to placate the evil demons, and so magic medicine evolved from practices which were instinctive and empirical.

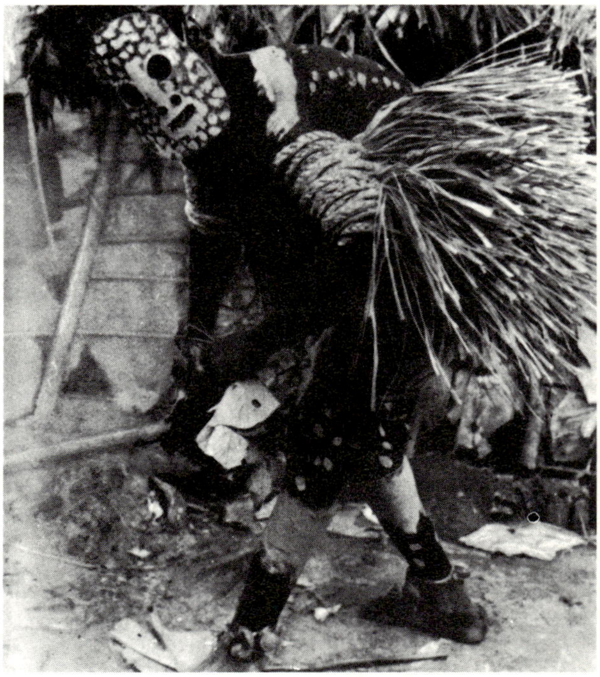

It is likely that the functions of doctor and priest were then inseparable, as they indeed still are today in primitive societies which in many ways reproduce the conditions of prehistory. In one cave in France, Les Trois Frères, a rock-engraving has been found which dates back 17–20,000 years. It shows a doctor wearing a monstrous deer-mask over his face. He represents the archetypal sorcerer of a primitive community in any age, and serves as proof of the antiquity of totemism. (Totem is the term for clan used by the Ojibwa Indians of North America, denoting the animal from which by magical transformation the men of a tribe were descended. In origin the totem was a tabu to stop incest; members of the same clan or totem were not allowed to intermarry.)

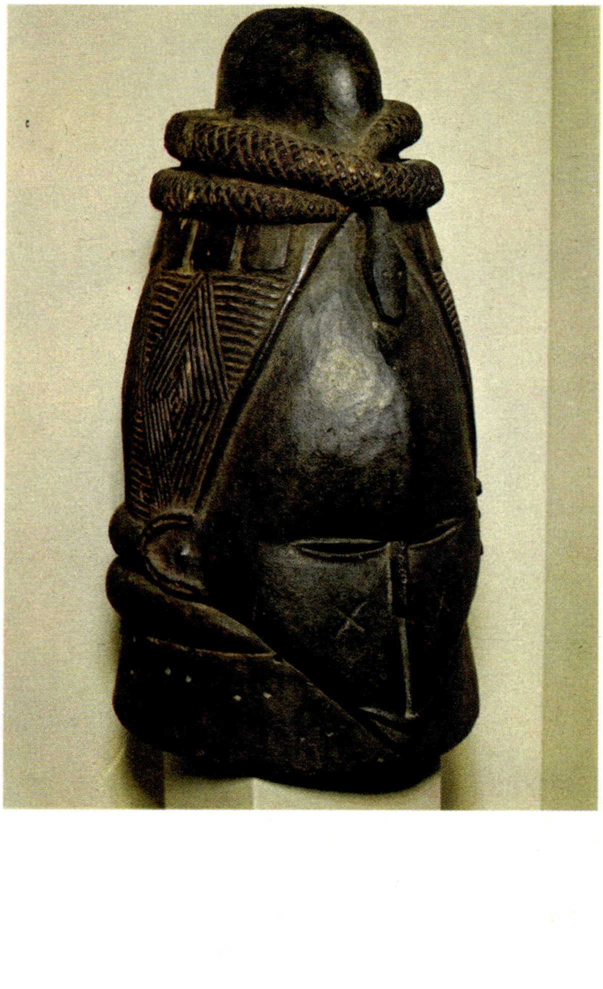

Animal-masks were worn to frighten away the demon causing the illness and to impress the patient, so that he would have faith in the spells, which were accompanied by suitably dramatic rituals, and in the medicines administered to him. The anthropologist Claude Levi-Strauss maintains that there is no ground for doubting the effectiveness of some magical practices, which depend basically on suggestion. The sorcerer must believe his

Prehistoric surgical instruments.

Primitive tribal wizard.

Mask worn by women during initiation ceremony. *Monde art, Congo Museum, Tervuren.*

Wizard with deer-head. *Prehistoric graffito in Trois Frères cave, French Pyrenees.*

Fertility goddess. *Red-glaze terracotta, second half of third millennium* BC. *Louvre Museum, Paris.*

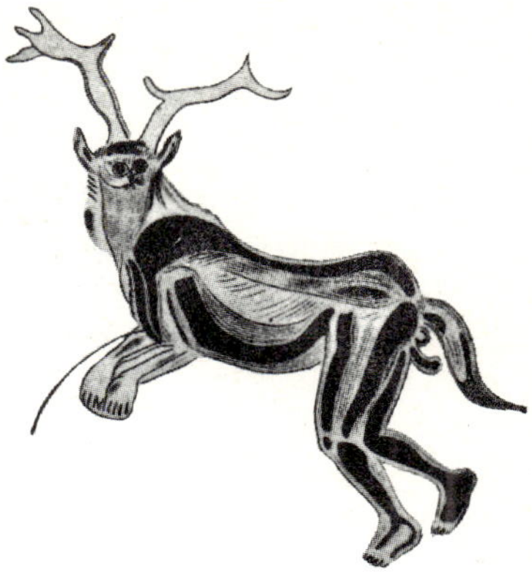

treatment works and in turn the patient, or the persecuted victim, must also believe in the sorcerer's power, and so must the community to which the sufferer belongs.

'Since the pioneering work of Cannon', writes Levi-Strauss in his essay on *The Sorcerer and his Magic,* 'we understand more clearly the psycho-physiological mechanism underlying the instances reported from many parts of the world of death by exorcism and the casting of spells. An individual who is aware that he is the object of sorcery is thoroughly convinced that he is doomed according to the most solemn traditions of his group. His friends and relatives share this certainty. From then on the community withdraws. Standing aloof from the accused, it treats him not only as though he were already dead but as though he were a source of danger to the entire group . . . the victim yields to the combined effect of intense terror, the sudden total withdrawal of the multiple reference systems provided by the support of the group . . . Physical integrity cannot withstand the dissolution of the social personality.

'How are these complex phenomena expressed on the physiological level? Cannon showed that fear, like rage, is associated with a particularly intense activity of the sympathetic nervous system. This activity is ordinarily useful, involving organic modifications which enable the individual to adapt himself to a new situation.

'But if the individual cannot avail himself of any instinctive or acquired response to an extraordinary situation . . . the activity of the sympathetic nervous system becomes intensified and disorganized; it may, sometimes within a few hours, lead to a decrease in the volume of the blood and a concomitant drop in blood pressure, which result in irreparable damage to the circulatory organs. The rejection of food and drink, frequent among patients in the throes of intense anxiety, precipitates this process; dehydration acts as a stimulus to the sympathetic nervous system, and the decrease in blood volume is accentuated by the growing permeability of the capillary vessels. These hypotheses were confirmed by the study of several cases of trauma resulting from bombings, battle shock, and even surgical operations; death results, yet the autopsy reveals no lesions.'

Sorcerers made magic, weaving spells to make people sick and spells to make people well, and

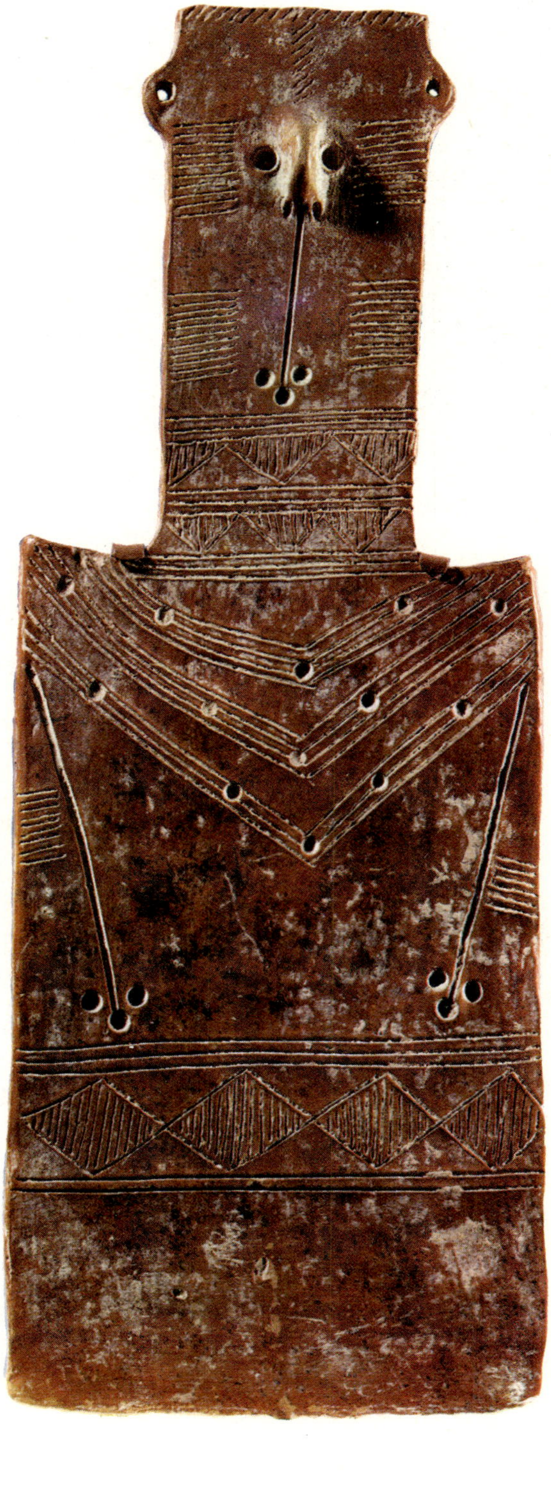

The earliest surgical instruments were sharp-edged pieces of stone, which were used to lance abscesses and to let blood as well as for trephining. Many of the works of art left by prehistoric man are recognized as fertility symbols. The instinct for the preservation of the race was at least as strong as that for self-preservation, and there was a pre-occupation with sexuality, birth and death.

Surgical instruments of primitive tribes.

Mask used by sorcerer to ward off illness. *African. Von der Heydt Collection, Rietberg Museum, Zurich.*

Pre-columbian goddess of childbirth and fertility. *Robert Wood Bliss collection, Washington.*

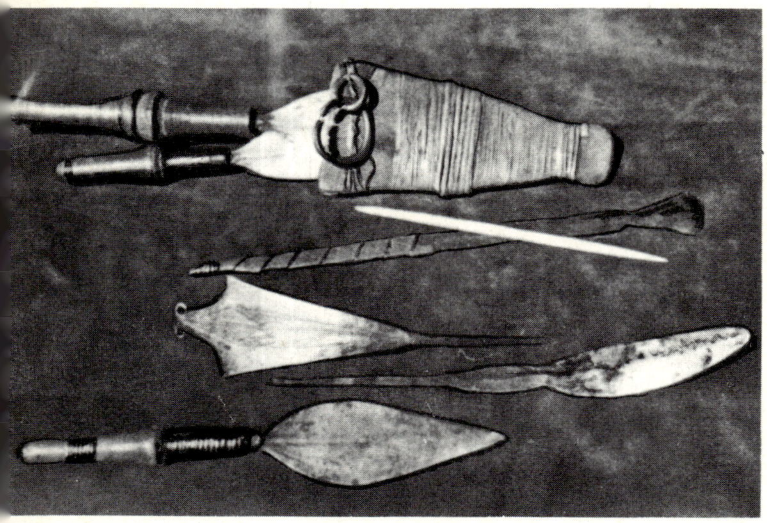

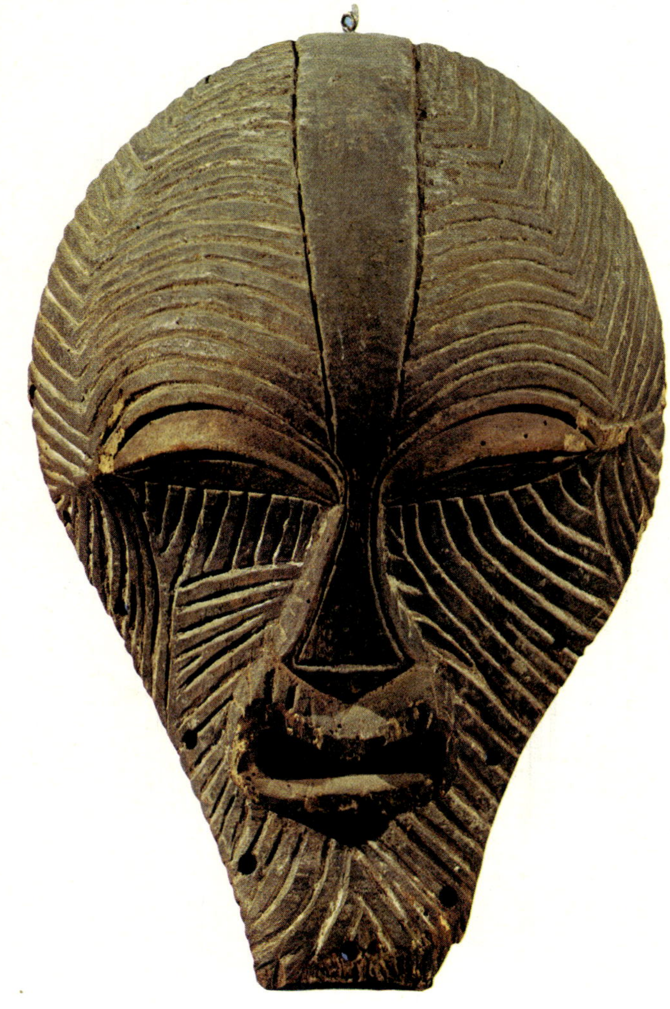

fashioning amulets to keep ill-luck and illness at bay. As guardians of such vital secrets, they eventually formed a class apart. The rites they performed may seem charlatan, but their work had a certain relevance to modern medicine, for their lore was often gleaned from a study of nature, and especially of the properties of plants and of animal poisons. The use, for example, of mandrake (which contains hyoscine) as a soporific and of antidotes to snake-bite goes back into the dim and distant past, preluding two of the developments of medical science: sedatives and vaccination.

Above all, sorcerers were the first to practise trephining or perforation of the skull on living subjects. That patients survived the operation is known, since in many skulls, found in various parts of the world, the rims of the perforations are blunted, indicating clearly that reparative processes later took place in the bone tissues. The sites of perforation tend to support the theory that surgery was practised for specific purposes such as relieving headache or epilepsy.

It is not impossible that the prehistoric sorcerer wanted to remove something from the skull, which was plainly the home of important secrets. Perhaps it was a demon tormenting the subject; the operation was probably both ritual and therapeutic.

Undoubtedly, some of the surgeons of prehistory had great technical ability. The oldest instruments were sharpened stones, used to lance abscesses and let blood as well as for trephining. According to the elder Pliny, the Roman naturalist, prehistoric man learned blood-letting from the hippopotamus: this animal on over-feeding was supposed to pierce a vein at the knee, by pressing against a sharp reed, and when enough blood had flowed to stop the bleeding by plunging its foreleg in the mud.

As we have seen, empirical medicine, based for example on observations of the properties of various plants or on primitive surgery, has existed from the earliest times. But the history of medicine has always been most closely connected with that of religion, for both after all work to the same end—the defence of the individual against evil forces—and as in the earliest civilizations religion took a more definite form, so medicine gradually became established in temples and sanctuaries and other priestly retreats.

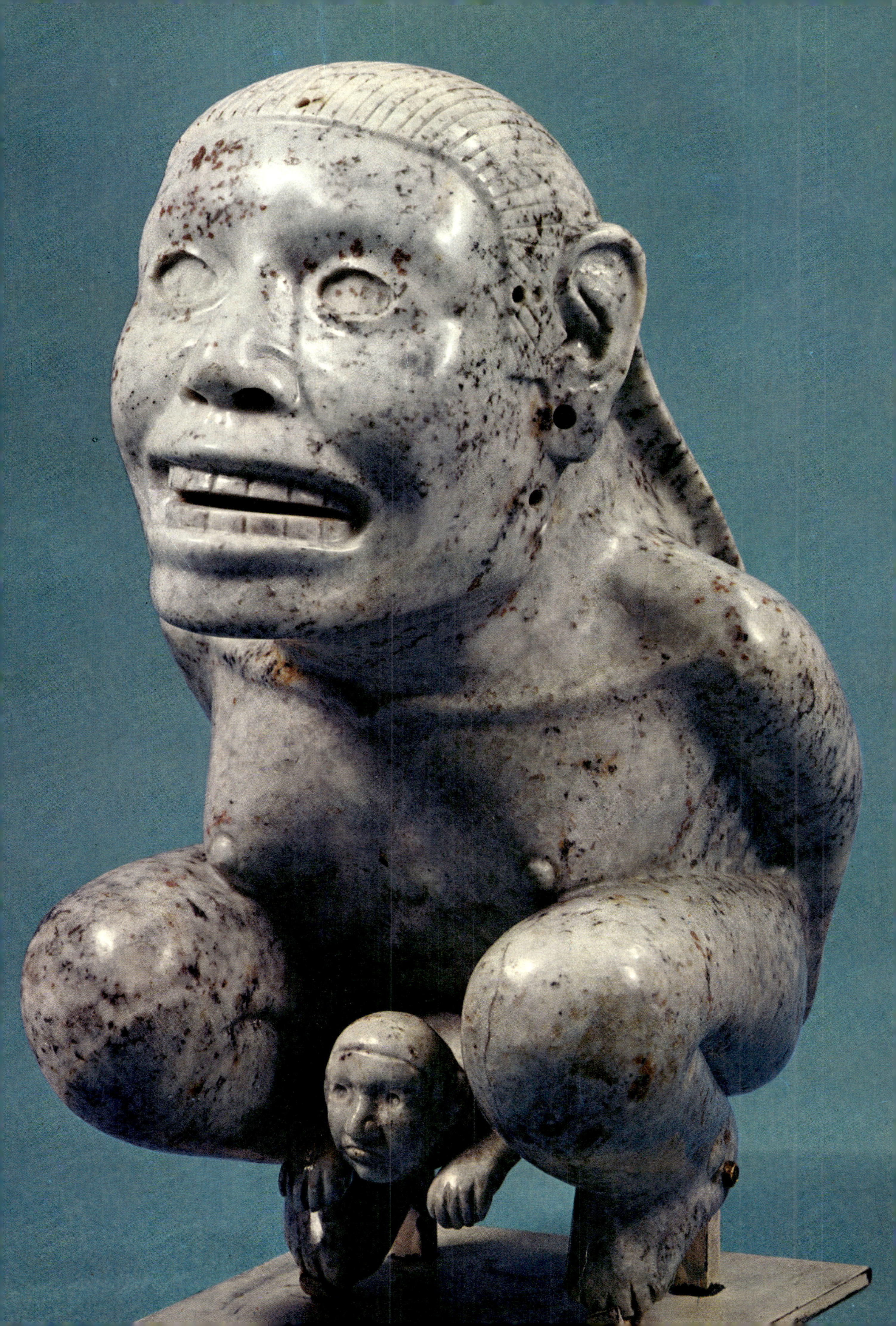

EARLY CIVILIZATIONS
Mesopotamia

The Sumerians

At Ur in Mesopotamia, long before the biblical patriarch Abraham was born, there flourished a great civilization, whose remains were found beneath eleven feet of silt, clearly deposited by some great flood. This discovery was made in 1929 by the archaeologist Sir Leonard Woolley. During the closing stages of excavating the tombs of the Sumerian kings, he decided to dig deeper despite his colleagues' persuasions that the clay stratum under the tombs was only the old bed of the Euphrates. Woolley's own instinctive feeling was so strong that he continued undeterred, and so brought to light the treasured relics of a civilization which dates back to about 4000 BC.

At the same time, he provided a basis of fact which accounted for the story of the Great Flood in the book of Genesis. Indeed, a flood capable of depositing such a layer of silt must have given survivors the impression that the whole earth had sunk below the waters. The biblical story of the Flood was based on a legend of the Sumerians, one of the first peoples of Mesopotamia; written versions have been found that date from at least 2000 BC.

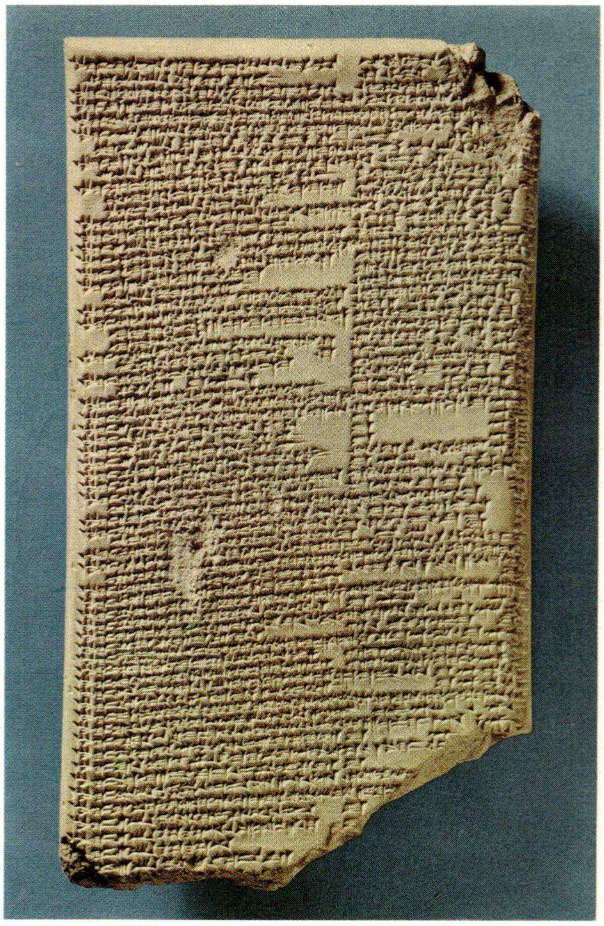

This civilization is the oldest of those of whose medicine we have knowledge, although archaeology may reveal that it was preceded by several others, and there are already signs to this effect. For the time being, Sumerian civilization serves as the point of departure in this attempt to pick out the main landmarks in the history of medicine.

Sumerian medicine was based on the study of astronomy; the Sumerians attempted to ascertain relationships between the movement of the stars and the seasons, and between changes of season and bodily disturbances. Astronomy may have begun as an exact and rational branch of learning, but it was soon transformed into astrology, for the Sumerians believed that from birth man's destiny was subject to the stars.

Archaeologists have recovered in Mesopotamia many clay tablets which were used by priests for writing out entire medical treatises in cuneiform script. From these we learn that the blood was thought to be the source of every vital function, with the liver as the collecting centre for the blood and so the seat of life; this explains why we read of

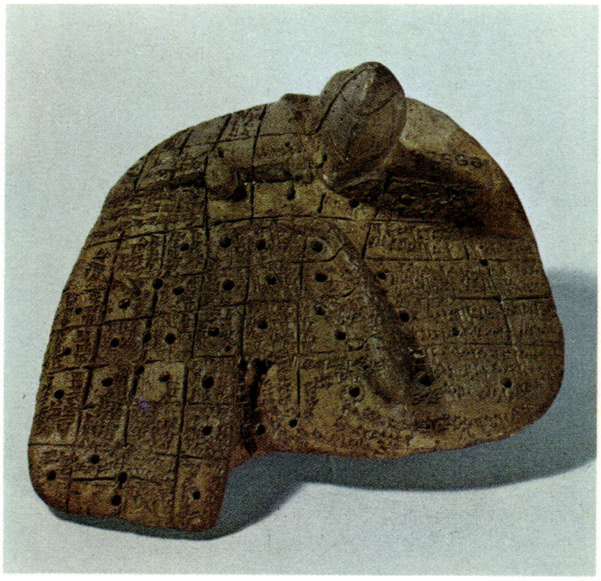

The Sumerians lived 6,000 years ago in the area later known as Mesopotamia, a fertile region between two rivers which is thought of as the cradle of our civilization. The Sumerians recorded their knowledge on clay tablets, inscribing the characters with a wedge-shaped stylus; most of the tablets belonged to the library at Nineveh, and many contain ancient medical remedies, some empirical and some magical, and case histories.

Omens from a baby's actions and health. *Tablet forming part of a large series of medical observations. Sixth century BC, from Borsippa. British Museum, London.*

Clay model of sheep's liver, used for divination. *First Babylonian dynasty, 1830–1530 BC. British Museum, London.*

Medical treatise giving remedies for stomach disorders. *Seventh-century BC tablet from Nineveh. British Museum, London.*

Assyrian astrolabe, used for astrological calculations. *Seventh-century BC, from Nineveh. British Museum, London.*

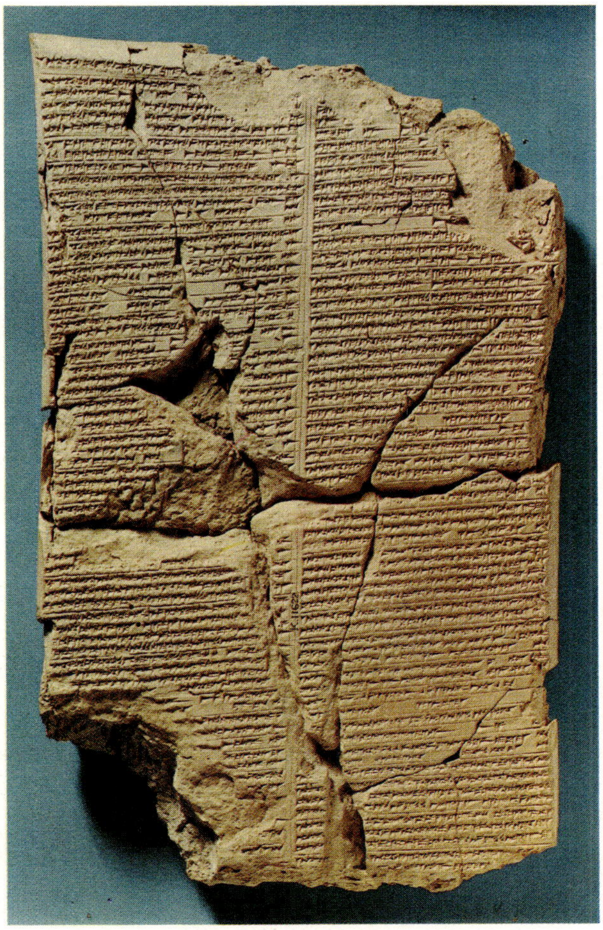

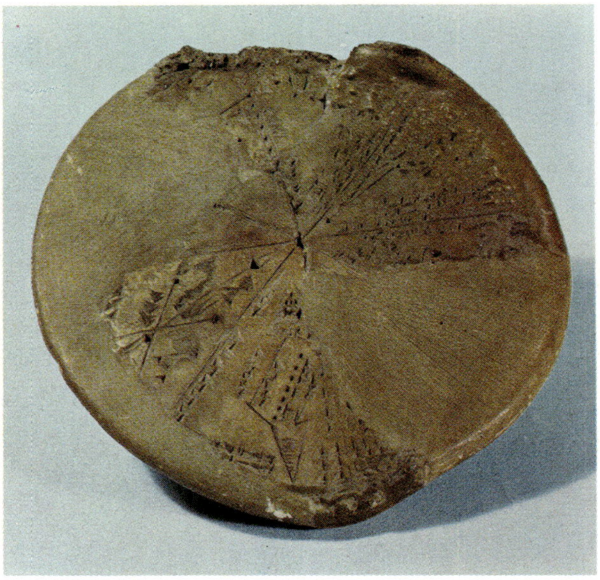

the ancient heroes consulting the omens in the lobes of an animal liver, before embarking on great undertakings. This concept also gave rise to the idea that the continuation of life depended on the renewal of the blood by nourishment.

More than forty of the tablets recovered contain information about interpreting dreams and avoiding nightmares. According to the Sumerians, dreams too depended on the state of the blood.

The Babylonian doctor

The Sumerian civilization was on the wane by about 2000 BC, and was absorbed by that of the Assyrians and Babylonians who conquered Mesopotamia. The region between the Euphrates and Tigris rivers became the centre of Old World civilization, with a political system rigidly dominated by kings who claimed to be the intermediaries between godhead and the people. Astronomy and astrology, already important under the Sumerians, soon took precedence over all other subjects of study, for it was essential to discover the will of the gods in order that the king might carry it out.

There was a hierarchy of some fifteen divinities, but this number multiplied as time went by and as studies of the stars progressed. The most ancient medical deity was the moon god Sin, who made herbs grow and was credited with the power to destroy evil spirits. Later the god Marduk, curer of all illness and inspirer of magical spells, watched over medicine. Then the gods too started specializing: under the goddess Ninchursag there were eight other divinities, each curing some specific complaint.

This proliferation of divinities was justified by the existence of the horde of demons which infested the air, earth and dwelling-places of the Assyro-Babylonians. The demons called *utukku,* sons of the gods, were divided into five groups of seven each. There were also evil spirits of human origin, as of people left unburied after death. Of all the ancient civilizations the Assyro-Babylonian seems to have been the most demon-conscious.

The king of the demon realm, god of death and destruction, was Nergal. When he visited mankind to sow grief and desolation, Nergal was heralded by Nasutar, the dreaded plague demon who in turn had a whole host of lesser demons at his beck and call, including *axaxuzu,* who produced jaundice,

The Assyrians and Babylonians, who conquered Mesopotamia and absorbed the Sumerian civilization around 2000 BC, laid even more emphasis than the Sumerians on astronomy. Disease was still believed to be caused by demons, the variety of which was matched by the numerous divinities revealed by studies of the stars. The doctor-priests alone could interpret the action of the demons and invoke the gods.

But at the same period the practice of surgery was acquiring a lay professional status: at the time of the great king Hammurabi, around 1900 BC, while the doctor-priests were answerable to the gods, surgeons as far as their professional conduct went were answerable to the civil authorities. The laws govern-

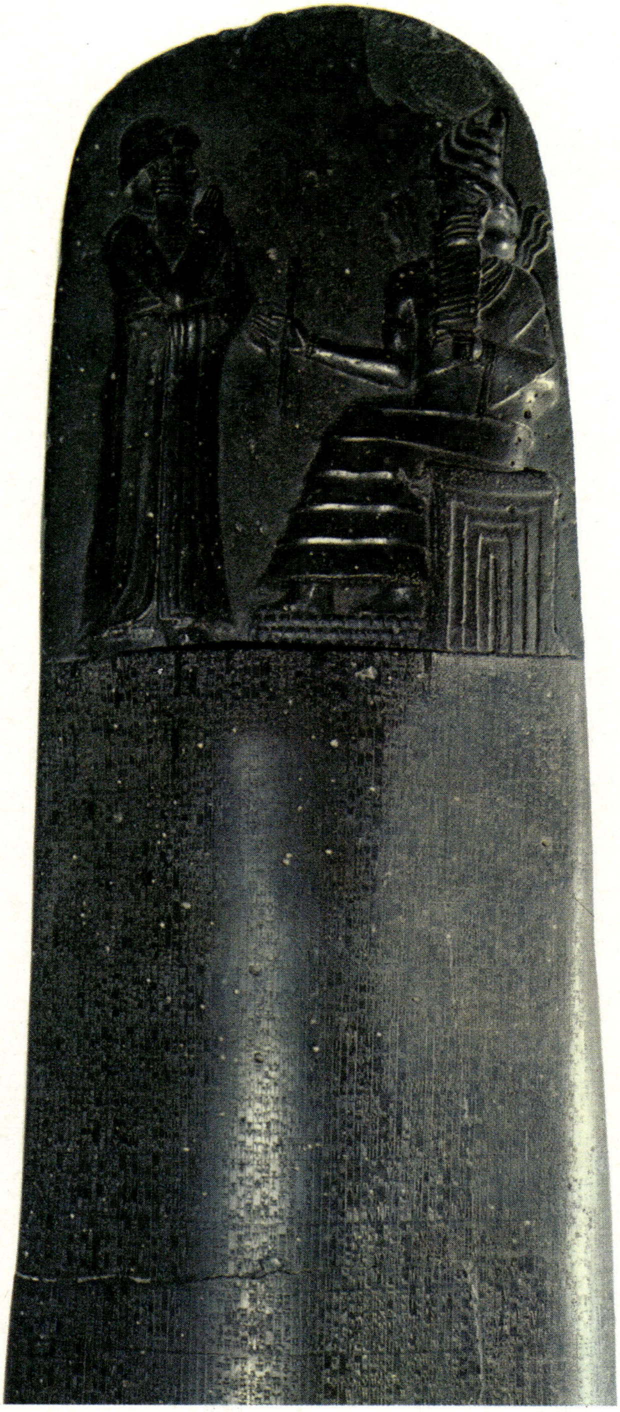

and *asukku*, who was the cause of consumption.

Many other illnesses were recognized, including different fevers, apoplexy and plague, and some clay tablets also bear descriptions of diseases of the eyes, ears, skin and heart, rheumatism and of various venereal diseases. Toothache was thought to be caused by the gnawing of a worm (which was a common belief in Europe up till the eighteenth century). It is also of some interest that Nergal appears in Babylonian mythology in the form of an insect, and it seems that the part played by insects and other small animals in the spread of infectious diseases was appreciated at this early period.

The demons were unleashed when the divinities gave them free rein, in anger over the sins of a man or a nation. When this happened, the doctor-priest stepped in and enquired into the exact nature of the offence to the divinity; when he had learned this he could proceed with the due rites of exorcism and expiation.

Medicine among the Assyrians and Babylonians

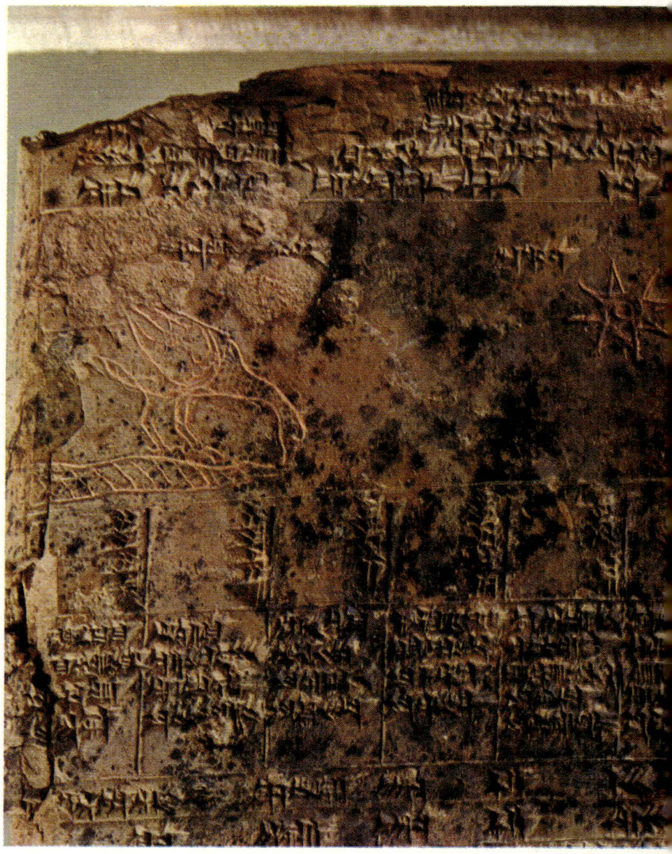

ing their work were contained in a Code which was incised on a great stele; from this it seems that surgical operations were quite frequently performed by the Assyro-Babylonians.

In addition, Babylonian doctors had considerable empirical knowledge and used many drugs derived from plants and animals.

Hammurabi's professional code for surgeons. *Stele in Louvre Museum, Paris.*

Babylonian astrological tablet. *Louvre Museum, Paris.*

Bird-women. *Clay figures from Ur. Louvre Museum, Paris.*

was the prerogative of the priesthood, who were answerable to the gods. But surgeons were laymen, answerable to the state for the operations they performed. The great king Hammurabi (1948–1905 BC) was the first in history to define the concept of the profession's civil and criminal liability; a copy of his Code is on a stele now in the Louvre in Paris. Some enactments laid down the scale of fees and the penalties for incompetence or negligence.

Article 215 ordained: 'If the doctor performs a major operation or cures a sick eye, he shall receive ten shekels of silver. If the patient is a free man, he shall pay five shekels. If he is a slave, then his master shall pay two shekels on his behalf.' But if the patient lost his life or an eye in an operation, then the doctor's hands were cut off. If the patient was a slave, the doctor was only bound to make good the loss by getting the owner a new slave. In the same code are listed the diseases which were disabling and so could lead to a sale contract for a slave being null and void.

Assyrian and Babylonian doctors were highly successful in their calling, and were often consulted and from as far afield as Egypt. Although they based their activity on magic symbolism, they were nevertheless acute observers of nature and so helped the advance of empirical medicine. For example, for eye trouble they prescribed a drink of beer and sliced onion. This is a perfectly valid prescription, since an onion produces tears and tear fluid contains a bactericidal substance, lysozyme. Then the eyes were to be massaged with olive oil on the palm of the hand. But lastly the priest-physicians added a touch of ritual to deal with the evil spirit: a frog's bile mixed with sour milk to be applied to the eyes.

A wide range of drugs were prescribed for various conditions, including the fruits, flowers, leaves, roots and bark of such plants as the olive, laurel, asphodel, lotus and myrtle; diverse organs

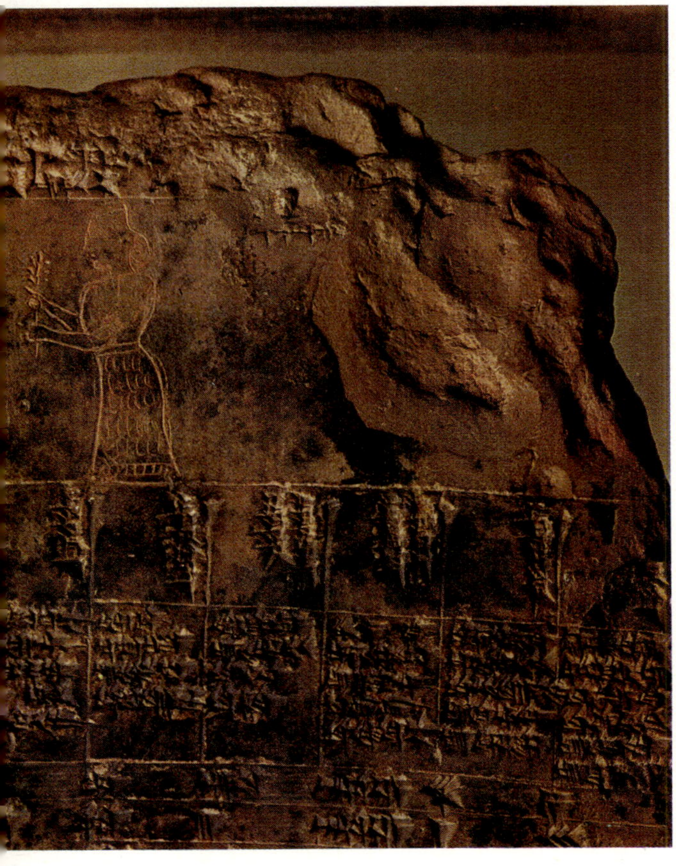

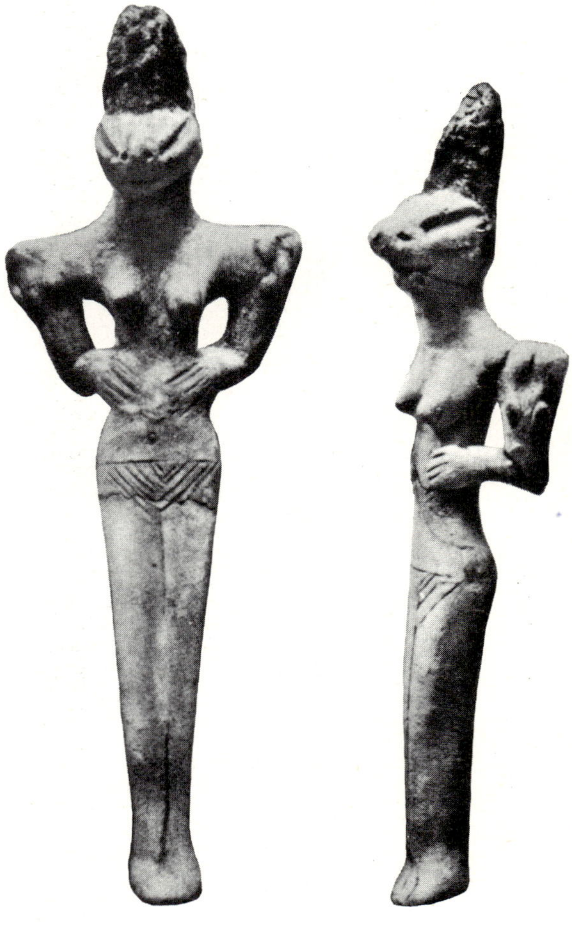

Assyro-Babylonian doctors were highly regarded and were often summoned to give their services as far away as Egypt, where another great civilization flourished on the fertile Nile valley.

Study of the papyri on which the Egyptians recorded their medical knowledge indicates the existence of something like a national health service. Other interesting features of Egyptian medicine were a high degree of specialization among doctors, if of a somewhat irrational nature, and an emphasis on hygiene in dwellings, diet, sexual relations and burial.

Votive hand. *Syro-Phoenician. Louvre Museum, Paris.*

Knife for circumcision. *Egyptian. Archaeological Museum, Florence.*

Circumcision. *From the tomb of Ankma-Lor, Saqqara necropolis.*

of domestic and wild animals; and also a number of mineral substances such as iron, copper and aluminium. In addition, much use was made of the excreta of animals, a practice common not only to primitive people, who perhaps adopted it to disgust and drive away the demon afflicting the sick patient, but also to European medicine until two hundred years ago. Thus a hospital pharmacopoeia published in London in 1718 prescribes an infusion of horse dung for pleurisy, and such treatments did not die out until the end of the century.

Medicines were administered by Assyrian doctors in the form of pills, powders and enemas, and pessaries and suppositories were also used. On his rounds the physician carried his case containing drugs, bandages and instruments, and after a consultation his findings would be recorded on clay tablets.

Descriptions of symptoms inscribed on the clay tablets are of some interest. A typical one is for pulmonary tuberculosis: 'The patient coughs a lot, his saliva at times contains blood, his breathing sounds like a flute. His skin is clammy but his feet are hot. He sweats profusely and his heart is in uproar . . .'

Most phenomena were still explained in magical terms; that much is clear from documentary evidence. But now, during this period of civilization, man's empirical knowledge had advanced to the stage where he had a degree of control over certain diseases. From archaeological evidence discovered in fairly recent excavations, we have concluded that the Assyro-Babylonians knew more medicine than was supposed by Herodotus when he wrote: 'The sick man is led to the market place and passers-by talk to him about his illness, to see if they have suffered from it in the past, mentioning what remedies they used or if they ever heard of anyone who knew an effective medicine for it. It is not lawful to pass a sick man by in silence, without taking an interest in his complaint.'

Excavations in Babylonia have also revealed large stone drains, probably part of a sewage system, and stone privies appear in the remains of this and other early Mediterranean civilizations. These primitive public health measures, which became more important as the complexity of civilization increases, indicate a growing awareness of the responsibility of the state for the health of its citizens.

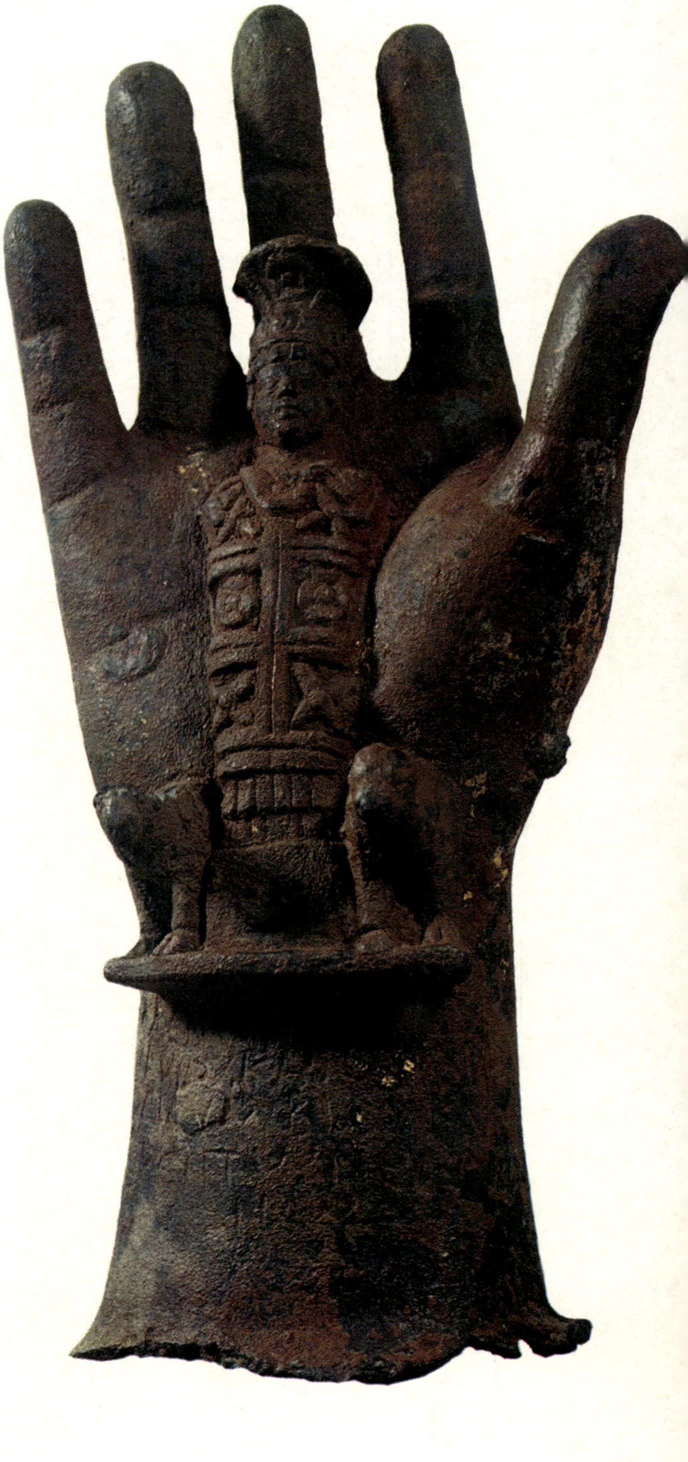

The Egyptians

In his *History,* Herodotus refers to the medicine of the peoples of the Nile valley, where civilization flourished in parallel with Mesopotamia. 'The art of medicine is thus divided: each physician applies himself to one disease only and not more. All places abound in physicians; some are for the eyes, others for the head, others for the teeth, others for the intestines, and others for internal disorders.'

Diodorus Siculus, another Greek historian, records a practice which in a way anticipated modern national health systems. 'In wartime and on journeys anywhere within Egypt, the sick are all treated free of charge, because doctors are paid by the state and scrupulous observance of the prescriptions drawn up by great doctors of the past is incumbent on them.'

Specialization and a national health scheme may seem the most noteworthy aspects of ancient Egyptian medicine. Of course, this is from the twentieth-century standpoint, and it seems more than likely, from what we know of other aspects of the history of ancient Egypt, that her law-makers did not indulge in anything like our social views.

The cause of medicine, as the centuries passed, made little appreciable progress in the Nile valley. It was initiate medicine, practised for the purpose of ridding patients of demonic powers. All cures were revealed by the gods and codified by Thoth, called by the Greeks Hermes Trismegistus, in secret books kept in the medical schools associated with the temples of Sais at Heliopolis. They were books for initiates, that is to say priests. According to tradition, Thoth invented the sciences and the arts, knew the secrets of the gods and how to cause and cure illness. He is said to have invented cursing by sympathetic magic, which is still used today. Hairs, threads of clothing or nail parings from the intended victim were kneaded with wax into a likeness in the form of a figurine; when this was cursed, the victim grew ill and succumbed.

The gravestones of the doctors of the old schools at Heliopolis carry inscriptions: 'superintendent of the secrets of health of the house of Thoth', 'the greatest of doctors' (the dean of the school of Sais, who lived around 3000 BC), 'eye specialist to the palace' (inscription of 3200 BC). From hieroglyphics on his tomb, we learn that a doctor Iry was entitled 'keeper of the king's rectum' around 2500 BC. There was a 'keeper of the king's right eye', and also a 'keeper of the left eye', which gives the impression

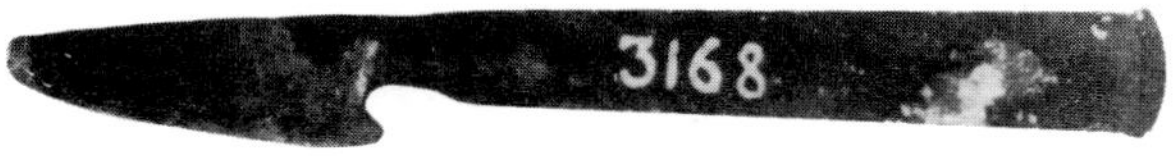

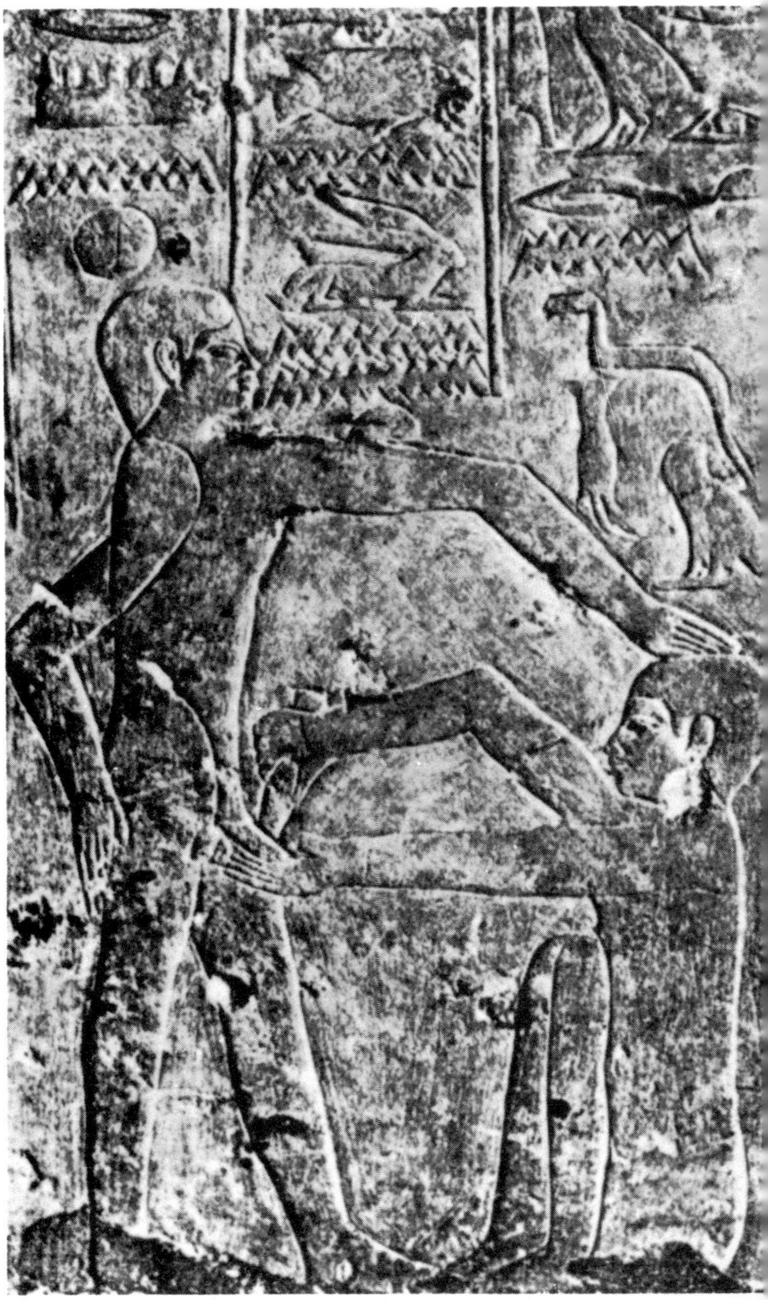

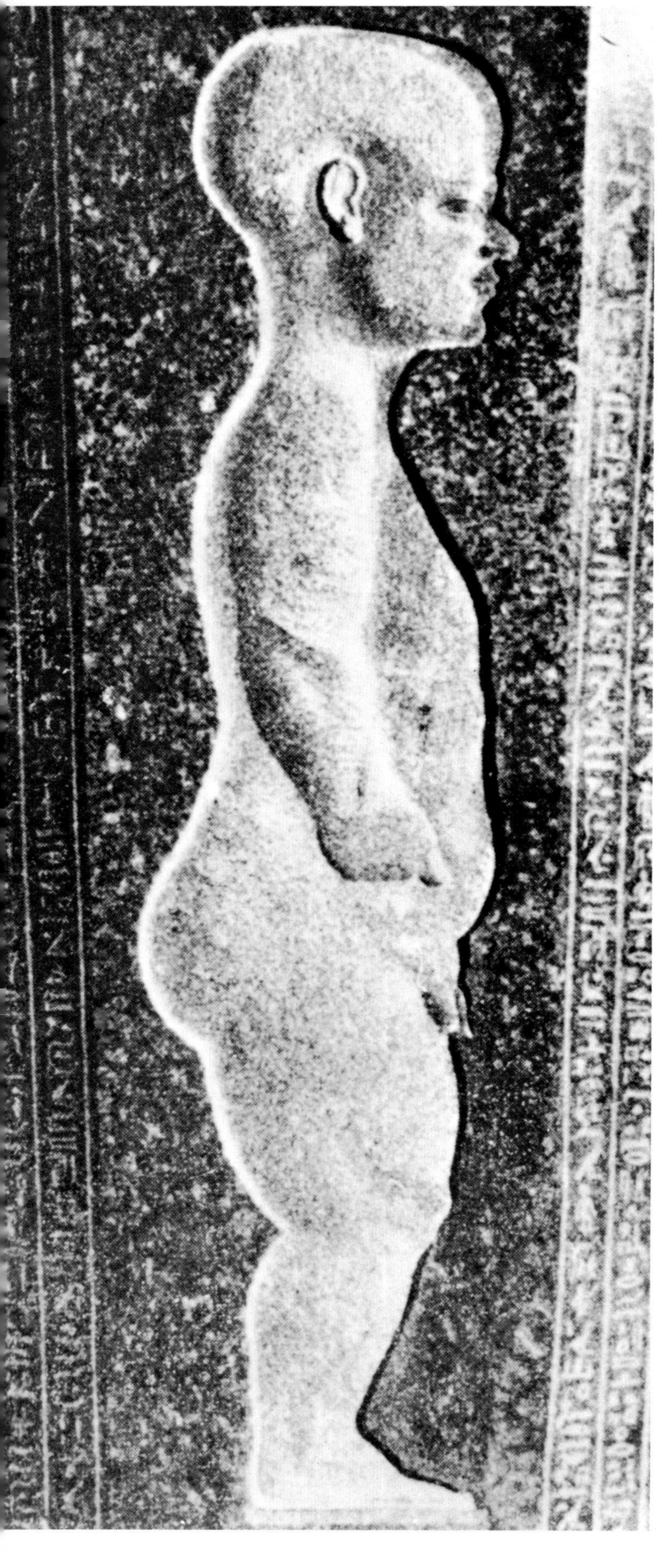

The first doctors in the Nile valley were priests. Disease was believed to be the work of evil spirits and remedies could only come from the gods, so that those best qualified to cure were the priests, who alone had access to the divine secrets guarded in the temples. The first stage in treating a patient was to seek out the spirit who possessed his body, confront it and then expel it, using magic rites and amulets.

that specialization, admirable in itself, was attributable more to the supremacy of the pharaohs than to any rational division of function.

Besides inscriptions in hieroglyphics and Greek and Roman sources, information derives in the main from what are called the medical papyri, writings exclusively medical in content. The papyri found by Georg Ebers and Edwin Smith are of most interest. That of Ebers, discovered at Luxor in 1873, which can be dated to the period 1553–1550 BC, is a collection of texts which probably originated in the old empire (3300–2360 BC), from the time of the first eight dynasties whose proud rulers built the pyramids of Cheops, Chefren and Mycerinus as testimonies to their power.

During the third dynasty (there were 26 dynasties in the period 3300–525 BC, before the Ptolemaic), lived Imhotep, famous as an architect and as a builder of pyramids, but who was also a great doctor; he was deified by the Egyptians and the Greeks identified him with Asklepios, now more commonly known by his Latin name Aesculapius, their god of medicine. It may well be that some of the prescriptions in this papyrus were originated by Imhotep.

The papyrus found by Smith, which predates Ebers, gives instructions for the treatment of wounds, fractures and dislocations. For fractures they used birch splints with bandages bound over them, and a method to reduce a dislocated jaw was not unlike that used by present-day doctors. Lesions on the right or left sides of the head were observed to be associated with paralysis on the opposite side of the body. Prognostic statements were also recorded: 'I will cure this disease' was usually recorded if the outcome appeared favourable; 'Nothing can be done in this case', if doubtful, or 'The patient will die', if hopeless. These and some other medical papyri (such as those of Brugsch) give an extensive and accurate picture of ancient Egyptian medicine.

Unlike the Assyrians and Babylonians, who thought of the liver as the seat of life, the Egyptians regarded respiration as the most important vital function. They knew that the heart was the centre of the circulation, but supposed that the circulation depended on breathing. The Egyptians recognized various complaints affecting the heart, abdomen and eyes, and also angina pectoris, disorders of the bladder and various kinds of swellings.

The dwarf Puoinhetef. *Representation of deformity, 341* BC. *Cairo Museum.*

Ebers' papyrus, showing medical recipes. *University of Leipzig.*

Magic amulet. *British Museum, London.*

Case of poliomyelitis (?). *Stele of Rem, 2000* BC. *Ny Glyptothek, Copenhagen.*

Imhotep, Egyptian god of medicine.

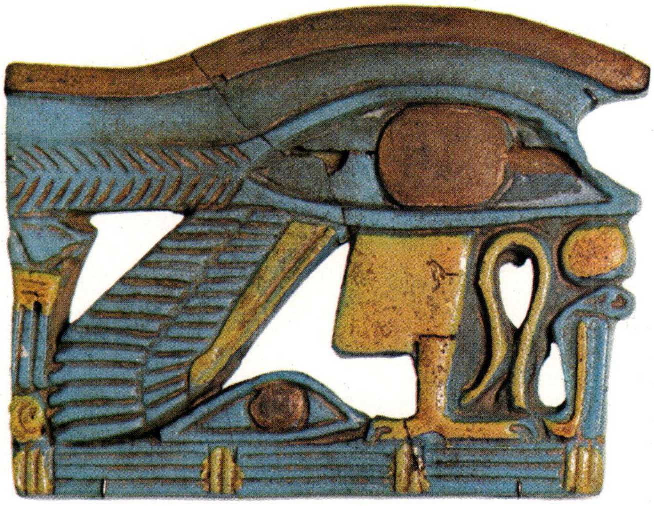

This is one of the many treatments in the Ebers papyrus: 'In the case of a tumour affecting a vessel in the form of a callosity which is stone-like to the touch, I would say it is a tumour of the vessels suitable for treatment by surgery. After surgery, cauterize the wound, lest it bleed too much.' When physicians went visiting, they took their patients' pulses, examined their bodies and went through a process of auscultation by laying an ear to the shoulder-blades and chest.

Considering the mummies and the refined embalming techniques used in the Nile valley, it might be supposed that Egyptian medical men were strong on anatomy. In fact they were, but only to a certain level; anatomy seems to have been learned from a study of animals, judging by hieroglyphs, that for 'heart' being shaped like that of a cow, 'throat' like the head and windpipe of cattle, and 'uterus' being bicornuate, unlike that of the human female. But embalming was not done by the priest-

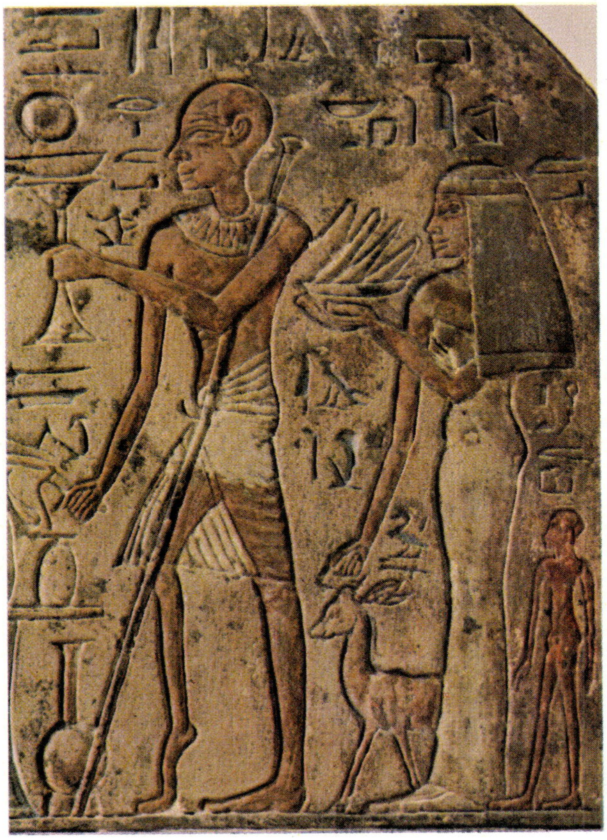

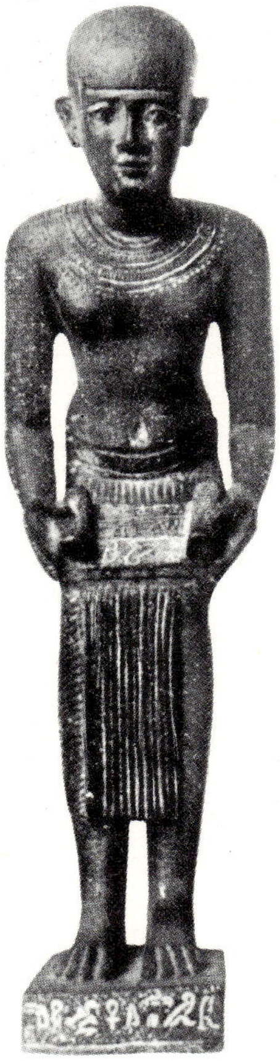

There was knowledge of various drugs, including opium and hemlock, used in ointments and gargles. Egyptian doctors recognized many diseases affecting various parts of the body and knew that the heart was the centre of the circulation. They also performed surgical operations, although their knowledge of anatomy seems to have been derived from a study of animals; the dissection of human corpses was forbidden (as it was and still is among many peoples believing in a life after death).

The embalming of the dead for their afterlife was carried out not by the doctor-priests but by expert laymen who formed a separate caste and kept their methods secret. To keep the corpses from decomposing

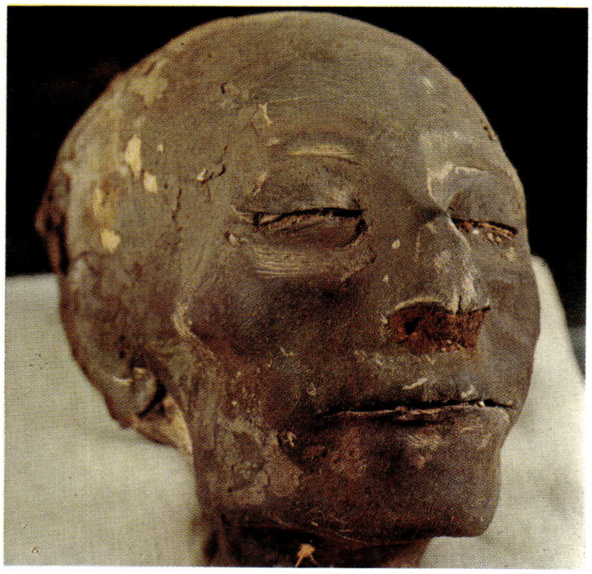

doctors, who ministered in the house of life; it was the work of those in the house of death, who formed another distinct class.

Herodotus describes the technique of embalming: the brain was removed by a hook inserted through the nose, and the brain cavity cleaned with the utmost care. The body was opened by means of long vertical incision, and when the internal organs had been removed it was washed several times over with infusions of aromatic herbs and then filled with spices of all kinds except incense. The opening was then sewn up and the body was immersed for a certain time in a special solution. After this, it was washed again and swathed in linen bands impregnated with bituminous substances, which ensured it would remain in a perfect state of preservation. In fact, preservation is often so perfect that study with the microscope of tissue sections shows fine detail and sometimes evidence of disease.

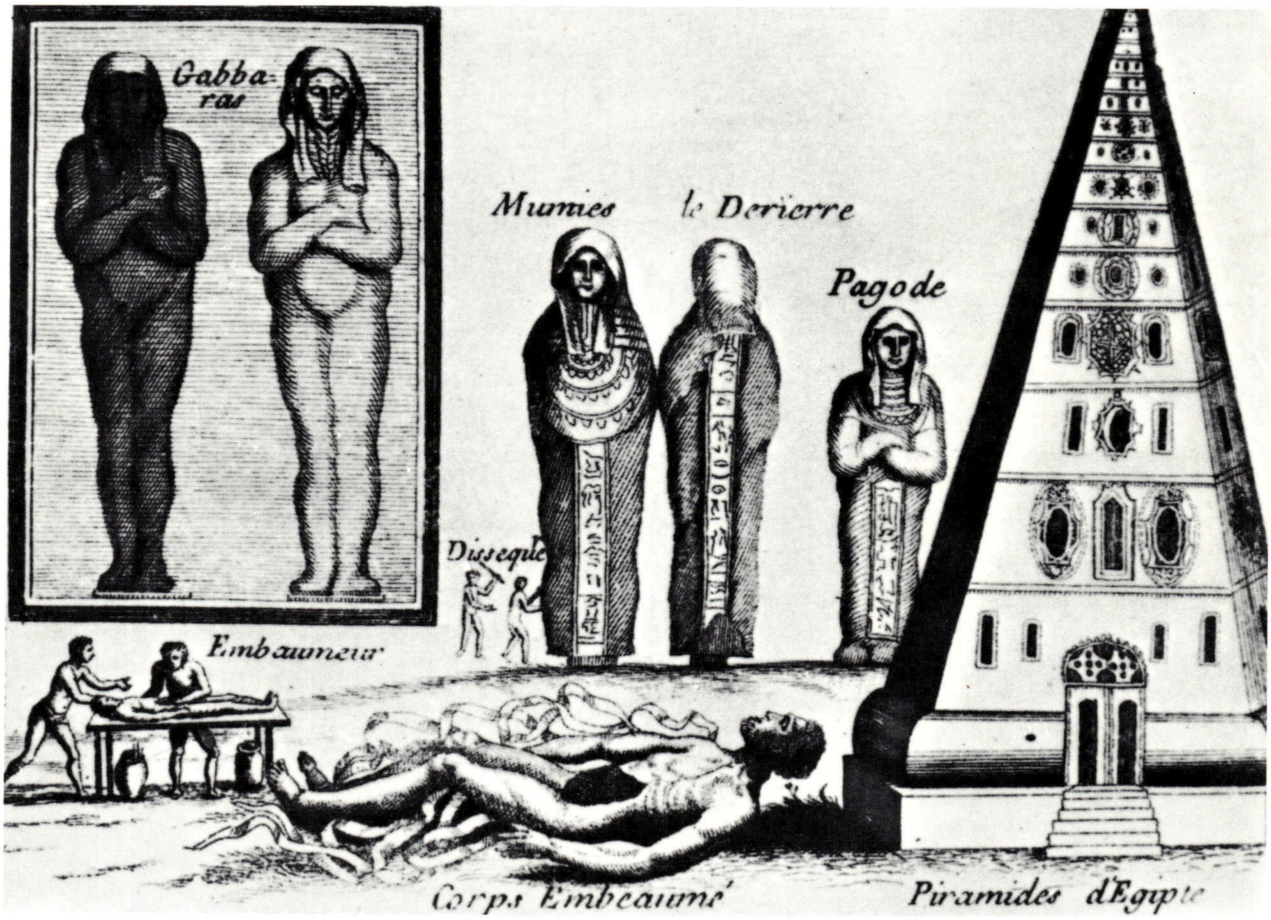

the embalmers took off as much fluid as possible, removed the internal organs, and applied special fluids. Their mummies remain intact and in a remarkably good state of preservation; examination under the microscope of tissues from mummies has provided clear indications of several recognizable diseases including arteriosclerosis.

Mummified head of high official Nebera (Ramesids). *Egyptian Museum, Turin.*

The embalmers. *Engraving from a History of Drugs by Pierre Pomet, 1694.*

Funeral, preparation of the mummy. *Theban necropolis, Sheikh Abd el Gurna, tomb of Menna.*

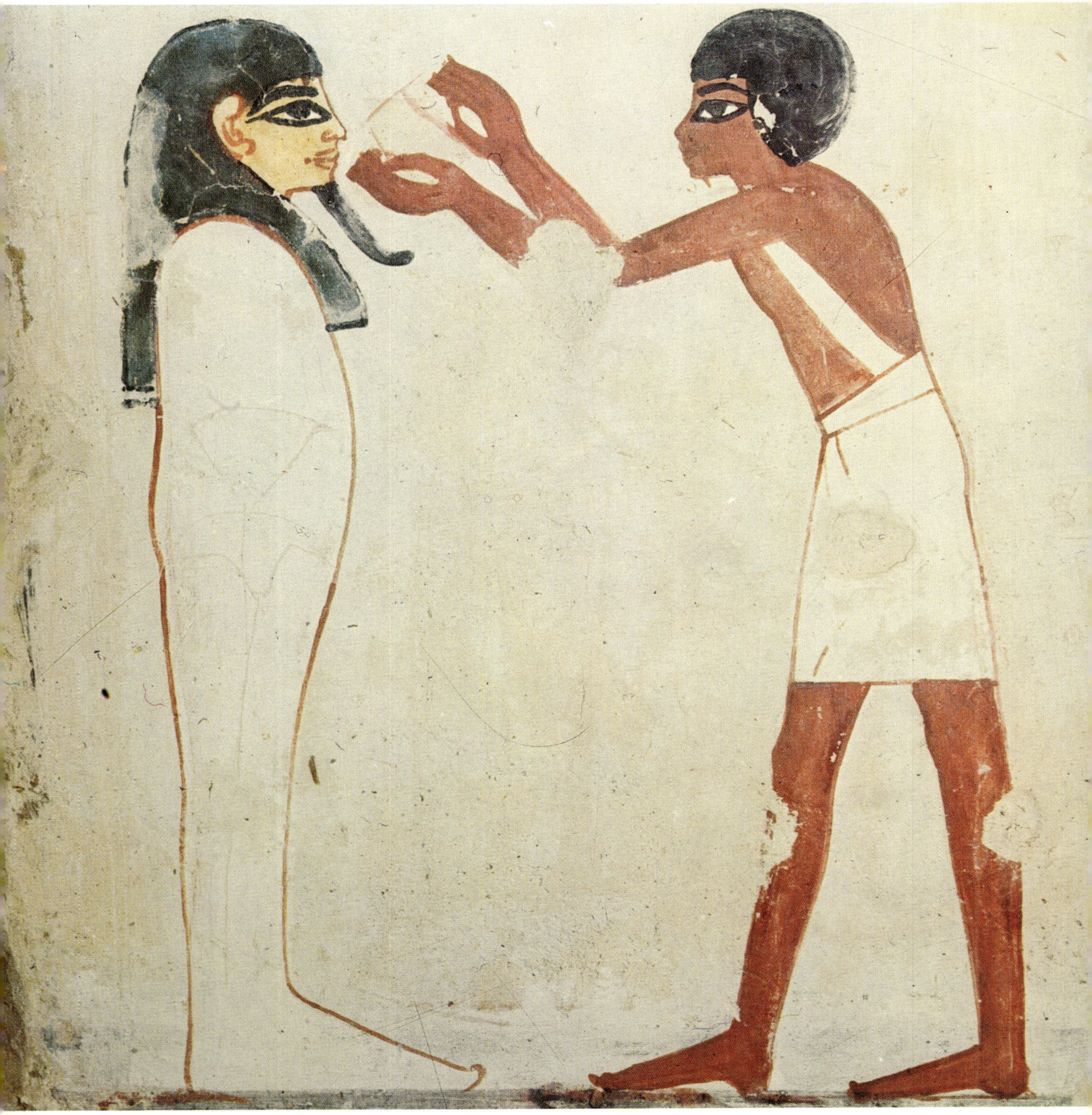

Ancient Indian medicine

With the Hindu invasion of the Punjab about 1500 BC began the first period of Indian medicine, the so-called Vedic period. It was during this period that the books of Veda (learning) were composed. These were truly books of science, the most ancient of which was the *Rigveda,* containing hymns to the gods. One of the latest was the *Ayurveda* (Veda of long life), which was concerned particularly with medicine. As these are sacred texts revealed by divine beings, the history in them is always interwoven with legend.

One of these legends recounts the miraculous birth of Dhanvantari, who is to Indian medicine what Aesculapius was to the Greeks: the god arose from the churning of the sea of milk, in company with the moon, Lakshmi, Surhabi the sacred cow, Varuni goddess of wine, Parijata the tree of paradise, and a winged horse rather like Pegasus. In later life, moved to compassion by the ills assailing mankind, Dhanvantari wished to be reborn on earth as a prince of Benares. He withdrew to woods, to live as a hermit according to the custom of ancient Hindu princes, and there wrote the *Ayurveda.*

The Vedic period was succeeded around the beginning of the ninth century BC by the Brahminical period, which marked the peak of development of Indian medicine. To this period belong the two greatest Hindu doctors, Charaka and Susruta, whose writings formed the groundwork for all the subsequent systems of Indian medicine. The *Charaka Samhita,* arranged in eight books, is in the form of a dialogue between master and pupil, and is to medicine what the *Susruta Samhita,* which is less accurate but shows fair knowledge of human anatomy, is to surgery.

Susruta's text is divided into six books. One of its requirements is that the doctor should resemble the god incarnate Dhanvantari. 'The doctor must be dressed in clean clothes, be clean shaven and cut his nails. He is to wear a white robe, go shod in sandals, with a staff or sunshade in his hand, showing gentleness to everybody and a benevolent look.'

Chapter thirty-four of the first book of Susruta contains a section on the duties of the doctor in battle:

'When the king leads his army out against rebels or foes to punish their transgressions, let him take a good doctor, a devout holy man whose prayers will be heeded (and a clever astrologer). The doctor will concern himself over the food, water, fuel and

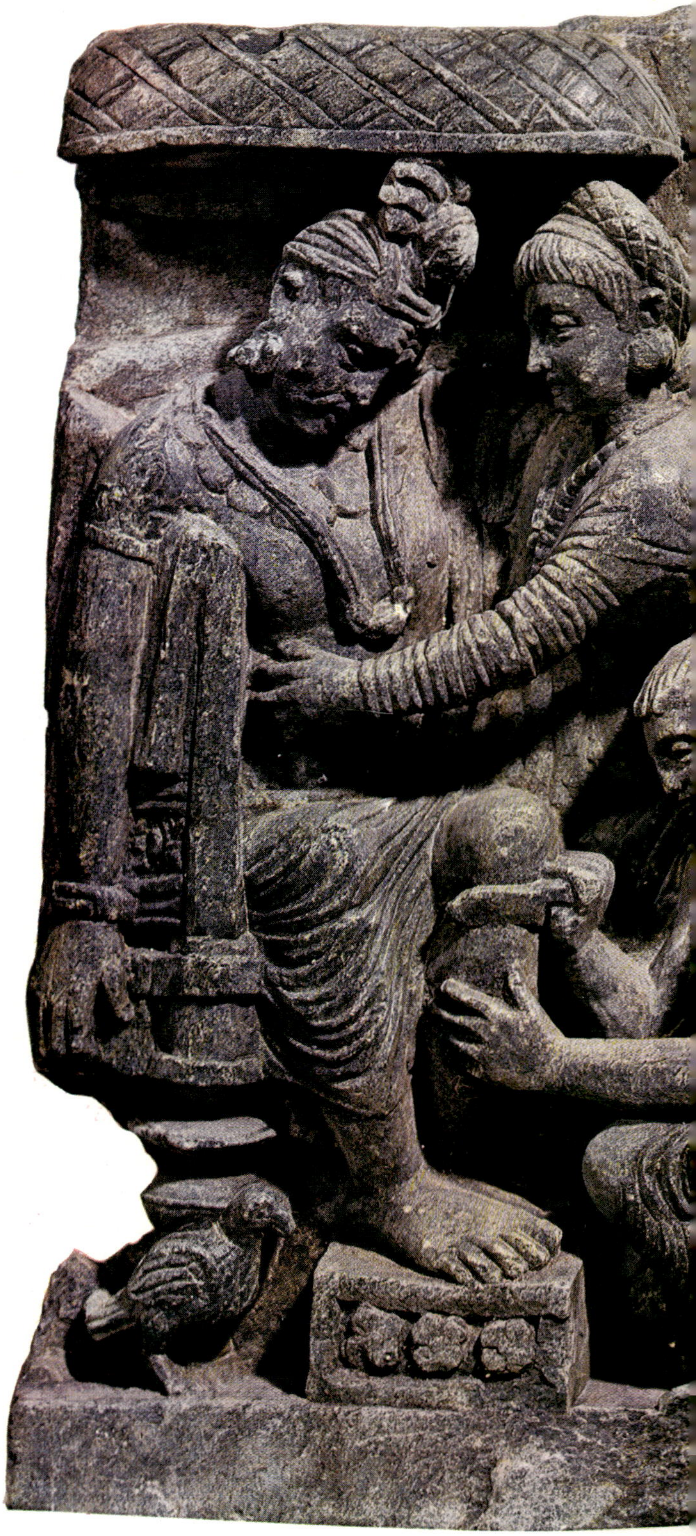

There were three periods in the development of medicine in India in ancient times. The medical knowledge of the first, or Vedic, period, which began about about fifteen centuries BC, was recorded in hymns and other sacred texts, while the second, or Brahmin, period, dating from around 800 BC produced the great doctors Charaka and Susruta, whose works form the basis for all later systems of Indian medicine. The chronology of these two periods is obscure, with legend, history and contemporary observations often inextricably confused.

The third period followed the Moslem conquest in the seventh century AD, which introduced Arab medicine into India.

Legend of King Sibi. *Gandhara-style relief, c. third century* AD. *British Museum, London.*

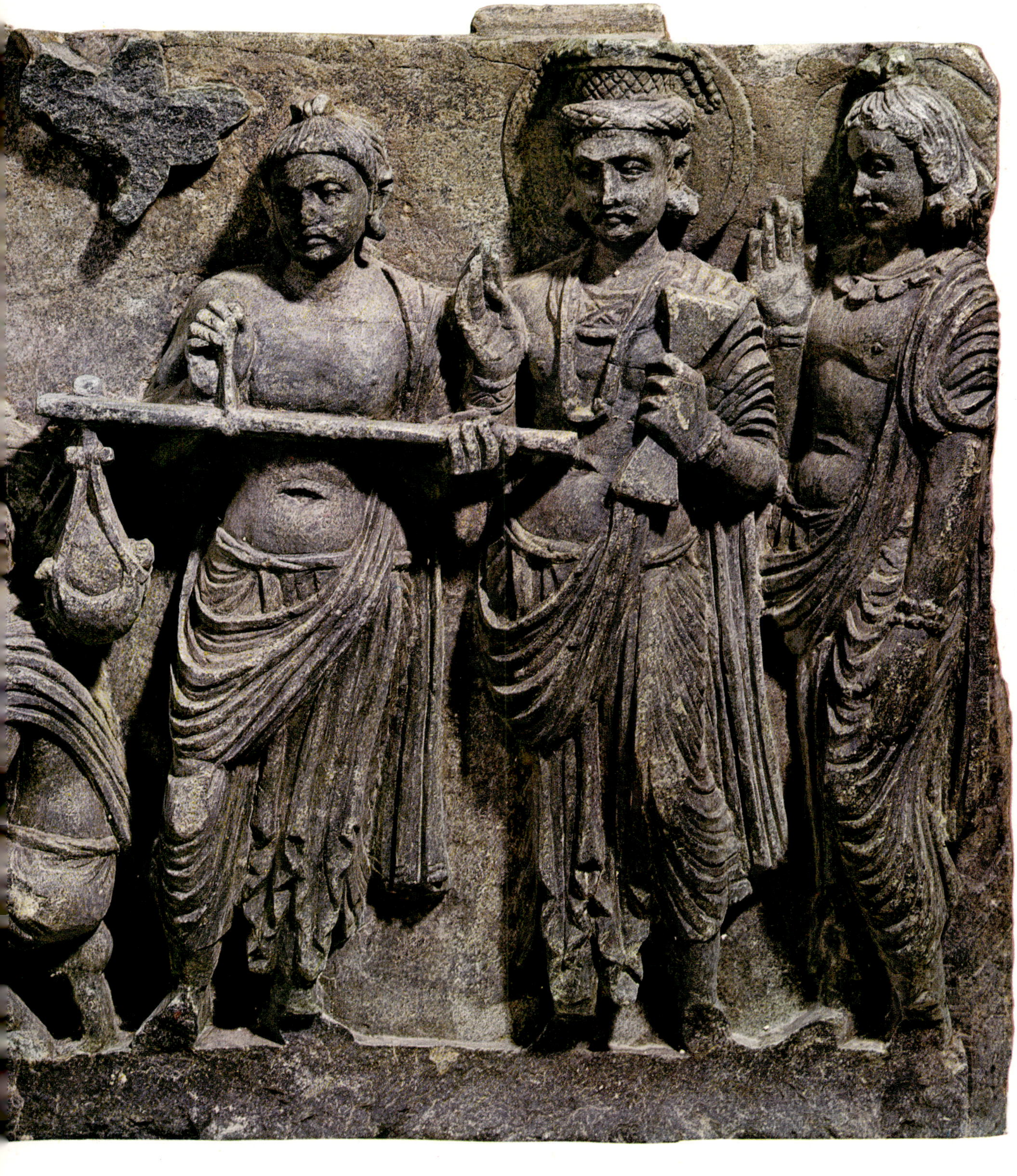

Ancient Hindu medical texts contain few references to anatomy, knowledge of which seems to have been poor, although Susruta pointed out that the teaching of this subject was of the greatest importance for surgeons. In spite of this, Indian surgeons were accomplished and performed a wide range of operations, such as tonsillectomy and amputations, using over a hundred different types of instruments including scalpels, saws, scissors and forceps. Perhaps their most remarkable achievement was the operation devised for the restoration of noses (at that time often cut off as a punishment), which involved the use of a skin graft from another part of the patient's body. One other subject which was carefully and accurately studied was the formation and development of the embryo, especially of its circulation.

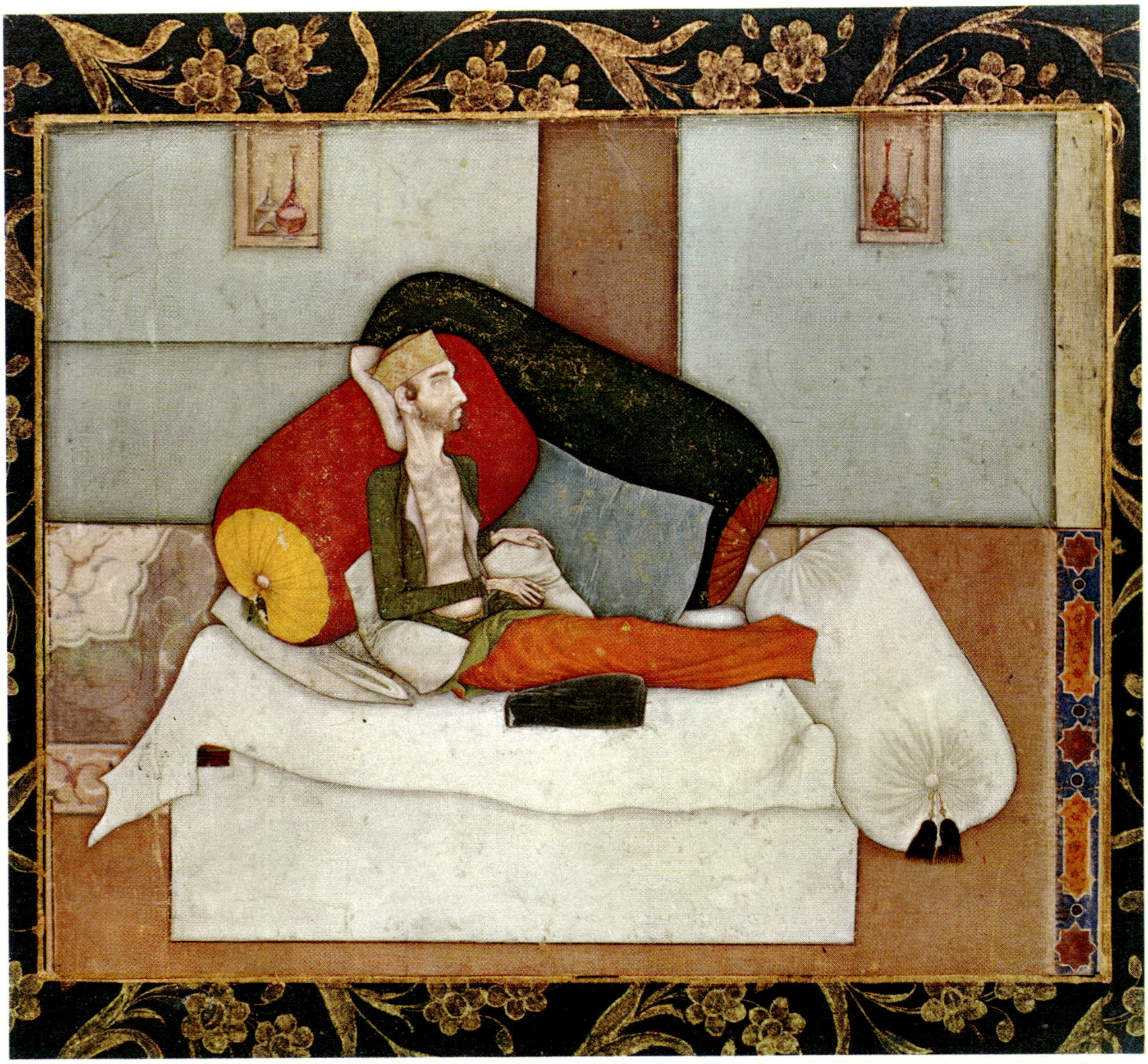

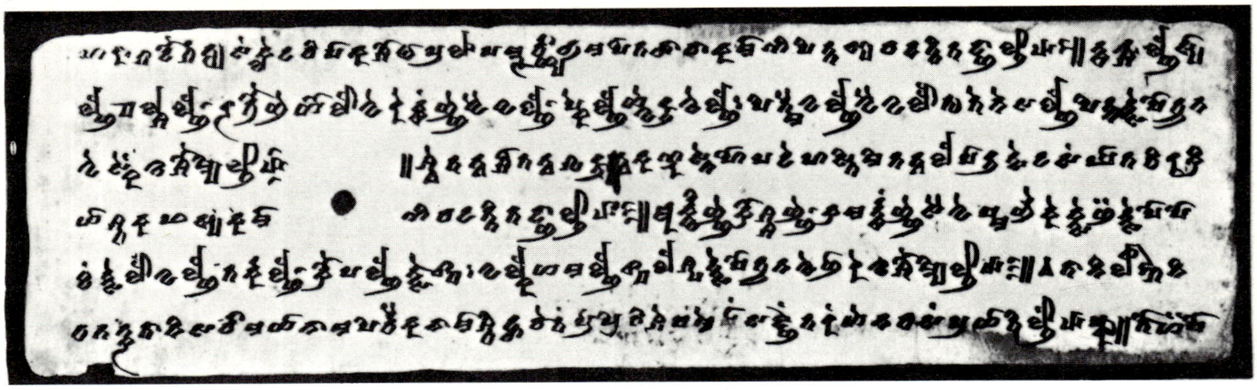

Jnyat Khan on his deathbed. *Mughal art. c. 1618. Bodleian Library, Oxford.*

Sanskrit medical text (Yogacataka). *Eighth-century Central Asian ms. Bibliotheque Nationale, Paris.*

Foot bath. *Seventeenth-century Indian miniature. British Museum, London.*

Rhinoplasty. *Plate from the Gentleman's Magazine of Calcutta, October 1794.*

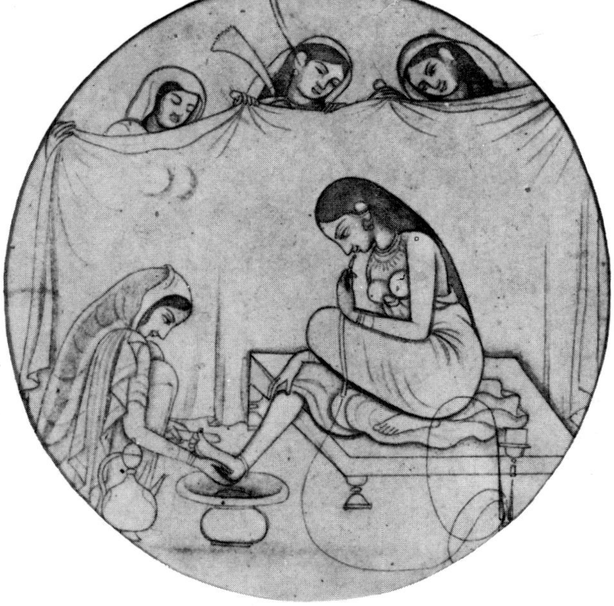

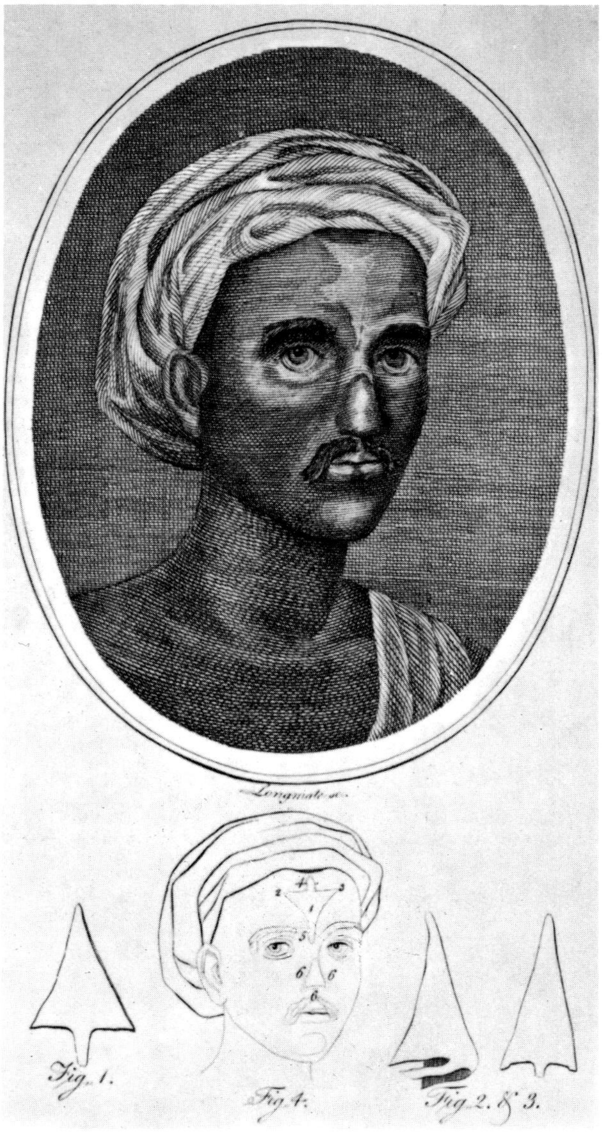

sites for encampment, making careful inspection of them in case they have been poisoned by the enemy. If he finds poison, he must eliminate it to save the army from death and destruction. Instructions about this are given in the chapter on poisons. The holy man's function, through his prayers, is to ward off evil influences arising from the breath of the strong, the sorrow of the oppressed and shame over sinning (while the astrologer staves off misfortunes written in the stars by announcing the correct sacrifice according to the instance). If there is sickness among the forces, the doctor must act with the utmost zeal, with especial care for the king's person because the fate of all the people depends on him; as the proverb puts it, "Where there is no king, subjects turn on each other". Let the doctor's tent be near the king's and let him always have his books and medicines to hand. Let a pennon be flown on his tent, so that the sick, poisoned or wounded can reach him in an emergency.'

This passage illustrates the main feature of medical thinking in ancient India: the tendency to build a system, with a niche for every concept in it. The medical works of ancient India are of composite nature, like encyclopedias. For this reason scholars have been unable to date the range of concepts and precepts that they contain, or to pick out the ideas indigenous to India from those that are derivative of other civilizations, for example the Assyro-Babylonian.

Ancient Hindu medicine presents a curious paradox in that it was strong in surgery and weak in anatomy, a subject which might be expected to be fundamental to surgery. This may have been due to the religious laws which forbade the use of a knife on a dead body. Susruta advised doctors to immerse the body in a basket in the river; after seven days of decomposition, the internal organs could be viewed simply by poking the overlying skin and other soft tissues away. Apart from this, ancient Indian texts are devoid of anatomical references.

A field in which the ancient Indians were centuries ahead of all other civilizations was that of plastic surgery. Rhinoplasty, for reshaping the nose, was very widely practised. It was not so much a question of aesthetics, to improve on nature, as a rebuilding operation. For adultery was punishable in India by cutting off the nose and surgeons devised the operation as an attempt to restore the normal

The understanding of illness was based on a concept of imbalance between various humours, both physical and moral, and Indian doctors knew and gave accurate descriptions of many diseases; it seems that as early as the sixth century BC connections between mosquito bites and malaria and between rodents and plague were recognized. Indian medicine was also strong in diagnosis, and in therapeutic techniques such as blood-letting, baths and the use of numerous drugs.

Giant having a tooth pulled. *Buddhist bas-relief from Bharut, second century* BC. *Guimet Museum, Paris.*

Birth of the hero Rustem. *Persian print. Wellcome Historical Medical Museum, London.*

appearance of those who suffered this terrible penalty.

Susruta explains in his book how the surgeon went about his work. From the leaf of a plant he cut a piece the size of the missing nose. This he laid on the patient's cheek and cutting round it removed a piece of skin the same size. Then the surgeon applied this piece to the nose stump, from which the skin had been removed, and sewed it on. After that, he put two pieces of hollow reed into the nostrils so that the patient could breathe easily. If the nose was now too big, he cut it off and started again. In a similar manner, a new ear lobe could be made from a piece of cheek. It is interesting that the ancient Indians recognized the need for a successful graft to come from the subject himself.

Many other surgical procedures are described in Susruta's book, including operations on anal fistulas and neck tumours, and tonsillectomy, lithotomy, lancing of abscesses and amputation of limbs. A painstakingly detailed list of 121 surgical instruments is given, including knives, scalpels, bistouries, saws, scissors, forceps for extracting teeth and others for extracting foreign bodies from nose and ear, twenty-eight different kinds of sound, three different kinds of needle for suturing, catheters and syringes. One section is devoted to the treatment of fractures with the use of bamboo splints.

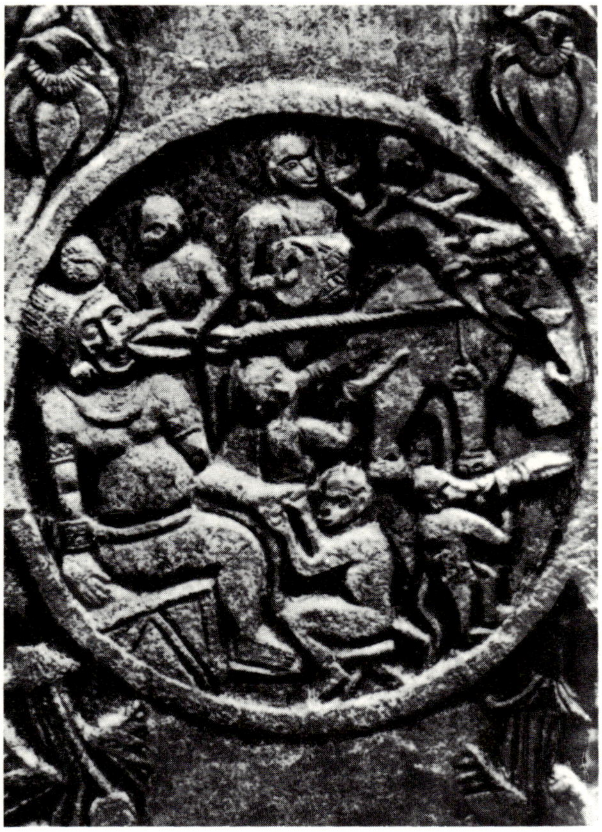

Diagnostic technique was also of a relatively high standard. Doctors inspected and palpated the patient, listened to his heart, lungs and abdomen, and noted the condition of the skin and tongue. Many illnesses were attributed to imbalance between the three physical humours—spirit, bile and phlegm. Besides these there were moral humours, disturbance of which could also underlie physical illness, an idea echoed in the present-day concept of psychosomatic disease. Ancient medical treatises give very accurate descriptions of the symptomatology of diabetes and tuberculosis, which then as now was rife in India, and of contagious diseases, especially smallpox. The Indians of that time knew that malaria was a consequence of mosquito bites, and in a Sanskrit text, predating Susruta, the role of plague carrier was ascribed to rodents.

Apart from a number of magical practices, Indian therapy was based on purgatives, enemas, emetics, blood-letting by leeches, steam baths, inhalations and sternutatories (preparations to cause sneezing—which was believed to clear the head). Susruta lists 760 medicinal plants, including *Atropa belladonna* (deadly nightshade) and *Cannabis indica* (Indian hemp) to induce stupor, and *Rauwolfia serpentina* for sedation.

An extremely important part is played in Indian medicine by the strict hygiene rules of the Brahmin religion. A largely vegetarian diet and the prohibition of alcohol are ordained, and there is great emphasis on cleanliness, with much bathing and the immediate removal of excreta and other waste from the house.

The third period of Hindu medicine was Mogul in origin, beginning in AD 664, after the Moslem conquest of India. It resulted in the introduction of Arab medicine into India. At the same time, Ayurvedic medicine persisted and in fact survives to the present day, being practised in innumerable villages and towns by doctors called *kaviraj.*

The health laws of the Israelites

'Never shall they fall on you, the many woes brought on Egypt; I am the Lord, and it is health I bring you' (Exodus XV, 26).

'Deny not a physician his due for your need's sake; his task is of divine appointment, since from God all healing comes, and kings themselves must needs bring gifts to him . . .' (Ecclesiasticus XXXVIII, 1–9).

For the ancient Hebrews, disease was not due to a demon or evil spirit or to spells cast by jealous fellow men, but represented a visible sign of God's wrath at the sins of men. Health could never fail as long as the Ten Commandments were observed. In order to get well, a sick man had to ask the priests to intercede on his behalf, since they were the arbiters of the law of Moses and did more health work than the doctors.

By attesting belief in one God, the giver of good health and bad, Mosaic law inevitably wielded the power of sanctions to overcome superstition and magic practices, though these did persist to a certain extent. It was faith and faith alone that brought health to the body and salvation to the soul. Since to be unclean was the worst sin of all, the rules of hygiene laid down in the scripture aimed to make men clean in the eyes of God. Physical purity and moral purity were thus equated.

In the book of Leviticus an exemplary code of health is given (V, 2–3): 'A man may have touched what has been killed by a wild beast or has fallen dead, or the carcase of a reptile, or some other unclean thing, unaware of his defilement at the time; yet he has incurred guilt by the fault. Or he has touched some defilement of the human body; there are many such; he may be unaware of it till afterwards, but he has incurred guilt . . .' The purifying bath would cleanse him of this guilt; otherwise a man would not be allowed to enter the Temple.

During menstruation, a woman was unclean and could not carry out religious duties in the temple, or have intercourse with her husband. When the menstrual flow ceased she had to be purified by a ritual bath, and before being immersed naked in the water, her body had to be carefully cleaned. Every community, no matter how small, always built a ritual bath as well as a synagogue. Naturally it was not only menstruating women who were unclean but also people with infectious diseases such as gonorrhoea and leprosy, who made anything or any individual they touched unclean also.

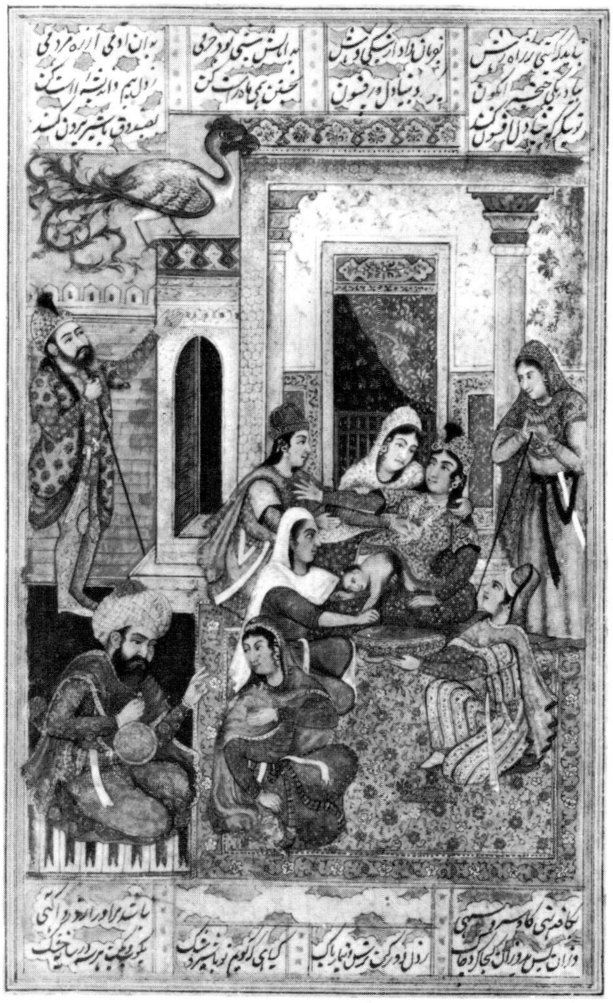

It was also a religious duty to wash the hands before meals; washing them after meals was regarded as a duty of respect to others rather than as a religious one. And another ritual practice of hygienic importance was circumcision, which may have originated among the Jews.

As has been described in previous chapters, regulations concerning hygienic and health matters, such as the prohibition of certain foods, personal cleanliness and circumcision, existed among other Oriental peoples, but here they applied only to the priest caste (which by the Middle Kingdom in Egypt, at least, had probably accepted the principle of monotheism). The Jews on the other hand, according to their scriptures, were a chosen people –a people of priests, with no different castes–and

The historical importance of ancient Hebrew medicine lies in its fundamental contribution to communal hygiene through concepts contained in the Bible and the Talmud, the book which forms the basis of Jewish civil and canon law. Principles of bodily cleanliness, nutrition and diet, obstetrics and child welfare were codified in the book of Leviticus. *Belief in only one god denied the use of magical practices.*

all religious and sanitary regulations were imposed equally on everyone among them.

Regulations for the control of contagious disease represent the first compulsory health enactments. When an epidemic was raging, the alarm was sounded on the shofar (ram's horn). People who caught the disease were isolated, and their clothing and dwelling disinfected. The steps taken in mediaeval Europe to counteract the spread of 'leprosy' were straight out of the Bible.

Some of the rules about food were based on specific medical observation. For example, the eating of pork was forbidden, as this meat can transmit tapeworms to humans. 'You are not to eat the fat of sheep or ox or goat; but you may keep the fat of anything that falls dead, or is killed by a wild beast, for various uses. Anyone who eats the fat which ought to be offered as part of the Lord's burnt-sacrifice is lost to his people.' (Leviticus VII, 24).

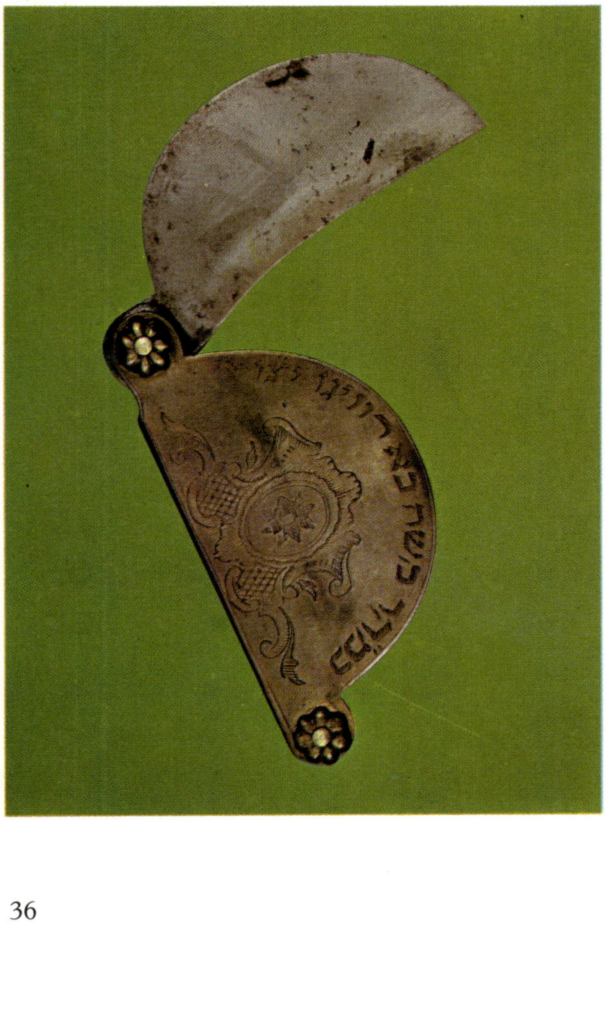

Ancient Persian medicine may have shared a common origin with Jewish medicine, and it too placed emphasis on personal and communal hygiene. Health depended on the god of light and good, Ahura Mazda, and medicine was in the hands of his worshippers.

Circumcision knife. *Eighteenth-century Jewish. Putti Collection, Rizzoli Institute, Bologna.*

Milah for circumcision. *Vogelmann Collection, Florence.*

The skill of ancient Jewish surgeons was considerable. They performed operations for anal fistula, for imperforate anus in the newborn, Caesarean section, and treated dislocations and fractures by rational methods. The practice of circumcision was so much a part of ancient tradition that it was done with stone tools even after metal had come into common use.

Our knowledge of Jewish surgery comes from the Talmud, books of learned rabbinical interpretation of the scriptures. The Talmud also contains information on anatomy and physiology, and accurate descriptions of many diseases, including jaundice and cirrhosis of the liver, various parasitic diseases and diphtheria; haemophilia is mentioned as an hereditary disease which permits circumcision to be omitted.

The most significant feature of ancient Hebrew medicine was its emphasis on prophylaxis–the prevention of disease. Besides the cult of cleanliness and the enforcement of health regulations, credit must go to the Jews for being the first to set aside one day a week for rest, to the inestimable benefit of all mankind. The law of Moses said: 'Six days for drudgery, for doing all the work you have to do. When the seventh day comes, it is a day of rest'.

Persian medicine

At this point, a few words should be said about ancient Persian medicine, as practised at the time when the great empire extended from the Mediterranean and the Caucasus to India. What is known of the medicine of this period comes largely from the sacred books of the *Avesta,* which belong to the ancient dualistic religion in which Ahura Mazda, the god of light and good, is in conflict with Angra Mayniu, the spirit of evil and darkness. Medicine was the weapon of good in the fight against demons; its nature was embodied in the myth of the marvellous tree of Gaokarena which conferred immortality and cured all ills. In the *Vendidad,* the sixth book of the *Avesta,* the medical rites of the primitive Persians are described; as in other magical systems, therapy is based on prayer and incantations to rid the sufferer of the malign spirit through the power of Ahura Mazda. Emphasis is placed on personal and communal hygiene, and it seems that ancient Persian and ancient Jewish practices shared a common origin, perhaps before the time when the

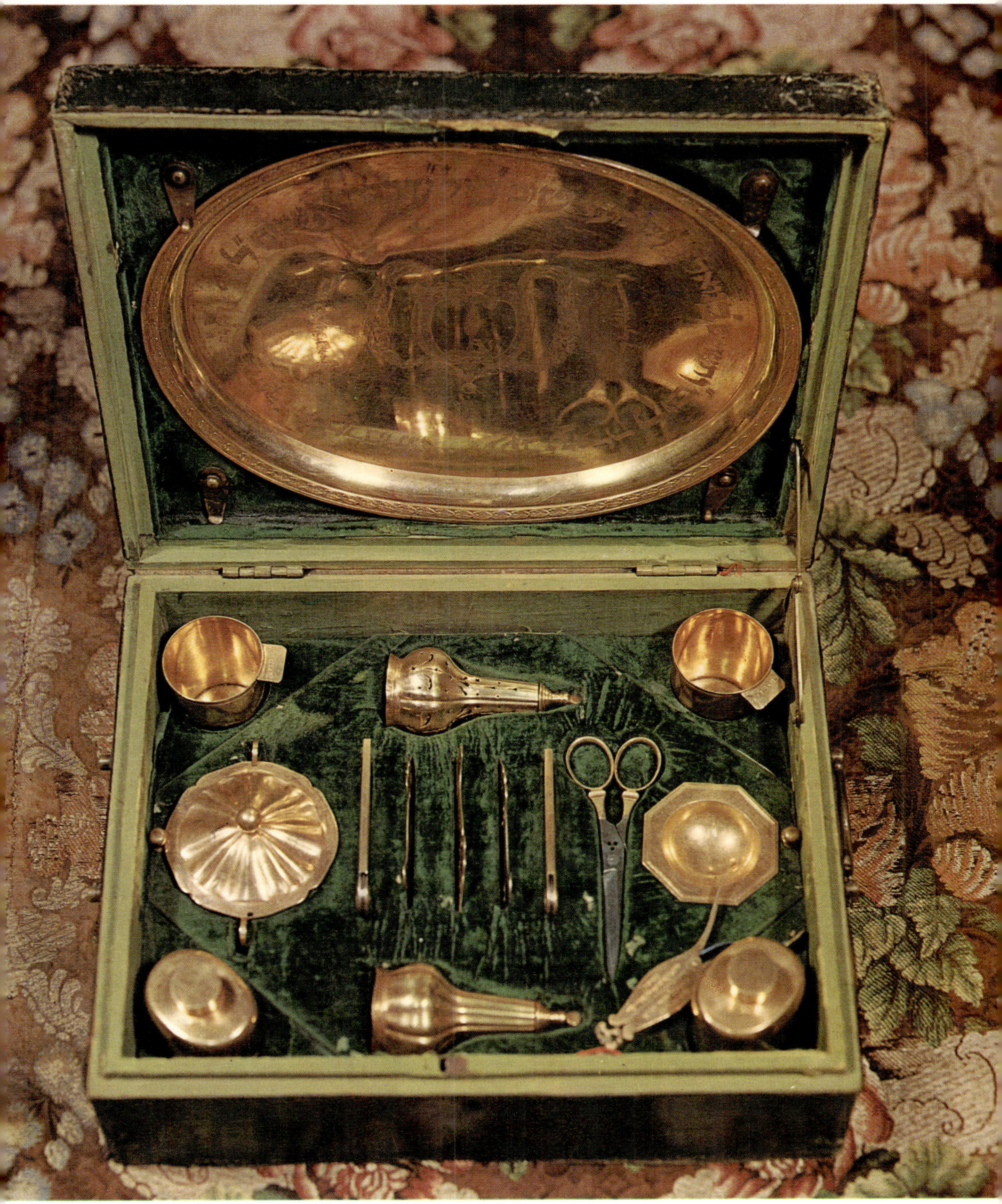

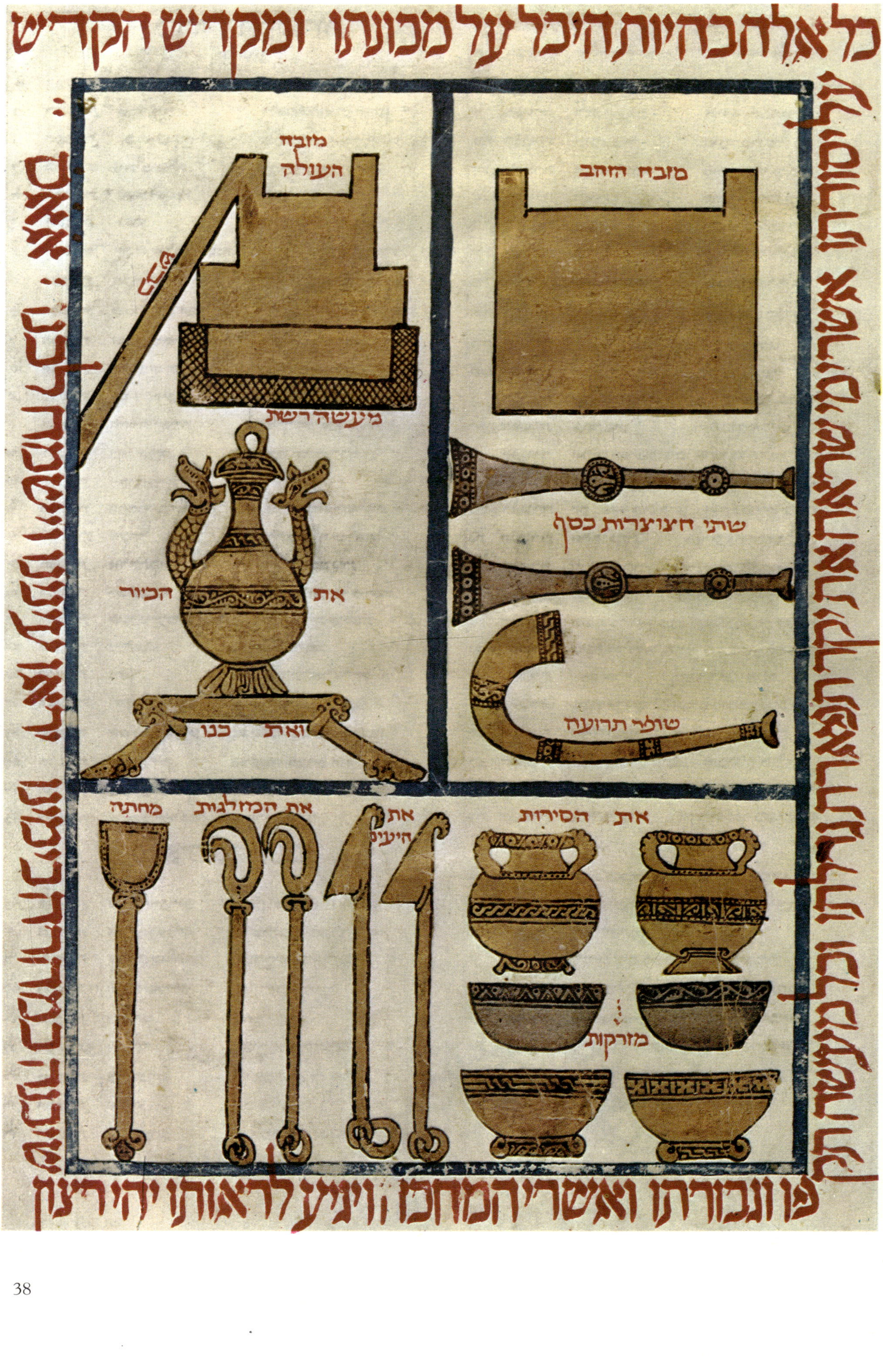
מזבח העולה
מזבח הזהב
מעשה רשת
את הכיור
ואת כנו
שתי חצוצרות כסף
שופר תרועה
מחתה
את המזלגות
את היעים
את הסירות
מזרקות

Knives, surgical instruments and sacrificial vessels. *From the Hebrew Bible written at Perpignan in 1299 by Solomon Ben Raphael. Bibliotheque Nationale, Paris.*

Cabala scheme. *From a Hebrew ms. Bibliotheque Nationale, Paris.*

Ritual bath of Jewish women. *Plate from Kirchner's Jewish Ceremony, Nuremberg 1726. National Library, Vienna.*

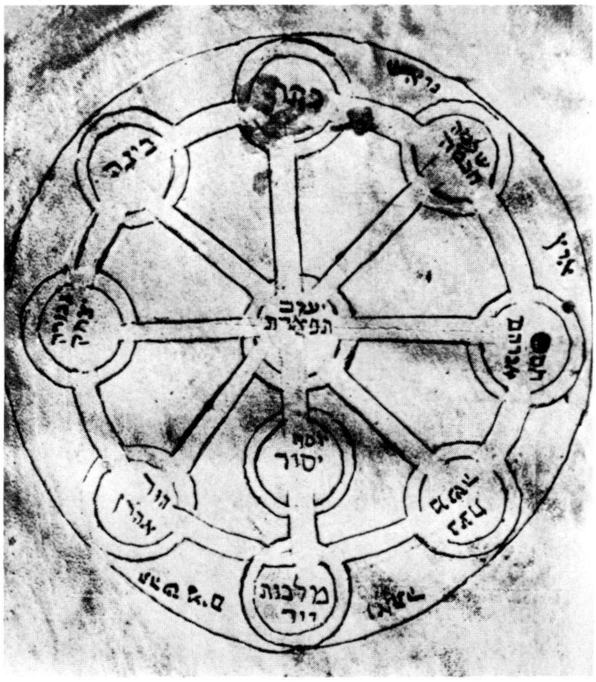

pastoral peoples of Mesopotamia assumed separate identities.

Medicine was in the hands solely of the worshippers of Mazda. A professional code is laid down in the *Vendidad,* with stipulation of training requirements, fees and penalties for malpractice. Surgeons as well as physicians existed at this period, for in the writings of Firdausi, who lived around AD 1000, are to be found descriptions of doctors in ancient Persia who healed with the knife, as well as accounts of successful Caesarean section. Herodotus recorded other practices, such as segregating the sick and those suffering from contagious disease.

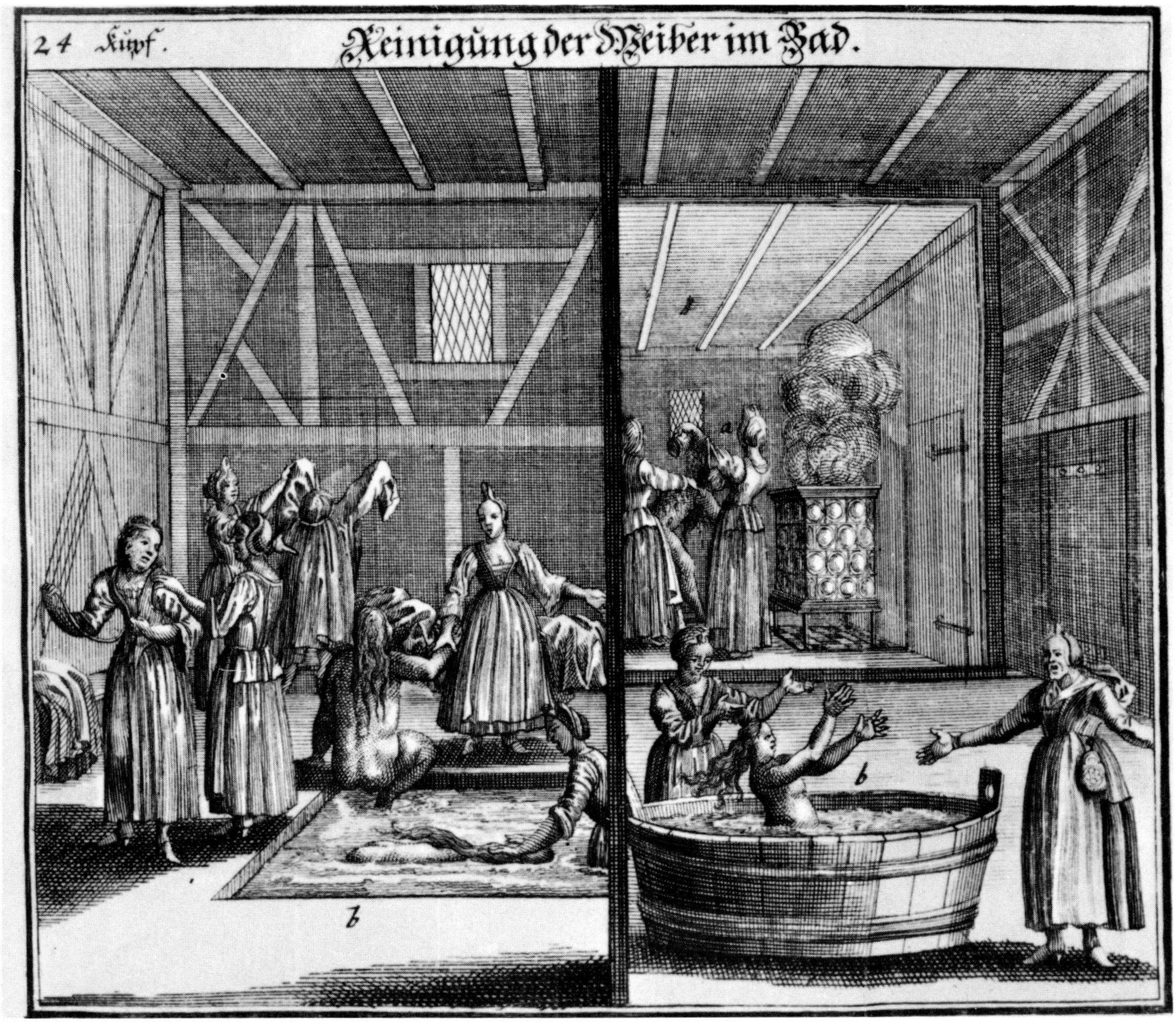

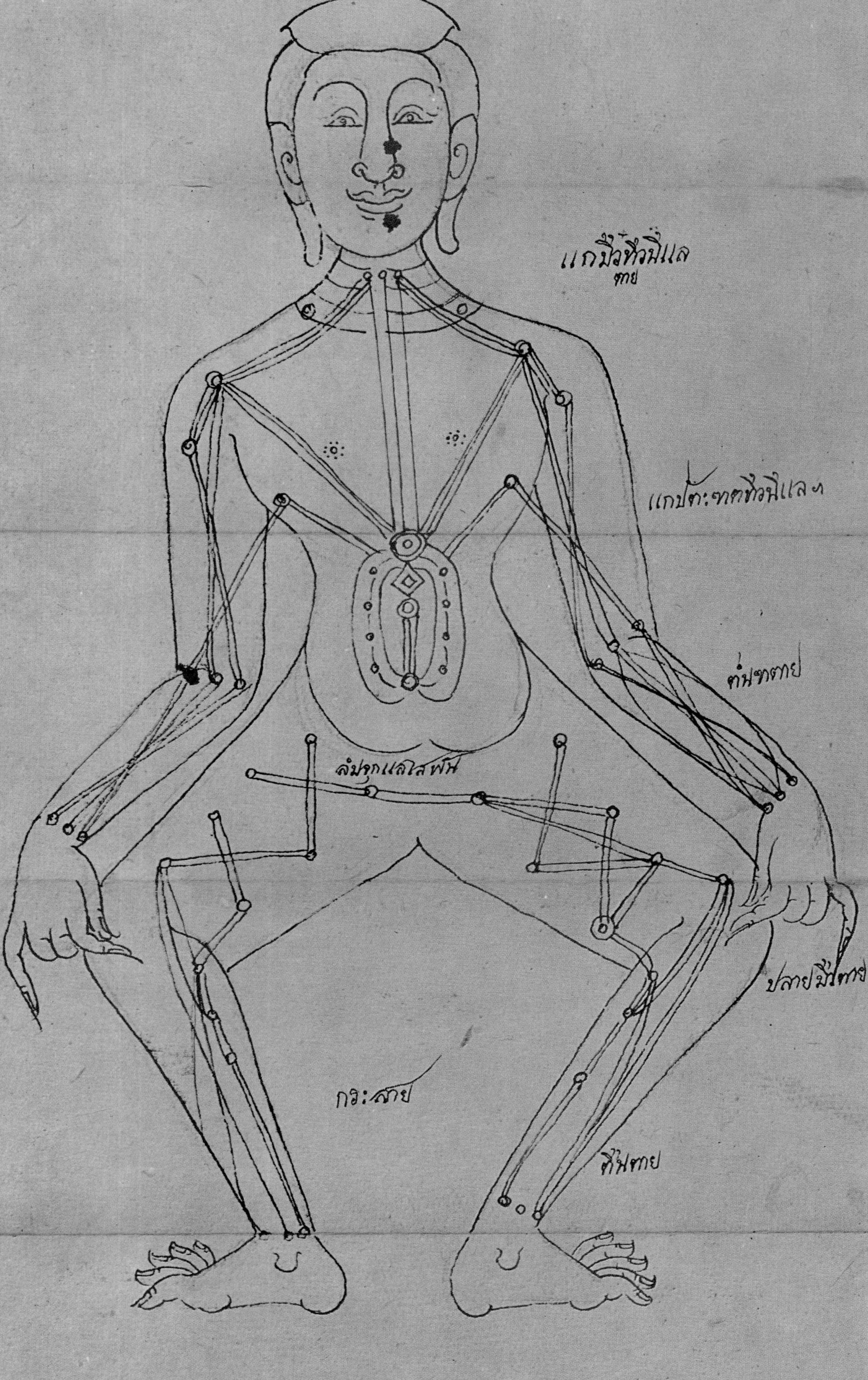
แกปิ้วหัวมิแล
ตาย
แกปัตะฆาตหัวมิแล ๗
ต่ำฆาตาย
ลำปรุกแลใสพัน
ปลายมิ้วตาย
กระสาย
ตีนตาย

Tradition and Chinese medicine

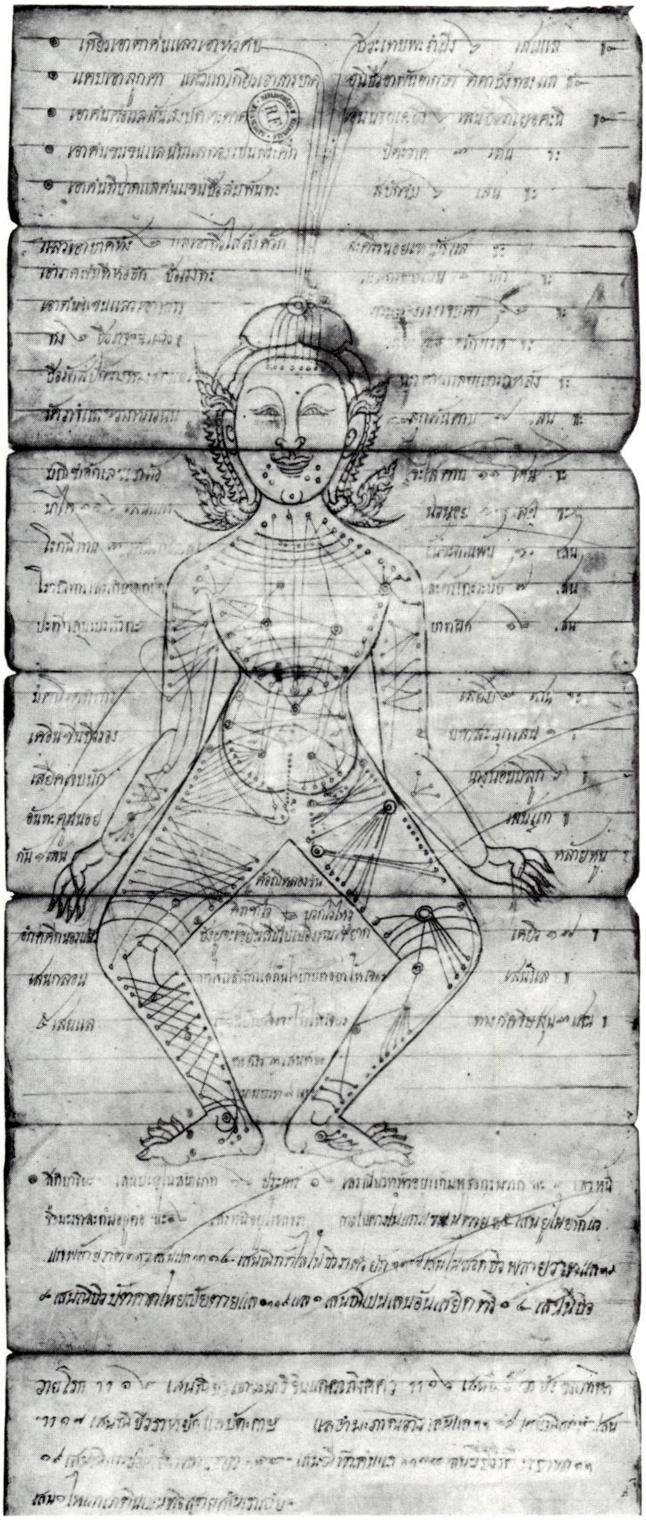

While the pharaohs of Egypt were engrossed in erecting pyramids, the ancient Chinese emperors were preoccupied with medicine. Yet the history of China bears some resemblance to that of Egypt, in that it embraced a series of dynasties dating back to Shen Nung, a legendary emperor who is said to have ruled from 2838 to 2698 BC. This enlightened ruler was looked upon as the inventor of agriculture and medicine, under the inspiration of Pan Ku, the god to whom the creation of the world was attributed in Taoist legend: chaos was overcome and order established on the basis of two opposite poles, *yang* and *yin*.

The *yang* principle was positive, active and masculine, as signified by the sky, light, might, hardness, warmth and dryness, and also the left side. The *yin* principle on the other hand was negative, being passive and feminine, as signified by the moon, earth, darkness, weakness, cold and moisture and the right side. Chinese medicine was based on these two principles; *yang* and *yin* together with the blood constituted the vital substance that circulated in the body. Illness was held to be caused by imbalance of the two principles, while death supervened when they ceased to flow.

One particular contribution of the emperor Shen Nung to Chinese medicine was his *Pen T'sao Ching* or Herbal. This little book lists 365 herbs, prescriptions and poisons in three volumes. Quite a few of the prescriptions found in this herbal and its successors are common to modern therapy, for example opium as a narcotic, rhubarb as a laxative, flowers of Artemisia for worms, Rauwolfia (already referred to in respect of medicine in ancient India), kaolin for diarrhoea, ephedrine for asthma and chaulmoogra oil for leprosy. Following it a succession of similar works appeared, culminating in the *Pen T'sao Kang Mu* or Great Herbal (AD 1552) of Li Shi-Chen, which describes 1,871 drugs in fifty-two volumes and took twenty-seven years to write.

In addition to the prescriptions derived from the legendary emperor Shen Nung, the ancient Chinese made use of other treatments which are still found in modern pharmacopoeias, such as sodium sulphate for purging, iron for anaemia and arsenic for skin disorders. They also took the first steps to immunize against smallpox, introducing pustular crusts in powder form into the nostrils (the left nostril for boys, the right for girls).

Another emperor with an important place in

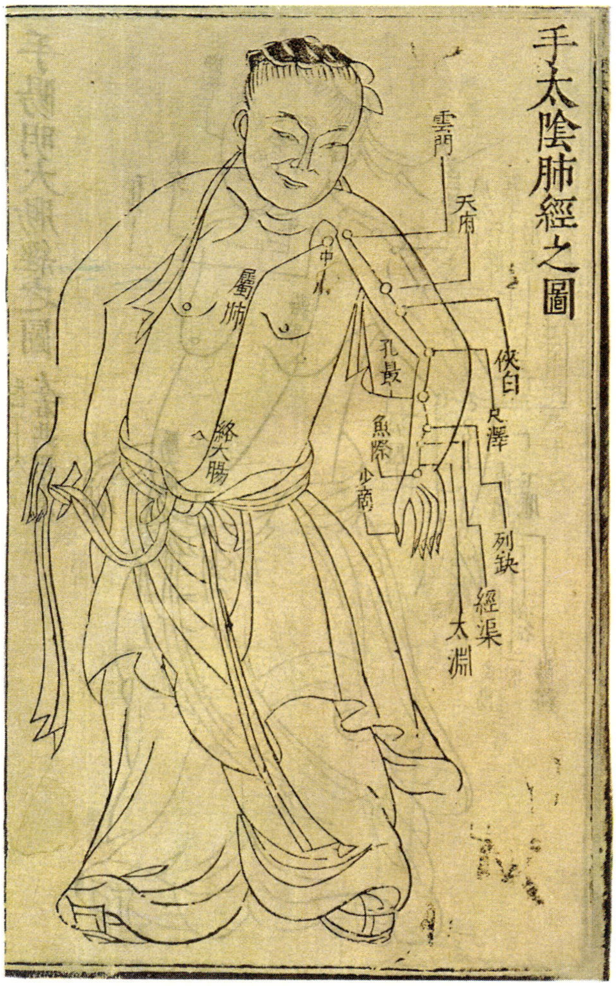

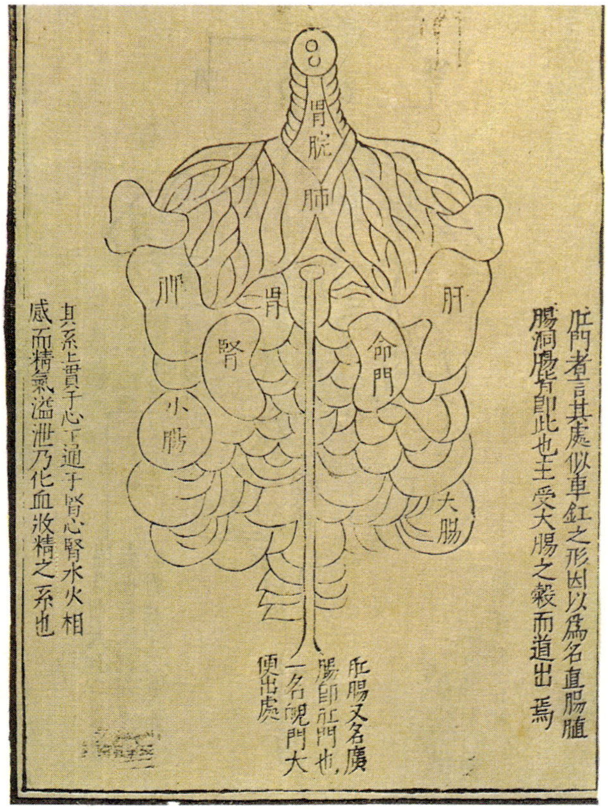

Previous pages :
Siamese drawings indicating points for acupuncture. *Bibliotheque Nationale, Paris.*

These pages :
Drawings: acupuncture points (upper) and anatomy of diaphragm and abdominal organs (lower). *From Trong Jin Tchou King, 1031. Chinese ms. Bibliotheque Nationale, Paris.*

Jade statuette used by Chinese ladies to show doctors their symptoms. *Dept. of History of Medicine, University of Kansas.*

Chinese instrument and drug cases. *Oriental Art Museum, Rome.*

medicine was Hwang Ti (2698–2598 BC), to whom is ascribed the *Nei Ching* (Book of Medicine), the most ancient as well as the greatest Chinese medical work, and one that is still studied in China. One passage from it states: 'All the blood of the human body is under the control of the heart and regulated by it. The blood current flows continuously in a circle and never stops; it cannot but flow ceaselessly like the current of a river or the sun and the moon in their courses'. These are superficially remarkable statements, considering that ancient Chinese understanding of anatomy was only fair. Dissection of the dead, while generally prohibited (for a man had to die with his body whole if he was to join his ancestors), seems nevertheless to have been attempted, judging by some anatomical measurements. The suggestion has been made that it was the prerogative of the Chinese emperors as absolute rulers to conduct anatomical investigations. More probably, Hwang Ti's categorical statement about the circulation of the blood should be regarded as a very near guess at the facts.

The *Nei Ching* also includes this picturesque presentation of physiology: 'The heart is king, the lungs are his ministers, the liver is his general and the gall bladder his justice, while the spleen governs the five senses and three hot cavities eliminate waste matter, namely thorax, abdomen and pelvis'.

Chinese doctors did not delve into the medical histories of their patients and their families, or go in for full physical examinations. In diagnosis, they concentrated on examining the pulse, taking it in a variety of ways and producing an endless list of

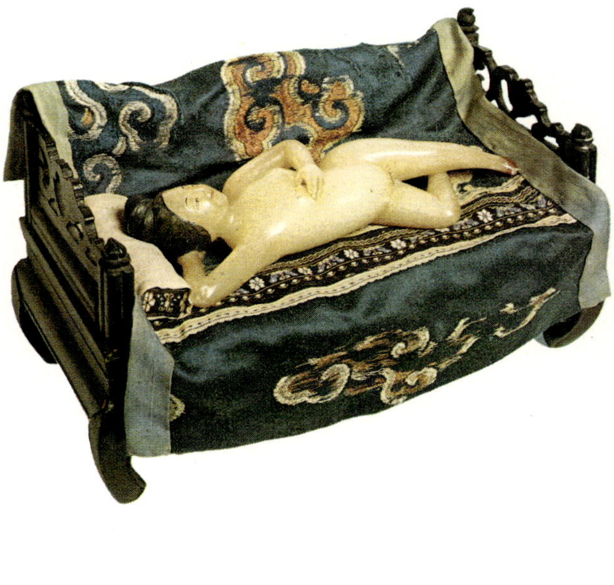

In the strongly traditional and dynastic history of China, the origins of medicine were attributed to a legendary ruler inspired by the Taoist god Pan Ku.

Knowledge of anatomy was limited by the forbidding of human dissection by Confucian teaching and the Chinese scheme of physiology also was scanty and imprecise. The well-known Chinese practice of acupuncture, in which the patient's skin is pricked with different types of needles, uses a system of surface anatomy based on the teaching of a legendary emperor of ancient times.

However, it was probably simple modesty rather than Confucian principles which led to the practice whereby Chinese ladies did not undress for examination by a doctor, but pointed out the site of their symptoms on special statuettes.

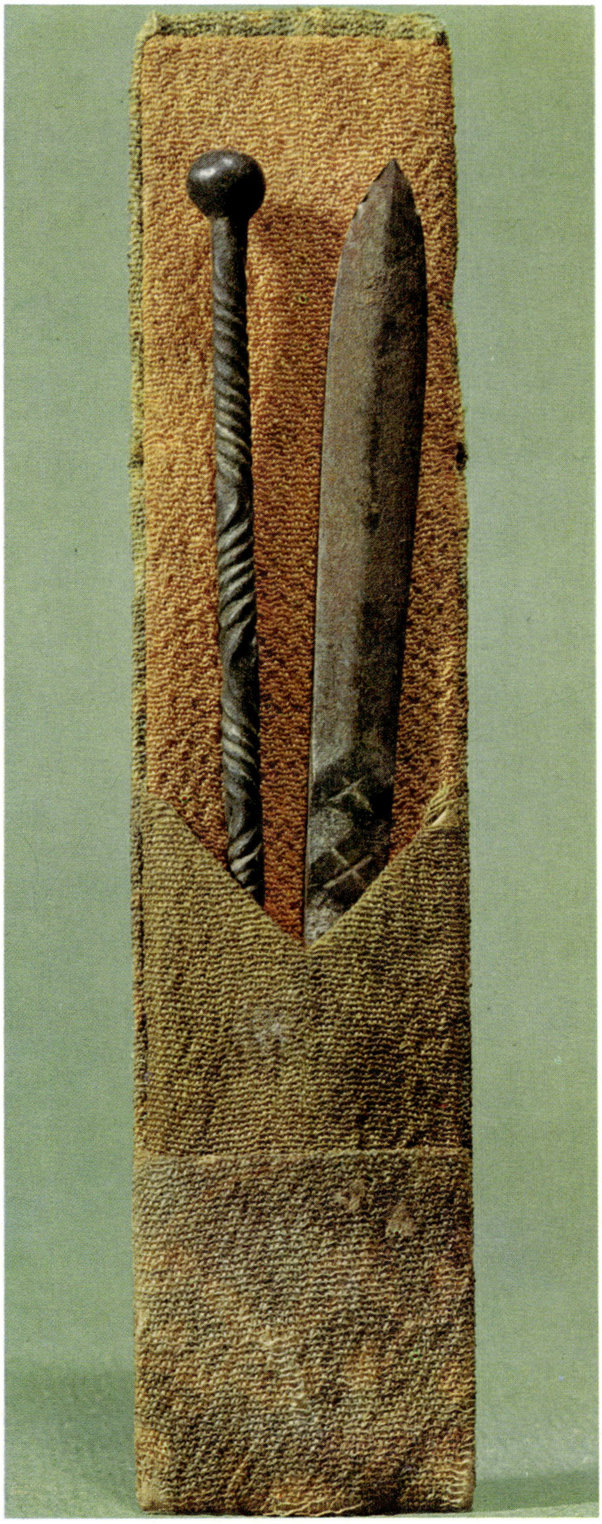

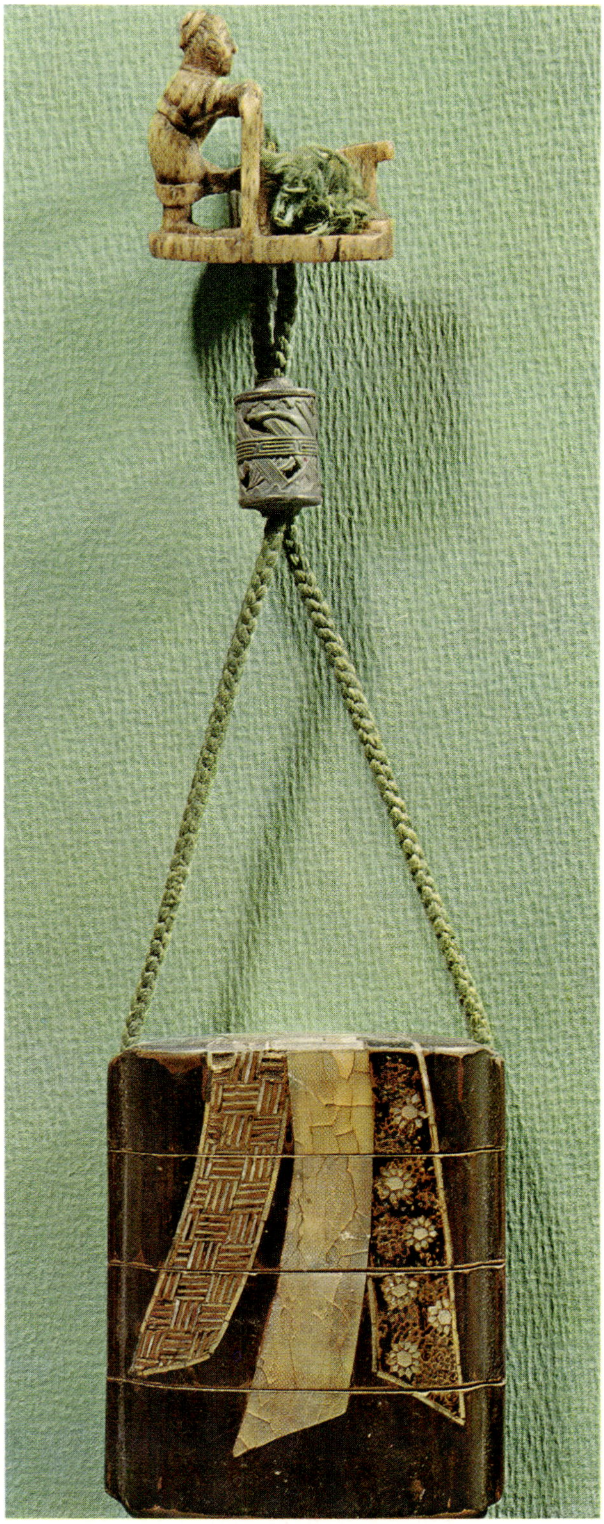

Surgery was practised, sometimes using primitive narcotics and anaesthetics, but the greatest achievements of ancient Chinese medicine were a series of herbals, culminating in the 52-volume Pen T'sao Kang Mu *of AD 1552 which described over 1,800 drugs. Chinese doctors also took the first steps to immunize against smallpox, using powdered pustular crusts introduced into the nostrils. The teaching of medicine was entrusted to a medical college controlled by the Chinese emperors, who introduced state examinations.*

Herbs with healing or magic properties. *Drawings from Chinese ms. Bibliotheque Nationale, Paris.*

Young girl with smallpox. *Eighteenth-century Chinese miniature. Bibliotheque Nationale, Paris.*

variations, each with its own prognostic significance. For the pulse indicated the flow of the vital element, formed as explained earlier from the union of *yang* and *yin* with the blood.

The most famous Chinese surgeon was Hua T'o, who lived about the second century AD. Before performing an operation, incision or amputation, Hua T'o is said to have made the patient insensible of pain by administering a narcotic brew he had made himself. Some eight centuries before Hua T'o the practice of castration was widespread in China and many doctors specialized in it, to provide eunuchs for the emperors' service. Then, too, surgeons used to dull pain before the operation by using anaesthetic substances; none of the old texts give details of the actual ingredients, but in more recent times a hot decoction of pepper pods was used, applied to the genitals. For the operation itself, the penis and scrotum were tied together with a strip of silk, and a semi-circular knife was then used to sever them in front of the pubis. To stop the bleeding, a styptic powder of rock alum and resin was applied. The surgeon next put a plug of wood in the urethra. If the patient survived, he was ready three months later for his duties as guardian of the imperial concubines.

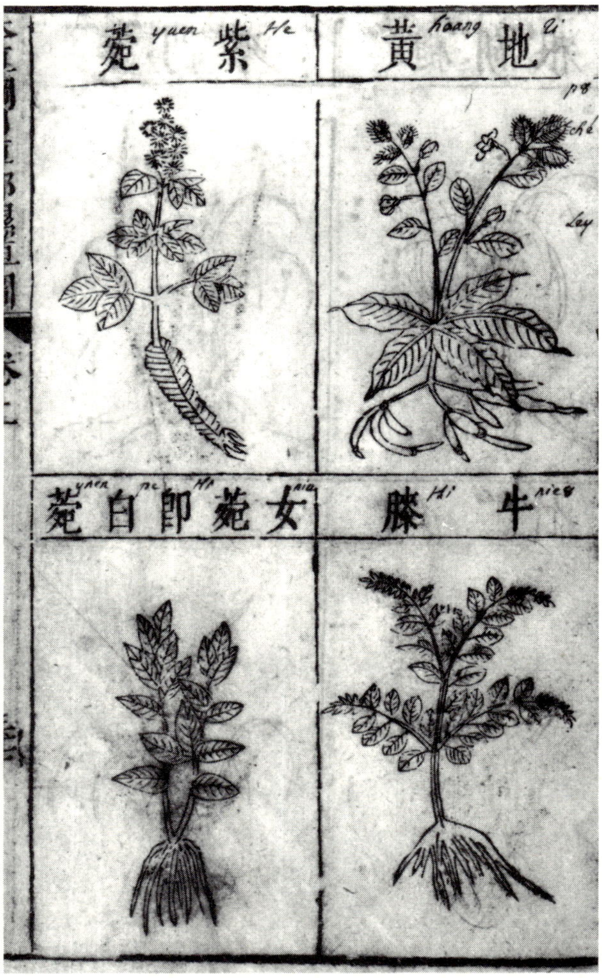

Another practice which persisted into this century was the binding of the feet of high-born women. The victims of this cruel custom, imposed from a misguided sense of aesthetics, were not given the option of refusal. While they were still small and powerless to resist, they had to undergo special bandaging, which was tight and painful, to turn the toes down and hold up the instep, with permanent deformity.

The most typically Chinese medical practice was acupuncture, still in use today and no longer confined to the Far East. It consisted in pricking the patient's skin with needles of gold, silver or iron, cold or hot, of various lengths from one to ten inches. The idea was to remove any obstruction in the *chin, loh* or *sun,* the vessels carrying the two vital principles, blood and air. Old treatises name some 365 points for acupuncture. Specialists taught their pupils by means of metal statuettes, pricked all over with holes at the points of puncture. Since this was their chosen training method, it seems that the Chinese did not learn their surface anatomy in a rational way.

Against that, the method lends support to the view that the emperors alone were knowledgeable about anatomy, since they were responsible for starting the practice of acupuncture; it may have been the legendary Shen Nung himself who was the originator. The pin-pricks on the statuettes were by no means random. The technique, well known in Europe since about 1930, is gaining ground in the western world as a treatment for some symptoms arising from joints and muscles.

In the following centuries, Chinese medicine was at a standstill because of people's veneration for the wisdom of their ancestors. It was not until the thirteenth century that another major advance took place. In 1247, the judge Sung Tz'u compiled

一女三歲

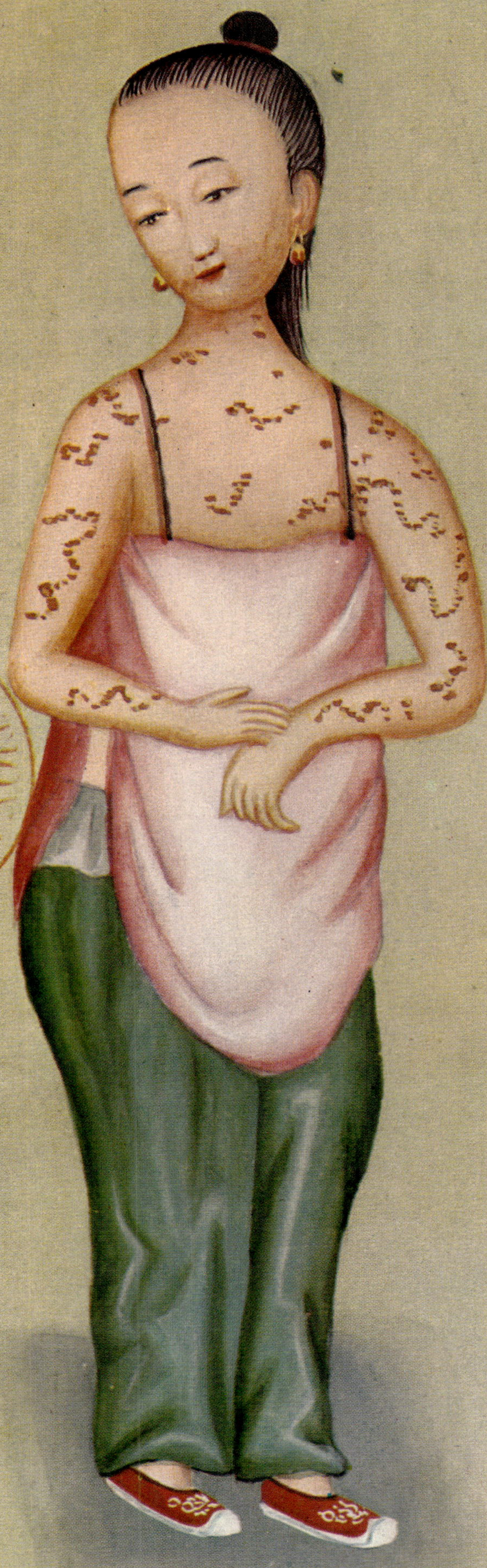

雁行痘形三十三

Chinese doctors based their diagnosis on the examination of the pulse in a variety of ways: the body was compared to a chord instrument in which the different pulses represent the chords, so that the harmony or discord of the organism could be ascertained by taking the pulse.

In the thirteenth century, after a long period of stagnation due to an excessive respect for traditional learning, appeared the Hsi Yuan Lu, *an important treatise on medicine and the law. It included methods of distinguishing death by drowning and poisoning, on artificial respiration and on antidotes to poisons.*

Treatment for reviving the drowned. *Japanese print.*

Chinese doctor taking pulse. *Photograph taken in 1890.*

the *Hsi Yüan Lu,* the standard treatise on law and medicine, or medical jurisprudence. It was intended for the magistrature and contained information on ascertaining the cause of death from a careful study of the deceased: accurate descriptions were given of signs to distinguish death by drowning, poisoning, strangling, stabbing and bludgeoning. As well as establishing diagnostic methods to distinguish murder from suicide, the work gave instructions on artificial respiration and antidotes to poisons.

Then, while science and learning advanced in Europe, Chinese medicine became dormant again. The teachings inherited from the ancients were so scrupulously revered that all progress was impeded. European medicine did not enter China until the nineteenth century.

Japan

About the fourth century AD Chinese civilization penetrated Japan, and for many centuries it entirely dominated the islands; its medicine supplanted native practices. The first attempts to reduce Chinese influence came in the sixteenth century, the greatest reformer being the physician Tokuhon Nagata (1512–1630), and the Portuguese landing in 1542 introduced European medicine, which was adopted as avidly as Chinese methods had been before.

Little is known of pre-Chinese medicine, although old legends indicate rudimentary anatomical knowledge and a theory of disease based on evil spirits and divine influences.

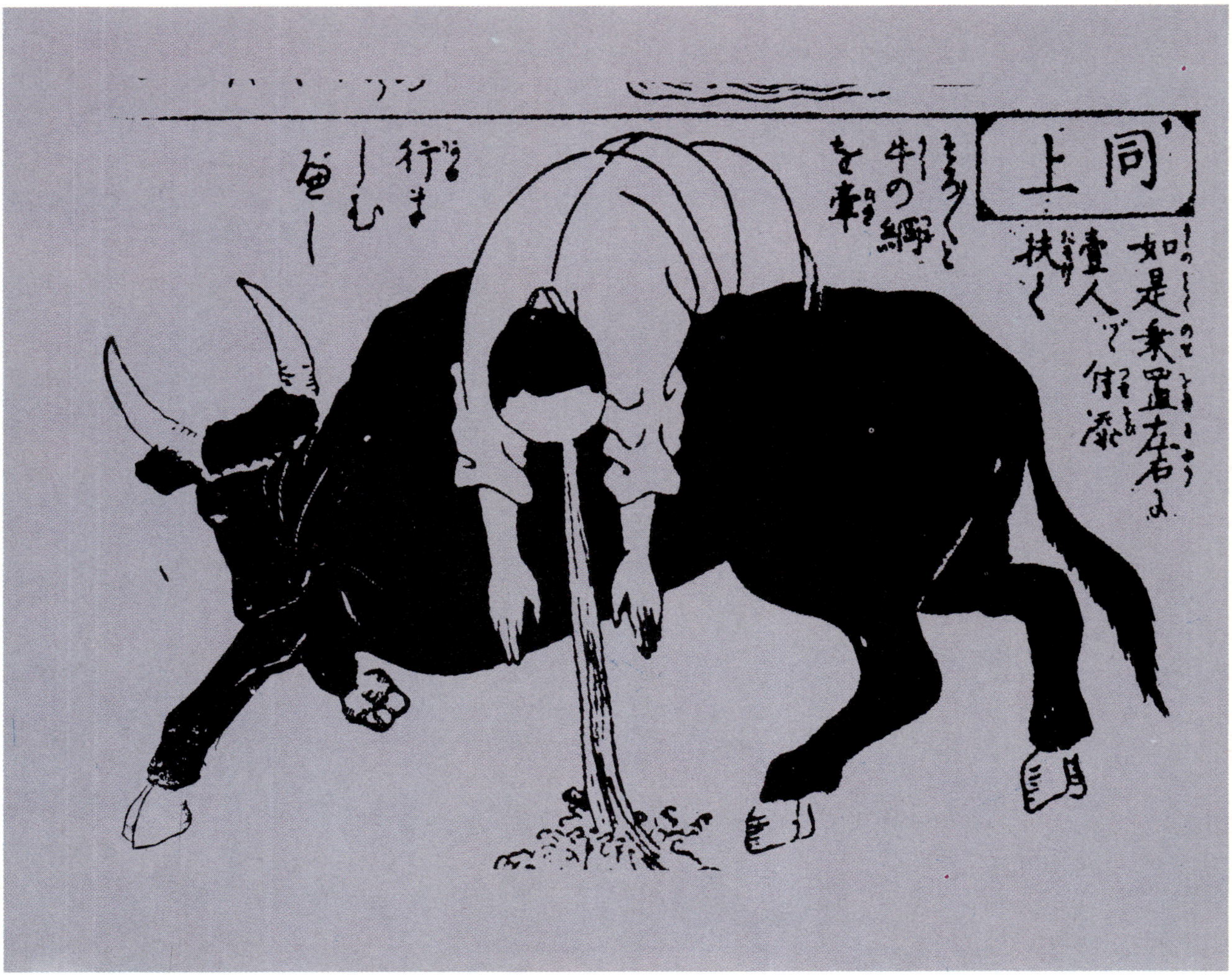

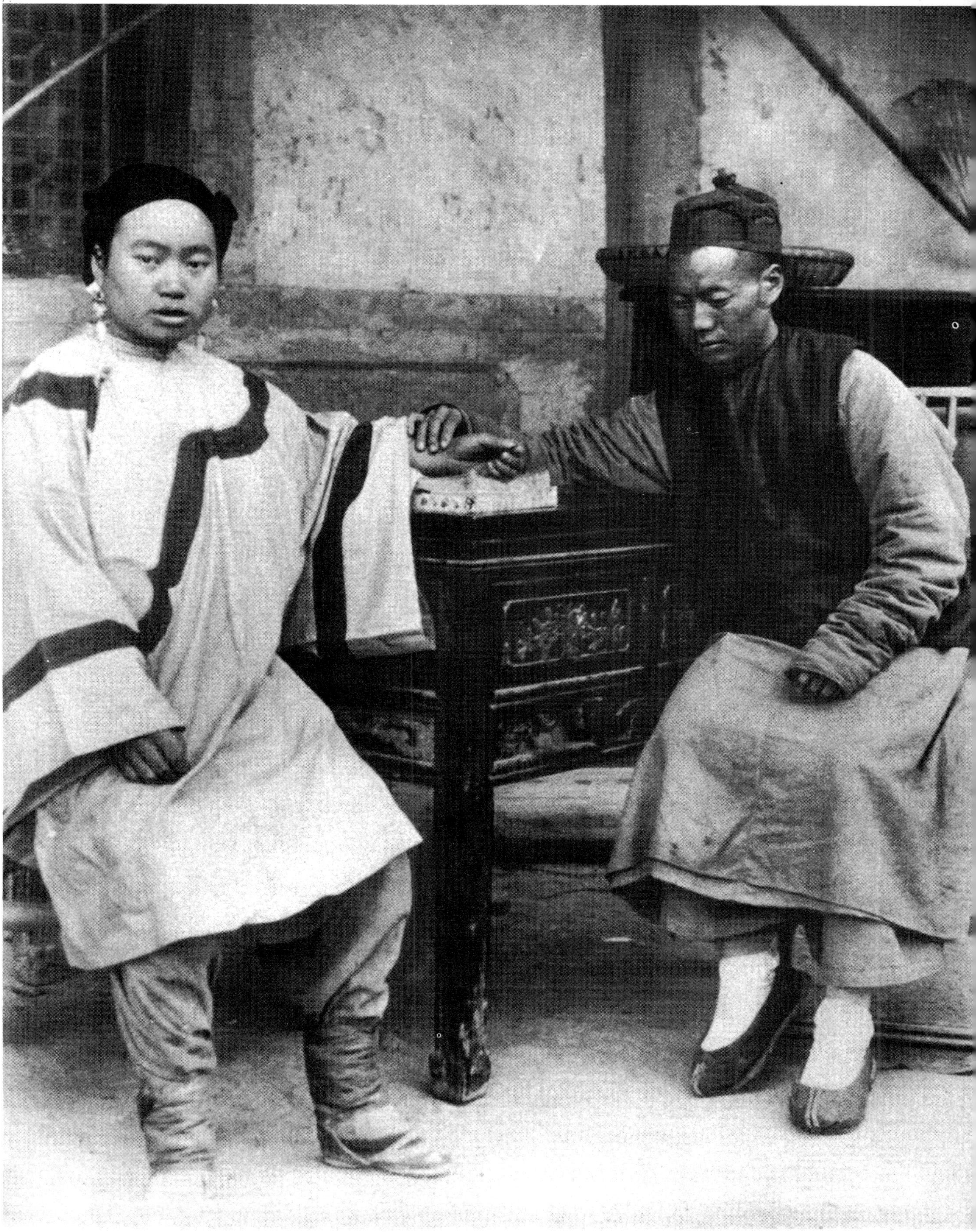

Hellenic civilization had its origins in the conquest of the Greek islands by races from the eastern shore of the Mediterranean. Various influences gradually moulded the unique culture of the ancient Greeks with its penetrating philosophical and critical methods. Medicine in Greece developed in this stimulating cultural climate and became for the first time a science, practised by laymen rather than priests.

The earliest references to Greek medical practice are found in Homer's epic poem the Iliad, *which includes descriptions of the work of surgeons on the battlefields of Troy.*

Achilles binding Patroclus' wound. *Sosia bowl, fifth century* BC. *Berlin Museum.*

Telephus wounded in the thigh. *From Grecian vase. British Museum, London.*

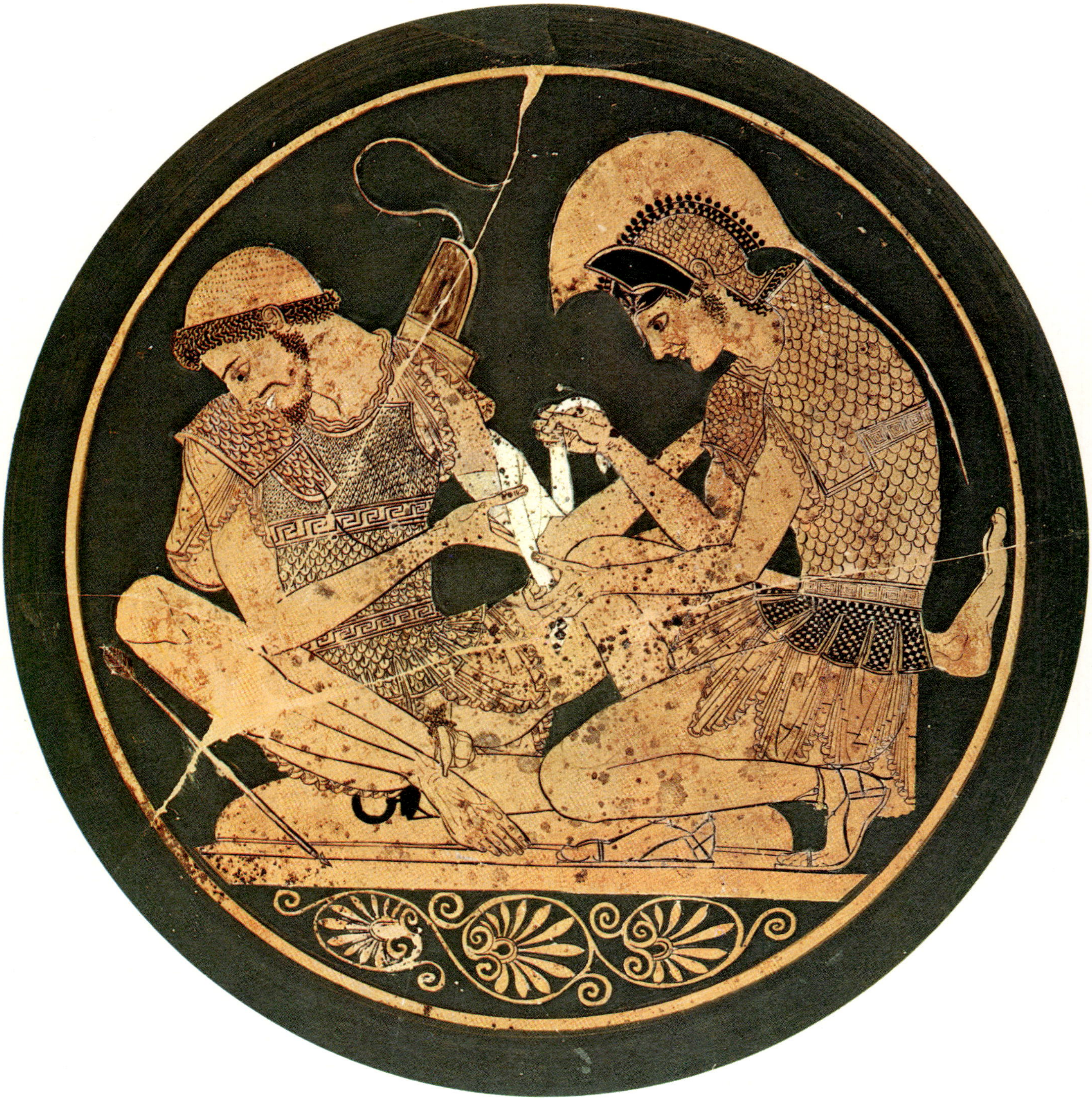

THE CLASSICAL ERA
Surgeons at the siege of Troy

Ancient Aegean civilization began around 3000 BC with the conquest of the Greek islands by the races inhabiting the eastern shores of the Mediterranean. Diverse oriental influences were fused into pre-Hellenic culture and at the same time transmuted by the process of separation from Asia, as can be seen today in the relics of Minoan civilization that survive at Knossos. Here sculpture and frescoes appear plastic and alive and are freed from the rigidity of Babylonian and Egyptian art. Not only art, but philosophy, astronomy and mathematics developed in the new environment, while medicine flourished along original lines: this is known from the palace at Knossos, where advanced plumbing is still to be seen, and from the attribution in later Egyptian texts of a number of remedies to 'the people of the islands.'

Hellenic medicine developed in company with philosophy, disciplined by strict criticism. Healing, for the first time, became a science as well as an art, practiced not by a priestly caste but by laymen who replaced magic by enquiry, and it was regarded as a noble science.

In the fifth book of the *Iliad* Homer recounts how in 1184 BC, during the Trojan war, Diomedes sought out his enemy Pandarus and killed him. Then he fought with the Trojan Aeneas, who was guarding the body of his fallen comrade in case the Greeks tried to rob him of it. Diomedes picked up a lump of rock, 'more than two men could lift today', but he wielded it easily on his own. Hurling it at Aeneas, he scored a hit 'at the point where thigh meets hip, at the socket of the hipbone. The rock is hard and lacerates the skin, severing the sinews and smashing the socket'.

Homer's epic also refers to the removal of foreign bodies–arrowheads and javelins–and to bandaging, compresses, methods of stopping bleeding and of curing wounds with balm, and to medicines made of herbal extracts. Wine and other liquids are also mentioned as used to revive the injured. Without a doubt the medical information Homer imparts must reflect the practice in the pre-Hellenic civilizations of Crete and the Aegean.

According to the findings of Fröhlich in a careful statistical study, the *Iliad* describes 147 wounds, 106 of them inflicted by spears, with 80 per cent fatalities, 17 by swords, all fatal, 12 by arrows and 12 by sling-shots, with respective fatalities of 42 and 66 per cent. The overall figure for fatalities due

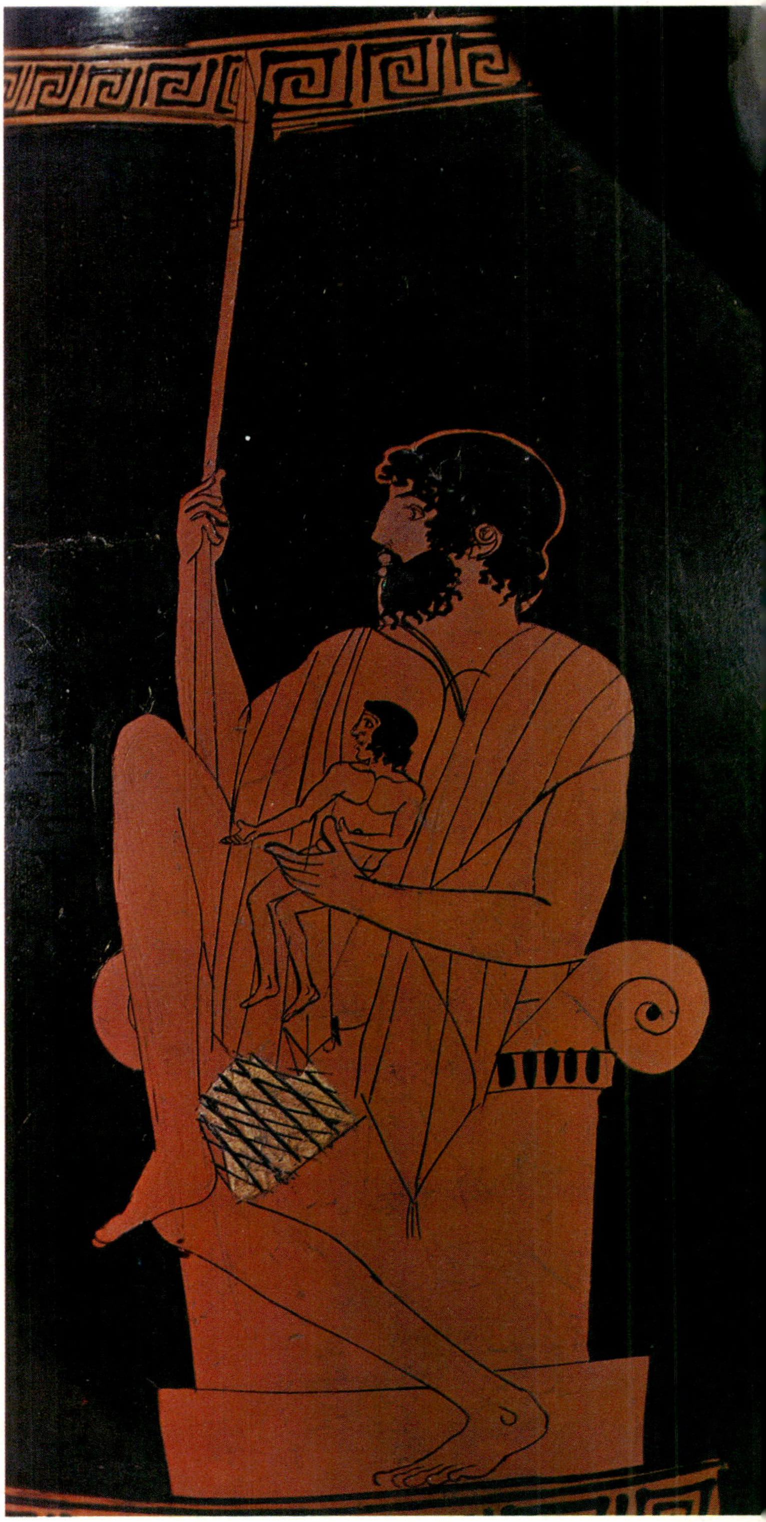

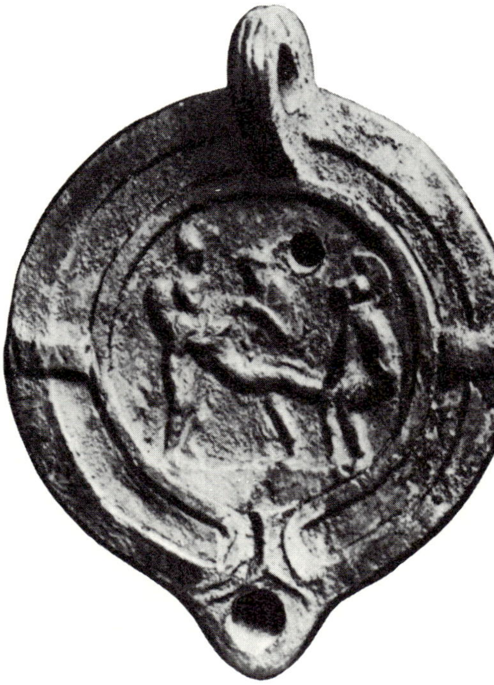

Like most early peoples, the Greeks recognized the importance of blood though not its true functions. The practice of bleeding was employed then and for centuries later for various complaints, either by cutting veins or by cupping; in this, heated cups were applied to the skin, the partial vacuum formed in the cup on cooling drawing blood to the area, which was sometimes incised first, sometimes not.

to traumatic lesions is of the order of 77.6 per cent. Of course Homer would not report deaths from dysentery, disease or any other commonplace cause, since the nature of his theme was after all heroic. Fröhlich was so struck by the anatomical references in the *Iliad* that he postulated that Homer himself was an army surgeon.

The most ancient source of information about the medicine of the Greeks is in Homer's work. Medicine is shown as something neither magical nor priestly, although in the *Iliad* the god Apollo and others sow the seeds of infection and act as healers, while the prayers of the dying are addressed to them. In Homer's time medicine was empirical and practised by laymen. A doctor was a respected figure; Homer wrote 'he is worth many lives, being unequalled in removing arrows from wounds and healing them with herb ointments'.

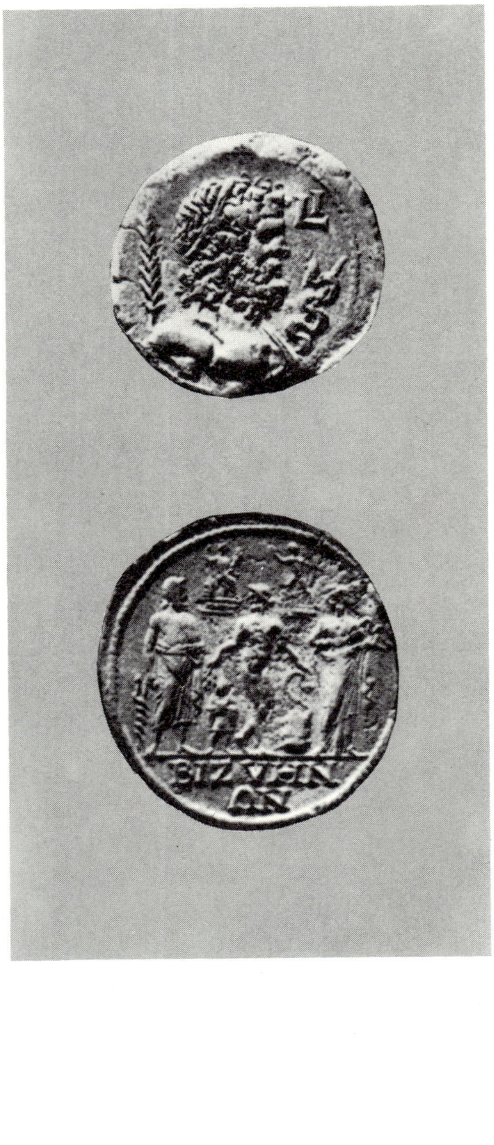

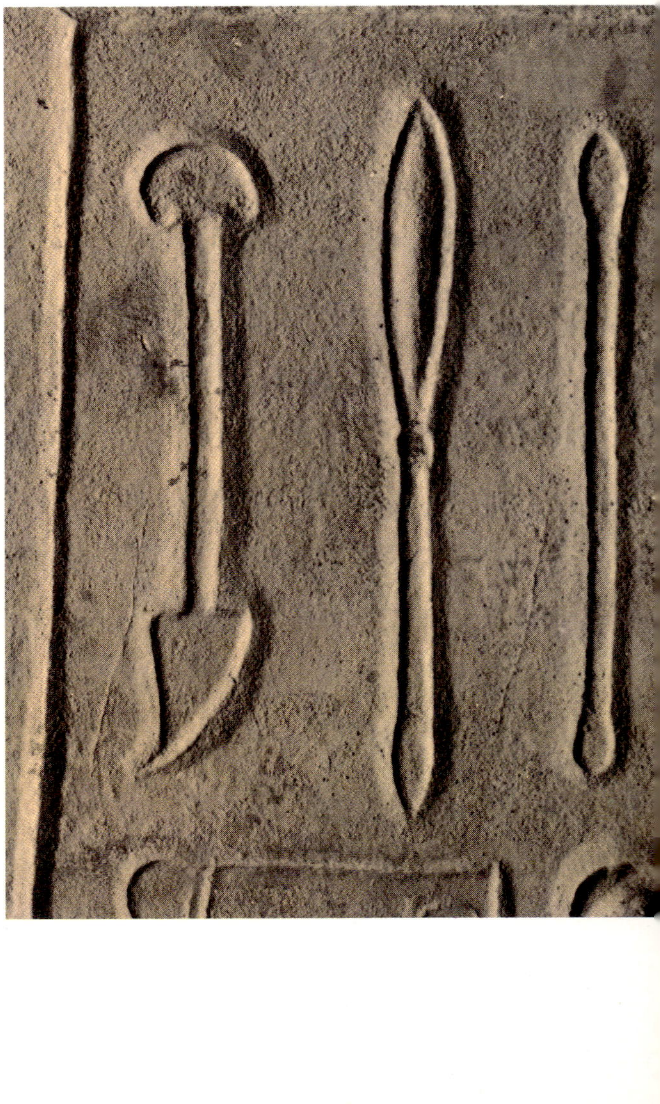

Melampus cures the daughters of Proetus. *Cabinet des Medailles, Paris.*

Bust of Aesculapius and figures of Apollo, Omphalos, Hygeia and Telesphorus. *Coins of third century* AD.

Surgical case with various surgical instruments and two cupping vessels. *Bas-relief from the temple of Aesculapius at Athens. Lateran Museum, Rome.*

Lame satyr with prosthesis for right leg. *Italo-Greek vase, fourth century* BC. *Louvre Museum, Paris.*

Machaon treating Menelaus' wound. *Paste-glass. Berlin.*

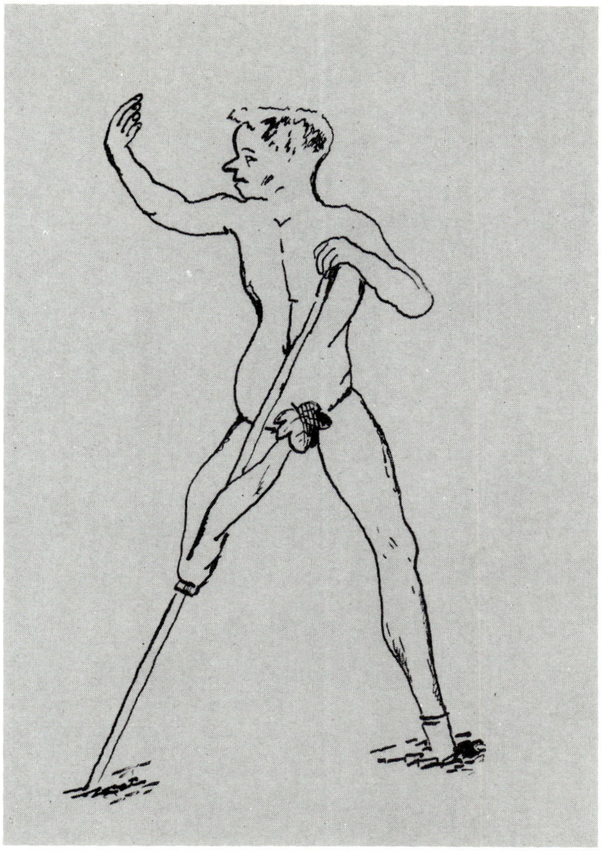

The reference here was to Machaon, son of Aesculapius, a surgeon serving like his brother Podalirius with the Greek expeditionary force besieging Troy. During the fighting, shortly before the wounding of Aeneas described at the beginning of this chapter, Machaon was summoned to attend Menelaus, who had been wounded by an arrow which pierced his body armour. The surgeon removed the arrowhead and sucked the blood flowing from the wound; then he applied to the wound some healing ointment, knowledge of which had lovingly been taught by Chiron to his father Aesculapius. According to legend Chiron, founder of Greek surgery, tutor of heroes like Achilles, was turned into a centaur, a creature half man, half horse. He was so famed for excellence that when he died, unlike the other centaurs, he took his place in heaven as the constellation Sagittarius.

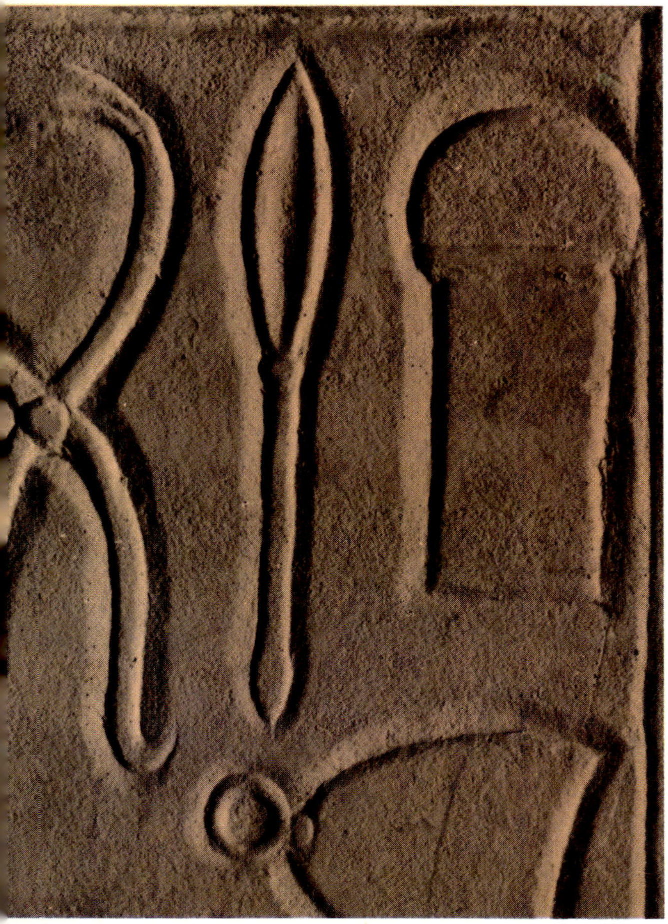

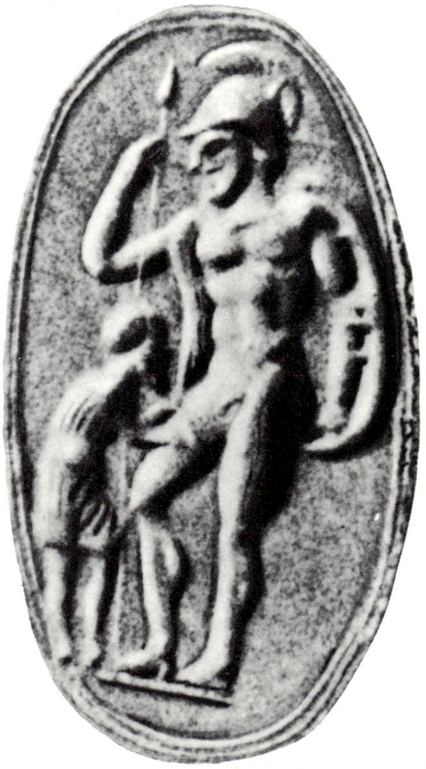

The temples of Aesculapius

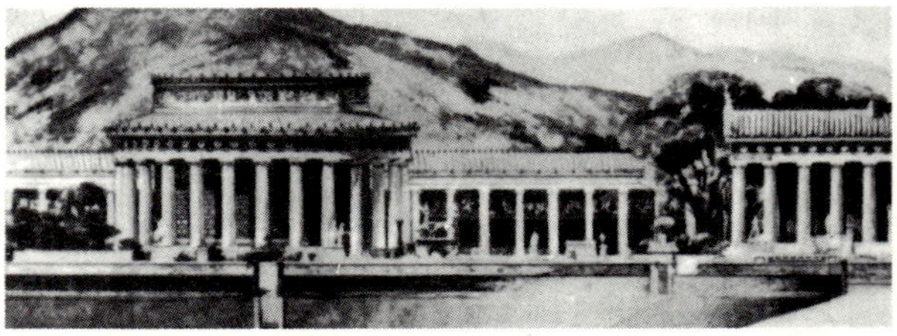

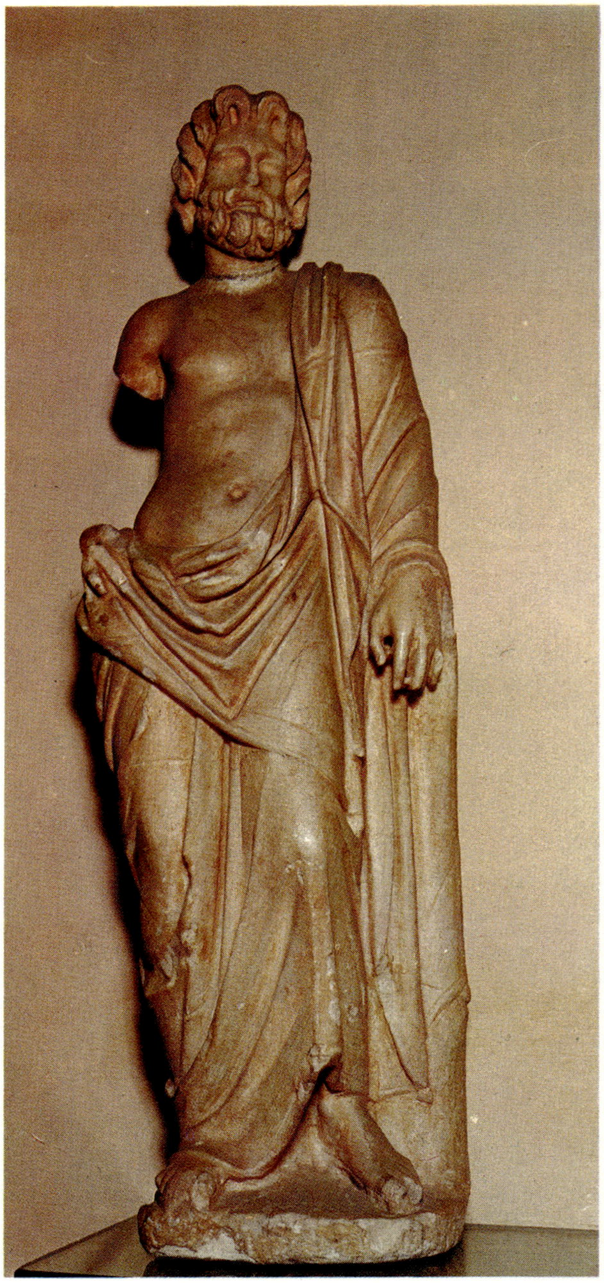

Despite the frequent references in the Iliad to the gods as healers of disease, and the invocations of deities by the dying, it is clear that medicine at the time of Homer was not based on magic, but was an independent discipline practised by experts who earned a living from it. But as time went by Oriental influences on Greek culture became increasingly marked and led to a spread of mysticism; in consequence medicine became more and more priestly and literature after Homer contains an increasing number of incantations, superstitious statements, and references to demons, soothsayers and omens.

Many of the Greek gods came to be identified with healing. Not only Apollo, Artemis, Athene and Aphrodite but also the divinities of the underworld, Pluto, Proserpine, Hecate and Cerberus, were regarded as being able to cure or avert disease. The cult of Aesculapius or Asklepios may well have developed from the worship of one such subterranean deity, for his symbol, the serpent, is a very ancient representation of underworld forces and was a sacred sign of the god of healing among the Semitic tribes of Asia Minor.

It cannot be said for certain if Aesculapius really lived and was a doctor deified after death like the Egyptian Imhotep. One story has it that Aesculapius was the son of Coronis and King Elatos of Thessaly; another relates that he was born of the union of Arsinoë and Apollo. Whichever may be the case, he grew up to become so great a doctor he could raise the dead. Pluto, ruler of the infernal regions, was afraid of a fall in the number of souls entering hell and so complained to Jupiter, who struck Aesculapius dead with a thunderbolt and then took him up to Mount Olympus, the home of the gods. Later, he returned as a hero among mortals.

While on earth, Aesculapius was father of a large family: Panacea, who had a cure for everything; Hygiea whose domain was public health and who fed the temple serpents; Telesphorus, always represented as a child, who cared for convalescents; Podalirius, the army surgeon and psychiatrist who diagnosed mental illness in the case of the hero Ajax; and lastly Machaon, the famous surgeon who died a hero's death on the battlefield.

Temples were built to Aesculapius as god of medicine. Among the Greeks, unlike other ancient peoples, religion was a poetic myth, never infringing freedom to criticize and explore nature. The

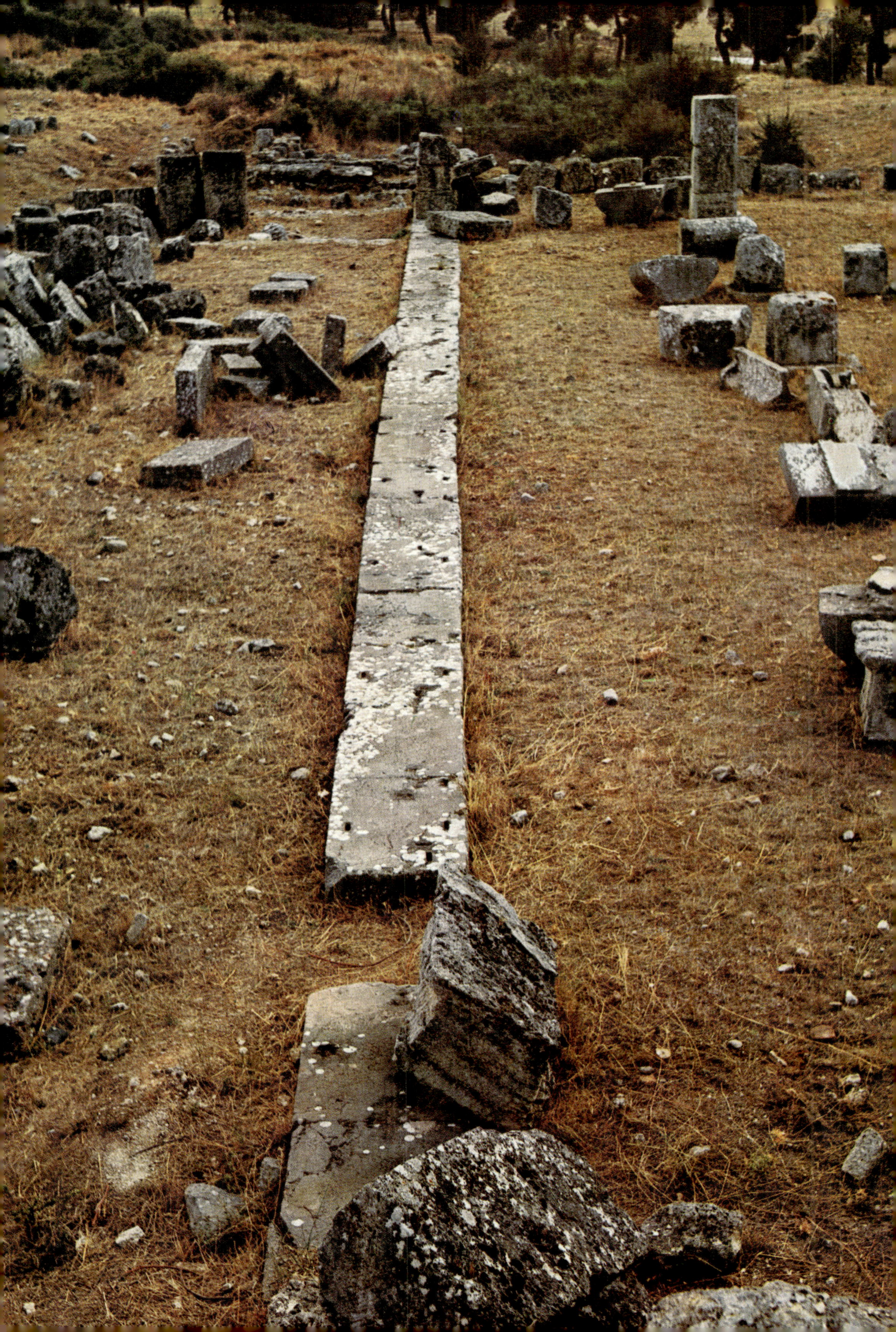

Previous pages:
Reconstruction of the temple of Aesculapius at Epidaurius.

Statue of Aesculapius. *Greek, third-second century* BC. *Archaeological Museum, Venice.*

Temple of Aesculapius at Epidaurus, the Abaton.

Facing page:
Case of phlebitis on votive tablet. *National Museum, Athens.*

Homer's medicine was not magical, in spite of many references to the gods. But in time the oriental influences in Greece produced a spread of mysticism, with numerous divinities thought to be able to cure and avert disease. The most successful cult was that of Aesculapius, whose priests healed at sanctuaries where patients paid with money or with votive tablets recording name, disease and treatment.

priests were never a special caste; they were not dogmatic, nor were they politically ambitious.

Artinos of Lesbos, one of the first documented Greek poets, who lived about 770 BC, ascribed supernatural powers to Aesculapius, and was the first to make the distinction between surgeon and physician. He said Aesculapius had in fact endowed each of his sons with an outstanding but different talent, giving Machaon good hands to take out arrows, perform operations and heal sores and wounds, and giving Podalirius insight to divine what was invisible and bring healing even when magic was of no avail.

It was probably in this period that the first Aesculapian sanctuaries, dedicated to the god of medicine, began to be built, and the serpent cult began to spread, although the serpent–signifying infernal powers–was already very important in magic medicine. The temple-building movement developed rapidly; over three hundred sites were named by classical authors. These temples were usually well situated with woods and springs of water, perhaps with mineral properties, and commanding splendid views, the most famous being at Epidaurus, Cnidus, Cos, Athens, Pergamon and Cyrene. People were still visiting them in the fifth century AD.

Patients came to the sanctuaries to seek the help of Aesculapius; the treatment they received was conservative and was based on bathing and fasting. Once they had been purified and made fit to approach the altar, a propitiation ceremony was held and the sick were admitted to the inmost precinct, the abaton. There, wrapped in covers, they lay down on sheepskins and slumbered, weary from fasting and drugged with sleeping draughts.

Then came the main part of the treatment: as soon as the patients were asleep, the priests started passing in and out among the beds, followed by the sacred serpents, which licked the sores of the sleeping patients. On waking, each patient had to give an account of what he had dreamed. A priest then explained the meaning of it to him and prescribed the appropriate treatment. A cure resulted sometimes, but the priests had a ready-made reply if there was no improvement; the patient had not done exactly as he had been told to, or had simply lacked faith in their treatment.

The priests worked for gain. Disease has always assailed man and the sick have always longed for health and hoped it would be granted. When the empirical medicine of lay doctors failed, people streamed to Aesculapian sanctuaries to ask the gods for help. In this way many temples to Aesculapius could be built, and the priests made a handsome living as a result.

The sick man, before he left the sanctuary, would offer money and a stele or votive tablet with his name, affliction and treatment recorded on it. The tablets were hung on the walls of the temple and no doubt imbued trust in newcomers to the sanctuary. Today they are of interest for their recognizable depiction of various diseases, including breast cancer, and for their accounts of cures.

According to one of the tablets, recovered by Kavvadias the Greek archaeologist at Epidaurus in 1883, a man came to the god for aid. He had only one eye, with eyelids covering an empty socket, and some of the other patients took him for a fool, since he thought he would be able to see out of the missing eye. He slept in the abaton, and a face appeared to him. He dreamed that the god made a special preparation and poured it into his open eyes. Day came and he departed, with sight in both his eyes. Clearly, this was a miraculous cure.

One account is of a cure effected by means of suggestion. A boy came to the sanctuary who was unable to speak. While sacrifice was being made ready and the rites performed, the fire-bearer of the god turned to the boy's father and asked if he would make sacrifice within a year, wherever he was. Suddenly the boy shouted, 'I promise'. His father was astounded and told the boy to say it again. 'I promise', the boy repeated. From that instant, he was cured.

Another tablet records how the priest, wearing the mask of Aesculapius, performed an operation while the patient was in a hypnotic trance. A man with an abdominal abscess had a dream in which the god told slaves to pick him up and then to hold him down, so that he could open up his abdomen. The man tried to get away but the slaves had a firm hold of him. Aesculapius removed the abscess with his knife and closed the wound, and the man went away cured, leaving the paving-stones of the abaton spattered with blood.

The account of Aristomides of Cheos, who came to the god to ask for sons, tells how when he was

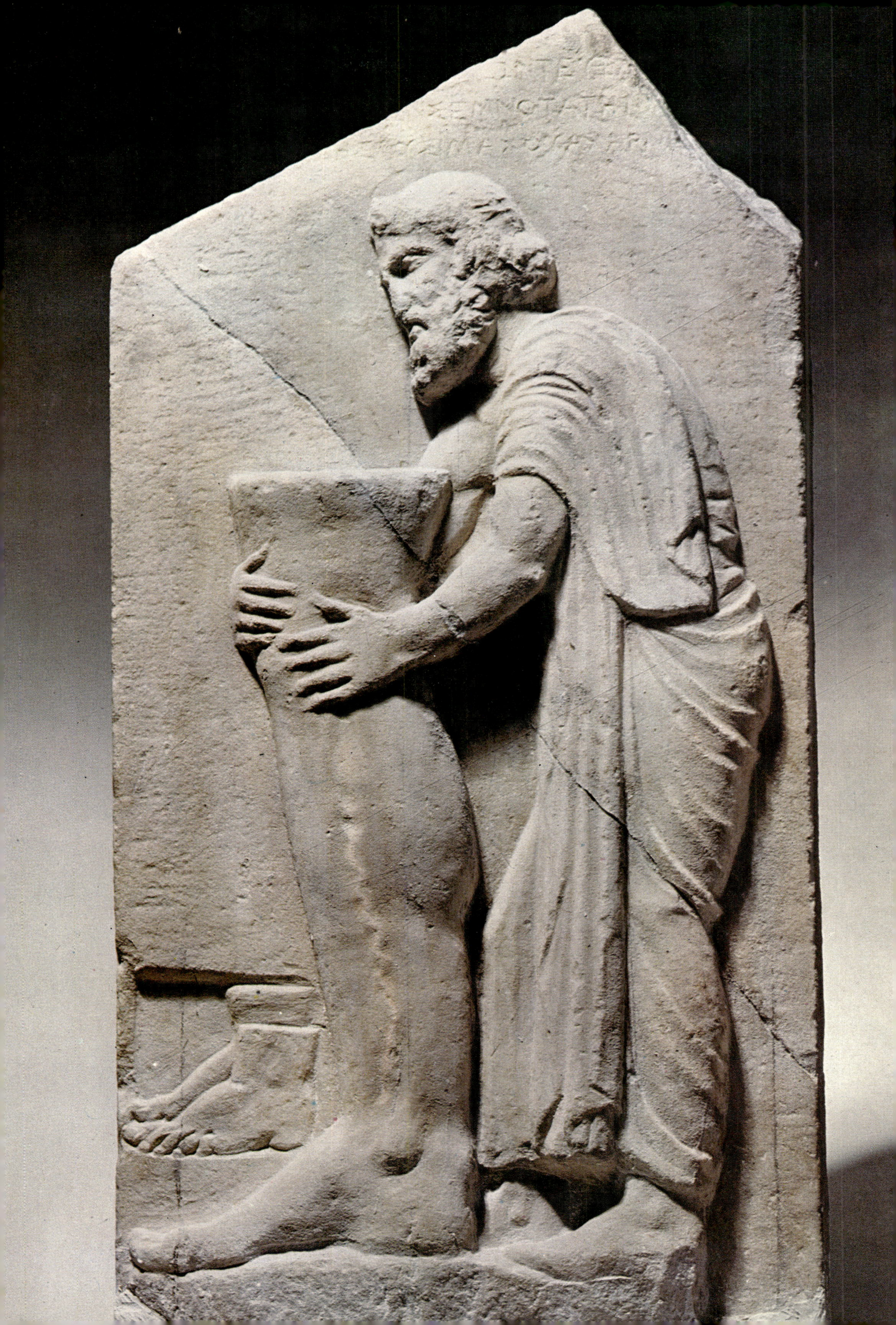

The cult of Aesculapius was very successful. The priests worked for gain, and temples were built in many places around the Mediterranean where Greek influence had spread, always on sites of great beauty and commanding magnificent views. The Temple at Epidaurus in Argolis in southern Greece became the centre of the cult. Parts of this magnificent building are still standing, including the abaton, the precinct where patients rested and a fine theatre in which were marble seats for more than ten thousand spectators. In spite of the success of the sanctuaries, many people were sceptical about their superstitious practices; Aristophanes satirized them harshly in his play Plutus. *Lay medicine was always practised alongside*

asleep he dreamed of a serpent crawling over his stomach; and how afterwards he had five sons. Lastly, another tablet with a Freudian touch. A man suffering from a bladder stone dreamed that he slept with a beautiful youth and in his dream he was able to get rid of the stone. He left holding it in his fist.

Some of the tablets served to warn anyone foolish enough to quibble over the fees. Thus the god cured Hermo of Pasos of blindness, but when he refused to pay the sanctuary the god made him blind again as a punishment. When he returned and slept in the precinct the god made him well again. From another source it seems that the priests of Epidaurus were so jealous of their colleagues and rivals at Troixene that they said they had made a serious mistake in diagnosis; apparently professional rivalry is a very ancient phenomenon.

Aristophanes satirized the practices of Aesculapian priests in his comedy *Plutus,* first performed in 388 BC. He picked on the element of quackery in treatment, parodying popular superstition in an amusing way. Plutus, god of riches, was going about among people in the guise of a blind man, indiscriminately scattering wealth. He helped a good old man, who was so grateful that he told his slave to lead the blind man to the temple of Aesculapius. Here Aristophanes, to whom nothing seems to have been sacred, describes the priestly ritual.

The blind god is given a cold bath then taken to the altar to make his offering to the god. He is bedded down with the other sick people waiting for the miracle of healing. The lights are put out and everyone is told to sleep and stay still, no matter what noises he may hear. In the play the slave reports: 'When the minister of the god had put out the lights and told us to sleep, saying we were to stay quiet whatever we heard, we lay there as good as gold. But I could not sleep because of a plate of food, near an old hag's head, which affected me and made me want to get near it. Then I looked up and saw the priest grabbing figs and cakes from the holy table, going round the altars one by one and stuffing whatever he found there into a sack'.

Aesculapius appears, feels the sick man's head and wipes his eyelids with a piece of linen. Panacea ties a red cloth round his head. 'The god whistled and two marvellous dragons came out of the cellar . . . creeping very slowly under the cloth and licking his eyelids, as far as I could make out. Before you could drink ten cups of wine, the blind Plutus got up and he could see'.

Aristophanes' irreverence typifies the Greek spirit of intelligent criticism, and reminds us that the independent mind even then saw through the superstitious tricks of healing. But Greek medicine did not start with Aesculapius. It was older than this cult and for a certain period developed in parallel to it. Greek medicine was based on reasoning, doubtless mistaken on occasion, but not on

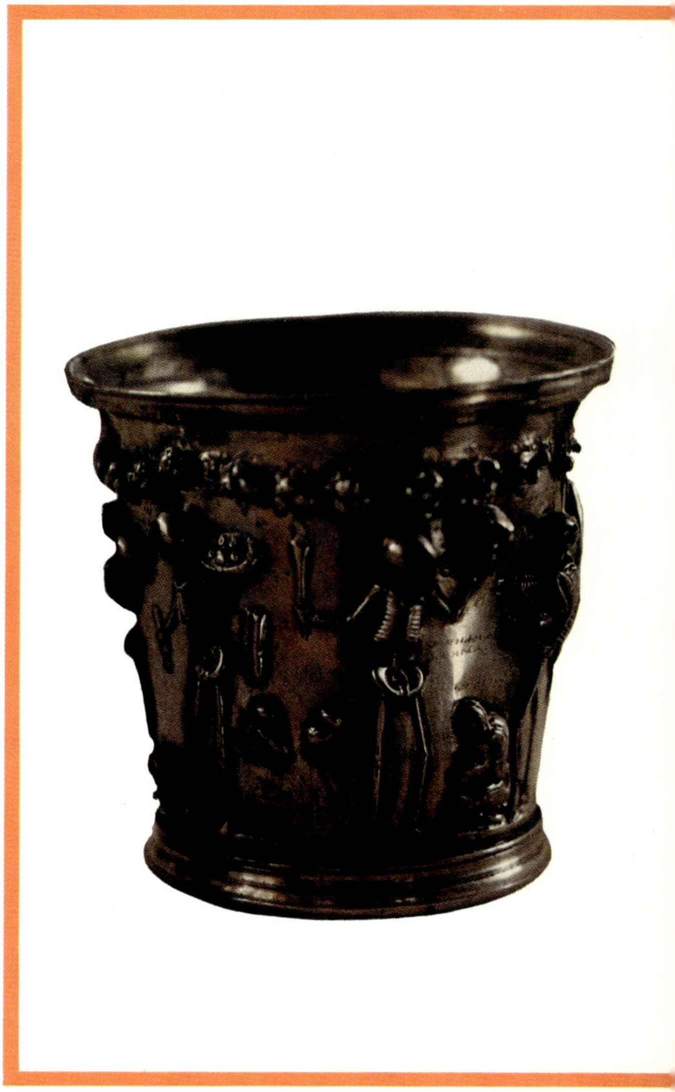

the Aesculapian system and in some places medical schools arose near temples; some, such as the school at Cos, were built earlier than the temples. But although lay medicine became more established and influential, and scientific thinking was evolving in the Italic school of Pythagoras, the Aesculapian cult continued to be followed well into the Christian era.

Skeletons, with Zeno and Epicurus, Menander and Archilochus. *Vases from Boscoreale. Louvre Museum, Paris.*

magic and miracles. The great virtue of the spirit of Greece, as far as medicine goes, lay in the awareness that therapy based on a demoniacal concept could not progress far, since supernatural forces could not be observed.

However, in spite of the criticism and the growing influence of lay medicine, priestly medicine spread throughout Greece in the fifth century BC and in fact was in common practice up to the fourth or fifth centuries AD, when the cult of Aesculapius is sometimes found mingled with that of Christian saints.

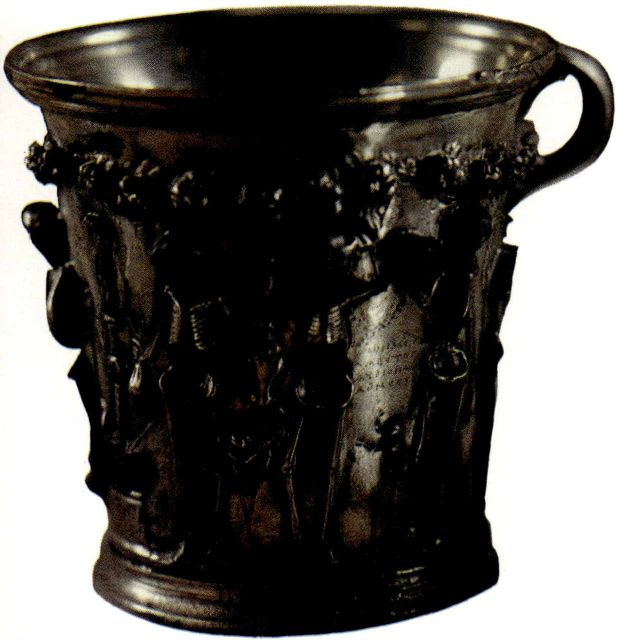

Lay medicine

It was the cult of Aesculapius that made the Greeks begin to lay particular stress on one aspect of illness – the hope and anxiety of patients about their recovery. It could be said that psychotherapy, freed from exorcism, was initiated in the sanctuaries. As time went by, the priests moved further and further from purely ritual treatment.

Lay medicine was practised from the earliest times alongside this temple system. The pupils of the non-priestly medical schools were called asclepiads, but the name had nothing to do with the Aesculapian sanctuaries. It came from Podalirius and Machaon, mentioned earlier, the sons of Aesculapius, who were both famous doctors. In the early days, medical lore was handed down from father to son. Later, with the growth of schools, students lived with the master like adoptive sons.

From the sixth century BC, medicine had professional status. The asclepiads applied for a licence to practise from a council and the licence was only granted when the standing of the school the student had attended had been duly taken into account. Practitioners could open a surgery or iatreion in which they could receive and treat patients for fees. The doctor often had an assistant, the rhizotome or cutter of roots, for preparing the medicines.

There were also army doctors and gymnasium doctors, the latter rather like today's medical advisers in sport. The locums or periodeutes were more lowly, and may have been less highly thought of, as they went about from place to place visiting the sick, operating and selling medicines. Midwives were numerous; and there is some evidence in writings of the period that they were sometimes called in for unorthodox purposes such as procuring abortions and providing aphrodisiacs.

These were the people practising medicine in Greece before the fifth century BC, when medical science was born, together with philosophy. Hellenic culture was not limited to the Greek peninsula, but extended through the Aegean and Ionian islands to the coasts of Asia Minor, southern Italy and Sicily, where Greek colonies were flourishing; southern Italy was in fact known as Magna Grecia. From this it will be understood what Aristotle meant when he gave the name of Italic to the great school of philosophy that laid the basis of medical science.

The Italic school — the dawn of scientific medicine

The Greeks were distinguished by their ever-enquiring minds, and they made a fresh approach to the problems life presented. Man and nature were the subjects of their scrutiny; thus the first philosophers were pre-eminently biologists and naturalists.

By philosophy, the Greeks meant the attempt to understand man and the world; their aim was to devise a fit and happy way of life and then to let everyone live it. Tradition has it that Pythagoras of Samos (580–489 BC) was the first man to use the term philosophy in this sense. Pythagoras based his teaching of geometry, arithmetic, music and astronomy on mathematics, and said that 'things are numbers', meaning that mathematics were not just a branch of knowledge but the essence of being.

He also formulated mystic concepts, including reincarnation. Man and his fate concerned Pythagoras deeply. He thought of man as a creature halfway between god and the other animals, subject to wrongdoing and death. God was the only being possessed of complete wisdom; man differed from the other animals in his desire not to remain in ignorance, but, erring and so unable to achieve utter wisdom, all that he could do was to love wisdom and strive to resemble the godhead.

Before Pythagoras the concept of disease was enmeshed in a magical and supernatural veil. With his advent, it began to be seen by the light of the rising star of science. The principle of harmony and proportion governing the universe, the macrocosm, was reflected in the microcosm of the human organism. Anxious mankind was filled with new hope of success in counteracting those disturbances in the balance of the organism with which disease came to be identified.

The Italic school, as already stated, was the name given by Aristotle to the great philosophic school, founded by Pythagoras, which provided the most important basis of scientific medicine. It is associated in particular with the town of Croton in southern Italy, which already had a flourishing and respected medical school before the arrival of Pythagoras from Greece.

Pythagoras, disgusted by the tyranny of Polycrates in his native city of Samos, had resolved to go and live elsewhere; he decided on Croton, for he knew of the good medical school there. Pythagoras was able to carry out enlightened research into animal organisms, studying the phenomena of procreation and formulating his theory of numbers. He infused new life into the Croton school and ensured its survival by instituting an association of very strict rules for initiates. Rather in the style of a secret society, adepts swore loyalty to the leader and promised not to betray any of their esoteric knowledge to the uninitiated.

The most famous doctor of the Croton school was Alcmaeon, a younger contemporary of Pythagoras, who gave medicine the true dignity of a science. He discovered the optic nerves and the Eustachian tube of the ear, and was the first to assert that the brain was the seat of the intellect and the senses. He recognized three main factors affecting the sight: external light, internal fire and liquid contained in the eye. This master of anatomy and physiology also made some early observations of the circulation and distinguished veins from arteries.

Alcmaeon of Croton investigated the functional disturbances caused by brain injuries. He also proposed a long-accepted explanation of sleep and death, apropos of which the Italian Nobel prize winner Camillo Golgi noted, as late as 1910, that Alcmaeon's theory was 'generally held to this very day, in the form of cerebral anaemia'. Alcmaeon in fact maintained that sleep occurred when the blood ebbed from the brain into the veins, and that when this outflow was complete and one-way only, death ensued.

The book *On nature* contained the sum of Alcmaeon's learning. Unfortunately the only parts extant are in quotation in the works of later authors, particularly Plato's *Phaedo*. One part is important because it offered the Greeks a plausible theory of the nature of disease and thus indicated possible means of prevention and cure, without recourse to explanations in terms of the supernatural. It dealt with a theory deriving from the Pythagorean concept of numbers, more properly perhaps called the theory of harmony. According to Alcmaeon, health and ill-health depended on pairs of elemental opposites, like hot and cold, wet and dry, sweet and sour, and so on; disease was due to some disturbance in their reciprocal relationships. The desire to conquer disease began to be embodied in concrete form when the famous physician from Croton indicated the potential sources of disharmony: the natural

By the time of Pythagoras, the great mathematician and philosopher, the centre of Hellenic culture had shifted from Greece itself to southern Italy and Sicily, which were known as Magna Grecia. This culture produced the Italic school, of which Pythagoras was the most important founder. The medical school at Croton, where Pythagoras settled after leaving Greece, became a brilliant centre for work which represented the first truly scientific studies on anatomy and physiology. Human dissection was still not permitted by the Greeks, and work was carried out on animals.

Representation of uterus and bladder on votive tablet from Cos. *400* BC.

Delivery with assistants on votive tablet from Oropos. *National Museum, Athens.*

tendency of the individual, malnutrition, irregular or inadequate diet, and external factors such as climate and altitude. Today this may seem rather meagre, but people then may well have thought that it needed only a few more discoveries for the battle against disease to be won. Alcmaeon had many followers, though none his equal or even rival in ingenuity, among whom Philolaus of Tarentum was the most important.

The teachings of Philolaus, who lived about the middle of the fifth century BC, contain the germ of Platonism. He maintained that there was a perfect analogy between the world and the individual: 'Just as the world has its central fire, so the human body has heat as its essence. The origin of all life is in the heat of the sperm and the womb. The body attracts into itself the outside air, and thus maintains itself by respiration in order to temper its heat by cold'.

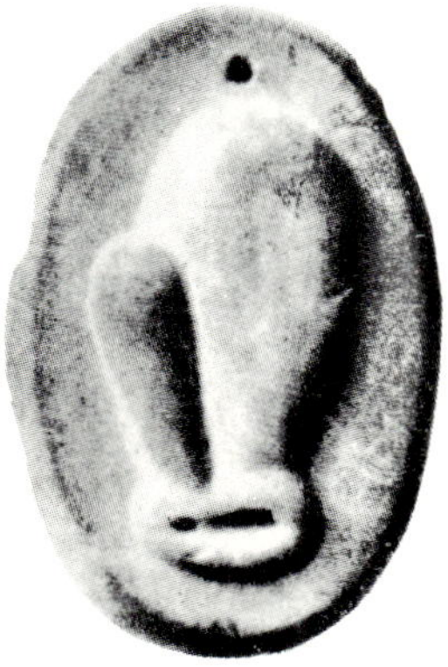

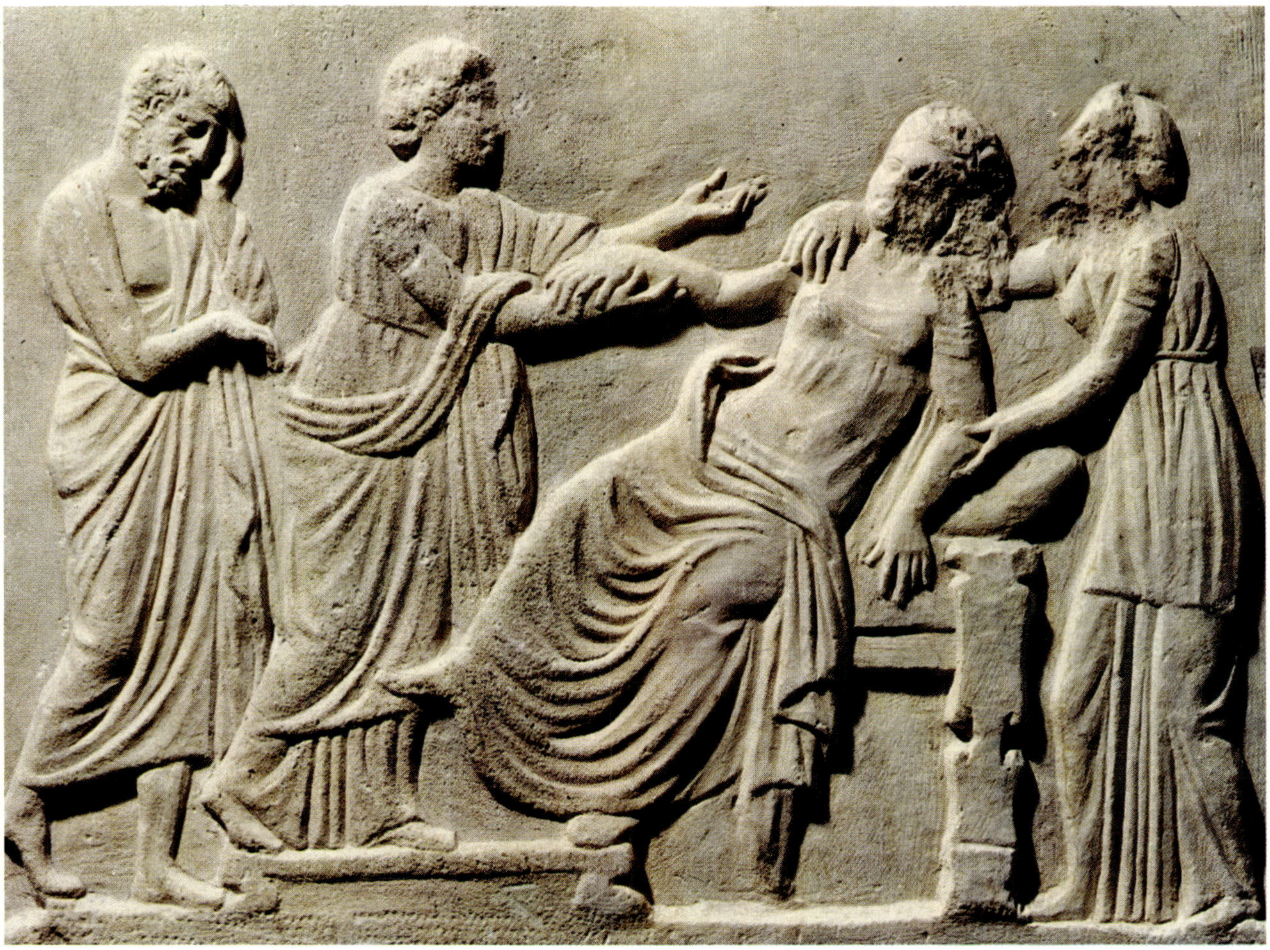

The school at Croton produced many outstanding doctors, the greatest of whom was probably Alcmaeon, a younger contemporary of Pythagoras, who stated that the brain was the seat of the intellect and senses, and made numerous anatomical discoveries. It also produced the most successful and best-paid surgeon of his day, Democedes, who served at the court of Darius, the great Persian king. The most remarkable figure of the Italic school was Empedocles of Agrigentum, who held that the world was made of four elements, earth, air, fire and water, and who contributed new ideas to the study of physiology.

Votive tablet for case of pustules. *National Museum, Naples.*

Representation of uterus. *Bronze amulet from Umbria. Dr M Grunwald Collection, Zurich.*

This exchange of heat and air produced changes in the blood, phlegm and yellow and black bile, and abnormal change in these humours was the cause of disease. As in other systems derived from Pythagoras, life was seen as a harmony, or balance of opposing factors.

Plato's *Timaeus* elaborated this doctrine within the framework of sketchy anatomy and physiology. The liver was regarded as the mirror in which was reflected the thought of the intelligent spirit, which might be disturbed by bitterness (an excess of bile) or calmed by sweetness; it thus had virtually a moral function, subordinate to the spirit. The spleen was thought to act as a sponge in mopping up the impurities of the liver.

Another doctor of Croton, Alcmaeon's contemporary but not his student, was Democedes, described by Herodotus as the best surgeon of his day. It seems that Hellenic cities vied with each other over their doctors rather as clubs do over good footballers today. Democedes was also the best-paid surgeon of his era, and when he left Croton for Aegina he received an appointment with the large annual fee of one talent. He then went to Athens as a private physician, and thence to Pythagoras' home Samos, where the tyrant Polycrates paid him the great sum of two talents per annum.

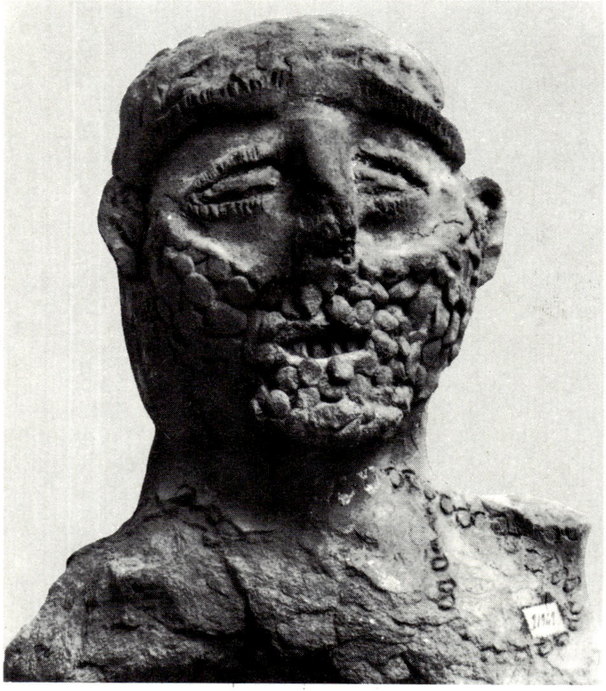

When Polycrates was assassinated by the Persians, Democedes was enslaved and served at the court of Darius. He treated the great king for a dislocated ankle, saving the lives of the Egyptian surgeons who had failed previously. Then the queen developed a breast abscess which he cured with ease. Darius was delighted and offered him whatever he wished, except of course his freedom. But freedom for an ancient Greek was everything, so Democedes suggested that the king should let him lead a mission to win over the rulers of Greece to the Persian cause. As soon as he set foot in Croton, Democedes deserted the Persian agents and with the ample funds from his career as a surgeon married a beautiful girl. The citizens of Croton, far from being shocked at their fellow-citizen's betrayal of his captors, made him head of the magistrature.

Democedes, for all his skill in the art of surgery, contributed nothing to progress in medical science. A noteworthy contribution was made, however, by another remarkable personality of the Italic school, Empedocles of Agrigentum. He lived around 500–430 BC and was one of the most arresting figures of his time. Philosopher, doctor, public speaker and mystic, he went round wearing a laurel wreath, his long hair curling on his shoulders, in a purple tunic with a gold chain for a belt. The crowds gathered everywhere he went, for he had a reputation as a wonder-worker. Being a poet too, he addressed the crowds thus: 'Greetings, friends. Everywhere I go, I go no longer a mortal but as one of the immortal gods. Everywhere I receive laud and honour, and indeed am crowned . . .'

Empedocles undoubtedly held an Olympian view of the laws governing the universe. He thought that the world was made of four elements, which were formed and unalterable and which he called the root of all things–earth, air, fire and water. His teaching led to the heart being regarded as the centre of the circulatory system: blood flowed continuously to and from the heart, and the pneuma, or breath of life, was distributed throughout the body by the blood vessels. He held the view that breathing was not confined to the lungs, but took place through the pores of the skin as well. Some have seen Darwin's concept of the survival of the fittest in Empedocles' statement that living creatures are composed of single organs, which subsequently unite in a combination, on the perfection of

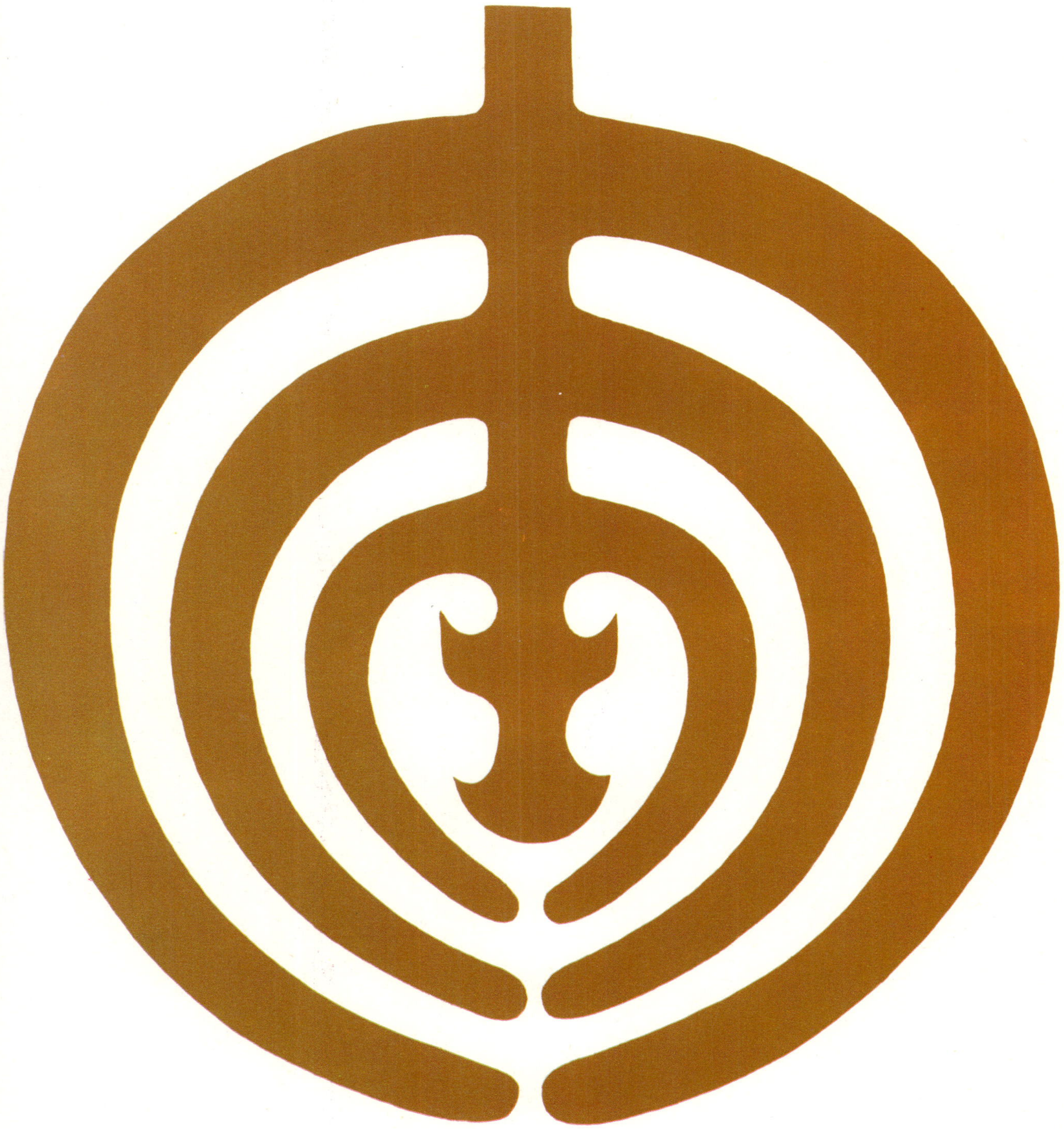

Patient cured by Aesculapius while another patient waits.
Tablet of Archinos from Oropos. National Museum, Athens.

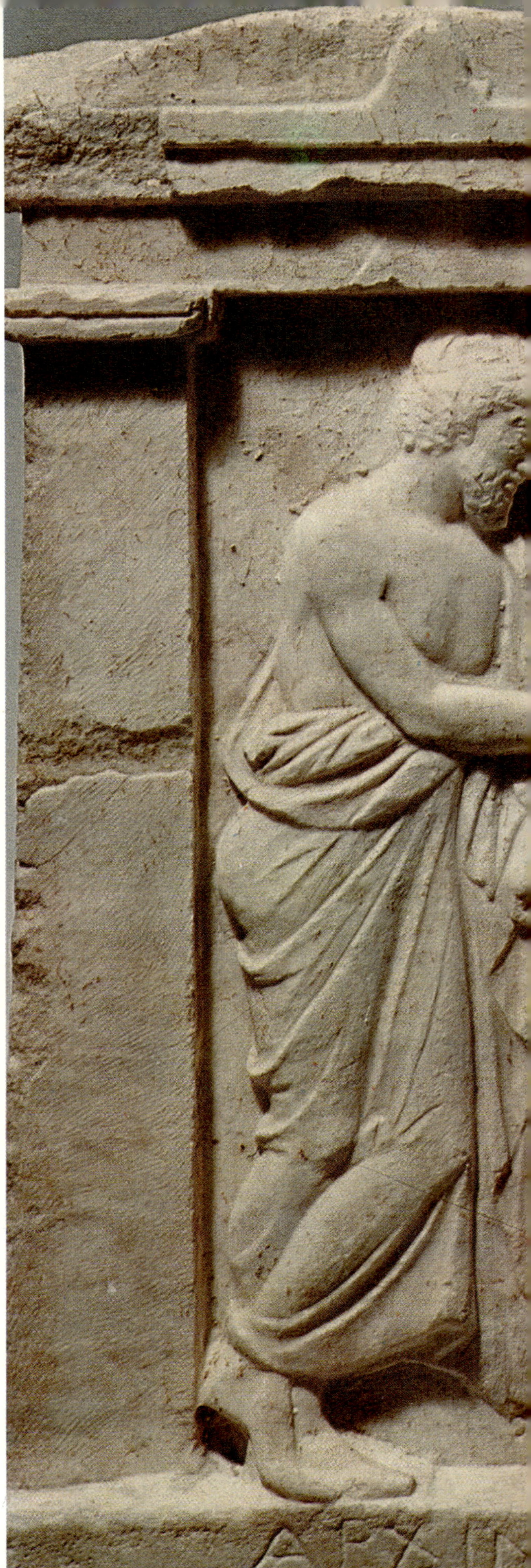

which their vitality and fitness to reproduce ultimately depends.

It is said that Empedocles delivered the city of Selinuntum from malaria by draining the Selinus marshes, and that he purified the air of his native city by fumigation when an epidemic was raging there. This is probably untrue, but these measures reveal the rational approach of the Greeks to problems of public health.

It can be said that the practicality of the Greeks in this and other medical matters was one of the results of the influence of pre-Socratic philosophy and in particular of the teachings of the school of Pythagoras. These placed especial emphasis on the direct observation of nature and inductive reasoning and on investigation into the cause and meaning of life. The Pythagorean school also elaborated the doctrine of the four elements and corresponding humours, which was to dominate pathology for centuries. Through this the Italic school prepared the way for Hippocratic medicine.

While the Italic school developed in southern Italy and Sicily, other important medical schools flourished at Cyrene in North Africa, at Cnidus at the southern tip of Asia Minor, and on the islands of Rhodes and Cos in the Dodecanese. The most ancient was that at Cyrene, while Cnidus, which was recognizably influenced by Mesopotamia and Egyptian culture, is known for its 'Cnidian maxims', a collection of its most important medical prescriptions.

But it was the school at Cos which was to become the most famous. Here teaching was based closely on diagnosis and examination and doctors concerned themselves not so much with discussion of the causes of disease as with the prognosis of the individual patient. Important too was the recognition for the first time of diseases as general conditions not limited to a particular organ or part of the body; while emphasis on diseases with a periodic nature led to the doctrine of crisis and critical days–reflecting the old Babylonian astrological concepts.

Thus various factors, including traditional empirical medicine, Assyro-Babylonian astronomy and Jewish and Egyptian sanitary laws, combined to form the foundations of the work of the greatest teacher of Cos–Hippocrates.

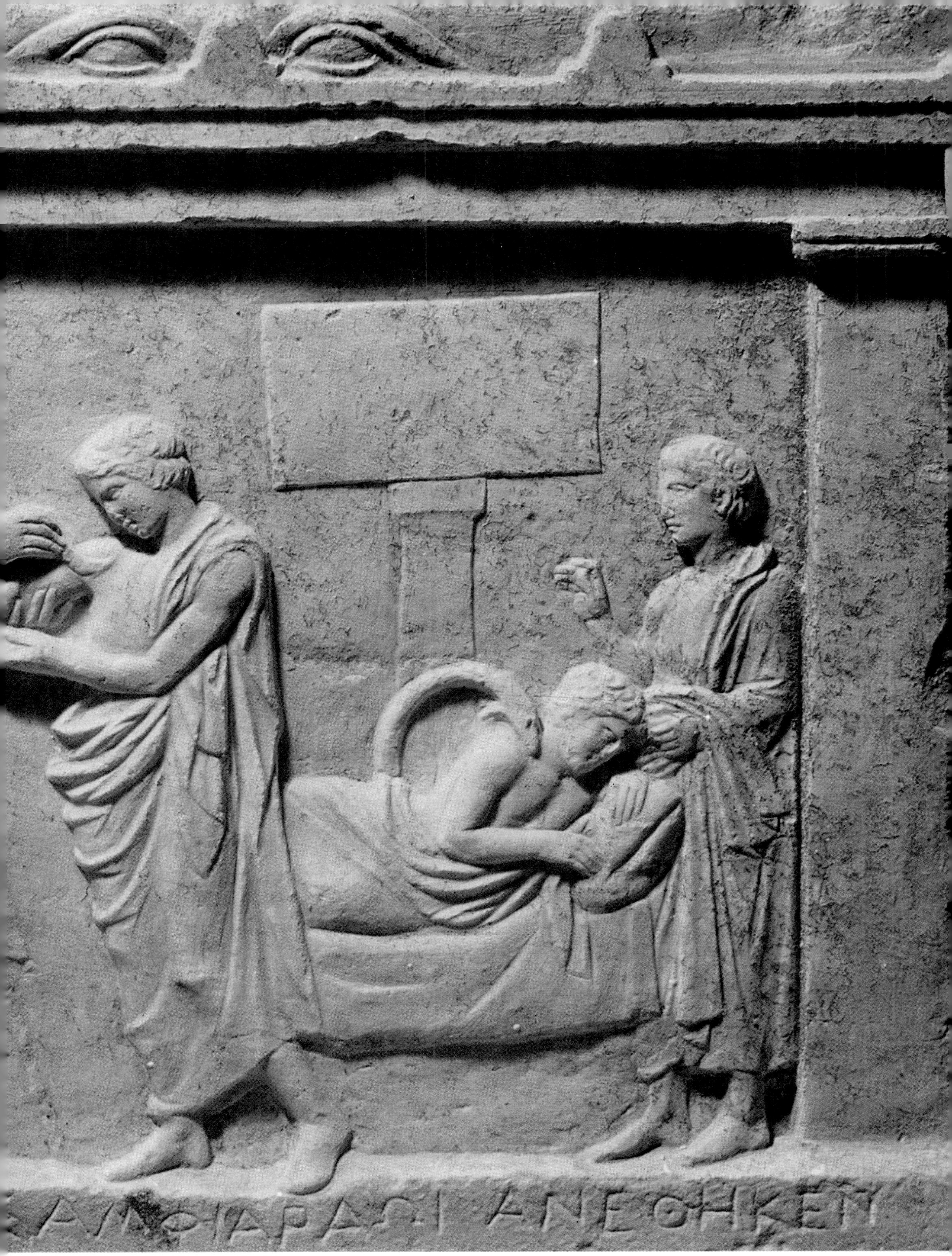
ΑΜΦΙΑΡΑΩΙ ΑΝΕΘΗΚΕΝ

Hippocrates, father of medicine

A great plane tree still stands on the island of Cos, in the Dodecanese not far from the shores of Asia Minor, under which, it is said, young men were formally initiated into the art of medicine as long ago as the end of the fifth century BC. With their fellows and elders clustered around, the men would take an oath:

'I swear by Apollo the healer, by Aesculapius, by Health and all the powers of healing, and call to witness all the gods and goddesses that I may keep this oath and promise to the best of my ability and judgement.

'I will pay the same respect to my master in the science as to my parents and share my life with him and pay all my debts to him. I will regard his sons as my brothers and teach them the science, if they desire to learn it, without fee or contract. I will hand on precepts, lectures and all other learning to my sons, to those of my master and to those pupils duly appointed and sworn, and to none other.

'I will use my power to help the sick to the best of my ability and judgement; I will abstain from harming or wronging any man by it.

'I will not give a fatal draught to anyone if I am asked, nor will I suggest any such thing. Neither will I give a woman means to procure an abortion.

'I will be chaste and religious in my life and in my practice.

'I will not cut, even for the stone, but I will leave such procedures to the practitioners of that craft.

'Whenever I go into a house, I will go to help the sick and never with the intention of doing harm or injury. I will not abuse my position to indulge in sexual contacts with the bodies of women or of men, whether they be freemen or slaves.

'Whatever I see or hear, whether professionally or privately, which ought not to be divulged, I will keep secret and tell no one.

'If, therefore, I observe this oath and do not violate it, may I prosper both in my life and in my profession, earning good repute among all men for all time. If I transgress and forswear this oath, may my lot be otherwise.'

This is the *Hippocratic Oath,* renowned through the centuries for setting a high standard of professional conduct. In the fifth century BC it symbolized the spirit informing the famous school of Cos under the inspired leadership of Hippocrates. That the oath, hieratic in style and avowing medicine as an initiate art, was derived from Pythagorean rites does not lessen it. There is every likelihood that Hippocrates took such an oath from his father and master Heracleides. But had it not then been formulated, the oath he took would not have been worded so very differently.

The spirit of the oath is that of the ethical works ascribed to Hippocrates or students very close to him. 'Regarding the art of medicine', he says in the work *On art,* 'I must first say what I believe its scope to be: to take away suffering or at least alleviate it. The fact that even those who do not believe in it can be cured by it is strong proof of its existence and power'.

Again, in the work *On the physician,* he says: 'For the physician it is undoubtedly an important recommendation to be of good appearance and well-fed, since people take the view that those who do not know how to look after their own bodies are in no position to look after those of others. He must know how and when to be silent, and to live an ordered life, as this greatly enhances his reputation. His bearing must be that of an honest man, for this he must be towards all honest people, and kindly and understanding. He must not act impulsively or hastily; he must look calm, serene and never cross; on the other hand, it does not do for him to be too gay.'

The ethical works and the oath are part of the *Corpus Hippocraticum*; this includes medical treatises of various schools and epochs, which were collected in the third century BC for the library at Alexandria through the Egyptian officials called the diadochi. As far as can be judged, the only works in the *Corpus* certainly originating from Hippocrates himself are: *On diet, Prognosis, The Coan Prognosis, The Prorrhetics* (books I and II), the famous *Aphorisms, The physician's establishment, On wounds and ulcers, On haemorrhoids, On fistula, On injuries of the head, On fractures, On reduction of dislocation, On airs, waters and places,* and two of the seven books *On epidemics.*

Writings of the Cos school at this period include the works *On the physician, On honourable conduct, On precepts, On anatomy, On the nature of the bones, On the humours, On crisis, On critical days, On the use of liquids, On the seventh-month foetus, On the eighth-month foetus,* and *On dentition.* The other

Hippocrates is perhaps the greatest figure in the entire history of medicine. His famous Oath laid down principles of professional behaviour which are still adhered to by doctors throughout the world. His system of diagnosis, based on observation and reason, formed the basis of medical practice for centuries, and in many respects is valid to this day.

Hippocrates had a deep understanding of human suffering and he emphasized that the place of the doctor was at the bedside of his patient. Although he knew many remedies, the great physician laid trust above all in the healing power of nature, clean air, good food, mild purgatives and baths.

Bust of Hippocrates. *Capitoline Museum, Rome.*

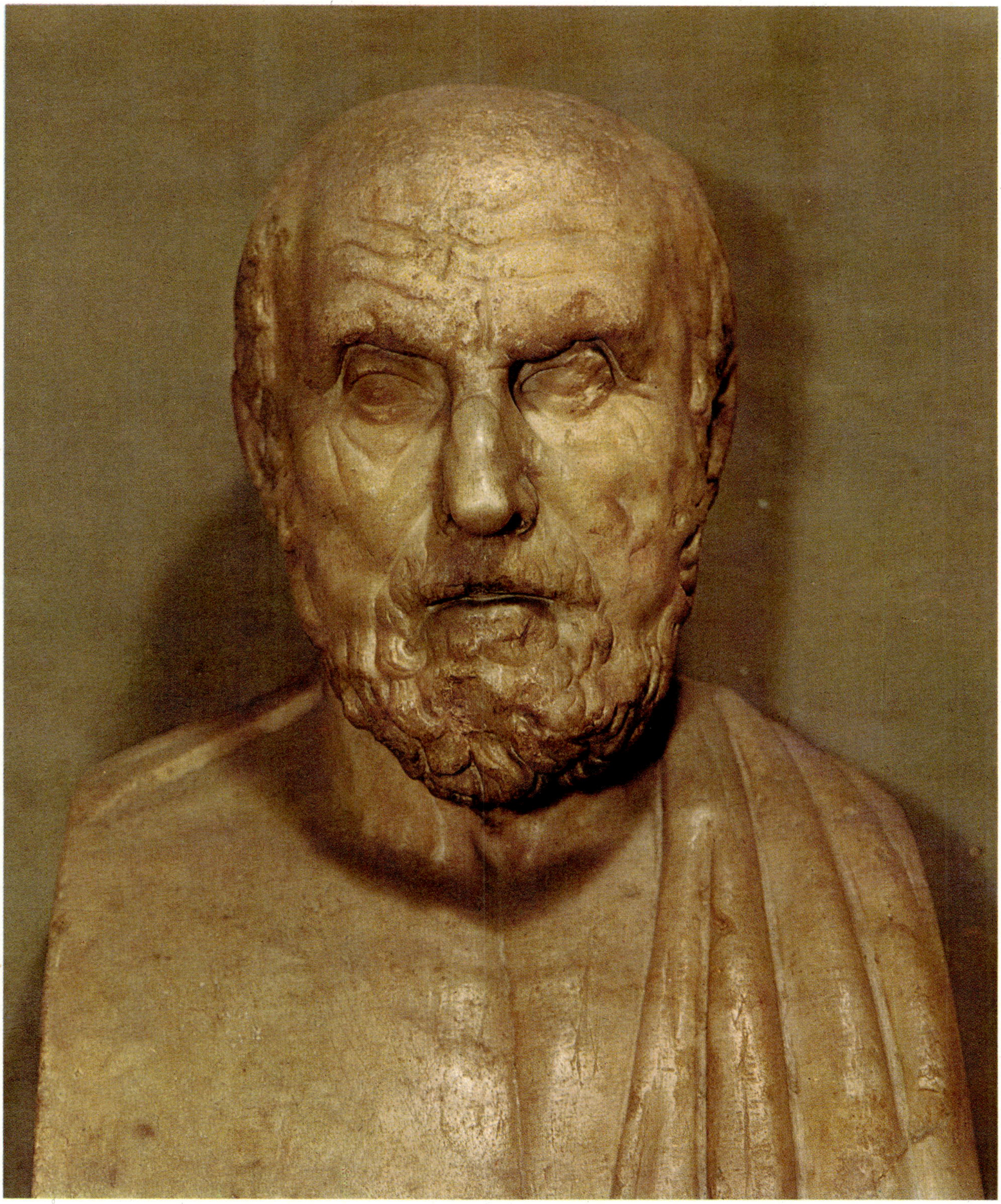

The weakness of Hippocratic medicine lay in its inadequate knowledge of anatomy and physiology. Nevertheless, it provided extremely clear descriptions of many conditions, including tuberculosis, diphtheria and mumps, and of many diagnostic and prognostic signs.

The body was believed to be formed from the union of the four elements, earth, air, fire and water, and of their attributes, hot and cold, wet and dry. Hippocratic pathology was based on a concept of the harmony or disharmony of humours, but Hippocrates was also well aware of the possible effects of external factors, such as climate, on the origin of disease.

The Oath states that the practices of medicine and surgery should be kept separate : 'I will not cut . . . but I will leave such procedures to the practitioners of that

72 works enumerated by Emile Littré, the authority on Hippocrates, are either of Cnidian origin and predate the school of Cos, or else belong to a later period with turns of phrase suggestive of the Sophist school.

The fact that only a few of the works included in the famous *Corpus* are from Hippocrates himself is of no importance, since what matters is the man and his masterly system. Hippocrates was undoubtedly the most eminent medical figure of ancient times, with elements of legend around him. Aristotle called him the great; Apollonius of Citium called him the divine; Plato compared him with Phidias, and Erotian with Homer; Galen termed him the 'marvellous inventor of all that is beautiful', and medieval authors described him as the father of medicine.

Hippocrates lived in the unique and brilliant century of Pericles, with many great names of history: Plato and Sophocles, Aristophanes and Thucydides, Phidias and Praxiteles. According to his first biographer, Soranus of Ephesus who wrote some time in the first and second centuries AD, Hippocrates was born on the island of Cos in 460 or 459 BC; his father was the doctor Heracleides and his mother was Praxitela, daughter of Phenaretis. He learned the art of medicine from his father, philosophy from Democritus the atomist and the art of eloquence from Gorgias Siculus. He travelled a good deal; it is known that he visited Thessaly, Thrace and the Propontis, while some sources say he went as far afield as Libya and Egypt.

For many years he taught in the school of Cos; among his students were his sons Thessalus and Draco, and his son-in-law Polybus. When he was accused of having set fire to the archives of the Aesculapian temple in Cos, he resumed his travels and died at Larissa in Thessaly at a very advanced age, possibly over a hundred. So great was his fame and the awe in which he was held that it was widely believed that honey from bees on his grave had extraordinary healing properties.

Many outstanding talents and abilities won Hippocrates this formidable reputation, during his lifetime and for centuries after his death. He had a profound understanding of human suffering, and put the doctor at the service of the patient, saying that his place was at the bedside of the sick. He

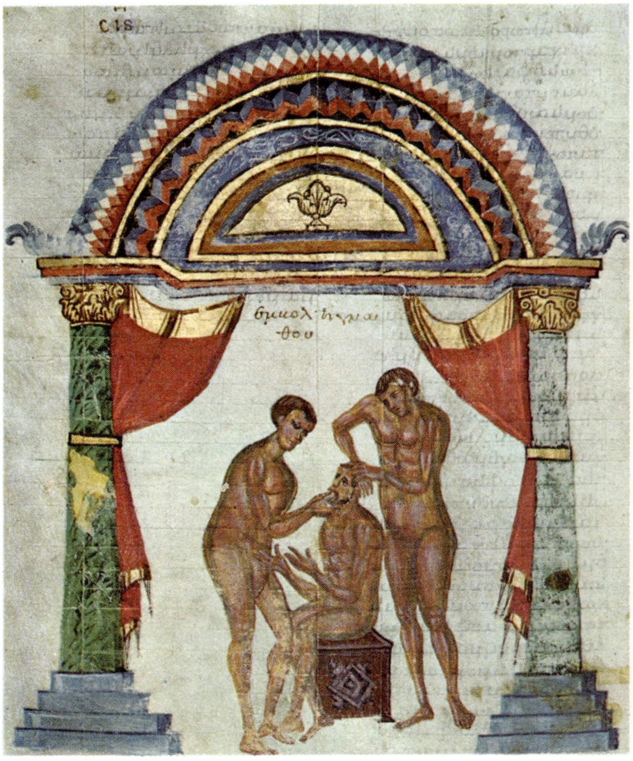

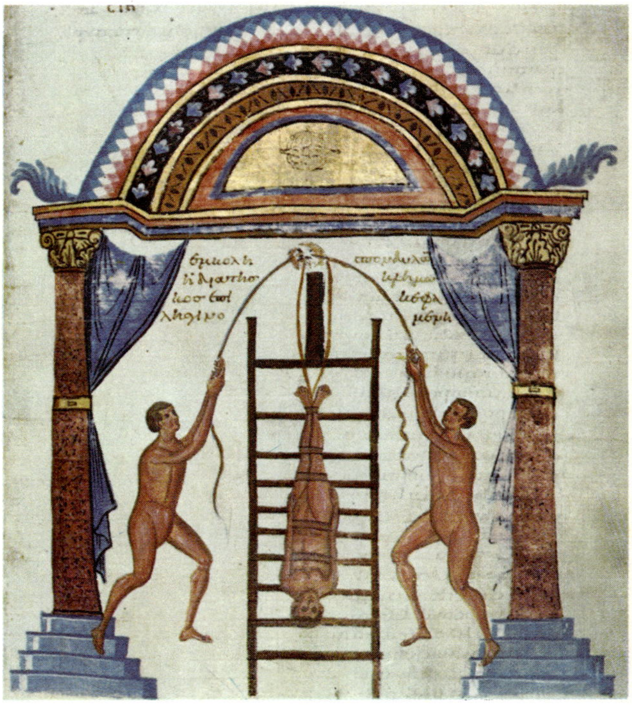

craft.' The writings of the Hippocratic school on the subject of surgery contain interesting information on the treatment of fractures. Instruction is provided on bandaging and on the positions in which fractured limbs should be placed. Dislocations of joints were reduced using ladders and stakes, and in the case of the hip with the Hippocratic bench, on which the patient could be bandaged and stretched.

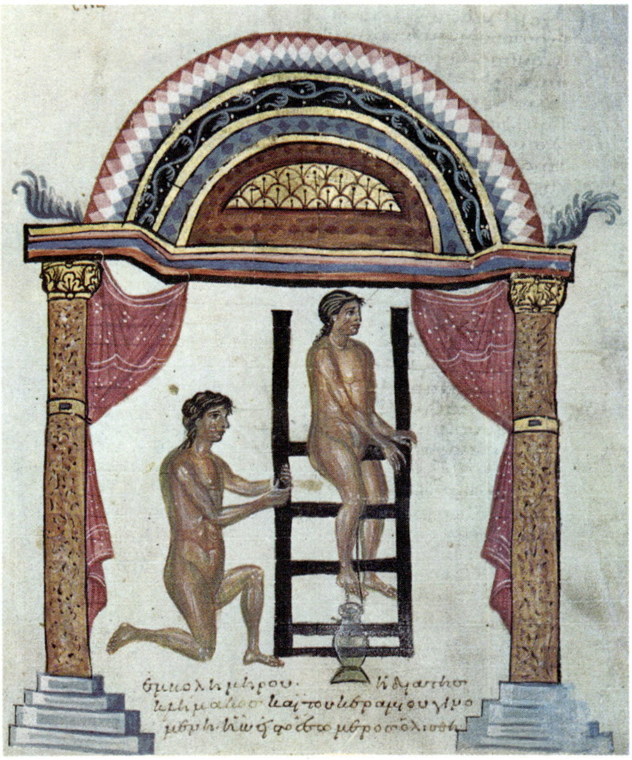

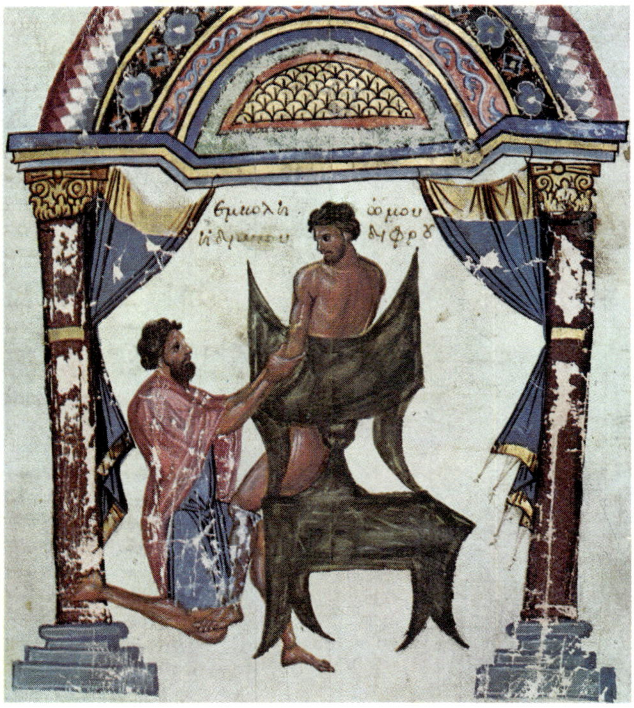

Reduction of dislocations of the jaw, vertebrae, hip and shoulder. *From an eleventh-century codex: Commentaries of Apollonius of Chition on the Peri arthron of Hippocrates. Laurentian Library, Florence.*

taught how suffering could be reduced not by any help from magic, but by hygiene and by proven cures. He set medicine on a new and historically decisive course, breaking away from the religious conception and towards the clinical method.

Besides giving specific orientation to treatment, Hippocrates related all the medical knowledge of his age to a concept of disease which, as will be seen, weathered the test of time and survived to the beginning of the present era. Lastly, he devised a method of diagnostic investigation based on observation and on reason which is valid today.

The weakness of Hippocratic teaching lay in its lack of anatomy and physiology, the very foundations of modern medicine. Knowledge of anatomy had to come from experiments on animals, since Greek respect for the dead meant that human dissection was banned. Again, Hippocratic medicine, fundamentally clinical and practical, focused wholly on the sick man and ignored the man who was well. The facts ascertained were therefore limited and inadequate for building up into a substantial mass of background knowledge. In spite of this serious drawback, doctors of the Hippocratic mould, with their splendid bedside manner, were of sufficient stature to command the admiration of successors.

Hippocrates' followers believed that the body was formed from the union of the four elements, earth, air, fire and water, and the union of their attributes, that is, hot and cold, wet and dry. Innate heat was the basic condition of life, and when it failed death ensued. For this heat to be maintained at constant level, pneuma must penetrate the body through the windpipe and circulate in the veins with the blood.

A passage from *On the nature of man* states: 'The body of man is composed of blood, phlegm, yellow bile and black bile; these are the things that make up its nature and lead to health and sickness; man is essentially healthy when these elements are correctly adjusted to each other, both in strength and amount, and are well mixed. Sickness occurs when one of these principles is present in an inadequate or excessive amount, or is isolated in the body and fails to combine with the rest. When one of these elements is isolated and ceases to follow the general rule, not only is there pain at the place that it has left but also at the place it floods into. Excessive

Hippocratic surgery. *From an eleventh-century codex: Commentaries of Apollonius of Chition on the Peri arthron of Hippocrates. Laurentian Library, Florence.*

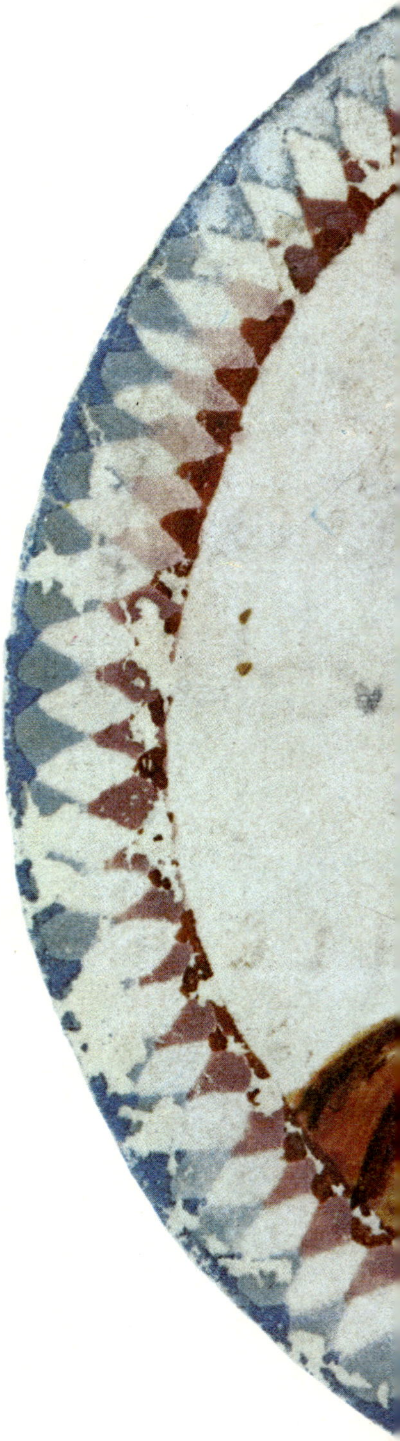

loss from the body of body humours makes for ill-being; but if the loss is internal the separation from other humours causes twice as much suffering, for pain is produced both in the place from where the humours have come and in the place where they have built up.'

If a concept of disease based on the harmony or disharmony of the humours seems fantastic today, it was nevertheless still regarded as valid in the first half of the nineteenth century. In fact, these concepts did not affect treatment, which as criteria of effectiveness used outward signs of disturbance, such as fever, inflammation, boils, abscesses and diarrhoea. These were thought of as timely and desirable means of purging, like any organic excretions. When body humours were in a state of dyscrasis or imbalance, the aim of nature was to restore the situation to normal.

Constitutional pathology is of far greater interest from the modern point of view. It forms the subject of the book *On airs, waters and places,* which can be attributed to Hippocrates with certainty. It represents the first real enquiry into the influence of external factors both on man's physical make-up and on the ethnological features of various racial types.

One of the main passages advises: 'Whoever intends to understand medicine aright must learn all that is written here. First he must consider the effect of each of the seasons of the year and the differences between them. He must take note of the winds, cold or warm, both those common to every country and those localized to one region. Lastly he must note the different qualities of water, varying in taste and in effects on the body . . . In the same way, he must observe how men live, what they like, what they eat and what they drink, whether or not they take physical exercise or are idle and gross. All this a doctor must know, in order to understand local complaints and be in a position where he can prescribe suitable treatments for them'.

Hippocrates makes these remarks about the river Phasis: 'It is the most stagnant and most sluggish of all rivers. The crops that grow in the country surrounding it are feeble, blemished and unripe due to the superabundance of water. A lot of fog comes from the river and covers the ground. The people

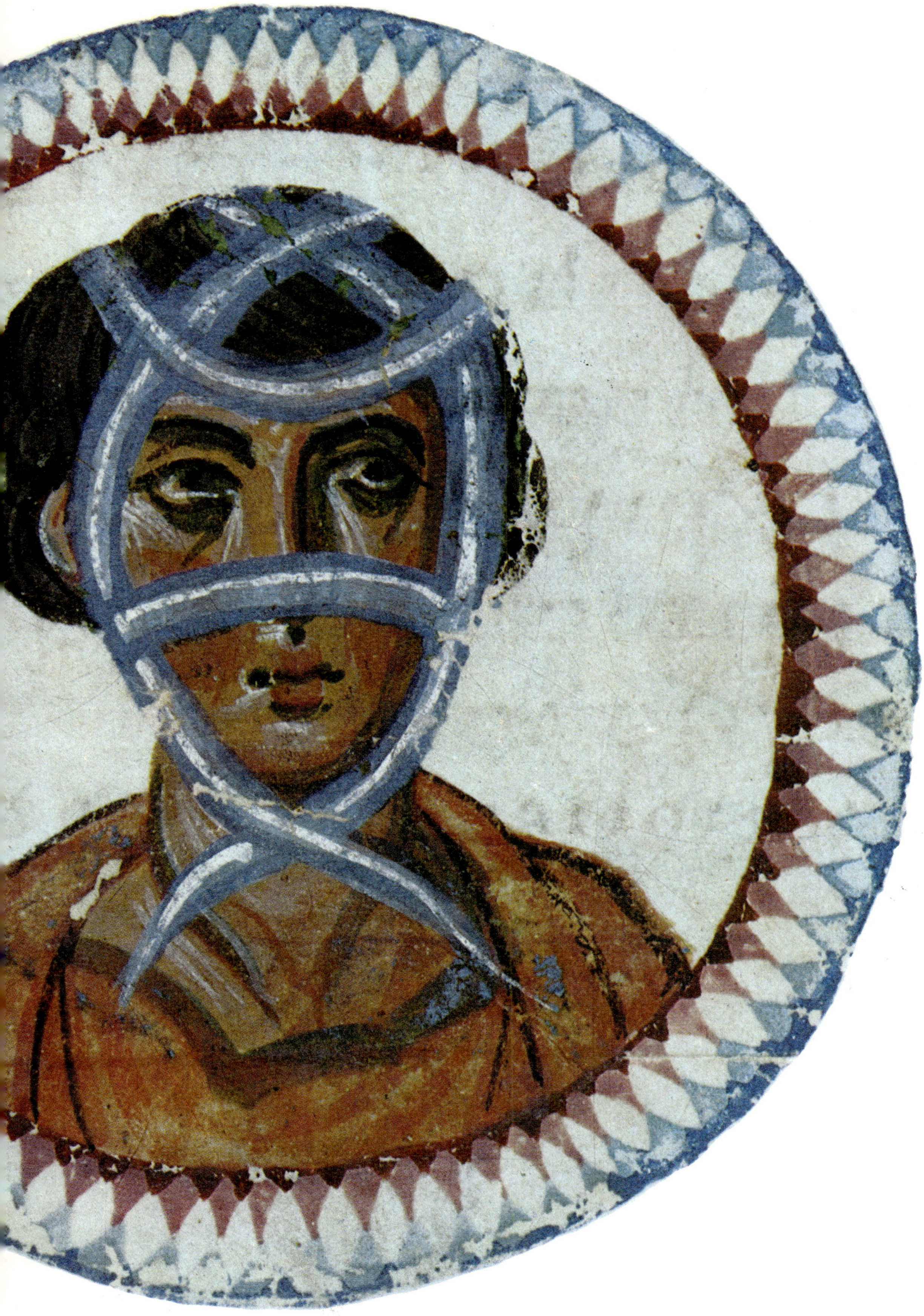

In his day, Hippocrates was respected not only as a great physician but also as an inspired teacher. Under his leadership the school at Cos produced many fine doctors who added their case-reports and other writings to the works of the master himself. All these works, together with the Oath, form the Corpus Hippocraticum, *which was collected in the third century BC for the library at Alexandria.*

The best-known writings of Hippocrates, the distillation of his clinical experience, are the 406 sayings or Aphorisms. *Many of these were incorporated in later works, particularly in the* Regimen *of the mediaeval school of Salerno, and in turn many had their origins before the time of Hippocrates, for example in the maxims of the school of Cnidus. Some of the aphorisms are still familiar to us today, such as*

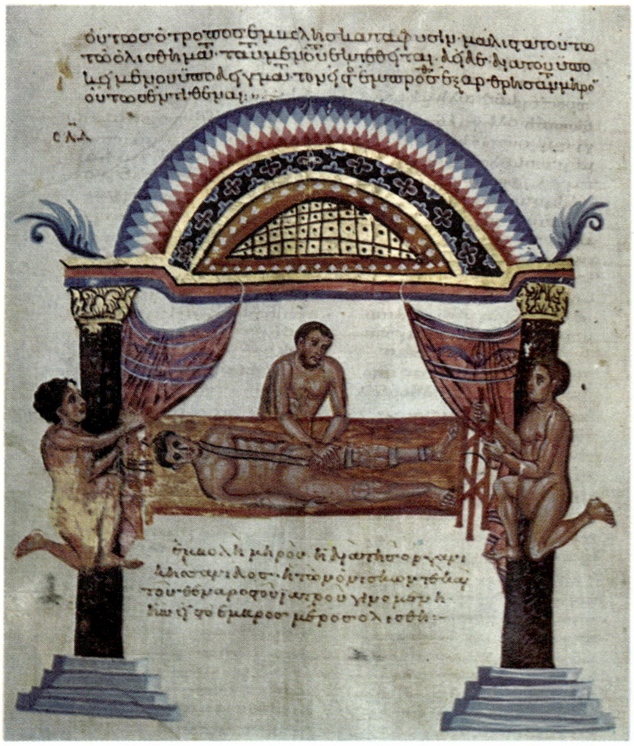

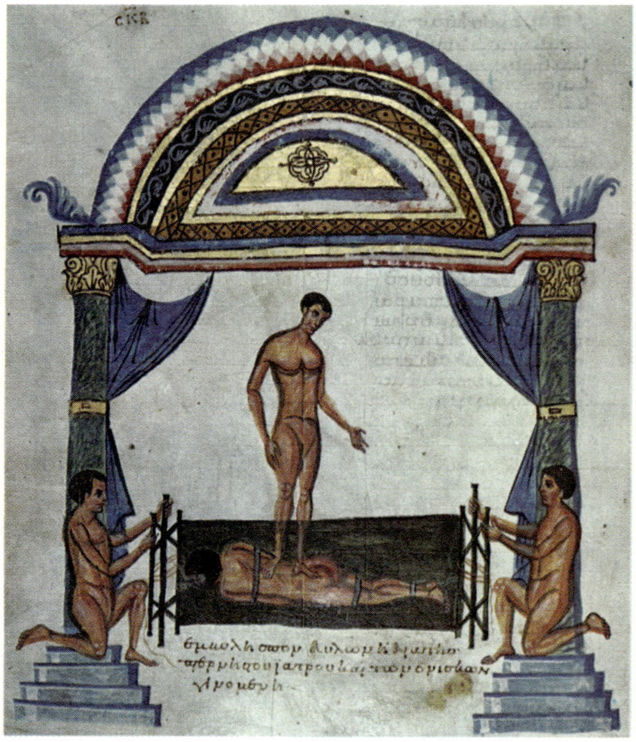

living there are affected by these things . . . they are tall and stout, and their veins and joints are covered with flesh. Their colouring is yellowish, like people with jaundice.' With reference to the Scythians he observes: 'Those who ride the most get varicose veins, sciatica and gout'.

For two thousand years this text remained as a unique collection of medico-geographic data. Another quotation from the same source serves to show how utterly Hippocrates dissociated himself from priestly and supernatural medicine. 'No disease is more or less divine than any other; they are all equally divine, in that each has its own nature and own cause out of which it arises'.

The Hippocratic practitioner did his rounds before noon, 'because in the morning both patient and physician are in a more tranquil frame of mind'. Having enquired about what sort of night the patient had passed and how his bowels were functioning, the physician proceeded to a careful examination of the body, respiration, sweat and urine of the patient. The temperature was taken by laying a hand on the chest; percussion revealed how hard and large was the liver, and also gave information about the spleen and lungs. Next the physician performed auscultation, bearing in mind the master's invaluable advice. Hippocrates' descriptions were precise and to the point. Of râles: 'In dropsy of the lungs, lay ear to thorax and listen for a while; it boils within like vinegar'. Again, of an attack of pleurisy: 'When the lung touches the ribs and the patient coughs, there is pain in the thorax, and a sound is heard like leather rubbing against leather'.

Prognosis was considered highly important. Every phenomenon was carefully recorded. The facies Hippocratica, as it is still called, gave cause for serious alarm. 'Nose peaked, eyes sunken, temples hollow, ears cold and contracted with lobes turned outwards, sweat clammy, yellowish hue . . .' This appearance signified impending death, as Shakespeare recognized; when Falstaff died, the hostess reported it in these words, '. . . For after I saw him fumble with the sheets, and play with flowers, and smile upon his fingers' end, I knew there was but one way: for his nose was as sharp as a pen . . .'

Besides the facies, some other prognostic signs are still linked with the name of the man who first *'life is short, the art long-lived, the chance soon gone, experience deceptive and judgement difficult'. The sayings are characterized by brevity and clarity, and by convincing observation and a commonsense method of reasoning: 'When the patient suffers two pains at the same time in different parts of the body, the stronger pain will have the effect of weakening the lesser'.*

Treatment using Hippocratic bench. *From an eleventh-century codex: Commentaries of Apollonius of Chition on the Peri arthron of Hippocrates. Laurentian Library, Florence.*

described them, such as Hippocratic succussion, a splashing sound heard when pus is on the chest.

The chief glory of the Hippocratic *Corpus* lies in the case-reports and aphorisms, which give a vivid illustration of the Greek genius for seizing on essential facts. The descriptions of tuberculosis, typhus, mumps and malaria, among others, are classics. Hippocrates included these case-histories from his three years practice on the island of Thasos in the first of the seven books *On epidemics.*

The following description probably refers to diphtheria: 'The woman who lived at Aristion's had angina of the throat; her trouble started with the tongue, then she lost her voice and her tongue became red and dry. She shivered on the first day and then felt cold. On the third day, she shivered and had a high temperature; both sides of the throat were red, inflamed and painful, her breathing was rapid and what she drank ran out through her nose; she was unable to swallow, and passed no excreta. On the fourth day, all symptoms worse. On the fifth day, she died'.

Hippocrates also gave a clear clinical picture of mumps: 'About the time of the autumn equinox and during the season of the Pleiades, there were frequent rain showers on the island of Thasos, and a southerly wind blew. The winter was mild with light winds from the north, and it was dry. On the whole, the winter was like spring. But the spring brought fresh southerlies and little rain. The summer was mostly overcast but rainless. The sailing winds were few and light, and then at irregular intervals. So the weather which seemed of dry southern type changed in spring to a northern type.

'Some people had high fever, in most cases benign, and nose-bleeds. No one died. But many people suffered from swellings near the ears, sometimes on one side only but more often on both. Most had normal temperatures and stayed up and about. A few had a slight fever. All the swellings disappeared and there were no harmful aftereffects; in no case was there suppuration, as is usual with swellings occurring in other disorders. The lumps were soft and large, diffuse, not inflamed and not painful. They disappeared in all cases without aftermath. The complaint affected mainly children and young people, and also adults in their prime, especially those given to gymnastics, but few women were affected. Many had a dry unproductive cough with a hoarse voice. At the onset in some cases, and later on in others, there were painful swellings of the testicles on one side or both'.

Hippocrates described what was probably Cheyne-Stokes respiration, which varies periodically in depth, so called after the Scot and Irishman who re-described it early in the last century: 'The wife of Delearces, who lived on the plain, took a high temperature with shivering. Ninth day: much random talking, but subsequently she calmed down and became silent. Fourteenth day: respiration infrequent, deep for a while and then the breaths would be rapid. She died on the twenty-first day, comatose with deep, intermittent respiration throughout.'

The day-to-day experience of Hippocrates is contained in the 406 sayings of the famous book of *Aphorisms.* It is surprising how many old saws and household phrases came first from the lips of this physician, like 'Extreme ills need extreme cures'.

The first aphorism is well known: 'Life is short, the art long-lived, the chance soon gone, experience deceptive and judgement difficult'.

The last aphorism, which is believed to have very ancient origins, and which was responsible for much suffering until centuries later, states:

'Those diseases which medicines do not cure, the knife does; those which the knife cannot cure, fire can cure, but what fire cannot cure must be deemed incurable'.

'Old people can readily do without food, adults less and young people still less readily, whereas children can ill do without especially if they are lively.'

'Growing bodies have most innate heat, and so need most feeding; if this is lacking, they do not do well. In old age there is little heat so little food is needed; more would go out. In the same way, the fevers of old age are not very violent, because old people's bodies are cold.'

'In acute cases purgatives must not be used except at the start, and then with prudence after painstaking examination.'

'When a sick man passes blood in the urine without apparent cause, it is a sign of lesion in a small vein of the kidney.'

'In jaundice, it is a bad sign if the liver hardens.'

'Those with hidden tumours should not be

λόγου· ἅτε προσεῖπον. Ἐπιμελείᾳ ἡρμοσμένῳ· ἐν ταύτῃ καταπαύσω· ἀξιῶ δὲ προξένοις ἡμετέροις καὶ τοῖς ἡμῖν συμμάχοις εἰθισμένοις εἶναι. Καὶ θεῶν καὶ ἡρώων ἕνεκα· καὶ χαρίτων· αἳ ἀνθρώποις παρ' ἀνθρώπων γίνονται· ἐχθρὰς μὲν [illegible] τὰς ἀλλήλων ἰδίας· εἰς δὲ φίλα προτρέπεσθαι· εἰ γὰρ μὴ ἐν τῇ ἡμετέρᾳ πόλει τούτων ἐξετασόμεθα· οὐκ οἶδ' ὅπου ἐλθόντες· [illegible] κυρήσομεν :–

Ἐκ τοῦ κατὰ τὸν Ἱπποκράτην ὅρκου
καθ' ὅσον οἷόν τε χριστιανὸν ὀμόσαι·

Εὐλογητὸς ὁ θεὸς καὶ πατὴρ τοῦ κυρίου ἡμῶν Ἰησοῦ Χριστοῦ ὁ ὢν εὐλογητὸς εἰς τοὺς αἰῶνας ὅτι οὐ ψεύδομαι· οὐ μελήσω τὴν τῆς ἰατρικῆς τέχνης μάθησιν· οὐδὲ δώσω τινὶ αἰτηθεὶς φάρμακον θανάσιμον· οὐδὲ ὑφηγήσομαι ξυμβουλίην τοιήνδε· ὁμοίως δὲ οὐδὲ γυναιξὶ δώσω φθόριον· ἄνωθέν τε καὶ κάτωθεν· ἀλλ' αὐτὴν δώσω τὴν τέχνην ταύτην ἢν χρήζωσιν αὐτὴν μανθάνειν· ἄνευ φθόνου τε καὶ ξυγγραφῆς· καὶ διαιτήμασιν ἐπ' ὠφελείῃ καμνόντων κατὰ δύναμιν καὶ κρίσιν ἐμήν· καὶ ἁγνῶς καὶ ὁσίως διατηρήσω τέχνην ἐμήν· ἐς οἰκίας δὲ ὁκόσας ἂν εἰσίω· ἢ εἰσελεύσομαι ἐπ' ὠφελείῃ καμνόντων· ἐκτὸς ἐὼν πάσης ἀδικίης· ἑκουσίοις τε καὶ ἀκουσίης· φθορίης τε· καὶ τῆς ἄλλης λοιμώσεως· καὶ ἀφροδισίων ἔργων· ἐλευθέρων τε καὶ δούλων· ἀνδρῶν τε καὶ γυναικείων σωμάτων· ὅσα δ' ἂν ἐν θεραπείῃ ἴδω ἢ ἀκούσω· ἢ ἄνευ θεραπείης συγκαταβίον ἀνθρώπων· ἃ μὴ χρὴ ἐκλαλεῖσθαι· σιγήσομαι· ἄρρητα ἡγούμενος εἶναι τὰ τοιαῦτα· ὅρκον μὲν οὖν μοι τόνδε ἐπιτελέα ποιέοντι καὶ μὴ ξυγχέοντι· ἐν θεοῖς μοι γένοιτο ὁ θεὸς καὶ βίου καὶ τέχνης· δοξαζομένῳ παρὰ πᾶσιν ἀνθρώποις ἐς τὸν αἰεὶ χρόνον εὐορκοῦντι μὲν μοι· ἀλλ' ἐπιορκοῦντι τάδε τἀναντία τούτου

τέλος

The Hippocratic Oath, which has provided the basic code of ethics for doctors right up to the present day, was probably in fact derived originally from the rites of Pythagorean and other initiate sects. It was thus in existence before the time of Hippocrates, who may well have taken a similar oath himself from his father and master Heracleides.

Oath of Hippocrates. *Twelfth-century Byzantine manuscript in the form of a cross. Vatican Library, Rome.*

The four elements: earth, air, fire and water. *From a sixteenth-century manuscript.*

treated. If they are they are liable to die quickly; if they are not, then they may yet live a long time.'

The *Aphorisms* were translated into Latin not later than the sixth century and by about the mid-thirteenth century a large proportion had been assimilated into the popular rhymes of the Salerno medical school, which were repeated in every household of western Europe; some of these rhymes are quoted later in this book (page 124).

It is clear that the *Aphorisms* lent themselves to repetition, since Hippocrates' style is succinct and stark. This is how he describes the requirements for operations: 'Required in the operating theatre for operations are the patient, the assistants, the surgeon, his instruments, and light. The surgeon, whether standing or seated, must be in a good light and in an appropriate position for the particular operation; he can use natural or artificial light, direct or indirect'.

Surgeons used bistouries and knives of various kinds, sounds of lead or bronze, straight or curving, the trepan for cranial operations, the cautery for haemorrhoids, the vaginal speculum for haemorrhage and fistulas and the syringe and forceps for tooth extraction. The most fascinating section of the writings of the Hippocratic school on surgery deals with dislocations and fractures; bandaging and resting positions for fractured limbs are described carefully. To reset the femur, the patient was laid on a 'Hippocratic bench' with a windlass for control. The writer of the treatise concludes by saying, 'In short, it is like modelling in wax; the parts must all be put in their correct positions, whether they are badly aligned or abnormally joined together, adjusted by hand and bandaged in the same position; but the job must be done with a gentle touch, not roughly'.

Hippocrates believed that the body had the means of cure within itself, and the healing power of nature is often invoked in his works–'Nature is the doctor'; 'Nature finds the way on its own' *(On epidemics)*; 'Nature acts without doctors *(On diet)*. His rational medical practice owed its greatness to this belief as well as to its encouragement of observation and experience and its avoidance of superstition and magic.

But almost immediately after the death of Hippocrates the school of Cos began to decline. The master's followers were not his equals and respect for his dicta was so great that no new contributions were forthcoming. Doctrines became ossified as dogma.

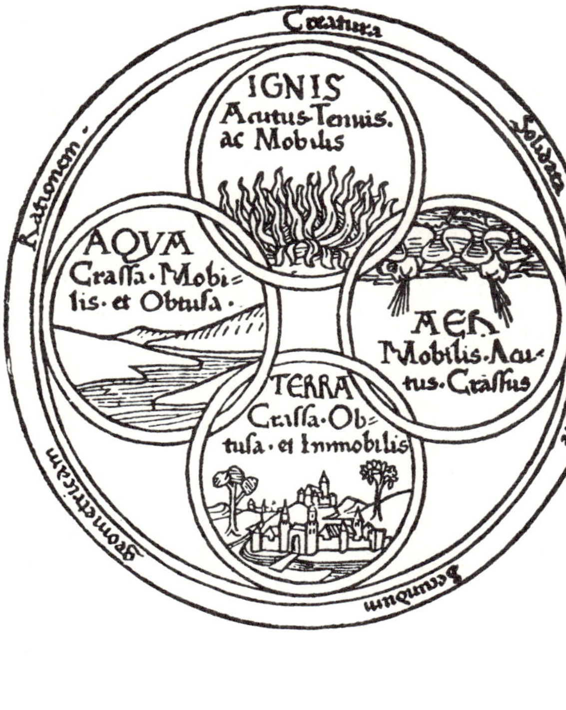

Alexandria—foundations of anatomy and physiology

The golden age of Pericles ended with the finish of the Peloponnesian war in 404 BC and the defeat of Athens by Sparta. Hippocrates had then reached the peak of his achievement. By the time that the father of medicine had died at Larissa the Spartans had in turn been defeated by the Thebans, and the young Aristotle had been sent to Athens to study under Plato.

Aristotle was born in 384 BC at Stagira; his father was Nicomachus, physician to the Macedonian court. In Athens he became Plato's best pupil and was appointed by Philip of Macedon as tutor to his son Alexander. Both master and pupil influenced medicine, the first as founder of biology and the second as founder of Alexandria. Aristotle was probably the first scholar to supervise and direct investigations that were carried out by a team of young people he had trained. He examined fundamental problems of biology – reproduction, heredity, nutrition, development and adaptation – and he gave an exact account of the stomach of ruminants, carried out a comparative study of the uterus in various mammals, and enquired into the development of the chicken embryo, and the natural history of bees and cetaceans.

The most gifted of Aristotle's pupils was Tirtanus, who came from Eresos on the island of Lesbos. His teacher renamed him Theophrastus, the divine orator, and it is by this name he has gone down in history. Theophrastus succeeded Aristotle as a teacher and inherited his library, and is said to have had 2,000 disciples, including the playwright Menander. He was the leading botanist of ancient times, and in fact remained unsurpassed up to the Renaissance. Through his studies of botany he also made some contribution to medicine, for his monumental *History of plants* and *Causes of plants* were major sources of pharmacological information and were used by the Romans as handbooks of treatment.

In 323 BC, Alexander – founder of a glorious but short-lived empire – met an early death from malaria. Aristotle retired to Euboea in Chalcis, since the anti-Macedon party was in power in Athens, and died within a year at the age of 63. Greece was involved in a struggle over Alexander's inheritance. In the sphere of art and culture, the star of Alexandria came into the ascendant. Under Ptolemy Soter, Alexander's general, Egypt became the hub of Hellenist civilization. Ptolemy was not only a soldier but also a patron of learning, and he instituted the famous library at Alexandria, where the *Corpus Hippocraticum* was brought and stored with tens of thousands of other manuscripts.

At Alexandria, the seed sown by the Coan medical school bore fruit of inestimable value, especially in the two fields not cultivated by followers of Hippocrates, namely anatomy and physiology. The most illustrious exponent of the next Alexandrian school was Herophilus of Chalcedon, who lived around 300 BC. He was a student of Praxagoras of Cos, who had made the first attempt to break free of the tenets of the decayed Coan school, dedicating himself, in contrast to Hippocrates, to anatomical and physiological observation and the study of the pulse.

Herophilus followed in the footsteps of his master, and his anatomical discoveries added up to a considerable whole. He studied the anatomy of the brain and spinal cord; he distinguished nerves from tendons and blood vessels, found that nerves determined and directed movement and that their centre lay in the brain. Within the skull, he distinguished the cerebrum from the cerebellum and described the meninges and ventricles. He noted the shallow depression of the fourth ventricle of the brain, known anatomically as the calamus scriptorius, and other small structures.

Modern medicine uses two terms coined by Herophilus: duodenum and prostate. Duodenum meant twelve digits long, and is the C-shaped part of the small intestine following the stomach. The word prostate refers to the position of this gland before the bladder. He described the part of the dura mater, the torcular Herophili, where several great veins from the brain join together. He observed and described the liver, pancreas, female genital organs and also the lymphatics; he did not appreciate either the origin or importance of these minute channels, which we now know absorb fluid from the limbs and chyle from the intestine, conveying it through the thoracic duct into the circulation. He enumerated the movements of respiration correctly, and stated that the arteries were six times the size of the veins and contained blood, not air. Lastly, he was the founder of the doctrine of the pulse in Western medicine, measuring it by means of a water-clock and distinguishing systole from diastole.

Perhaps Herophilus was able to make such a

At the time of Hippocrates' death, Aristotle was a pupil of Plato in Athens. Later he was to be responsible for much original work on the fundamental problems of biology. Aristotle himself became tutor to Alexander, son of Philip of Macedon, who founded the town that bore his name.

After the ruler's death, Alexandria became a new focus of Greek culture, with the most famous library of its time. At the medical school great advances were made in the neglected fields of anatomy and physiology, notably by Herophilus, who was said to have been the first man to practise human dissection.

Anatomy class. *Sixteenth-century woodcut from an edition of the works of Hippocrates, 1523 by Ugo Senensis. Bertarelli Collection, Milan.*

range of anatomical discoveries, far exceeding the achievements of his predecessors in number and importance, because of a degree of detachment and scepticism in his approach to the subject, a feature not shared by other anatomists of ancient times. The cult of the dead meant nothing to him; according to Galen he was the first man to practise dissection on human corpses, and if what Celsus says is true, he got his knife into the living too. The famous Roman, in the foreword to *De medicina*, reported that Herophilus and Erasistratus practised vivisection; their subjects were prisoners, who had been handed over to their keeping on the orders of the sovereign so that the parts hidden by nature could be seen before the men breathed their last.

Erasistratus of Chios was a younger contemporary of Herophilus. He was a physiologist, considered by some authorities as the founder of this subject, who rejected the theory of the humours, stating that blood and pneuma of two kinds were the essentials of bodily well-being. Erasistratus believed that every organ was equipped with three kinds of vessel–veins, arteries and nerves. He improved anatomical knowledge of the heart, observing and describing the mitral and tricuspid valves and commenting on their function. He also recognized the association between fluid in the abdomen and hardening of the liver, and correctly described the function of the epiglottis in preventing food and liquid from going down the windpipe during swallowing.

Erasistratus could be said to be an advanced scholar in that he adapted for his purposes the experimental method, to which doctors in his day were unaccustomed. This is how he described one of his experiments: 'If you take an animal, a bird, for instance, and weigh it, then put it in a cage without food and weigh it again with its excrement, you will find that an appreciable weight loss has occurred.' Whether Erasistratus was thinking in terms of the concept of metabolism is doubtful, but nineteen centuries passed before Sanctorius (1561–1636) conducted a similar experiment and found the effect of 'insensible perspiration' on man's body weight.

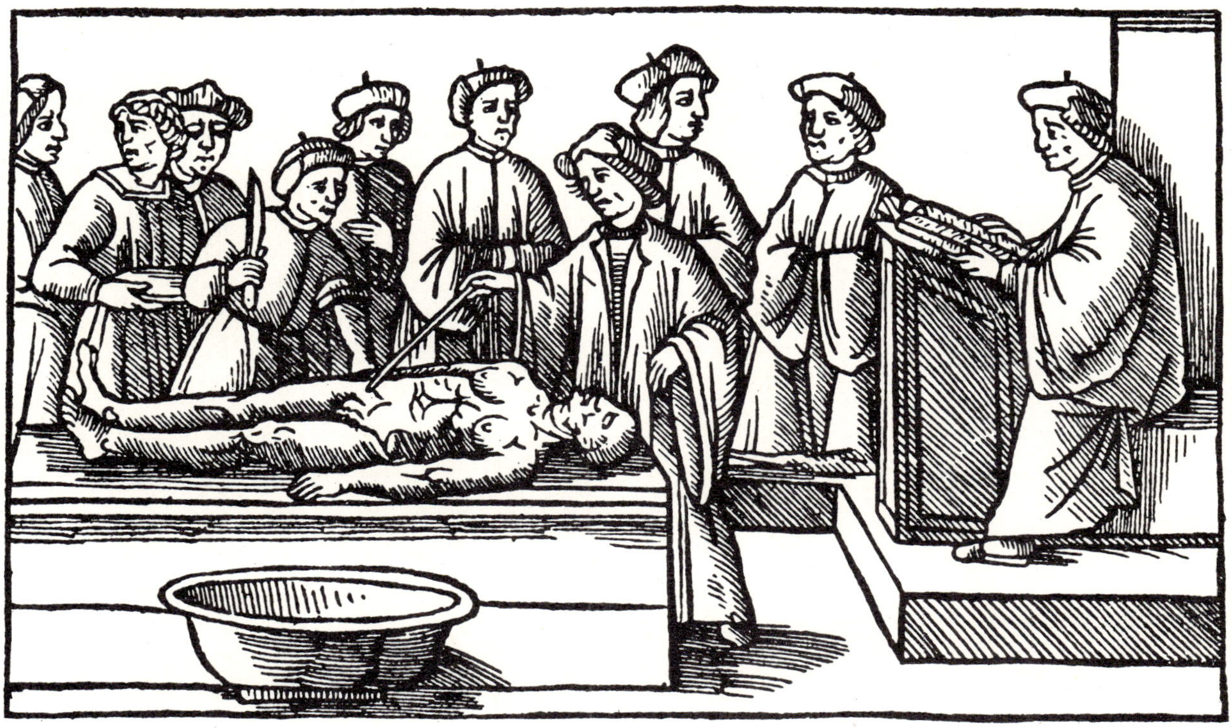

Rome–professional standards and public health legislation

The school of Alexandria achieved much in the study of physiology and anatomy, by organizing the teaching of medicine on a rational footing and by opening its doors to students of all races and countries. No diplomas were granted to graduates, however, with the result that many quacks and impostors were able to capitalize on the fame of the school.

Numerous Greek doctors, of greater or lesser ability, went to Rome, where they incurred the wrath of Cato (234–149 BC), who admired only the austerity of old and raged in the Senate against the effete way of life derived from Greece. He viewed Greek doctors with loathing; indeed, according to Pliny he accused them of constituting a threat to Roman health. In a letter to his son Mark, Cato put him on his guard against the Greeks, a race of rogues, writing, 'If that pack pass on to us what they know, it will mean the end of Rome, especially if their doctors come here. For they have sworn death by medicine to barbarians, and the Romans are barbarians to them. Beware of doctors!'

Unfortunately Cato had no plan of action against 'graeculi delirantes', the raving Greeks, as the Romans nicknamed them. The only cures Cato the censor could offer were magic words, which were farcical, and cabbages, cooked and raw, which were his universal remedy. Thus the best treatment he had for a dislocation was to hold a swallow in the hand and recite the nonsense words 'huat hana ista pista, sista domina damnaustra luxato'. To cure a polyp in the nose, Cato advised smelling a cabbage.

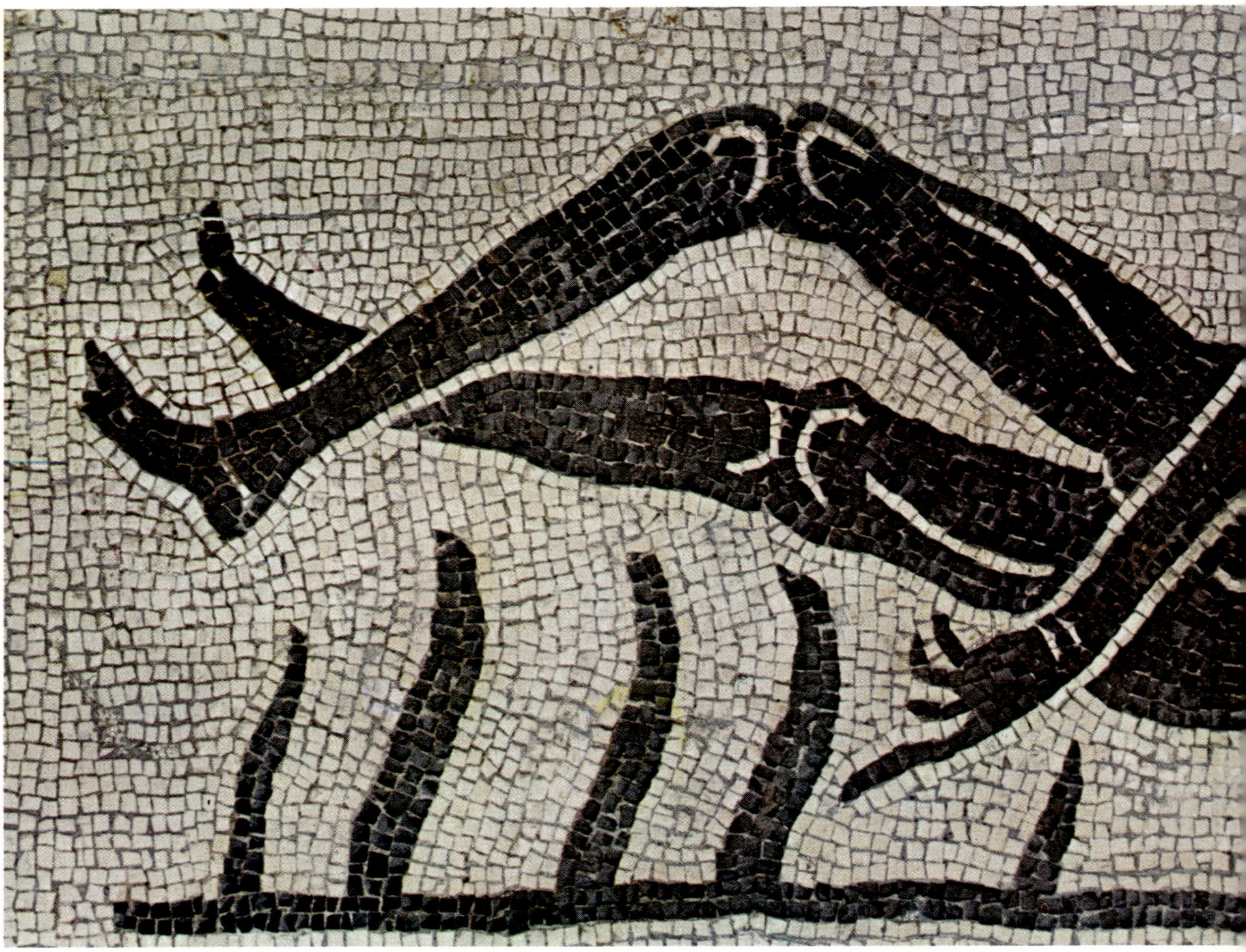

Representations of the skeleton. *Roman mosaics. National Museum, Naples, and Museo delle Terme, Rome.*

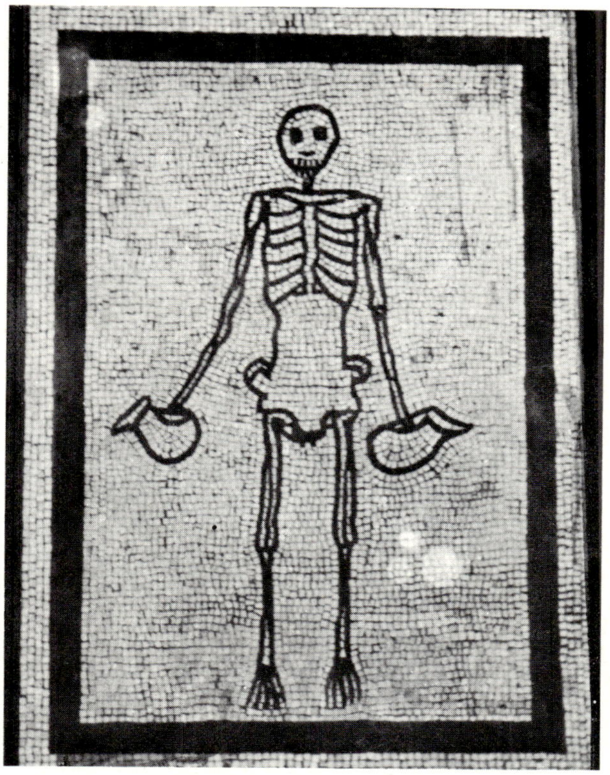

Infused in wine, and taken as ear drops, he believed the cabbage would cure deafness, too.

Pliny states that before the arrival of Greeks in Rome, that is for the first six centuries of its history from its foundation in 753 BC, the Romans managed without doctors at all. This may not be true since the so-called period of the seven kings (753–510 BC) can be equated with the Etruscan era in Rome. The town would therefore have been founded by Etruscans and subject to their colonial rule. This people, although relatively little about them is known, undoubtedly possessed knowledge of medicine. Theophrastus remarks in his *History of plants* how 'Aeschylus in his elegies says Etruria is a land rich in remedies and that the Etruscan race make medicine'. Etruscan priests would have served as

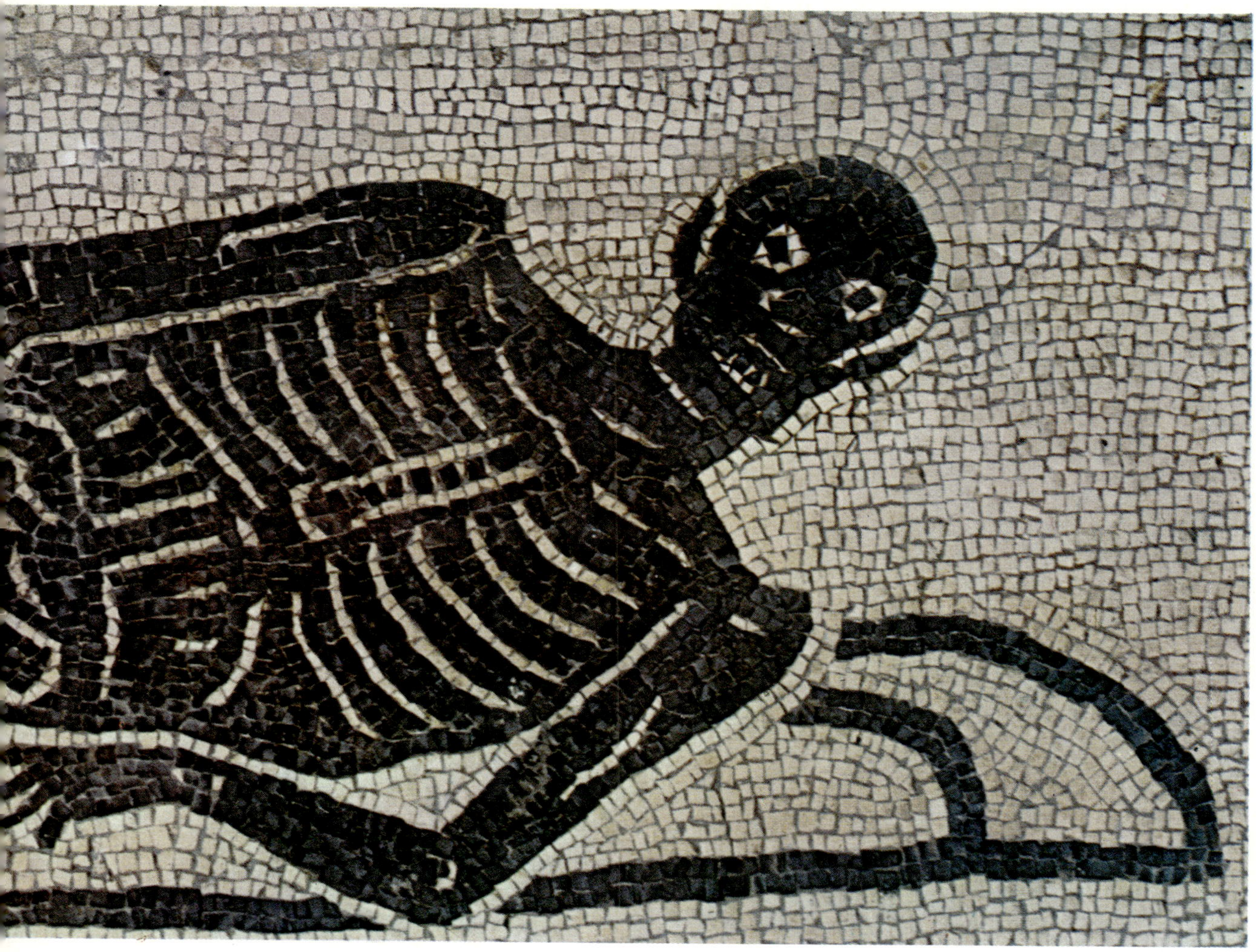

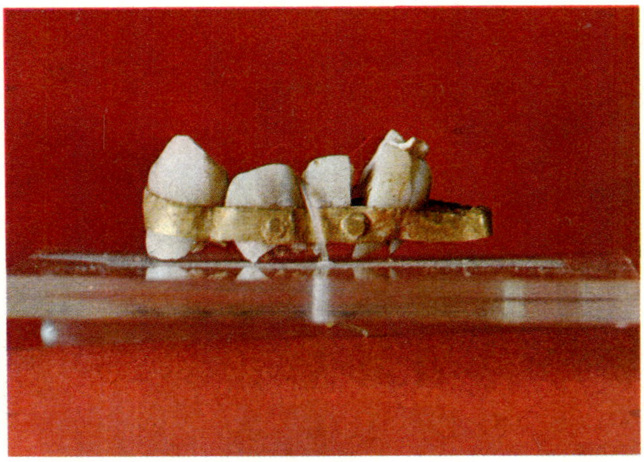

The early Romans considered the practice of medicine ignoble and had an extremely low opinion of Greek doctors, the most famous of the day, perhaps because many charlatans came to Rome.

On the other hand, the Romans made outstanding contributions in the field of public hygiene. From their predecessors the Etruscans they learned about building sewers, and how to combat malaria by draining marshy

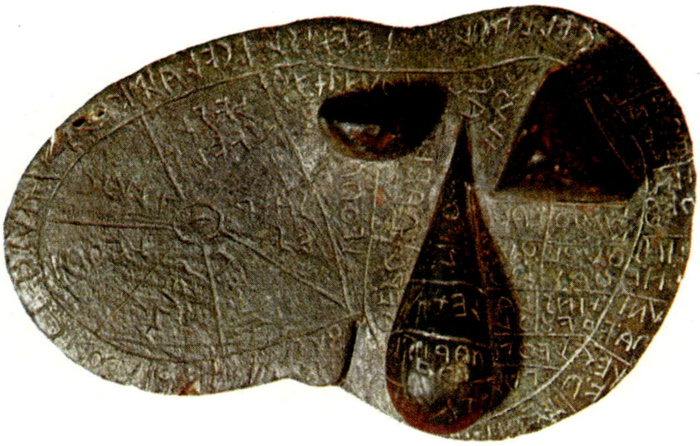

doctors. In the ruins of their temples, in fact, votive tablets representing organs of the human body and resembling those unearthed in the Aesculapian sanctuaries have been found. Dental crowns and gold fillings have also been unearthed and show the skill of Etruscan dentists.

The Etruscans cultivated the ancient art of divination from the viscera of animals, and especially the liver—in fact the word haruspex (soothsayer) comes from the Chaldean *har*, which means liver. Clay models of this organ have been found in Hittite and Babylonian settlements (see also page 20), while an Etruscan bronze in the form of a sheep's liver was found at Piacenza. This is divided into compartments, each corresponding to a region of heaven and its appropriate god: thus there was a pars familiaris (propitious part) and a pars hostilis (adverse part) corresponding to the soothsayer's right and left, both circumscribed by a limiting fissure.

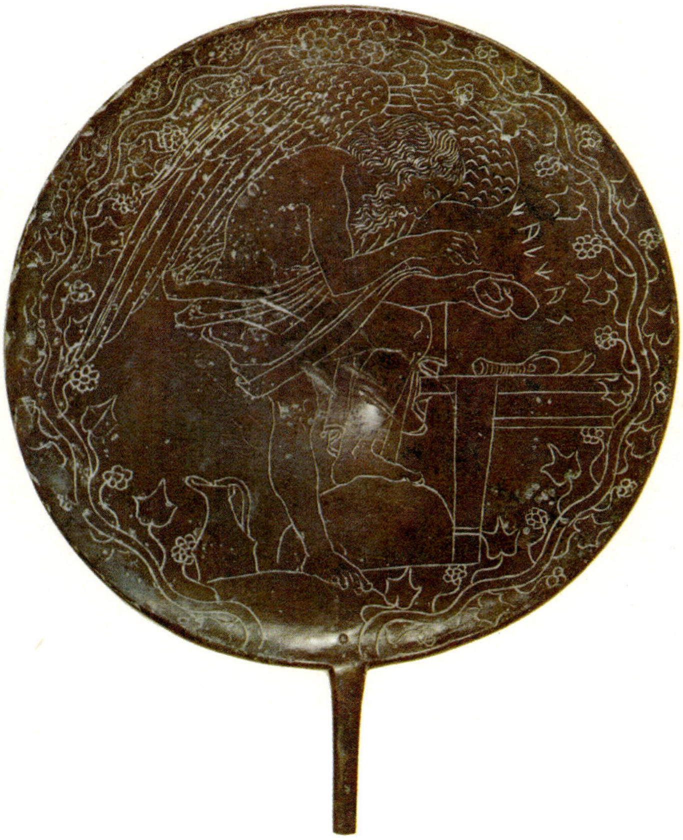

From the Etruscans the Romans inherited knowledge of the therapeutic properties of certain waters and of building for public health purposes. The Cloaca Maxima or great drain was finished under the rule of Tarquinius Priscus in the sixth century BC. It drained stagnant water from marshy ground and emptied it into the Tiber; it was later adapted for sewerage, in the modern sense. The first aqueduct bringing a water supply into the city was built later and completed in 312 BC.

It is clear that in the earliest times Roman medicine must have been both magical and supernatural. Various gods were responsible for the protection of health. Women in childbirth called on Opigena; people with fever called on Febris; those who feared marshes invoked Mephitis. Aesculapius was a latecomer to the banks of the Tiber; in 293 BC the Romans consulted the sybilline books and a mission was despatched to Epidaurus to seek deliverance from an outbreak of the plague. In Epidaurus, a sacred serpent left the temple of Aesculapius and took ship with the Romans of its own accord. When the mission arrived back home, the serpent left the ship and reached an islet where the Romans, in gratitude for their deliverance, built a temple. Long afterwards, the islet became dedicated to St Bartholomew.

The *Lex Aquilia* furnishes more evidence con-

ground. They also built a series of great aqueducts, which brought into the city a copious water supply.

The Etruscans, a race of obscure origin, placed great importance on the practice of divination from animal organs, especially the liver, and seem to have used magic incantations against disease. But they also had surgeons and skilful dentists, who devised a method of binding teeth with gold wire.

Etruscan false teeth. *Villa Giulia Museum, Rome.*

Model of liver for divination. *Etruscan bronze. Piacenza Museum.*

Etruscan bronze mirror showing the haruspex Kalkas examining a liver. *Vatican Museum, Rome.*

A surgical operation (?). *Roman bas-relief at Herculaneum. National Museum, Naples.*

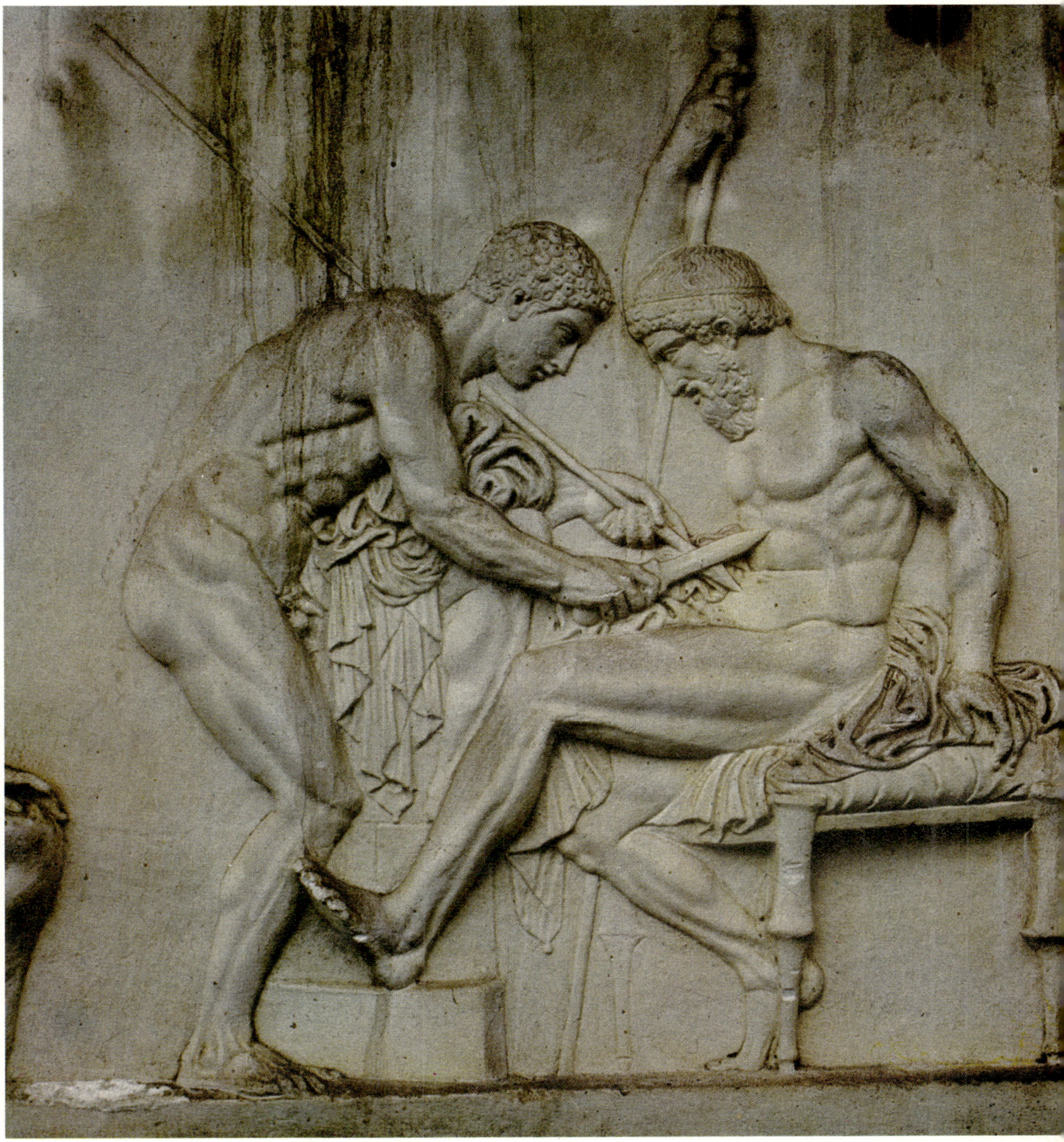

The cult of Aesculapius did not reach Rome until 293 BC, when a serpent from the temple at Epidaurus was said to have embarked of its own accord on a Roman ship and delivered the city from a plague. But Latin literature took many of the Greek legends as its subjects and sometimes contains medical descriptions. Vergil's Aeneid, *the story of the defender of Troy, Aeneas, tells how the hero was treated by Iapyx for a wound in his thigh with dittamy collected by Venus on Mount Ida. The story of the serpent from Epidaurus is related by Ovid in his* Metamorphoses.

Aeneas receiving treatment for a wound. *From a fresco from Pompei. National Museum, Naples.*

tradicting Pliny. It was issued in the fourth century BC and imposed severe penalties on any doctors who caused death by negligence. Doctors must have been practising even earlier, for a law of Numa Pompilius, the legendary second king of Rome, decreed that Caesarean operation was to be performed on women who died in childbirth. Bearing Cato in mind, one imagines the doctors of those days to have been ignorant and inexperienced. Anyhow, the first Greek doctor of whom we have knowledge (from Cassius Emina, an ancient author quoted by Pliny) arrived from the Peloponnese in 219 BC during the consulate of L. Semilius and M. Livius. He was known as Archagathus, that is 'the one who makes a good start'. He was well received and was given citizenship and a place to work. His patients called him at first 'vulnerarius' (healer of wounds) but then 'carnifex' (slaughterer) because his cures were swift and cruel.

Unfortunately, Archagathus was followed by many others of comparable ability, who came to Rome perhaps because of a lack of success at home in Greece.

Asclepiades

The Romans were at first too proud to practise themselves for they considered it beneath their dignity, but they learnt that in Greece the profession of medicine was respected, entailed rigorous training at a recognized school, swearing a solemn oath and the granting of a licence only after candidates' credentials had been duly weighed and considered. So later they became more discriminating and master physicians began to arrive in increasing numbers.

Asclepiades of Prusa arrived in Rome in 91 BC from Bithynia. Of humble birth, he had studied rhetoric at Athens and worked for a miller in his youth to pay for his education. He attended the school of Alexandria, and then came to Rome. He cut a fine figure, with his impressive features and noble bearing, and soon found his way into influential circles. He became a fashionable doctor; the great names of the day were among his patients and he counted Cicero, Mark Antony and Crassus as friends. A man of great insight, he knew what would captivate the gluttons of Rome, spoiled by their wealth and oblivious of the uncomfortable austerity preached by Cato. It was useless to prescribe foul-tasting medicines; indeed, he did not even believe they worked. Instead, he prescribed diet, exercise, walking, baths and massage.

Asclepiades was the most fashionable doctor of ancient times, and he became so famous that he was credited with a miraculous cure. The story was written down long afterwards by Apuleius (*Florida*, IV, chapter 19). One day Asclepiades was on his way back to his luxurious villa when he met a funeral procession. The pallbearers were tired of carrying the body and set it down at the side of the road to rest. The doctor went up to them, asked the causes of death and receiving no satisfactory answer stooped over to inspect the corpse for himself. Asclepiades persuaded those present to delay the rites for a while and carry the corpse into a nearby house, and there he revived the man taken for dead. The news of the event and the prowess of the Greek doctor spread all over Rome.

Pliny's opinion was that Asclepiades was an adventurer whose sole concern was to publicize his success in order to get the maximum number of patients possible. Galen wrote of him, 'He had no respect for the great thinkers or for truth, but was guided by a boasting spirit, arrogance, false reasoning and base obstinacy to behave in a shameful manner'.

Perhaps Galen found it hard to be objective about a very successful colleague; nevertheless history, more often than not, praises men for qualities their contemporaries regarded only with disparagement. Asclepiades, in the opinion of Celsus, was 'in the forefront of doctors, and apart from Hippocrates the foremost'. What Galen disliked was his refutation of the Hippocratic theory of humours, for Asclepiades, who played a leading part in developing the atomic theory of Democritus and Epicurus, cast a critical eye on the blind subservience to Hippocrates of those people who practised his precepts.

The pathology of Asclepiades was based on the concept of the body as made up of atoms, elementary corpuscles imperceptible to the senses and continually moving through the pores and canals of the body. If liquid substances flowed through the cavities of the body without meeting obstacles, the body was in a state of health. Illness resulted if the circulation of liquids was impeded through some obstruction caused by the corpuscles. The obstacles could arise out of mass, number or anom-

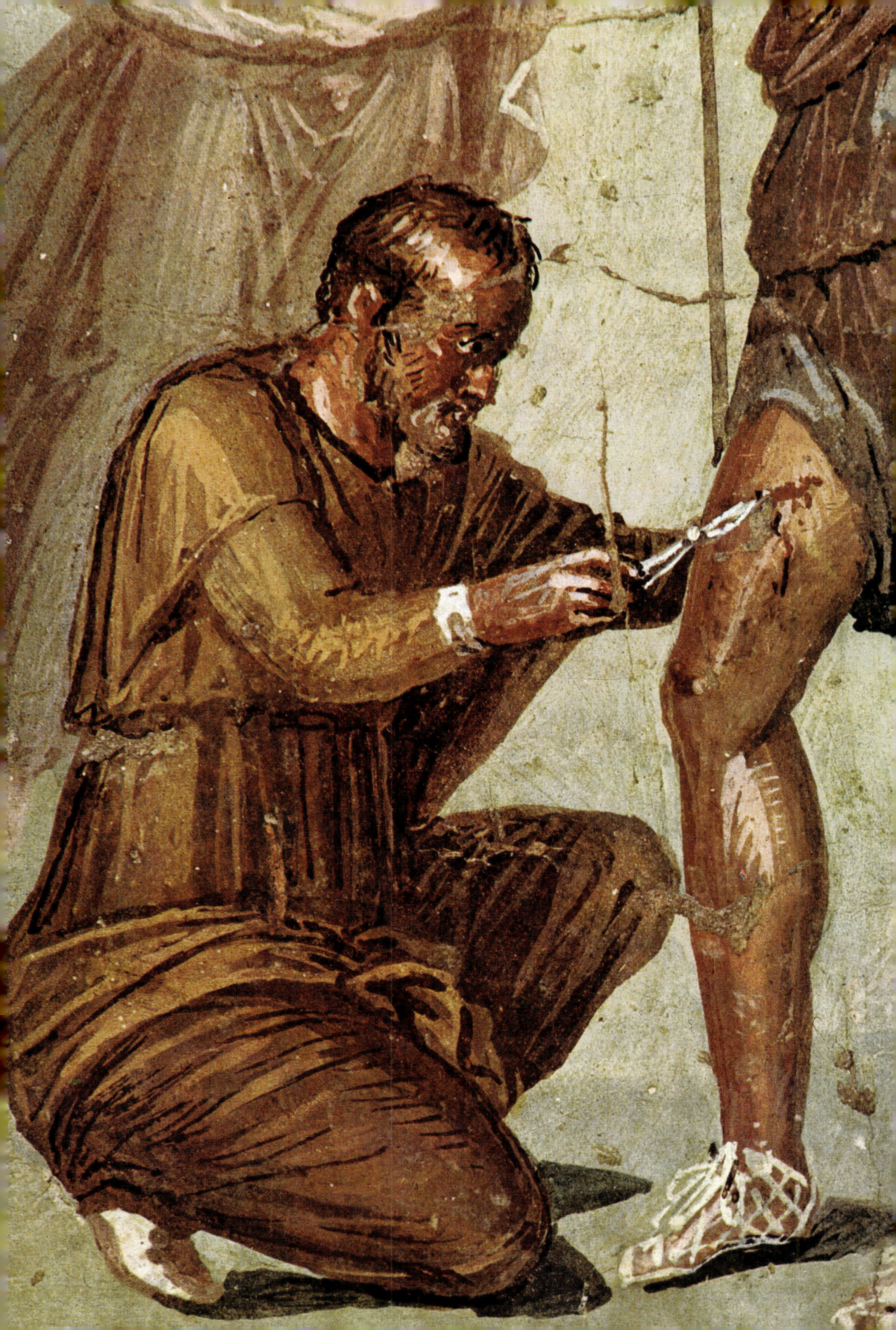

When the Romans learned of the professional qualifications and licences required by Greek doctors in their own country, they became more selective about those they allowed to practise in Rome.

Asclepiades, who studied at Alexandria, was the most successful and fashionable of these. His patients included many of the great statesmen of Rome, and his success was undoubtedly due to his ability to deal with

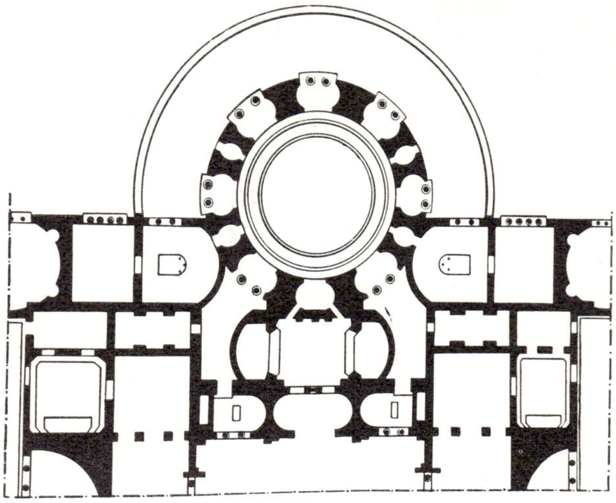

alous movement of the atoms. Themison of Laodicea, a pupil of Asclepiades, added that illness, besides arising from the quality and movement of corpuscles, also occurred when the pores through which the atoms moved were unduly restricted or relaxed–diseases were thus of two types: those with a state of tension and those with a state of relaxation.

For this reason the Methodist school, following Asclepiades, laid great stress on taking baths to induce sweating when the pores were restricted and astringents and tonics when they were dilated. The Methodists held that illness could also be of a

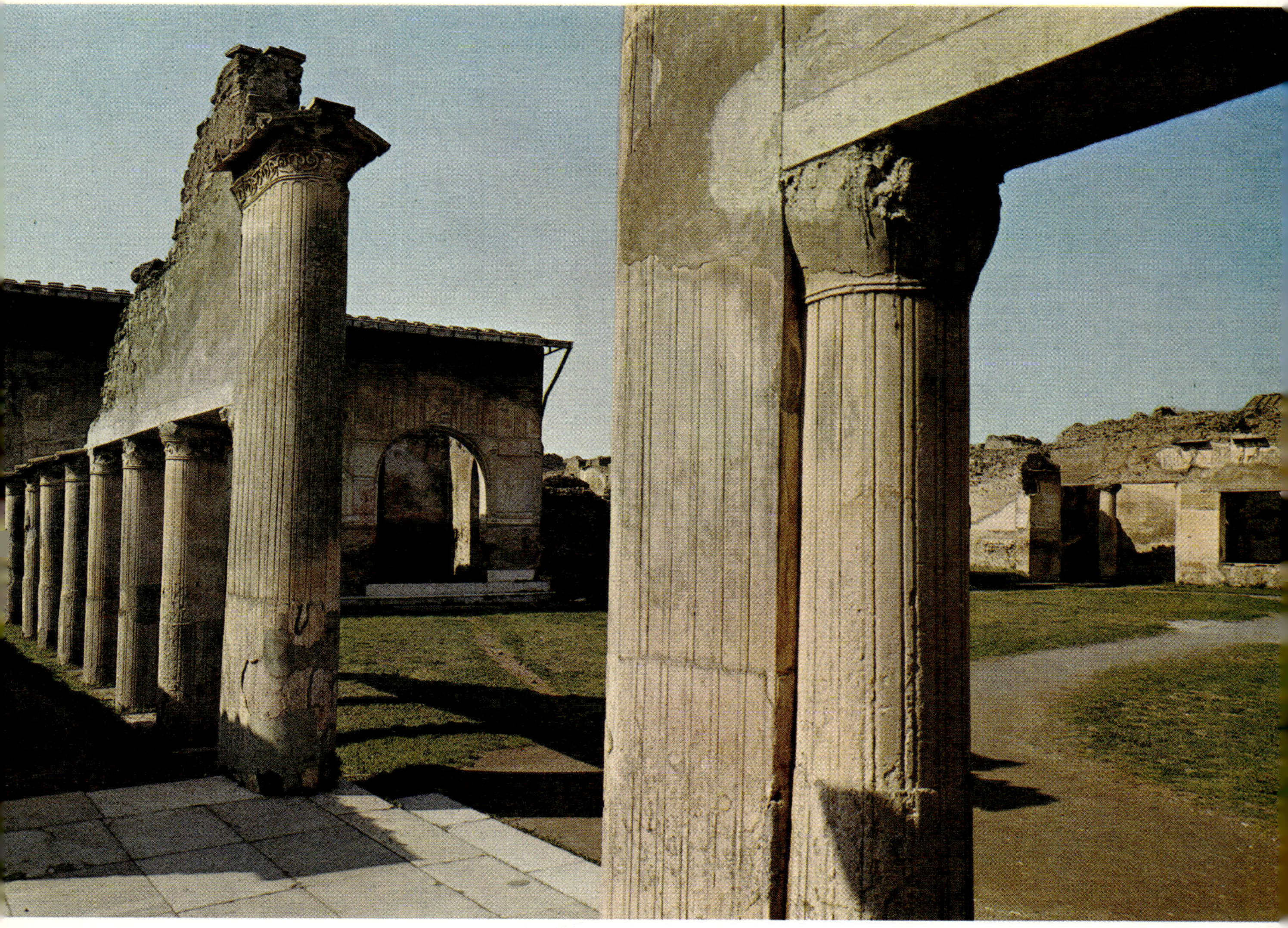

such figures: treatments were based not so much on medicine as on diet, exercise, baths and massage.

Thermae, the great public baths, were constructed by leading citizens and by emperors; they comprised the apodyterium (dressing-room), frigidarium (cold bath), tepidarium (warm bath), calidarium (hot bath), laconicum (sweat bath), sphaeristerium (exercise room) and unctoreium (oil room).

Plan of the Caracalla baths, Rome.

The Stabian baths, Pompei.

The death of Seneca. *Roman statue. Louvre Museum, Paris.*

mixed type, in which case treatment of the dominant pathogenic factor was advised. Asclepiades did not share the faith of Hippocrates and his school in the healing powers of nature. Indeed, he believed doctors should act 'cito, tute et iucunde'– in a fast, safe and pleasant manner. His material contributions to medicine include distinguishing between acute and chronic diseases and observing the periodicity of some diseases. He described malarial fevers with accuracy; he was the first to carry out tracheotomy, probably for diphtheria; and he introduced humane methods in the treatment of the mentally deranged, transferring them from dark places, where they were commonly hidden away, to well-lit quarters, where they carried out therapeutic exercises.

His prestige seems well-earned. His students included, besides Themison of Laodicea, Antony Musa, who achieved fame as the personal physician of the emperor Augustus. Musa also treated Maecenas, Horace and Virgil, and was most noted for the introduction of a new method of treatment, based on cold baths and diet. One of his manuscripts was a work in the form of a letter addressed to Maecenas, the patron of the arts, which gave medical advice; another was a treatise called *De herba vettonica,* giving 47 prescriptions for use of the herb betony in various disorders.

Lucretius

The cause of science was advanced by a younger Roman contemporary of Asclepiades, the poet and philosopher Lucretius Carus, who was born in 95 BC and died in 55 BC. His great work *De rerum natura* (The nature of the universe) discussed the meaning of existence with the clarity of genius, and stands today as the most important Latin scientific writing of classical times. At a time when personal and political feuds signalled the impending collapse of the power of Rome, Lucretius had to look beyond the confines of society for a meaningful way of life, for as an Epicurean he sought ideals that were totally freed of any dogma and superstition.

According to Lucretius, the world was infinite and composed of invisible atoms, minute particles which were always moving and coming into contact with each other, both in a harmonious and a discordant manner. Life and death followed one another in a continuous cycle without beginning or end. Although its author was not a doctor, *De rerum natura* contains a number of advanced statements about anatomy, physiology, hygiene, diet and the influence of environment, and it is therefore an important landmark in the history of medicine as well as of science.

These statements were set down in a framework of the highest idealism, for the poet was concerned with the purpose of life, the contrast between materialism and the freedom of the spirit, the mysterious workings of the natural world and physical and emotional problems.

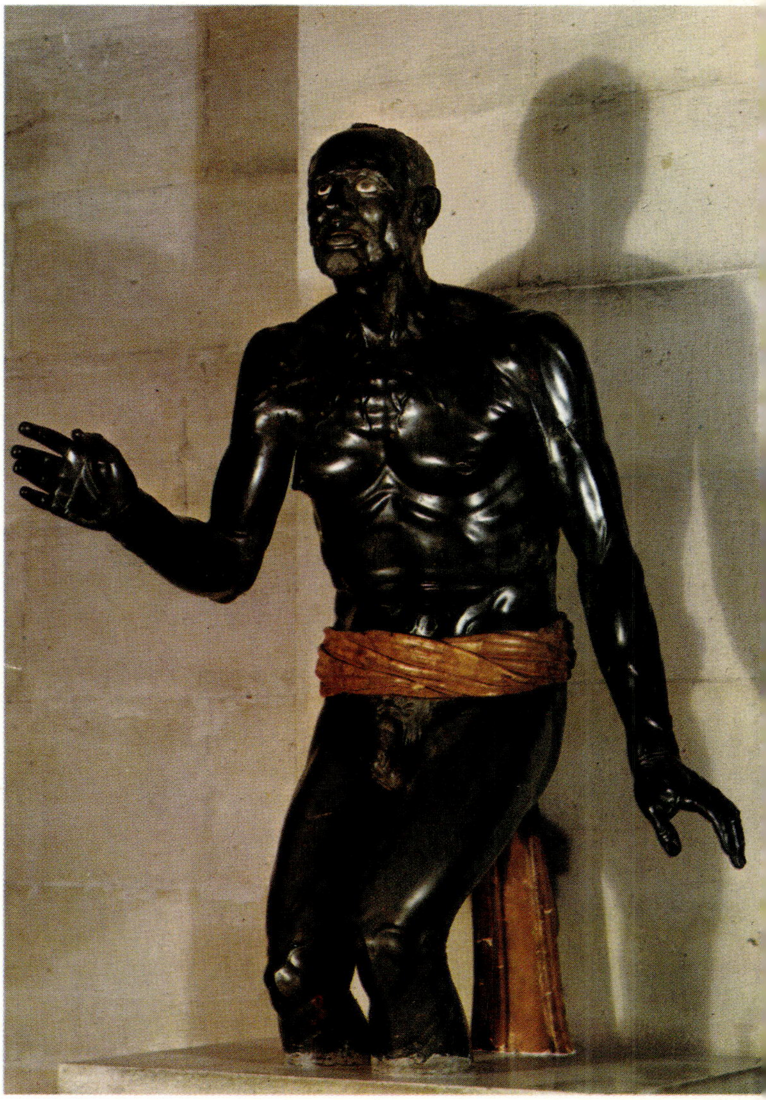

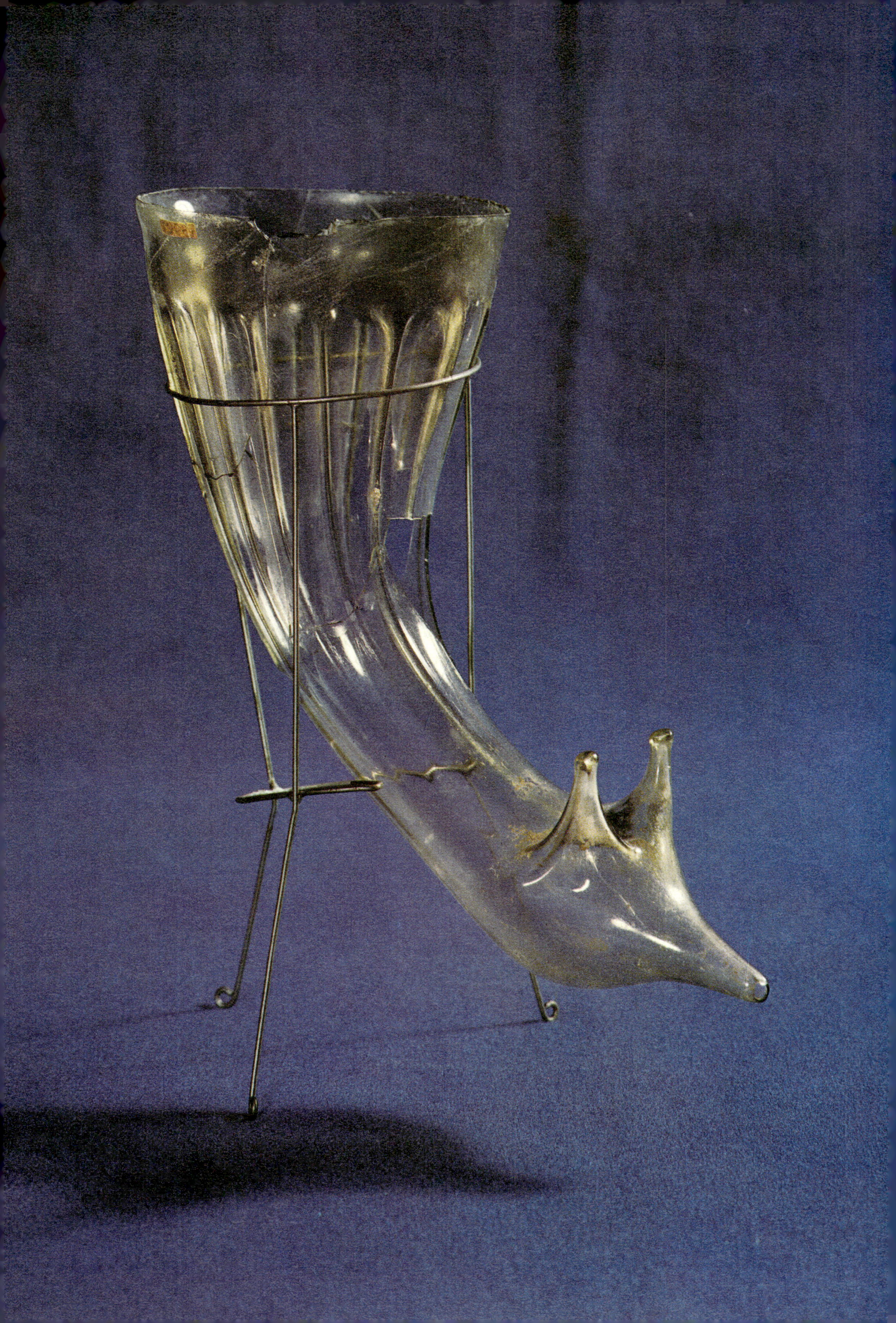

Celsus and Pliny, medical encyclopaedists

Aulus Cornelius Celsus, who lived at the start of the Christian era, was the most famous Roman medical writer. It is not known for certain if he practised medicine, and some experts think that he was not in fact a doctor, but a rich man of leisure who aimed to record all the knowledge of his time in a great encyclopaedic work. This work, entitled *De artibus,* embraced agriculture, military theory, philosophy and law, as well as medicine, the section on which, *De re medica,* is the only one to survive. Little known when written and forgotten in the Middle Ages, it was discovered in 1426 by a distinguished scholar, Guarine di Verona (1374–1460). In 1443 Tommaso Parentucelli (1397–1455), later Pope Nicholas V, found a tenth-century codex in the Basilica of St Ambrose in Milan. *De re medica* may have been the last ancient manuscript on medicine to be discovered, but it was the first to be printed: the *editio princeps* was published in 1478 in Florence.

In this work Celsus avoided doctrinal disputes and arranged material systematically. He subdivided diseases not by cause but by treatment, which might be by diet, drugs or surgery. Celsus may have been faithful to the Hippocratic concept of pathology but in this work, which represented the first attempt at producing a complete textbook of medicine, there was considerable advance over the viewpoint of the great Greek physician.

Much new information was to be found in *De re medica.* Celsus described nutrient enemas; 'To sustain the patient as a last resource oatmeal or boiled wheat-flour may be introduced into the intestine from below'. Descriptions were given of plastic surgery on the nose, lips and ears; this was developed by the Sicilian Branca fourteen centuries

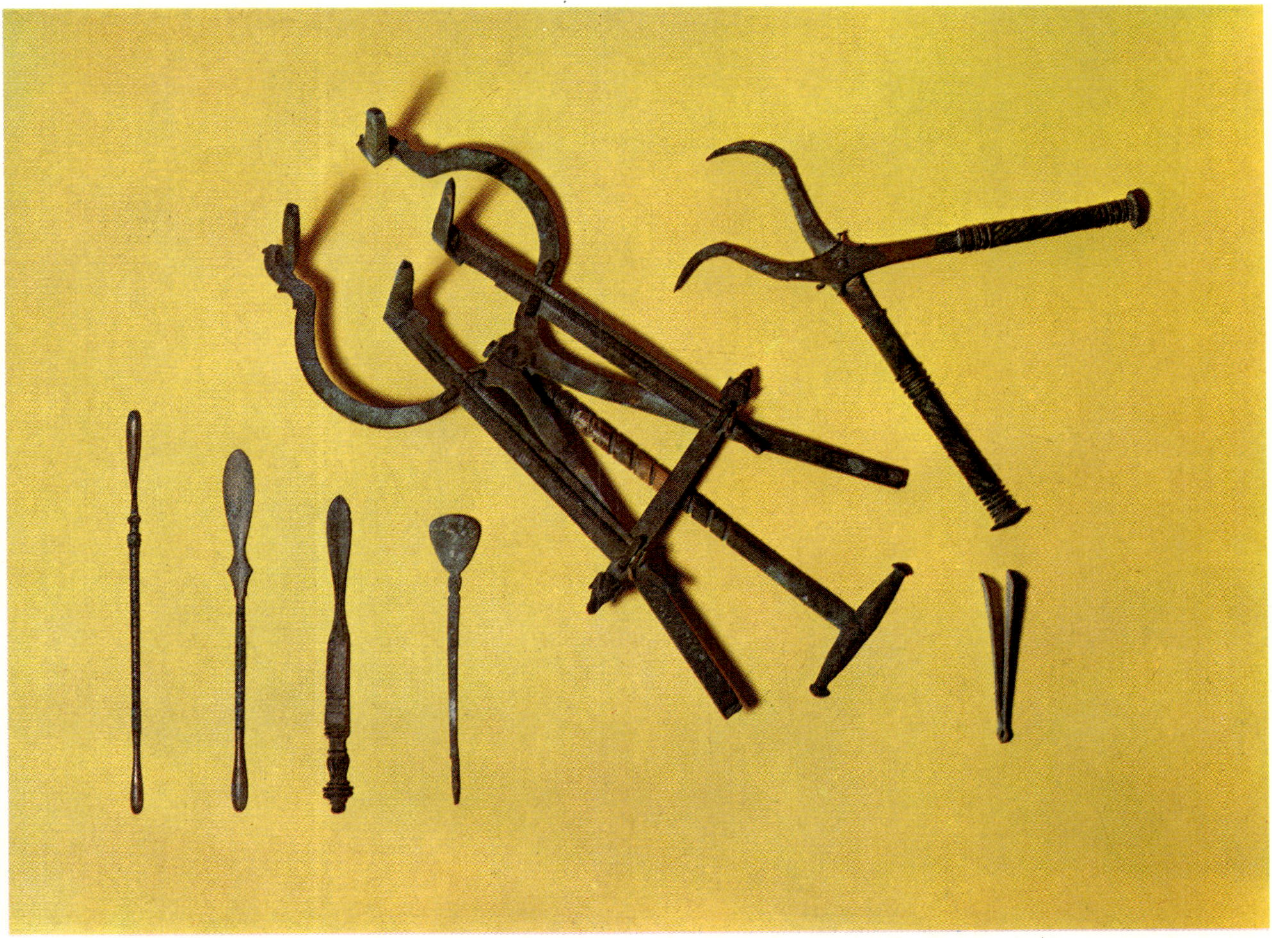

Previous pages :
Roman dropping glass. *Archaeological Museum, Aquileia.*

Roman surgical instruments from Pompei. *Archaeological Museum, Naples.*

These pages :
Medicinal clay tablets, early pharmaceutical preparations. *Louvre Museum, Paris.*

Serpent of Aesculapius. *National Museum, Athens.*

later and perfected by the Bolognese surgeon Tagliacozzi in the sixteenth century. Celsus wrote at length on the care of wounds and advised the use of compresses to stop bleeding, and exerting pressure on and tying vessels. He understood the complications of wounds: 'Let nothing be undertaken until the inside of the wound has been cleaned, lest any congealed blood remain within it. For this will turn to pus and cause inflammation which will prevent the wound from healing'. Lastly, the edges of the wound were to be sewn up with thread or better still held together by means of clips. Celsus stated the four cardinal signs of inflammation–'rubor, calor, dolor, tumor' (redness, heat, pain, swelling)–which are still memorized today by every medical student.

Treatment for broken bones is clearly stated. First the fracture was reduced, and then immobilization of the affected part was achieved by means of splints and bandaging, stiffened by wax and flour paste; the bandages were to be changed after one week or at most nine days, when the swelling had gone down. For open fractures, Celsus advised resection of the protruding fragment. For abdominal lesions, he suggested sewing up the large intestine, but excluded all possibility of effective treatment for lesions of the small intestine.

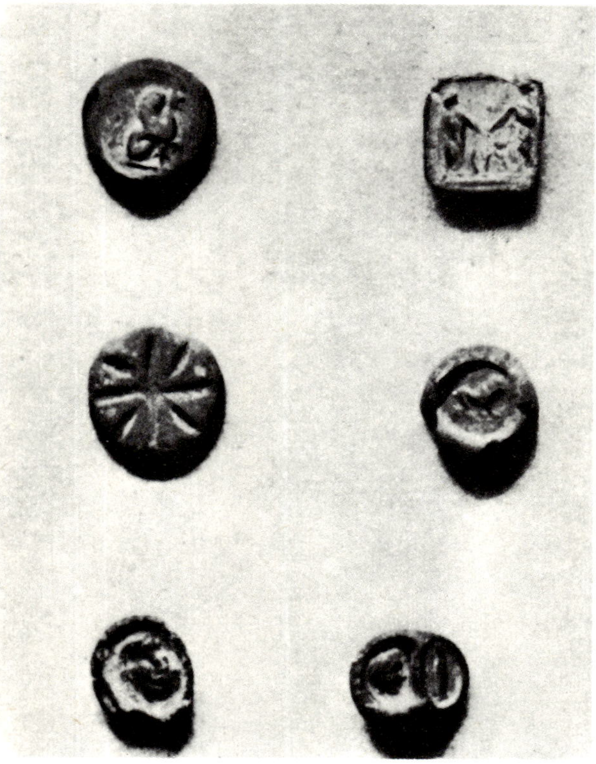

Surgical instruments found during archaeological excavations at Pompeii, now in Naples national museum, fit exactly the descriptions of Cornelius Celsus. Besides various types of forceps, scalpels, hooks, sounds, probes and tongs, there were ingenious devices new to the surgical armoury: one, called meningophylax, was used after trephining the skull to hold back the meninges; another, like an iron V, was used to keep a wound open while removing an arrowhead; a lithotome was used for surgical removal of stones; and special forceps were employed to remove bone fragments after trephining.

Caius Plinius Secundus (AD 23–79)–Pliny the elder–was the greatest Roman naturalist and an encyclopaedist like Celsus. He lived on intimate terms with the emperor Vespasian's son Titus, to whom he dedicated his massive *Natural history*, a work in 37 books which revealed no original thought but a wealth of scholarship. He wanted to know about everything, and he was lucky enough to be able to satisfy his inclinations by travelling. He spent some years on military service in Germany, and then held the office of proconsul in Spain; on returning to Rome, he became a close adviser of the emperor.

Pliny, like Cato the censor, disliked physicians, but his work is of interest from the medical standpoint since he dealt with drugs obtainable from vegetable, animal and mineral sources, and there are many references to public health in his time and to names and events which would otherwise be unknown to us.

The story of how he paid for his curiosity is well known. In the year 79 he was at Cape Misenum in his capacity of Roman naval commander. This was at the time of the disastrous eruption of Vesuvius, which was to obliterate Pompeii and Herculaneum, and Pliny was anxious to examine the remarkable phenomenon at close hand. He got into a galley, shouted 'fortune favours the brave' to encourage the steersman and managed, despite a high sea, to come ashore at Stabiae. His last day was described by his nephew Pliny the younger in a letter to Tacitus; after a bath, a meal, and a night's sleep he went on to the beach beneath the smouldering volcano, where he was overcome by sulphurous fumes.

Celsus was the most famous Roman medical writer. Of his great work De artibus, *which originally included sections on agriculture, law and strategy, only that on medicine survives. Celsus kept to the Hippocratic concept of disease, but arranged the material in his work, the first complete medical textbook, according to treatment–diet, drugs or surgery. It was used for years as a valuable source of information on pharmacology, and the descriptions of numerous surgical procedures are also very full; the operation for bladder stones–lithotomy–still bears Celsus' name on the Continent.*

Pliny was the greatest Roman naturalist, a man who travelled very widely and produced an enormous work of scholarship in 37 volumes, which includes many references to animal, vegetable and mineral drugs, as well as to public health measures.

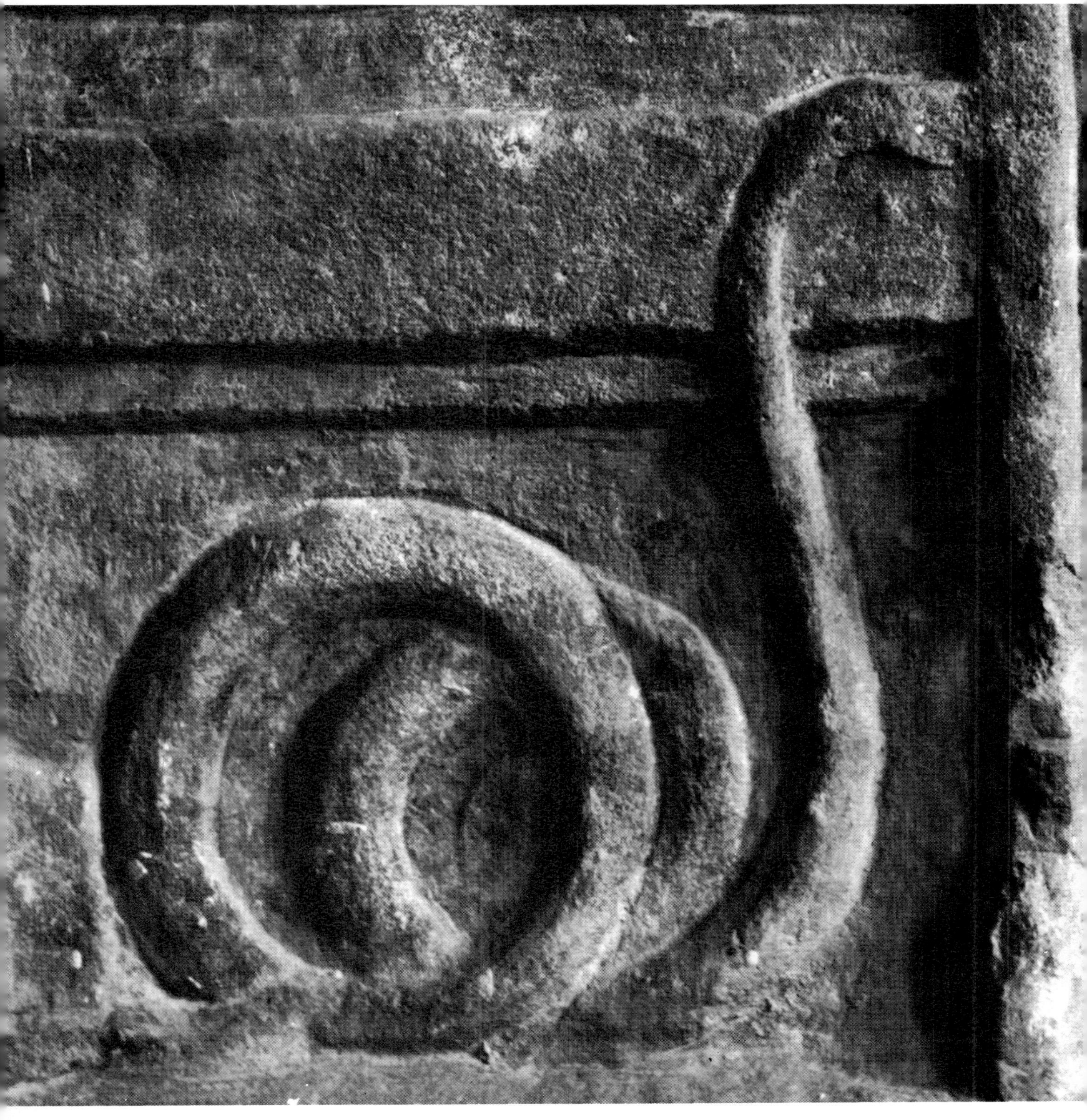

Soranus, father of obstetrics and gynaecology

As we have seen, the Methodist school dominated Roman medicine at the time of its greatest achievements. Many followers of the school were held in high esteem and confidence by the emperors; of these physicians the most renowned was Soranus, who is today regarded as the father of obstetrics.

At childbirth in Roman times the skill of midwives was of most importance, together with various magical rites. Parturition, as a physiological process, does not on the whole need medical intervention, and so the part of the doctor has always been small. The ancients devised Caesarean section, but used it only on the dead or dying woman, and they knew of no other obstetrical procedures. One reason was that the anatomical ideas held by the Hippocratic school about genital organs were incomplete. They thought that the position of the uterus in the body was variable and they had no knowledge of the clitoris or Fallopian tubes. With such vague notions of anatomy, their ideas about the physiology of fertilization were also vague. They knew, however, about the different positions of the foetus and how some of these made delivery difficult.

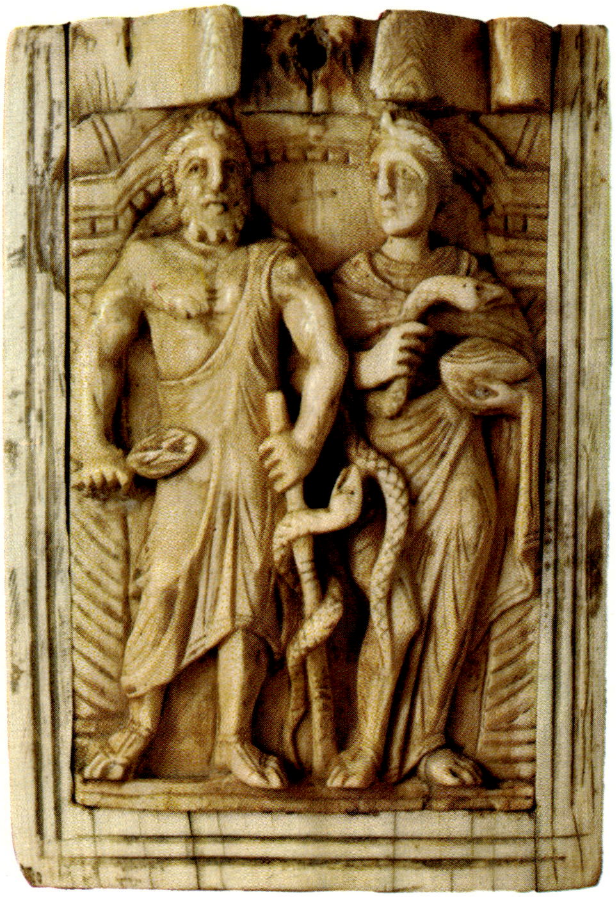

Soranus of Ephesus lived in the first century of the Christian era. Before settling in Rome in the time of Trajan, he practised medicine at Alexandria. His main work, *On the diseases of women,* was a textbook which remained in use for fifteen centuries. He described the female genital system in detail, and likened the uterus to a cupping instrument, open during coitus and menstruation. He advised contraception by means of cotton, ointments or fatty substances, but disapproved of abortion by mechanical means.

Soranus described menstruation, conception, and amenorrhoea, which could have physiological causes such as child-bearing and breast-feeding, or pathological causes, such as inflammation of the genital tract or debilitating disease, and he prescribed treatment for uterine bleeding and for dysmenorrhoea.

The most famous obstetrician of ancient times paid particular attention to the difficulties that could attend childbirth. They could be due to defects or infirmities on the part of the mother, such as a contracted pelvis, lordosis (an abnormal curvature of the spine), tumours and so on. In obstetric intervention before birth, Soranus advised protection of the perineum, the soft parts closing the pelvis in its lower section, and emptying the bladder by means of a catheter.

Difficulties in childbirth could also be due to the foetus, which might be too large or in an abnormal position. In this case, the doctor must intervene; Soranus illustrated various abnormal positions and explained how to manoeuvre the foetus into a suitable position at the mouth of the uterus. If manual assistance was of no avail, the doctor was advised to use forceps or hooks to extract the foetus. Embryotomy was only advisable in a desperate situation.

Having taken care of the mother, Soranus went on to deal with the survival, health and growth of the newborn child. He advised cutting the umbilical cord after two knots had been tied, recommended washing the baby's eyes with oils, and indicated how to clean the baby and swaddle him. Breast-feeding was not to start until the third day; on the

Ivory box for medicines, with sliding lid showing Aesculapius and Hygeia. *Fifth-sixth century* AD. *Sion Museum, Switzerland.*

Birth of Aesculapius. *From De re medica of Alessandro Benedetti, Basle 1549.*

Delivery with a midwife. *From the tomb of Scribonia Attice Amerimno, in the Isola sacra burial ground. Ostia excavations.*

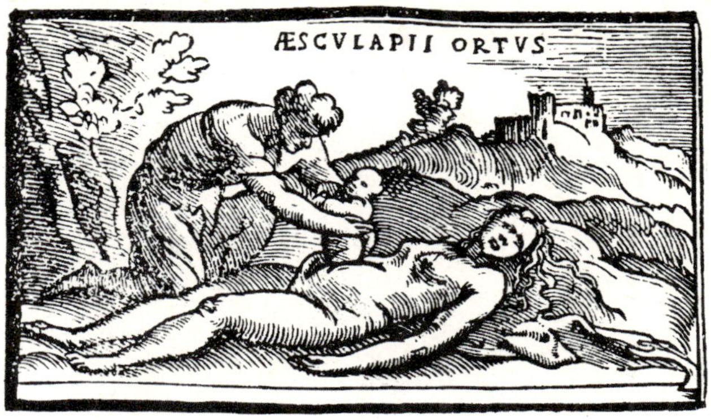

first two days, the baby was to be fed on honey, diluted and boiled. Soranus also suggested what to do if the breast-feeder's milk failed or was bad, and gave advice on weaning, teething and teaching infants to walk. Lastly, he gave some account of childhood diseases, and how to avoid and how to treat them.

Soranus also wrote treatises on acute and chronic diseases and on fractures. His works were plagiarized in succeeding centuries by writers who went so far as to claim authorship of them, like Aurelianus Caelius and Moschus, whose borrowings were not exposed until the late nineteenth century, when a codex of Soranus' work came to light in Paris.

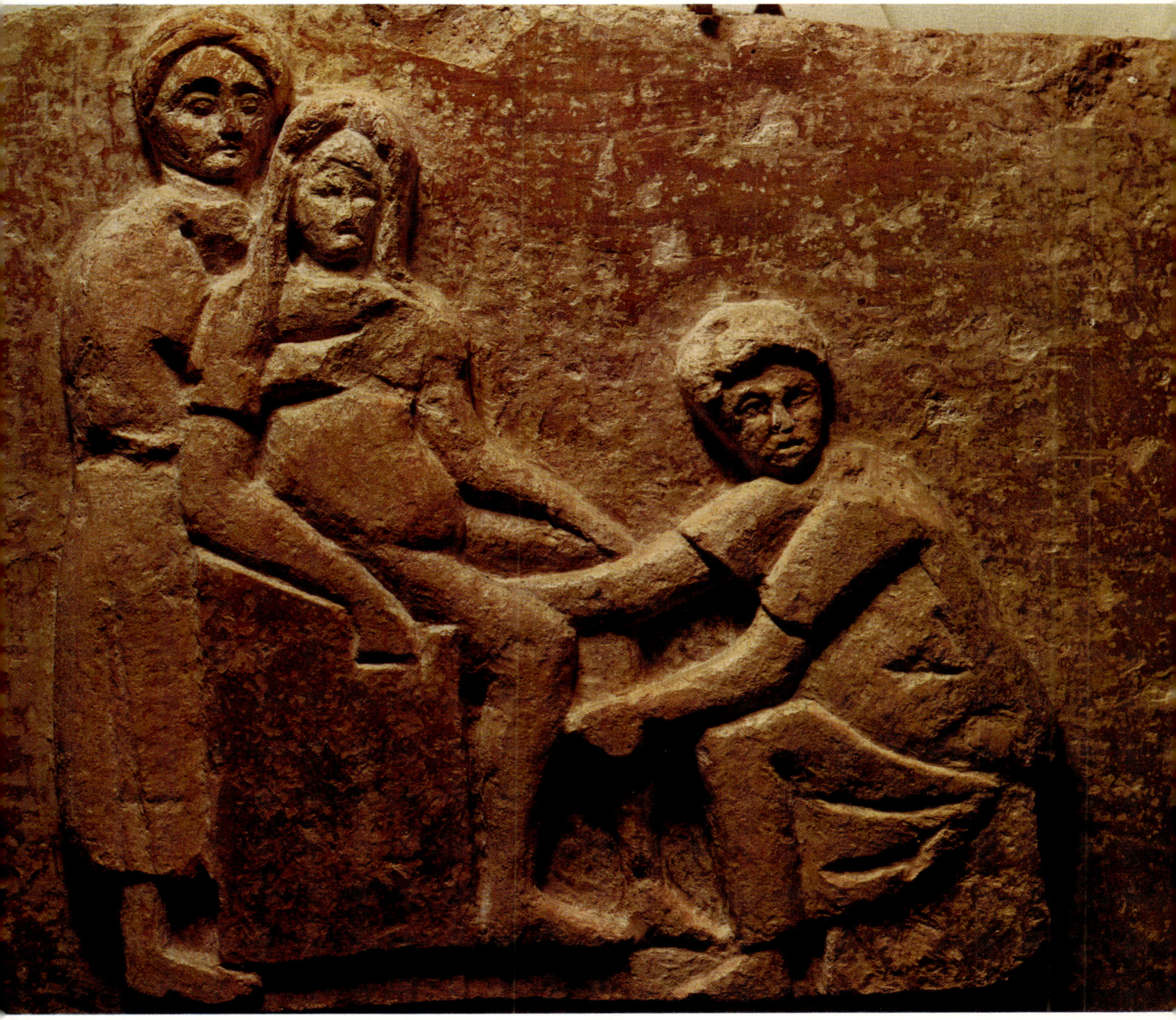

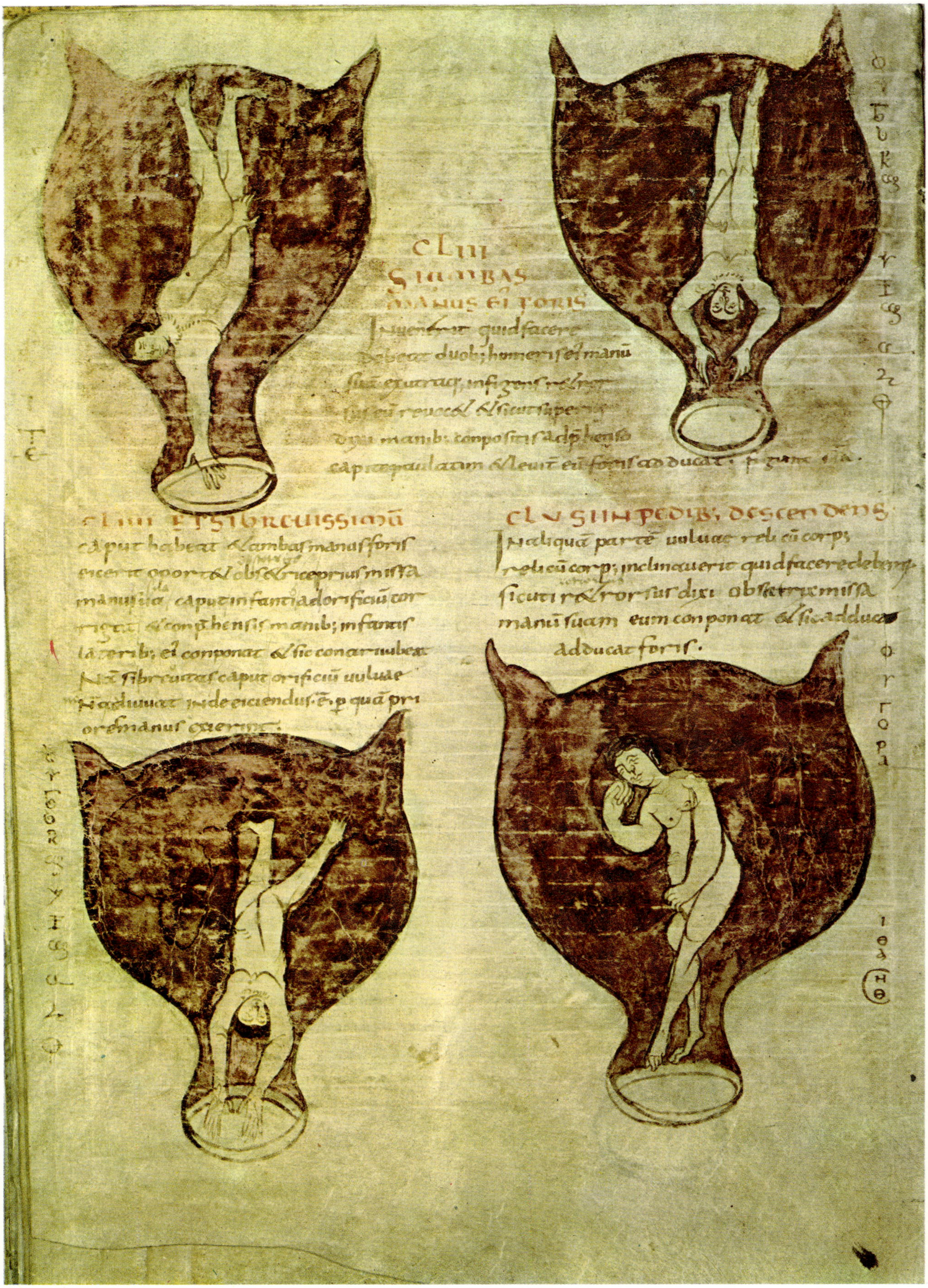

Soranus was the most renowned physician of the Methodist school which dominated Roman medicine during the period of its greatest achievements, and which followed the teaching of Asclepiades. At this time there were doctors of numerous kinds practising in the Empire, from those who treated slaves to the court doctors and the highest of all, the Palatine doctor. In addition there were doctors for the poor, employed by municipalities, and doctors to the army and the gladiators. In a similar way, there were also several kinds of hospitals, some caring for slaves, some for athletes and gladiators, others for the military.

Gynaikeia by Soranus, illustrating various presentations of foetus. *Ninth-century manuscript. Royal Library, Brussels.*

Just as the work of Soranus remained standard in obstetrics and gynaecology for centuries, the work of Dioscorides was used as a textbook in pharmacology until the Renaissance. Born about AD 40 at Anazarbos in Cilicia, Pedanius Dioscorides became one of the best known and respected army surgeons at the time of the emperor Nero. His chief work, *Materia medica,* in five books, contained all the pharmacological information available under the empire, with an appendix on poisons and antidotes. He was aware that he was no great stylist, for he warned his readers to concentrate on the facts and forget the frills, but his work was original, small part being derived from earlier sources such as the treatises of Theophrastus and of Crateuas, physician to the king of Pontus, Mithridates VI Eupator (120–63 BC), a renowned experimenter with poisons who gave his name to an antidote. The first book of *Materia medica* was devoted to herbs, ointments and oils; the second to food products from animals such as honey and milk, and from agriculture such as wheat; the third and fourth books dealt with plants and roots; the fifth with wines, and medicines from the mineral kingdom such as lead acetate, copper oxide and calcium hydroxide. The original Greek text was soon translated into Latin and illustrations were added; many copies of these versions have come down to us from a ninth- or tenth-century codex dedicated to a Byzantine princess, Juliana Anicia.

Dioscorides was not an army surgeon with a flair for botany, but rather a pharmacologist. In order to learn more about plants, and to visit as many countries as possible, he joined the legions.

The greatness of Rome rested largely on its invincible army, thus it is not surprising that the Empire fostered important developments in military medicine. The formation of stationary armies in large garrisons gave rise to the establishment of a medical service, with physicians ranked as noncombatant officers, called principales, who took their orders directly from the camp commander or, in his absence, from the tribune of the legions. It is known that at the time of Hadrian every legion, including the cavalry, had its own medical personnel. Naval units, too, had physicians aboard every trireme; these were called duplicarii, which indicates that they received double pay. Military doctors enjoyed other privileges, such as the *jus restitutionis,* which insured them against any loss of property incurred by absence from home during service with the army. In addition, the Justinian Code notes that a physician of the legion is exempt from all civil obligation during his military service.

Excavations have uncovered the remains of Roman military hospitals near Vienna, at Baden in Switzerland and near Bonn and Dusseldorf in Germany, indicating that the army was well cared for even in the provinces.

Hospitals were not only for the military: valetudinaria were for slaves, and there were others for athletes and gladiators. The slaves' doctor was called medicus commensalis, while the gladiators' doctor bore the title vulnerarius. The top rank a doctor under the Roman Empire could hope to achieve was an appointment at court, if not the chief post of Palatine doctor. Townships throughout the empire also enjoyed the right of electing special civic doctors, whose task was to care for the poor free of charge; these were known as archiatri populares. In addition, there were in Rome a number of physicians without official positions or definite titles who nevertheless enjoyed such privileges as exemption from all taxes and the right to denounce before the judges those patients who had not paid their fees. These were often large: Galen sometimes received more than a thousand pounds for a case.

The Roman doctors may not have excelled as theoreticians but their laws for hygienic regulation of baths and aqueducts were exemplary; the system of drains and canals was properly supervised; conditions for food sales in the market places were subject to certain controls; and orders were in force in respect of the burial and cremation of the dead, and so they could be said greatly to have advanced public health.

But it was not only in the field of hygiene that their influence was felt, for as the Roman Empire declined the status of the doctors increased. Physicians became more and more respectable and respected: instruction of Romans in medicine became systematized and at the same time the political power of doctors emerged and was increasingly felt, so that by the time of the later emperors the physicians were often the most important members of the court and the trusted friends of the ruler.

This new respectability did not keep the medical

One of the best-known army surgeons at the time of Nero was Dioscorides, who was more famous for his Materia medica, *a collection in five volumes of all the pharmacological ideas of the time, which was regarded for many centuries as the foremost textbook on the subject. Dioscorides' work, originally in Greek, was translated into Latin and illustrations were added; the Latin text was produced in many versions.*

Among Dioscorides' sources was the herbal compiled by Crateuas, who was the first known illustrator of plants; some of his work may have been used in the Iuliana Anicia codex, one illustration in which shows Dioscorides describing a mandrake, and in the foreground depicts a dead dog. It was long believed that mandrake, the root of which may grow in a somewhat human form, had magical properties and would kill

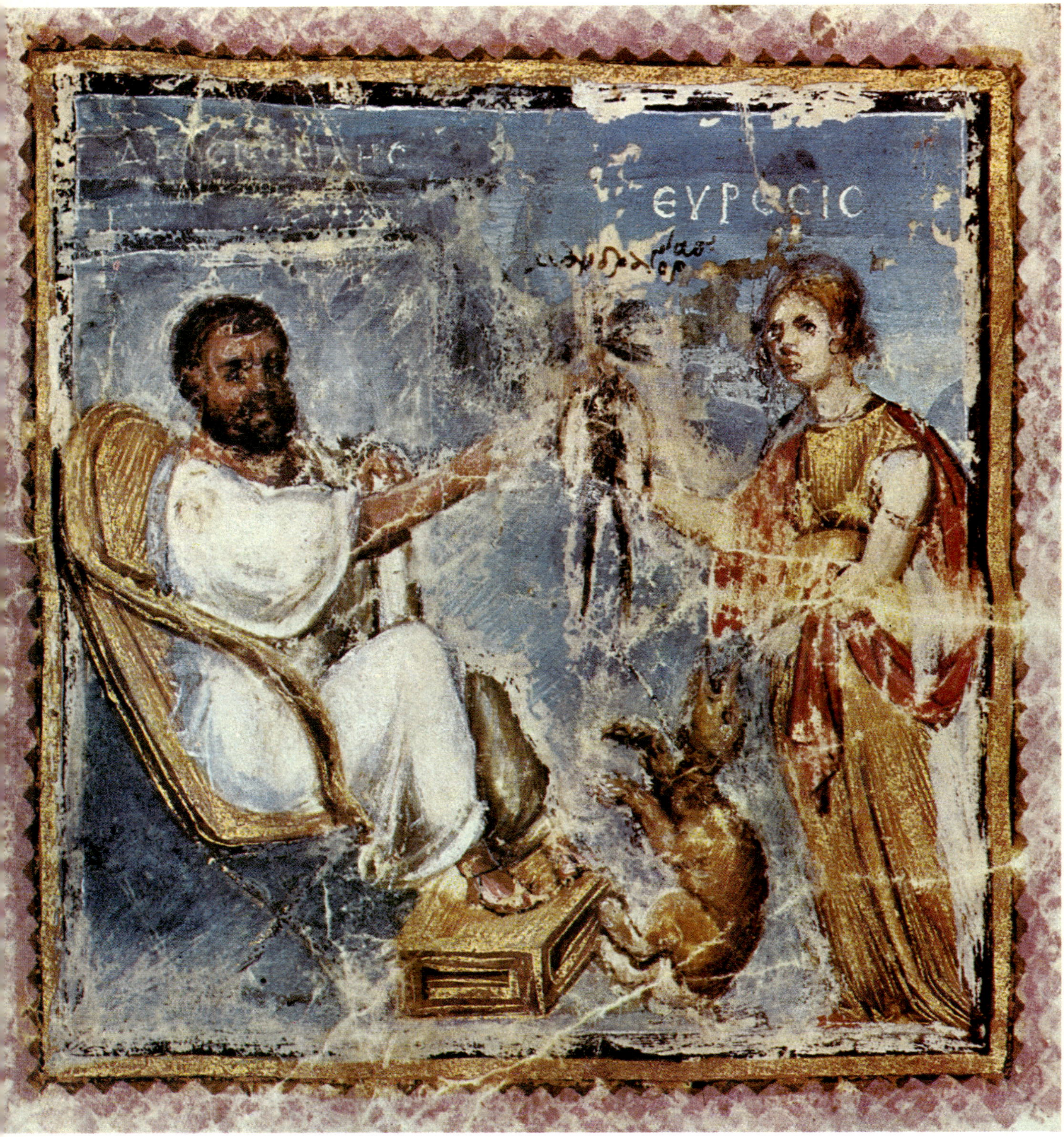

anyone who took it from the ground. Thus dogs were used to gather it, by tying them to the plants and making them run; when the dog was dead it was safe for a man to touch the plant. It is interesting that mandrake contains the drug hyoscine, although modern scientists do not recognize pharmacological properties in more than a few of the hundreds of plants used in ancient times.

Dioscorides describing the properties of mandrake. *From Iuliana Anicia, fifth-century Greek ms. National Library, Vienna.*

Medicinal plants described by Dioscorides. *Page from a seventh-century Neapolitan codex. National Library, Naples.*

profession from receiving its due measure of insults from anyone with a real or imagined grievance or merely with a harsh wit. Bad doctors continued to suffer in the way that a former eye specialist suffered at the hands of Martial:

Hoplomachus nunc es: fueras ophthalmicus ante:
Fecisti medicus quod facis hoplomachus.

Now you are a gladiator; you were formerly an ophthalmologist.
You did as a physician what you now do as a gladiator.

Martial was particularly scornful of medical quacks and charlatans, and elsewhere in his writings are to be found interesting passages which throw light on doctors and patients in the first century AD.

Eximit aut reficit dentem Cascellius aegrum,
Infestos oculis uris, Hygine, pilos,
Non secat et tollit stillantem Fannius uvam,
Tristia servorum stigmata delet Eros,
Enterocelarum fertur Podalirius Hermes.

Cascellius draws or repairs the diseased tooth.
You, Hyginus, burn the hairs that affect the eye.
Fannius does not cut, but raises the dropping uvula,
Eros removes the slaves' sad marks,
Hermes is called the Podalirius of hernias.

But Martial's most cutting epigram was that he wrote against the physician Symmacus, who on one visit was accompanied by a hundred of his pupils; Martial had to suffer the touch of a hundred cold hands and later complained:

'Before, I was quite well; since your visit, I have the fever.'

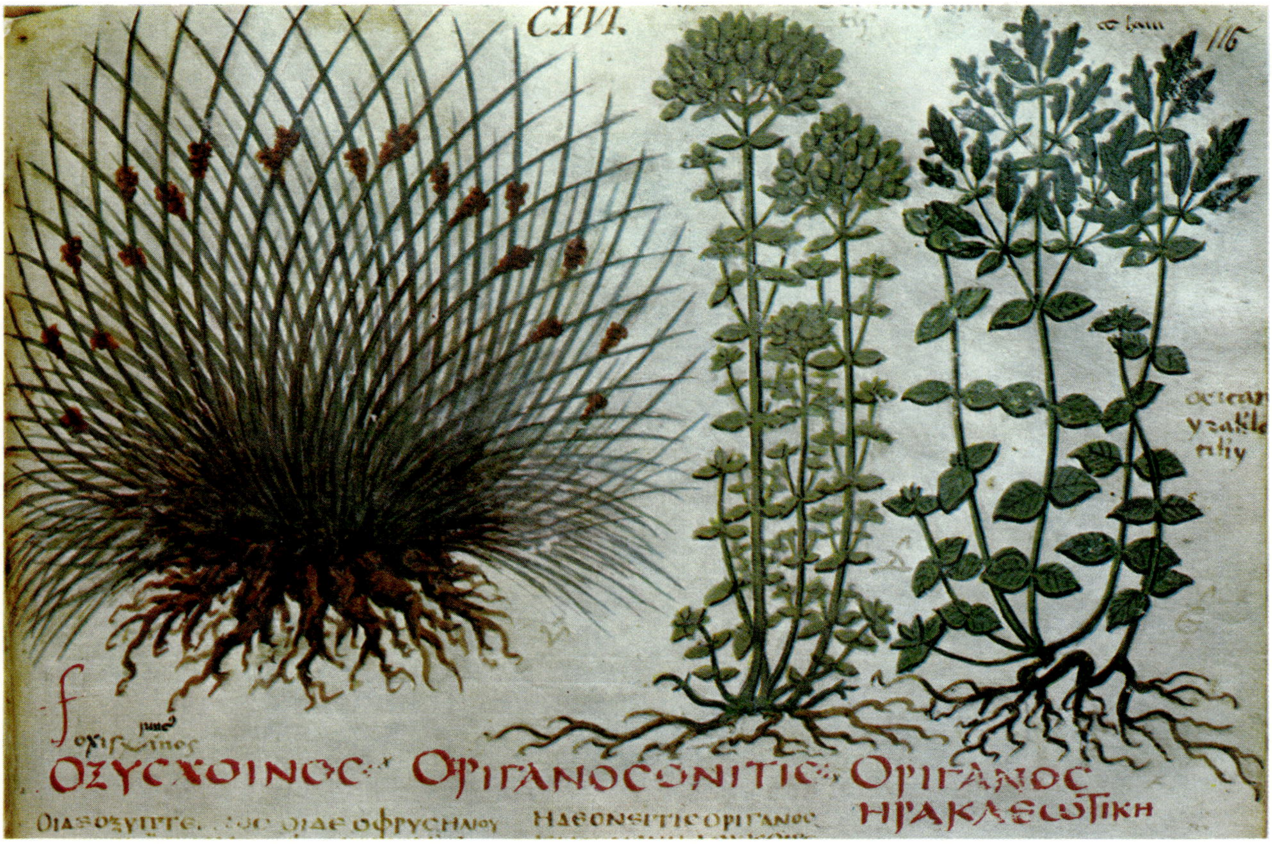

Imaginary portrait of Galen. *Sixteenth-century engraving. Bertarelli Collection, Milan.*

Frontispiece to a collection of works by Galen, Venice 1565. *Bertarelli Collection, Milan.*

Galen

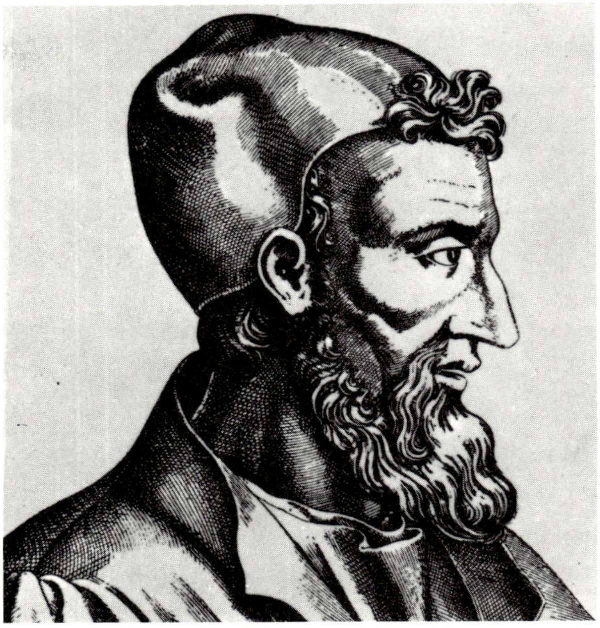

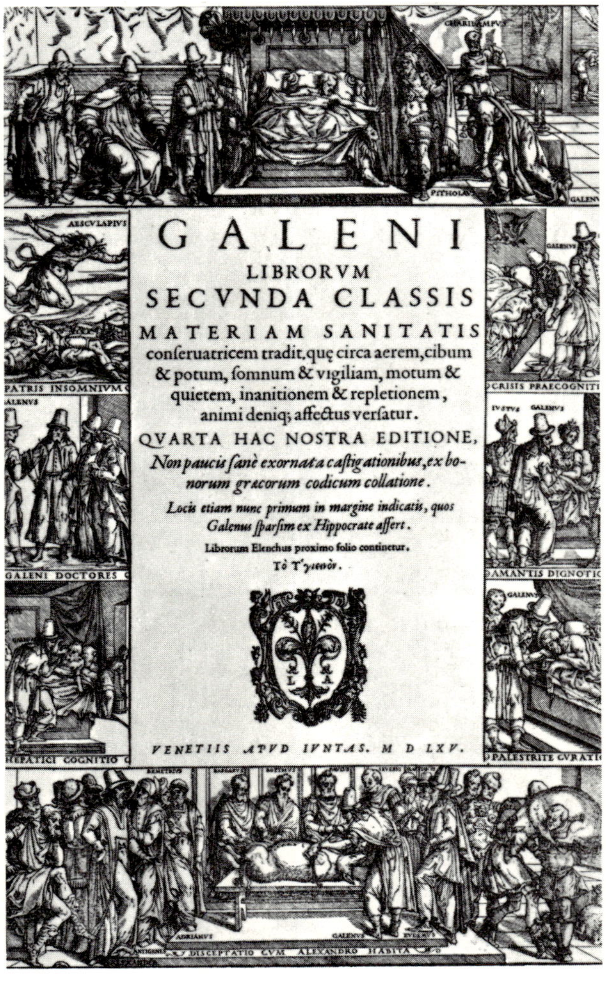

Claudius Galen is a giant in the annals of medicine. Without the bias of post-Hippocratic schools, yet loyal to the teaching of the master of Cos, Galen summarized and systematized medical knowledge of ancient times, with reasoning always based on observation and experience. The *editio princeps* of his work filled twenty-two massive volumes, equivalent to approximately one half the bulk of extant Greek and Roman medical literature. It is not easy to read, being verbose and teleological; but the work of Galen–together with the *Corpus Hippocraticum*–represents the sum of medical achievement in antiquity.

Galen was born at Pergamon about AD 130, the son of an architect who dreamed of a glorious medical career for the boy and so supervised his education carefully. He studied philosophy at Smyrna, where he was a pupil of Pelopides, and medicine at Alexandria, where he worked very hard at anatomy. When he was twenty-eight, he went back to Pergamon and was made doctor to the gladiators of the arena.

In the year 162 he went to Rome and soon earned a reputation as a practitioner and writer. He could behave with the utmost decorum with eminent patients and achieved great popularity, becoming the physician and confidant of two emperors, Marcus Aurelius and Lucius Verus, as well as gaining an enormous practice. What personality defect he suffered from is difficult to decide at the distance of two millennia, but he certainly had one, for he was always attacking his colleagues, suggesting that they were inept and that his own therapeutic and diagnostic ability was unparalleled. It seems strange that a man whose professional skill was so widely acknowledged should have felt compelled to behave like this.

Galen wrote some four hundred treatises, most of which were lost in a fire. Eighty-three were saved and are known to be genuine, because Galen was prudent enough to make a list of his works. This great and most industrious of doctors employed a whole team of scribes to write down his every dictum. His thoughts on anatomy, mostly contained in the sixteen books of the work *On anatomical preparations,* were drawn from studies of the human skeleton, from his experience as surgeon to the gladiators and especially from dissection of animals, but were marred by false deductions, since he applied to man what he learned from

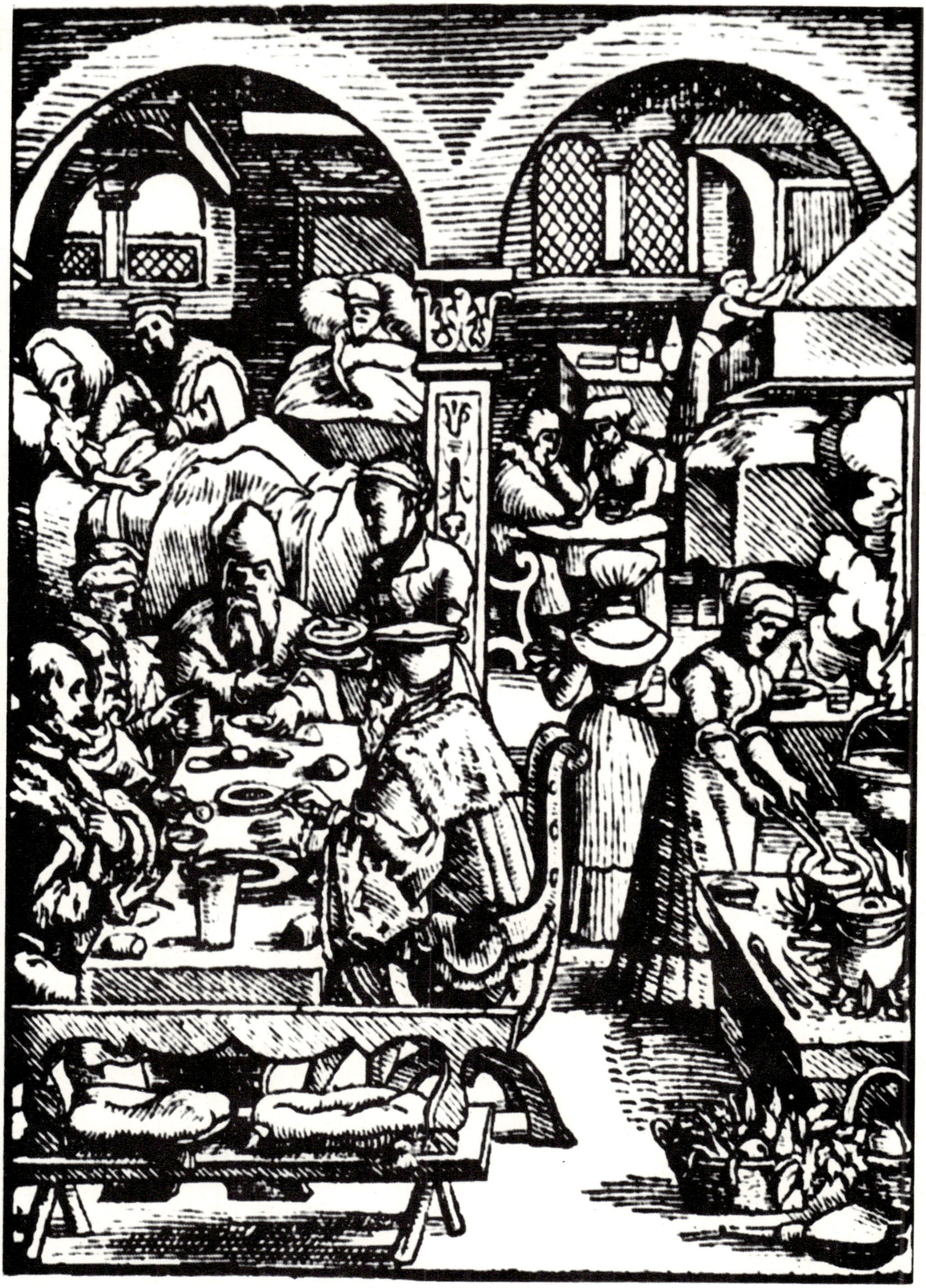

Previous page:

Illustration from De conservanda beata valetudine, Frankfurt 1553, a collection of dietary precepts. *Bertarelli Collection, Milan.*

These pages:
Medicatrina or surgery. *From the Isagogic books of Galen, printed by the Giunta Press, Venice 1576. Bertarelli Collection, Milan.*

Claudius Galen, one of the greatest physicians of antiquity, practised in Rome during the second half of the second century AD. He had a very high reputation both as a practitioner and as a writer, and he completed about 400 treatises on medicine. His work was the great medical synthesis of ancient times; the system known as Galenic embodied concepts of other writers.

the animals. Thus Galen found the rete mirabilis in the brain of a calf and assigned to this structure a vital physiological function in man–who does not possess it. Galen's descriptions of bones were admirable and his work on muscles accurate and he described in minute detail the brain, nerves and vascular system.

Galen's work on anatomy was an imposing structure and contained the seed of rapid progress, which might have been achieved if only students of the Middle Ages had thought to verify his findings. No checking was done, since dissection of human corpses was not allowed among Christians or Arabs, and so his observations stood unchallenged until the Renaissance and the revival of anatomy at the hands of Vesalius and others.

Galen's genius was evident in experiments conducted on animals for physiological purposes. The work *On the use of the parts of the human body* comprised seventeen books concerned with this topic. To study the function of the kidneys in producing urine, he tied the ureters and observed swelling of the kidneys. To study the function of nerves he cut them, and thereby showed paralysis of shoulder muscles after division of nerves in the neck and loss of voice after interruption of the recurrent laryngeal nerve. He also produced cardiac arrest by cutting the nerves to the heart and so dispelled the ancient misconception that nerves come from the heart rather than from the brain. He declared that every alteration in function resulted from an organic lesion and conversely that every organic lesion led to alteration of function. This concept remains substantially valid.

The fundamental principle of life, in Galenic physiology, was pneuma, which took three forms and had three types of action: animal spirit (pneuma psychicon) in the brain, centre of sensory perceptions and movement; vital spirit (pneuma zoticon) centring on the heart regulated the flow of blood and body temperature; natural spirit (pneuma physicon) resided in the liver, centre of nutrition and metabolism.

Pneuma entered the body through the arteria aspera, that is the trachea, passed to the lungs and thence through the arteria venalis (the pulmonary vein) to the left ventricle, where it met the blood from the liver. In the liver, blood was impregnated with pneuma physicon and received, through the vena porta, the nutritive substances which the intestine had transformed into chyle. The blood was distributed from the liver to the veins, which ran from it like arteries from the heart. Through the vena cava, blood entered the heart on the right side.

Blood was held in the right ventricle for a while to free it of impurities, which were then expelled

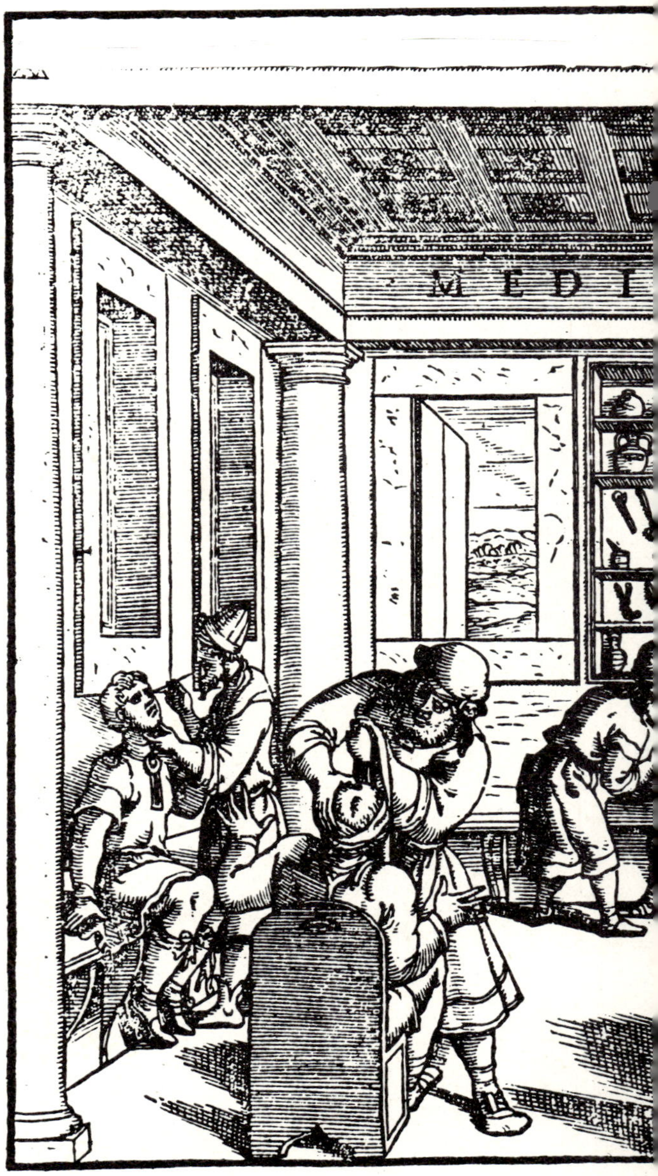

Galen studied the anatomy of the respiratory system, and of the heart, arteries and veins. But he did not discover the circulation of the blood throughout the body, and believed that blood passed from one side of the heart to the other through invisible pores in the dividing wall. Galen reached his conclusions on anatomy mainly by dissecting animals and applied what he learnt to man. He made many important discoveries but inevitably made several false assumptions. His work went unchallenged for more than a thousand years, including these errors.

One of Galen's most important discoveries was the basic principle that every change in function of the body results from some kind of injury, and that every injury leads to a change in function. He also completed original studies of the nervous system.

from the lungs with the breath. But a small amount of blood passed from the right to the left ventricle through minute, invisible pores in the interventricular septum. The intake of vital spirit was then distributed to the whole body through the arterial system, some of it reaching the brain where it split into the intricate network of the rete mirabilis already mentioned. In the brain, vital spirit was transformed into animal spirit and distributed throughout the body by means of the nerves, which Galen envisaged as empty ducts.

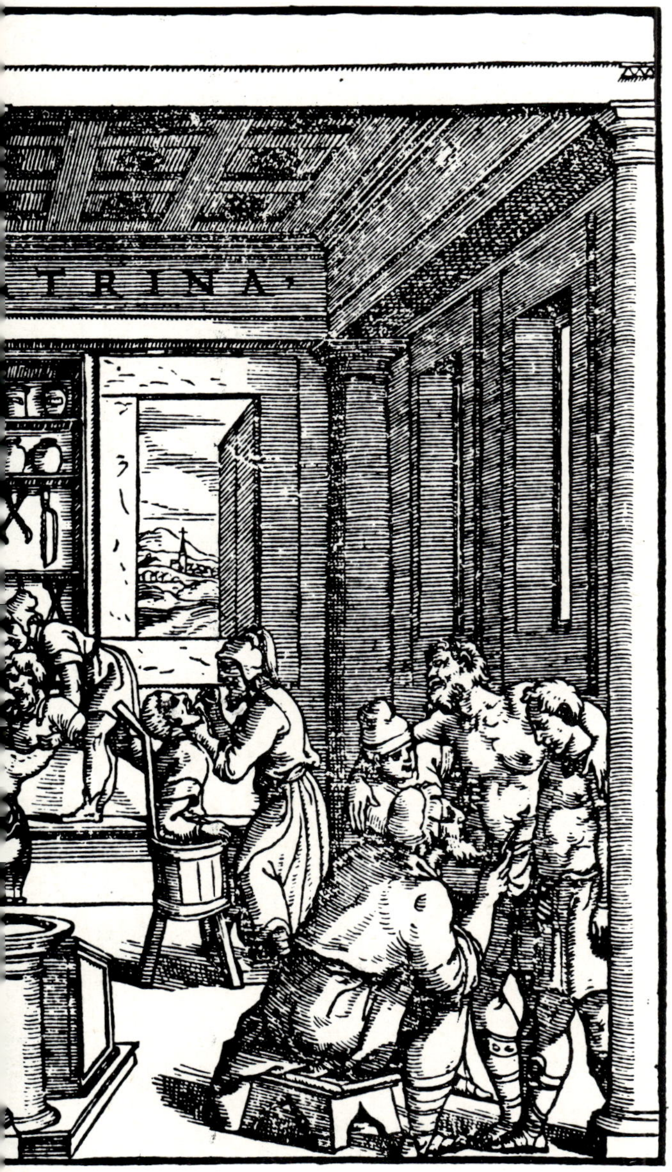

Galen was therefore convinced that the venous and arterial systems were each sealed and separate from each other. William Harvey, discoverer of the circulation of the blood, wondered how Galen, having got so close to the answer, did not himself arrive at the concept of the circulation. Perhaps this great doctor from Pergamon was not content merely to collect the results of his observations; if he had a theory in mind, he probably tried to make results of experiments fit it.

We possess in the writings of Galen and others numerous testimonies to his diagnostic acumen and therapeutic skill, as well as his considerable anatomical knowledge. One of his cures, a typical example of his methods, created a great stir in Rome:

A Persian Sophist lost sensation in the ring and little finger and half of the middle finger of one hand. He first called in some physicians of the Methodist school, who tried emollients in the first place and then astringents. When the patient discovered that these remedies had produced no improvement whatsoever he consulted Galen, whose first question was 'Have you been injured in the arm?'

The Persian replied that he had fallen on a sharp stone and had suffered a hard blow between the shoulders with the immediate onset of a violent pain which rapidly decreased. Galen diagnosed a lesion of the spinal cord and prescribed rest in bed with soothing applications to the upper part of the back. The patient recovered.

Afterwards Galen explained that he had been led to implicate the region of the seventh (lowest) vertebra of the neck as the source of the trouble because he knew that every nerve had a distinct origin from every other nerve, even though nerves bunched together to form plexuses, and that the ulnar nerve, which carried sensation from the affected fingers, came from the spine at the level of the seventh cervical vertebra.

He added that there was subsequently a heated controversy among physicians over the reason for loss of sensation without loss of power in the involved part of the hand; Galen maintained that there were separate nerves for the skin and for the

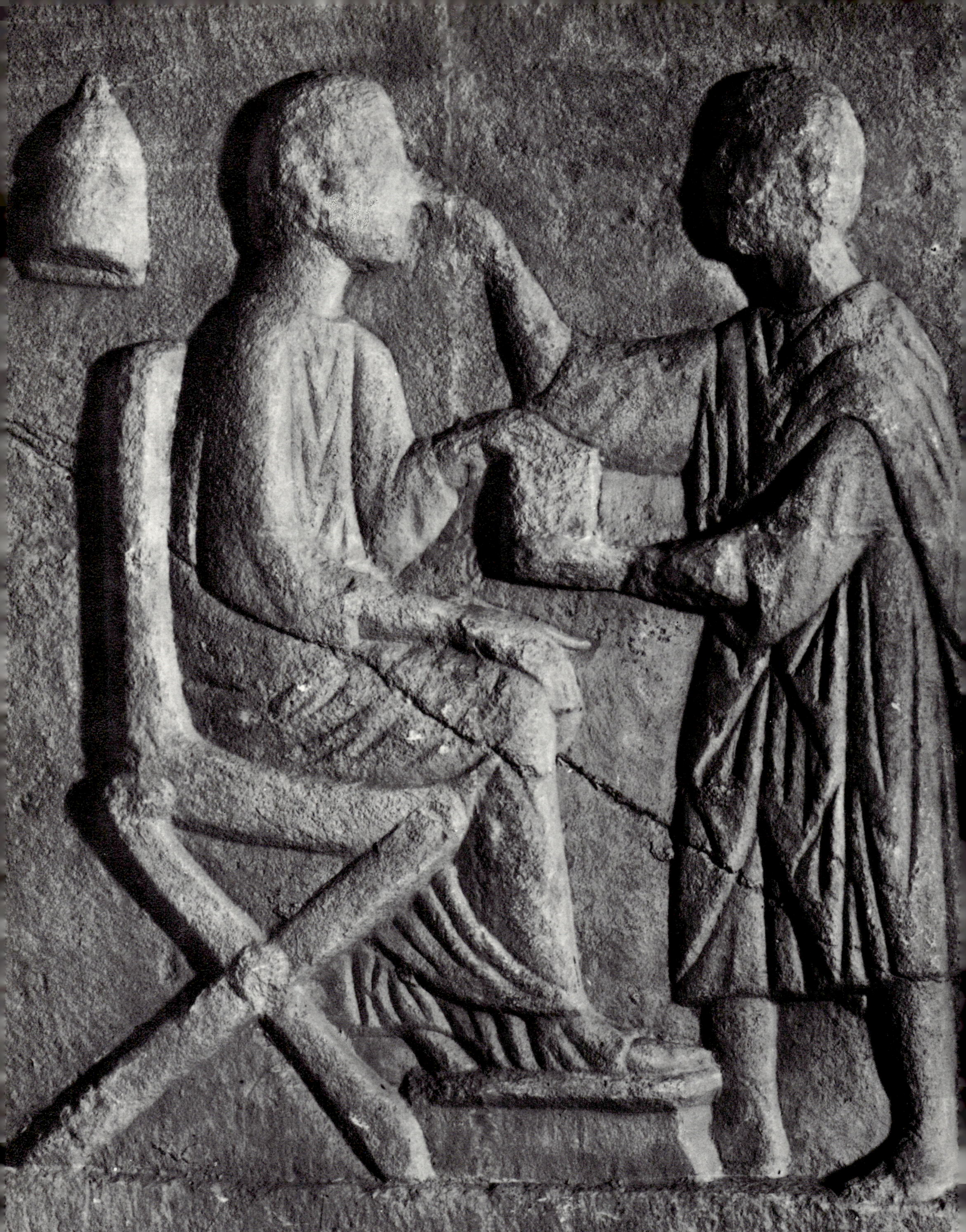

The Romans were the first to enact regulations to safeguard the medical profession. Under the Empire, the long-despised doctors became respected by citizens and rulers, while the highest public offices became open to them. Galen himself was the personal physician to two Roman emperors, and had many eminent patients.

The decline of medicine coincided with the decline of the Roman Empire and with the rise of Christianity; men seemed to wish to invoke the will of God to cure their illness rather than look upon illness as a natural phenomenon. But in the Christian world Galen became the unquestioned medical authority.

Visit to the optician. *From the sarcophagus of the Sosia family. Third-fourth century. Church of S Vittore, Ravenna.*

Galen dissecting a pig. *Detail from frontispiece to a collection of works by Galen, Venice 1565. Bertarelli Collection, Milan.*

muscles, and that damage to the former had occurred in the Persian without the latter being affected.

Galen's diagnostic supremacy lay partly in his recognition of physical signs, some of which he showed to be pathognomonic, or characteristic of specific conditions. Time and again he impresses by the acuteness of his observations, as when he notes that the escape of air from a chest wound indicates that the lung has been pierced, and when he distinguishes accurately between bleeding from the kidneys and from the bladder by the appearance of the urine.

Galen also showed great skill in sorting out malingerers from those with real disease; he wrote, a propos of this:

'People may pretend to be ill for many reasons: it is thus desirable that the physician should be able to arrive at the truth in such cases. The ignorant imagine that it is impossible to distinguish those that are simulating from those that are telling the truth.'

He then proceeded to distinguish skin lesions, swellings, haemoptysis and delirium in the malingerer from the real thing.

The treatments employed by Galen were derived from the concept of 'contraria contrariis'–the therapy of opposites–and so he applied heat if disease resulted from cold, and purgatives for conditions where the body was thought to be overburdened. In addition to diet and drugs, some of which were thought to have specific effects and indications, Galen also made great use of physiotherapy and other ancillary measures.

Why then did Galen, for all his mistakes, remain an unchallenged and unchallengeable authority for over a thousand years? How was it that after he died in 203, serious anatomical and physiological research ground to a halt, because everything there was to be said on the subject had been said by Galen? Although he was not a Christian Galen believed in one god, and declared that the body was an instrument of the soul. This made him most acceptable to the fathers of the church and to Arab and Hebrew scholars. Since God did nothing by chance, there must be a relation between cause and event. Animated by this doctrine of final causes, he sought the why and the wherefore of everything; his explanations made it look as though he had all the answers. Yet this man, whose authority and mistakes perpetuated fundamental errors for nearly fifteen hundred years, was a physician, observer and experimenter of so high an order that today it is impossible not to regard him with esteem.

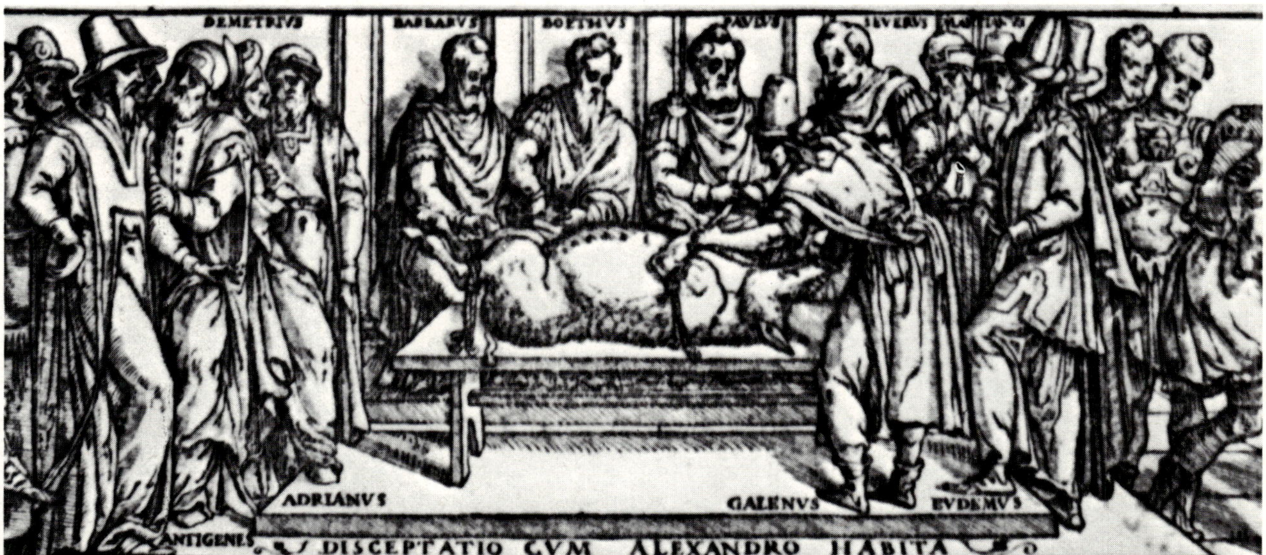

THE DARK AGES
The decline of Rome

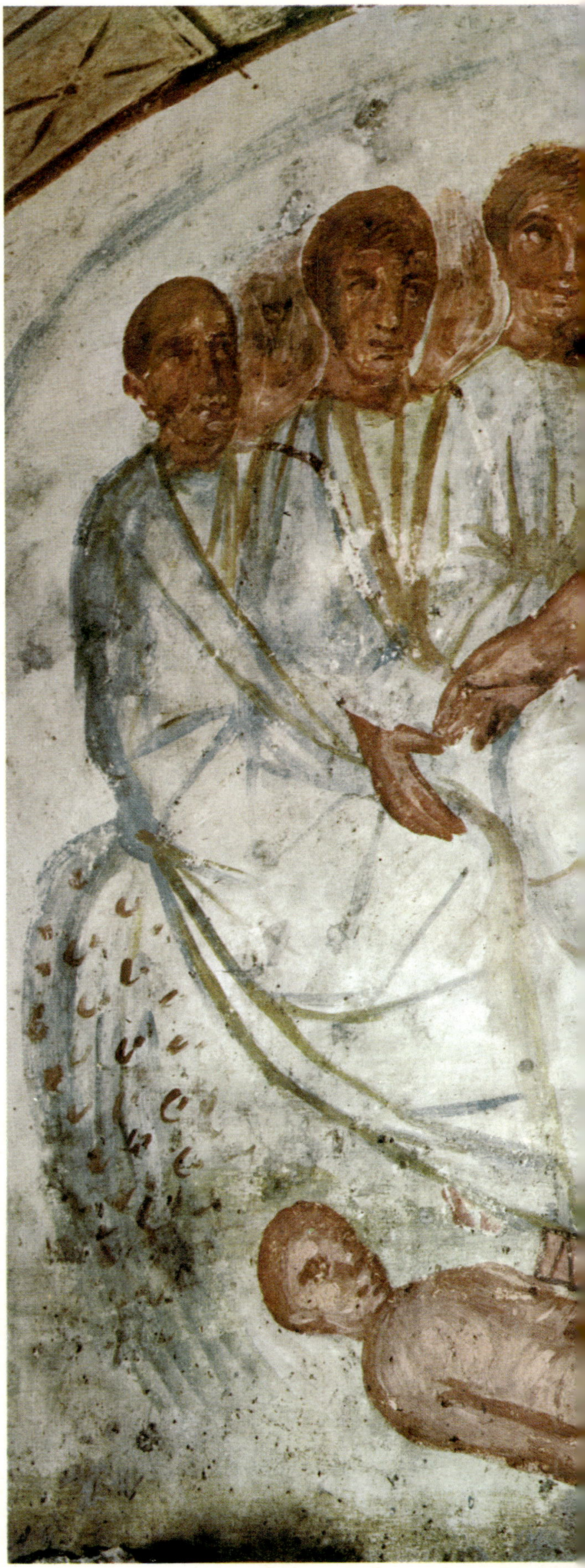

Galen wrote at a time when the Roman Empire was at its zenith; the culmination of Graeco-Roman medicine coincided with the greatest extension of the power of the Caesars. But Galen's works, which synthesized all the scientific thought of the ancient world, marked the beginning of the decadence of medical science.

A number of the reasons for the break-up of the empire – private and public corruption, oppression of minorities and poverty of much of the population, and incursions by the barbarians on the borders of Roman territory – obviously relate to what happened to medicine, for under such conditions rational, objective thought would become impossible. Another cause, the epidemics and plagues that ravaged the empire, implicated doctors directly; and, as happened in Europe in the Middle Ages, the powerlessness of medicine to do anything but observe the pestilence carried everyone away from science and reason.

Some of the epidemics are well documented. One raged through the province of Campania after the eruption of Vesuvius in AD 79, which destroyed Herculaneum and Pompeii, and according to the chroniclers people died daily in their tens of thousands. Another epidemic occurred in North Africa in AD 125, when Carthage and Numidia (now Tunisia and Algeria) were hit by a plague of locusts which destroyed the crops and by a disease that was said to have claimed one million victims. The plague of Antoninus, which made Galen flee from Rome in AD 166, lasted fifteen years and swept across the empire from its eastern frontiers to the west. Two other epidemics, which began in the years AD 251 and 312 and which both lasted a number of years, are thought to have been smallpox.

Today it is known that bubonic plague is the result of infection by a bacterium, *Pasteurella pestis,* and thus effective treatment and prophylaxis are possible. In ancient times there was of course no clear idea of the nature or cause of the disease; 'plague' was a generic term for any epidemic which took a heavy toll of human lives. Descriptions of the

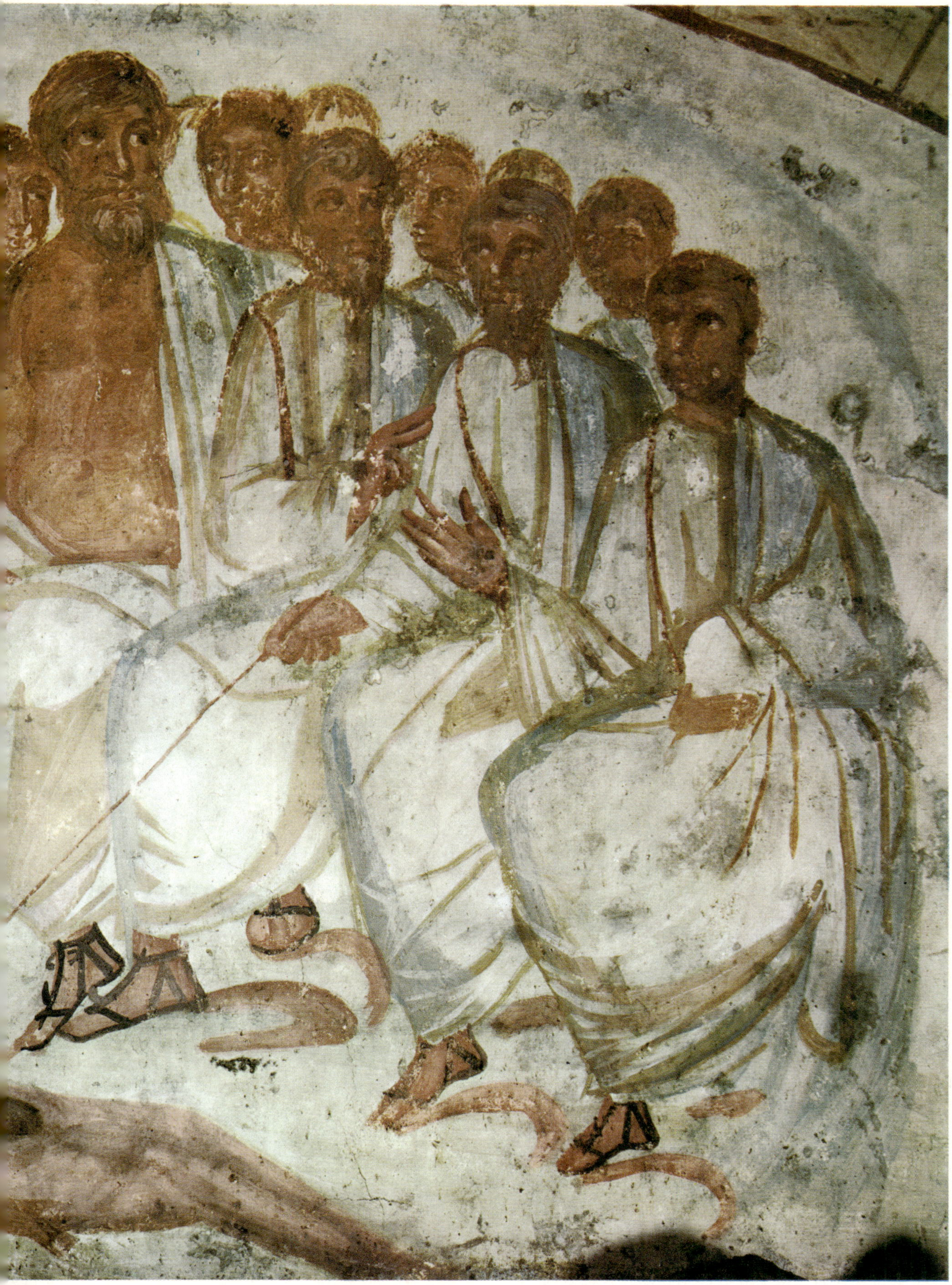

Previous pages:
Anatomy lesson. *From the New Catacomb on the Via Latina, Rome.*

Facing page:
Remedies against exhalations from the ground. *From Theriaques et Alexifarmaca by Nicander, eleventh century. Bibliotheque Nationale, Paris.*

One of the immediate causes of the fall of the great Roman Empire was the occurrence of a series of epidemics and plagues. The doctors of the day were quite powerless in the face of these disasters, which led to a popular reaction against the scientific and rational approach to disease which was still slowly evolving, with a resurgence of superstitious practices.

symptoms of plague can be found in such reliable sources as Thucydides and Galen. Thucydides recorded the terrible outbreak at Athens in 430 BC and Galen the epidemic that brought death and desolation to Rome in AD 164.

In many of the outbreaks of what was described as plague by several ancient authors, less authoritative perhaps but no less credible than Thucydides and Galen, the only common characteristic was a high death-rate. The physical features of a number of different diseases seem to be recorded; thus there are descriptions of blisters and pustules, erythema and pallor, haemorrhages and asphyxia—smallpox, bubonic plague, scarlet fever, cholera, exanthematous typhus and diphtheria were clearly all covered under the generic description of plague, although some of the features noted by ancient historians have still not been specifically identified with known diseases. Presumably some diseases have disappeared or at least changed. With reference to bubonic plague, it seems clear that the ancients recognized the disease and knew that it was spread by rodents; what they did not know was that fleas carried the plague bacillus and infected men and rodents. Bubonic plague produces swelling of the lymph nodes in the groin, arm-pits and neck, with discharge of pus and blood, in contrast to the obscure epidemic that rocked Athens in 430 BC, when Thucydides recorded gangrene of hands, feet, genital organs and eye-balls among the signs.

But, for medicine, these epidemics caused as much long-term harm as immediate devastation for men, threatened by scourges so terrible as to make the therapies of the day seem worthless, turned back again to supernatural powers for aid. Thus epidemics had the effect of fostering superstitious and magic practices, thereby enhancing religious faith.

Historical circumstances had prepared the way for a rise of the mystical element of Christianity, the religion which offered brotherhood and charity to the humble and the afflicted, and gave consummate meaning to earthly life. Bodily ills could only be made well with divine aid, as was demonstrated in the gospel accounts of miraculous healing by Jesus, achieved by invoking the help of God the Father. Instead of medicaments, use was made of anointing with holy oil, prayer and the laying on of hands. Two of the first Christian doctors to practise healing by faith were twin brothers, Cosmas and Damian, who were martyred under the Emperor Diocletian and in whose honour Justinian built a church.

Some authorities have asserted that Christianity was the cause of the decline of medicine, but this is not entirely true. It may reasonably be maintained that Christianity did nothing to halt the process of decline, since primary consideration had to be given by converts to problems of ethics and religion, rather than to those of natural philosophy. Christianity, following the teaching of the Lord, was bound to regard medicine as a work of charity. Religion reaped untold advantage from having instilled the idea of helping the sick as a bounden duty, from which neither the individual nor the community was exempt.

In practical terms, the Christians did much to relieve suffering. Hospices, called xenodochia, were built to shelter pilgrims and in time became proper hospitals. The first great Christian hospital was built by St Basil at Caesarea in the year 370. It had as many wards as there were diseases to treat, and resembled a little township on its own; it included a leper colony. The rule of love, implying also the care and comfort of the sick, thus embraced even lepers, who previously had always been kept in isolation.

The first hospital in the western world was built in Rome about AD 400 by the Roman lady Fabiola, a disciple of St Jerome, who returned from the Chalcis desert in 381. She was a penitent who sought absolution by spending her wealth on charitable works.

In the year 326, the Emperor Constantine moved the capital of the empire from Rome to Byzantium, and proclaimed Christianity as the religion of the empire. He had been a pagan all his life and was baptized only shortly before he died. Most of his subjects were still pagan; it has been estimated that perhaps fifteen or twenty per cent of the population of the empire were Christian. But the emperor decided that this minority was more powerful than the majority because of its moral and intellectual qualities, strength of character and resolute belief that pagans could not equal.

The leading Byzantine doctor was Oribasius, the son of a nobleman from Pergamon, who lived from 325 to 403. He studied medicine at Alexandria and

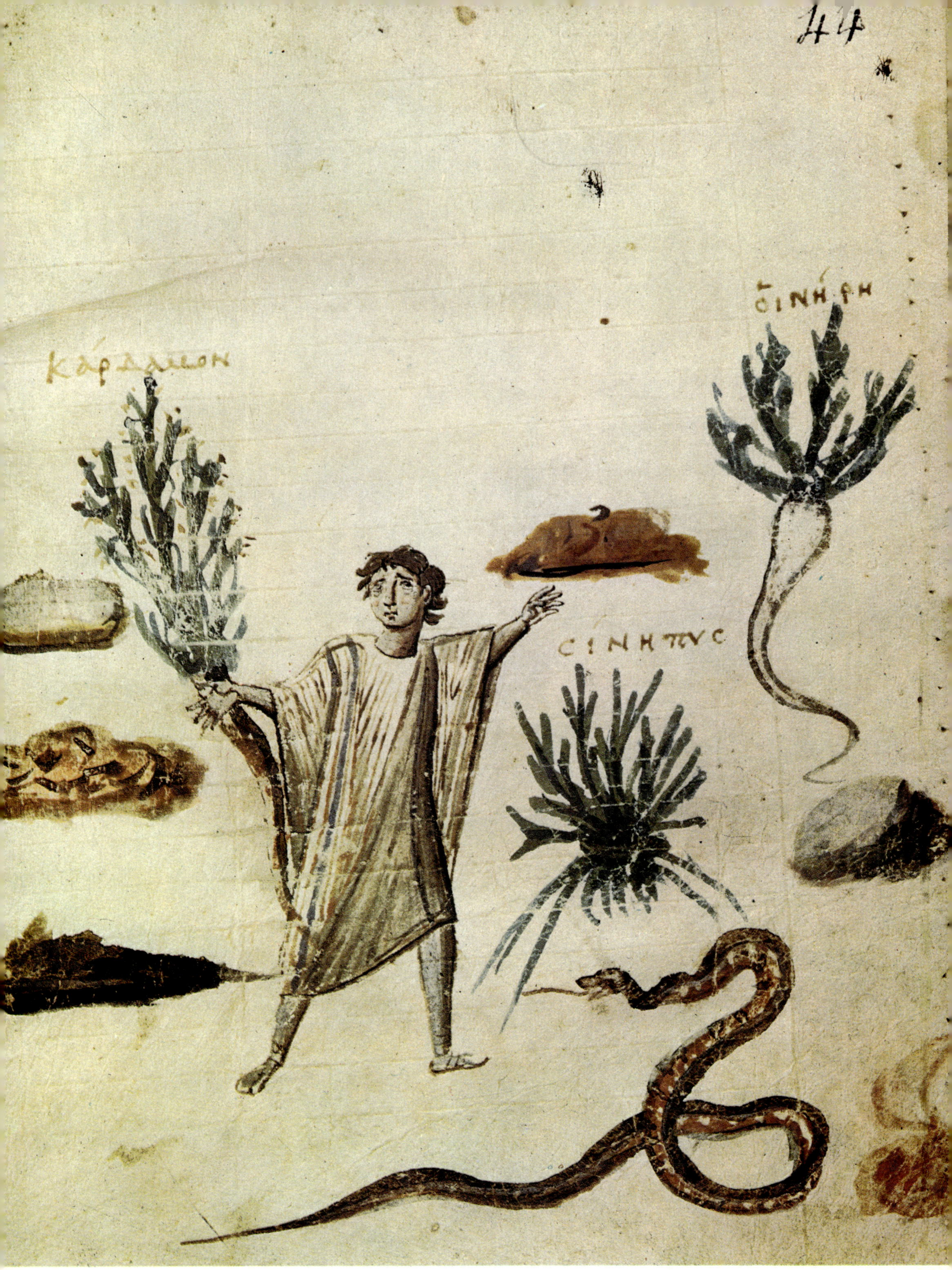
44
κάρδαμον
CINHPH
CINHπυC

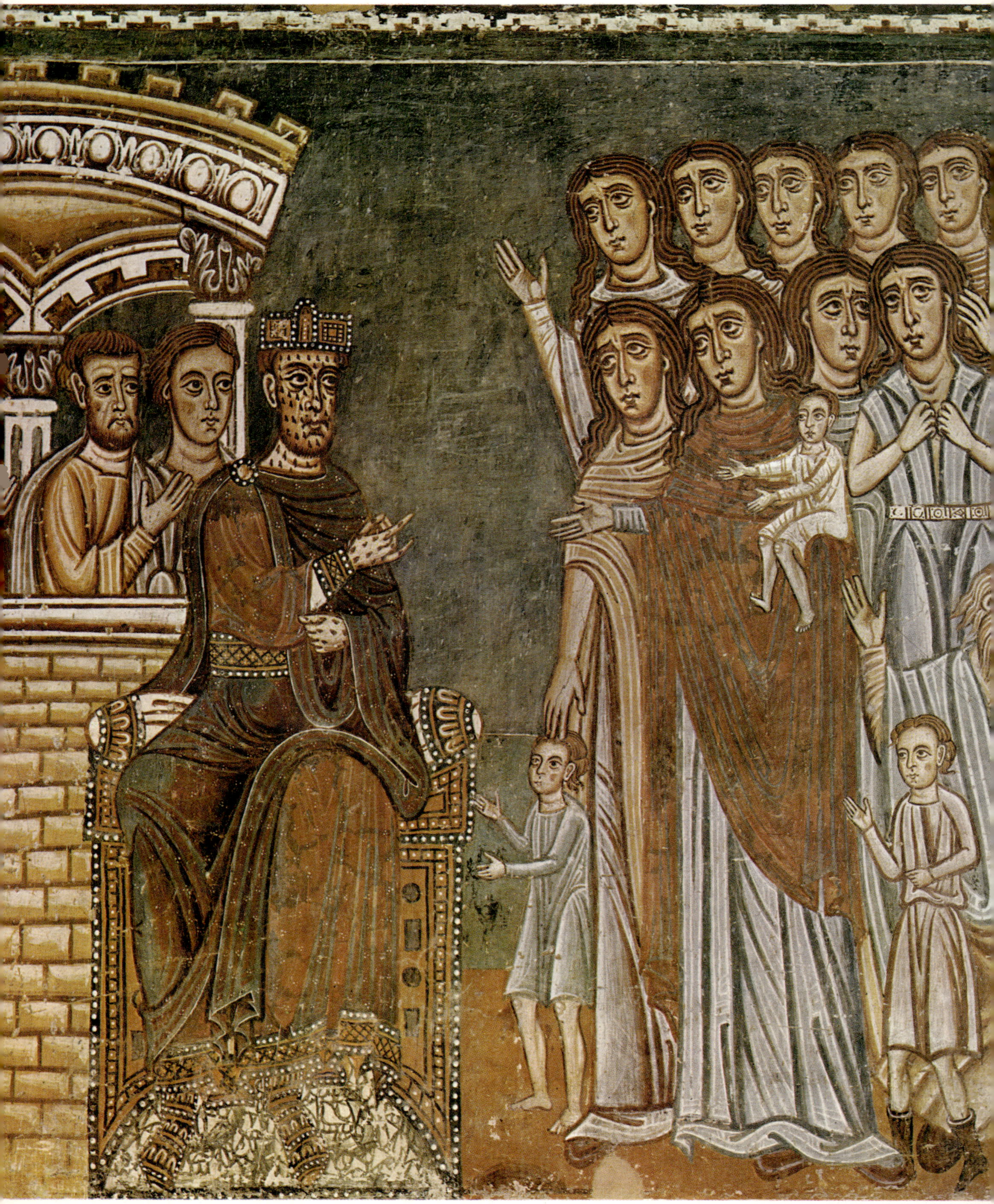

This period also saw the rise of Christianity and religious faith was enhanced by the widespread despair produced by the terrible epidemics.

There was much scholarship and some advances in medicine and surgery, but treatment often rested heavily on faith. Pliny related that Pyrrhus cured disorders of the spleen by touching the sick with the big toe of his right foot; Tacitus wrote that Vespasian used to cure the blind by touching their eyes; Hadrian also cured dropsy by touch. Ancient tradition merged with Christian practice when Christ laid hands on the leper.

Constantine the leper comforting women. *From a thirteenth-century fresco. Quattro Santi Coronati, Rome.*

became the physician and friend of the emperor Julian, who was known historically as Julian the Apostate because he did not share the religious views of his uncle Constantine. Oribasius added little or nothing to Galenic medicine, but holds a place in medical history for his anthology entitled *Synagogae medicae*. But for this work, a number of ancient and eminent medical authors might be unknown to us.

After the terrible plagues and earthquakes that devastated the eastern empire at the time of Justinian (482–565), two other notable Byzantine doctors became prominent: Alexander of Tralles (525–605) and Paul of Aegina (625–690). Alexander was the author of *Libri duodecim de re medica* (The twelve books of medicine), which were subsequently translated from the Greek into Latin and Arabic. His knowledge of anatomy and physiology was modest, but his experience, which was the fruit of nearly sixty years' practice, enabled him to deal authoritatively with such conditions as diseases of the nervous system, diphtheria, goitre and intestinal parasites.

The medical encyclopaedia of Paul of Aegina, which was also translated into Arabic, was of particular importance as it gave information about surgical progress since the time of Celsus, although it showed only a fair knowledge of anatomy. Until the seventeenth century, Paul's description of the radical operation for inguinal hernia was regarded as a classic: 'An incision is made three fingers long on the tumour of the inguinal region. Skin and fat are laid aside to reveal the peritoneum, and the intestines are pushed down with the end of a sound. Bulging bits of the peritoneum on either side of the sound are sutured together and the sound is then extracted; the peritoneum is not cut nor is the testicle touched in any way. The procedure is simply to treat the wound thereafter'.

The works of Oribasius, Alexander of Tralles and Paul of Aegina are evidence of the stagnation of scientific thought and the decline of original observation and experiment in the centuries that followed Galen, although medical practice and surgery in particular continued to show signs of appreciable progress. But the figure of the lay doctor was on the decline, for the church viewed the care of the sick as a moral obligation incumbent on its members, and as a calling rather than as a paid profession.

Healing the blind. *Sculptured ivory of the sixth century. Christian Museum, Vatican, Rome.*

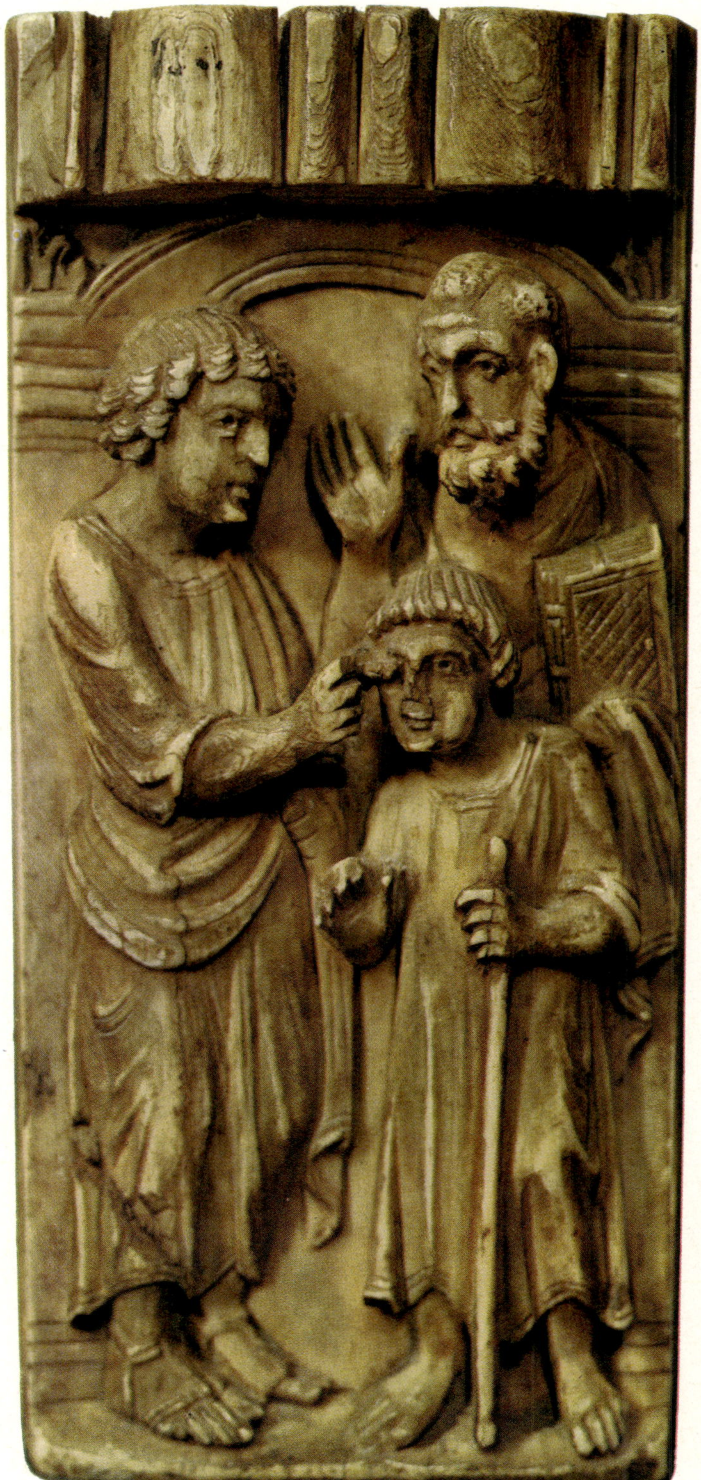

The rise of Arab learning

The Christian spirit of charity went so deep that it even pervaded a number of movements that had been declared heretical by the church. The church that derived from the members of the Nestorian sect provides an example. Nestorius was a patriarch of Constantinople who was deposed in the year 431 for having asserted that the Virgin Mary could not be held to have been the mother of God. He was condemned by the council of Ephesus, and as a result the Nestorians had to leave and go to Syria and Mesopotamia, where they founded a medical school at Edessa which became as famous as the one at Alexandria. But in 489 Bishop Cyril contrived to get the Emperor Zeno to close the school and expel the heretics from the empire. The Nestorians went to Persia, and their physicians and pupils then founded the school of Gondishapur, which flourished for several centuries.

When Khalid, the great general of Abu Bakr (successor of Mahomet and first caliph), destroyed the army of the eastern emperor Heraclius, the Nestorians, the Hellenized Persians and the Hebrew scholars of Gondishapur feared the imminent end of their school. This happened in 636; only four years had gone by since the death of Mahomet, the messenger of Allah, who had enlarged the tribal concept and welded the nomads and marauders of the barren wastes of Arabia into one nation.

But the Moslems were not destroyers, as was widely feared, for they sought to take over the civilizations of conquered nations and to preserve the ancient learning. They were immediately influenced by the works of Euclid, Plato, Aristotle, Hippocrates and other writers; and a Byzantine emperor was amazed to learn that the most acceptable gift for a Moslem leader was a copy of the *Materia medica* of Dioscorides. And Gondishapur, far from being destroyed, became the cradle of the Arabian school of medicine.

At Gondishapur (as at a number of other sites in the Middle East) the Nestorians had built a great hospital, the staff of which became justly famous. The doctors of the family of Bukht-Yishu (servants of Jesus) were in particular very highly regarded. One of them, Jurjis, who was the head of the hospital, was summoned in 785 to the new capital Baghdad to attend the Caliph al-Mansur, who was suffering from some type of serious abdominal complaint. The caliph kept Jurjis at court for four years. When the doctor fell gravely ill at the end of

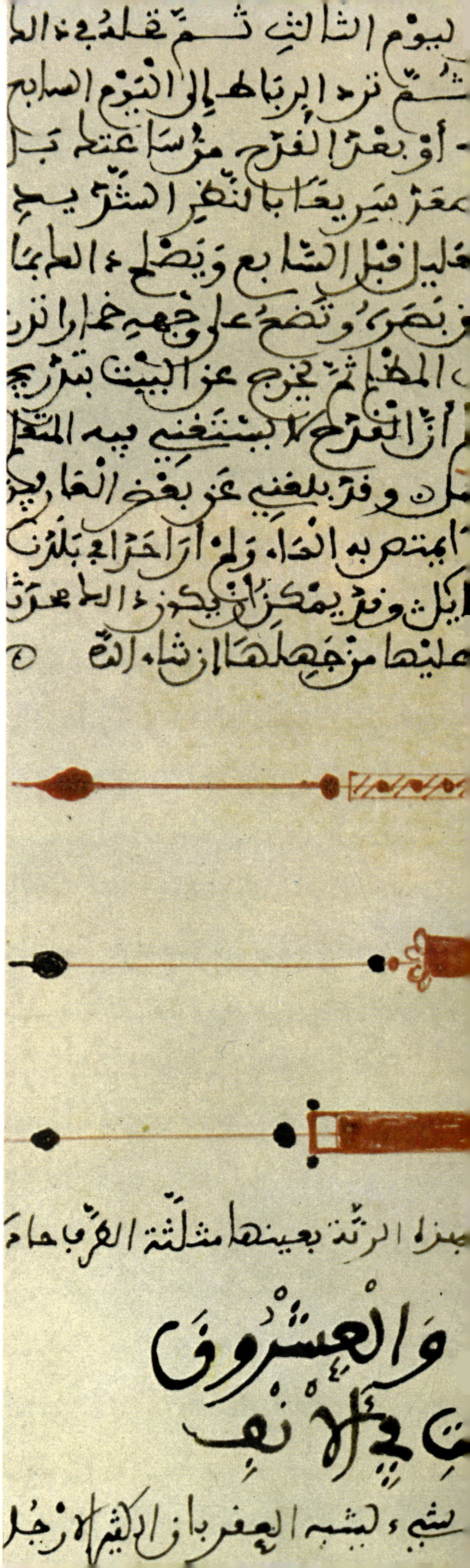

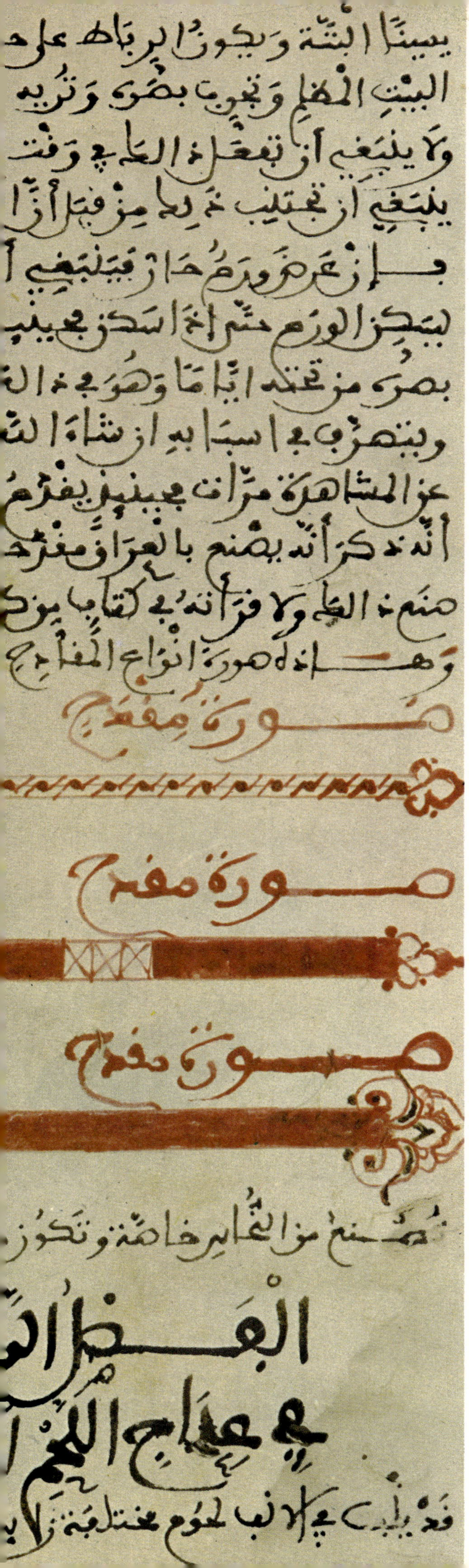

Surgical instruments. *From the treatise on external diseases by Abul-Khasim Khalaf ibn Abbas al-Zahrawi, copied in Morocco in the sixteenth century. Bibliotheque Nationale, Paris.*

this time and asked to be allowed to go home to die, the caliph tried to convert him to the faith of the Koran, promising him bliss in the Moslem paradise as vicar of Allah upon earth. Jurjis replied that he would rather join his own ancestors, whether they were in paradise or in hell, at which al-Mansur gave way and allowed him to return to Gondishapur. But the son of Jurjis became a court doctor, and his grandson became the personal physician to the celebrated Caliph Harun al-Rashid.

The first two hundred and fifty years after the Hegira (Mahomet's flight to Medina on 16 July 622) saw the development of a young and vigorous Arab culture. In this period, medicine was led by men of the Bukht-Yishu family, and by translators who rendered into Arabic the works of the great medical men of the west, from Hippocrates to Galen and Paul of Aegina. The new golden age of Hellenic culture came with the Abbasids, who succeeded the dynasty of the Omayyads, which had been preoccupied with military conquest. In a series of lightning campaigns within the space of a few years, not only the Middle East but Egypt, North Africa and Spain had been conquered by the Arabs. They crossed into France and might have advanced into northern Europe had it not been for Charles Martel and his Frankish knights, who stopped them at Poitiers in 732, thereby destroying the myth of their invincible might.

The first two Abbasid caliphs, Harun al-Rashid (763–809), who was a brilliant legislator and the founder of the first hospital in Baghdad, and his son al-Ma'mun (786–833) gave a great impetus to culture. Al-Ma'mun acquired manuscripts of Greek works from every possible source. The great Baghdad library was built up in this way, and a translators' centre was founded under the guidance of his doctor Yuhanna ibn Masawayh (latinized as Mesue or Johannes Damascenus). A student of Gabriel Bukht-Yishu and a Nestorian, Mesue the Older was the author of good translations and also of original writings; those on dietetics and gynaecology remained important works until the early Renaissance.

The most outstanding pupil of Mesue the Older was Hunain ibn Ishaq, a Nestorian who was born at Hira in Mesopotamia in 809, and is known in western literature as Johannitius. With his Baghdadi

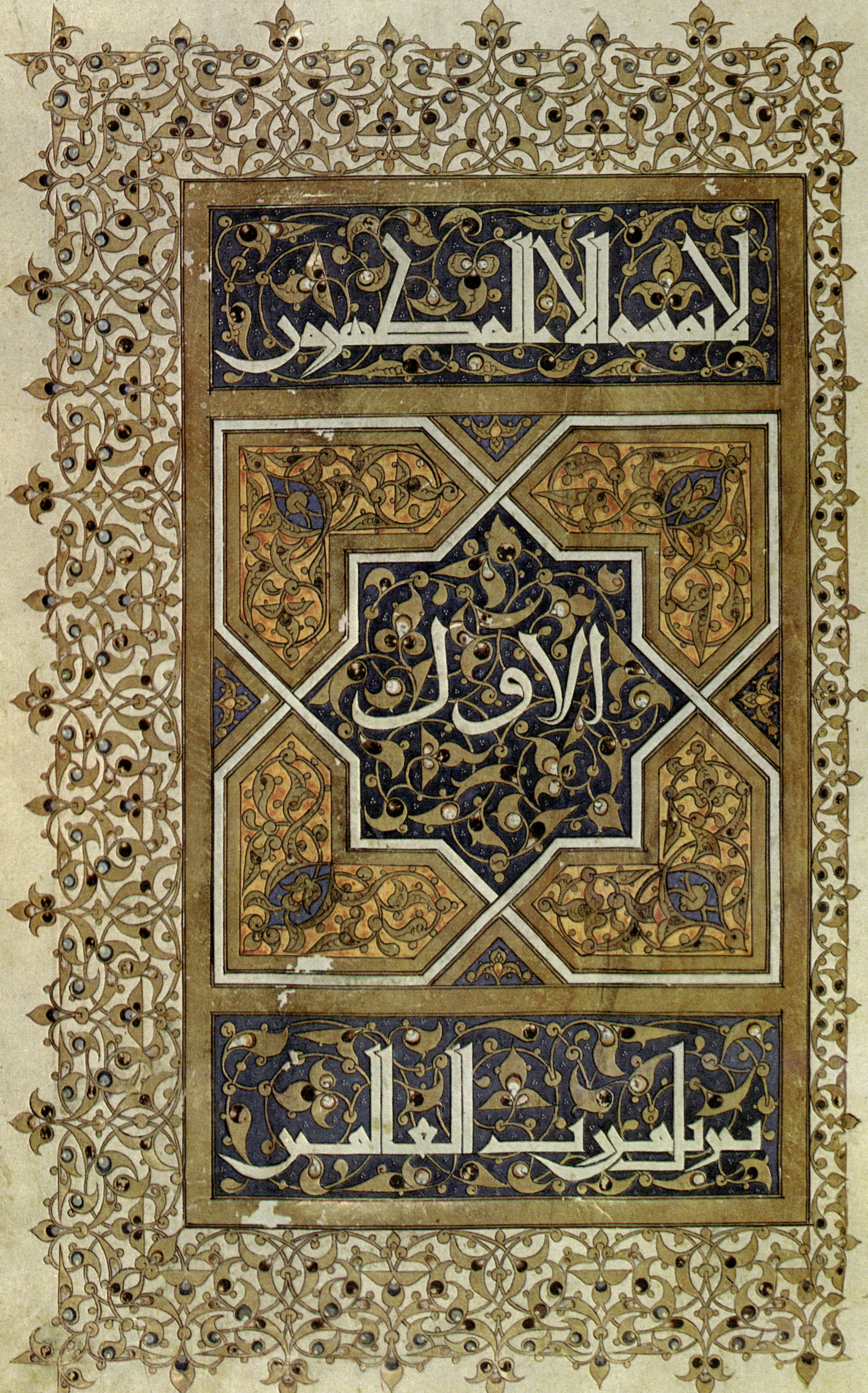
لا يمسه الا المطهرون
الاول
تنزيل من رب العلمين

Page of the Koran. *Seventeenth-century edition. British Museum, London.*

Celestial globe. *Fourteenth-century Arabic art. Capodimonte Museum, Naples.*

Miniature from a mediaeval Arabic herbal.

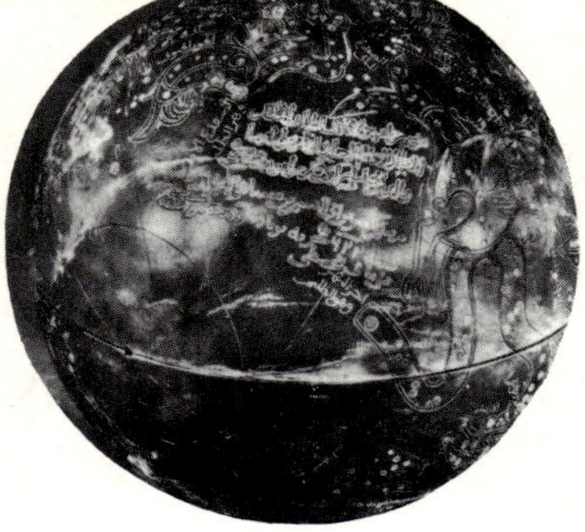

colleagues, he not only translated into Arabic the entire Hippocratic *Corpus,* all the works of Galen, those of Oribasius and of Paul of Aegina and the *Materia medica* of Dioscorides, but also created an Arabic scientific language, coining new words or creating Arabic forms for Greek and Syriac terms. Hunain wrote many original works including the *Quaestiones medicinae* (a textbook set out as questions and answers) and the *Ten dissertations on the eye,* which is the oldest systematic treatise of ophthalmology.

Many Arabic scientific terms have Greek or Syriac roots. On the other hand, many chemical terms of modern western civilization, such as alcohol, alkali, alkaloid, aldehyde, alchemy and alembic come from Arabic. The man who laid the basis of chemical science and devised the alembic or retort (in Arabic, al-anbiq) was Jabir ibn Hayan, who lived in the ninth century. Jabir may have been the first to make use of the procedures of filtration, sublimation and distillation; he was certainly the first to examine the blood and faeces.

Rhazes and Avicenna

The best known Arab medical authors were Rhazes and Avicenna, who were both associated with the eastern caliphate, and Avenzoar and Averroes who belonged to the school at Cordova, the capital of the western caliphate. Abu Bakr Muhammad ibn Zakaria, known as al-Rhazes, was a Persian from near Teheran who lived from 865 to 965. He studied medicine in Baghdad, where later he became established as the greatest Arab clinician of his time. Although he commanded high fees, he impoverished himself in order to help the poor. He was blind when he died, having refused an eye operation, saying that he felt nothing but repugnance for the sights of this world (and also knowing the surgeon's ignorance of the anatomy of the eye). His blindness is said to have come from blows on the head received on the orders of al-Mansur the Persian prince, who had become angry at Rhazes' failure to transform a base metal into pure gold; he was to be beaten on the head with his own book until either one or the other had been broken.

Rhazes was also interested in mathematics, astronomy, religion and philosophy; but over half his 237 works treat of medicine. The most widely known were *al-Hawi,* known in the west as the *Liber Continens,* an encyclopaedia of medical practice and treatment, and the *Liber medicinalis ad Almansorem,* a compilation from various sources, but mainly from Hippocrates, Galen, Oribasius and Paul of Aegina, which contains such aphorisms as: 'Ask many doctors, make many mistakes'; 'when Galen and Aristotle agree about something, then it is easy for doctors to make a decision, but when they differ it is very difficult to arrive at agreement'; 'truth in medicine is an end that cannot be reached and all that is written in books is worth much less than the experience of a wise doctor'.

The treatise on smallpox and chicken-pox, the *Liber de pestilentia,* is his most important work, because it is entirely original and based on direct experience and observation, from which he drew very perceptive conclusions. Exact description was given of the clinical picture of both conditions, as well as information on differential diagnosis.

'The eruption of smallpox', wrote Rhazes, 'is preceded by continued fever, pains in the back, itching in the nose and delirium in sleep. Then acute prickling is felt and this goes all over the body, the cheeks go red and the eyes are inflamed. The patient has a sense of heaviness and general discomfort, he sneezes, yawns, feels pain in the throat and chest, and breathes and coughs with difficulty. His mouth is dry and he has a headache, feels sick,

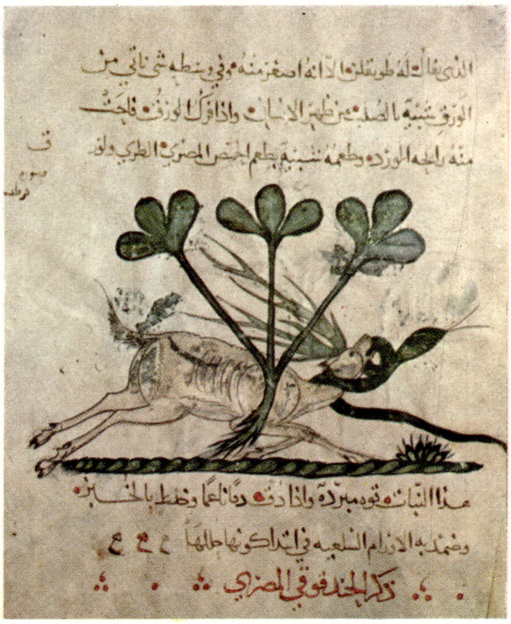

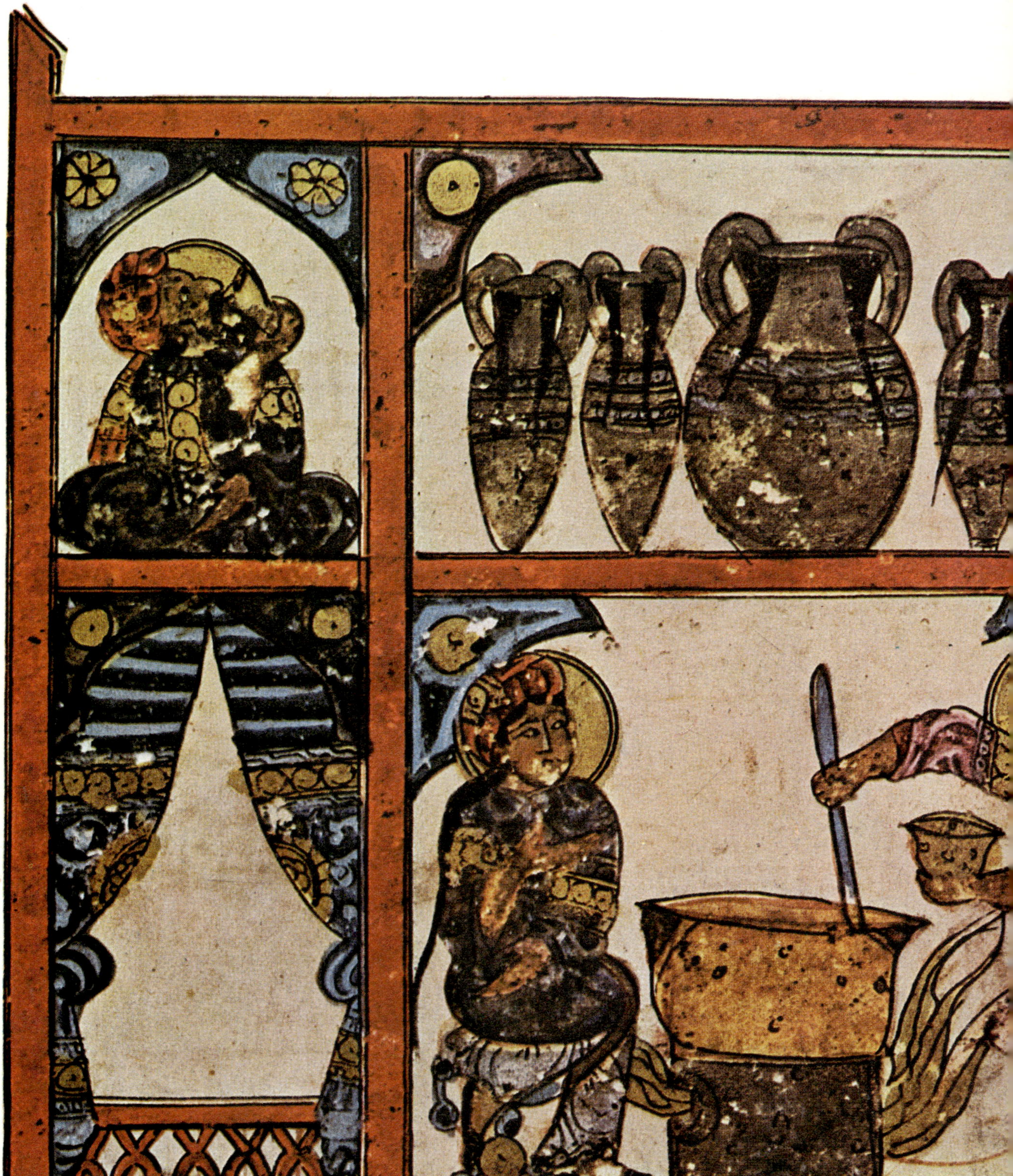

The pharmacy. *From De materia medica by Dioscorides. School of Baghdad. Metropolitan Museum, New York.*

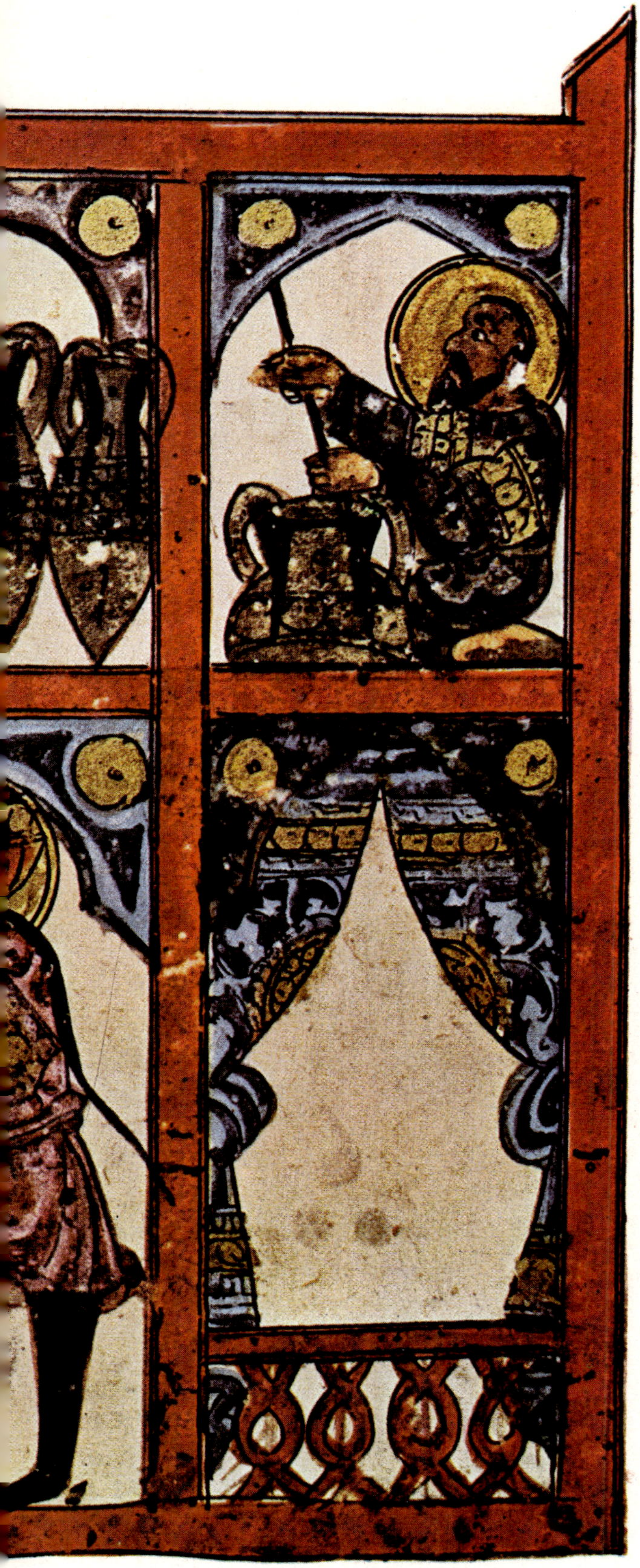

restless and troubled. Note that feeling restless, sick and troubled is more frequent in chicken-pox, while pains in the back are features of the smallpox. Other signs are fever and marked reddening of the gums. When the pustules appear, care must be taken first of the eyes, then the nose and ears: very small white pustules coming up in contact with each other, hard and without fluid, are dangerous, and if the patient remains ill even after the eruption it is a fatal sign. When fever increases after the appearance of greenish or black pustules, and there is palpitation of the heart, it is a very bad sign indeed.'

Rhazes also had something to say about skin care, indicating how pustules could be prevented from leaving bad scars. Smallpox was known in antiquity, but Rhazes was the first to advocate a definite regime of treatment for this infectious disease.

Abu Ali al-Husain ibn Abdallah ibn Sina, known to us as Avicenna, was the giant of this era of Arab learning, a polymath who captured the imagination of his own and later ages. Born in 980 at Afshena near Bukhara in Persia, the son of a tax-collector, Avicenna was a precocious boy; at the age of ten he could recite the entire Koran, and he went on to learn logic and grammar, philosophy, geometry and astronomy. At sixteen, he began to study medicine, and by the age of eighteen he was already an experienced practitioner. He was called upon to treat Prince Nuh ibn Mansur and as a reward asked only to be allowed to consult the prince's great library of rare texts. He read Aristotle's *Metaphysics* no less than forty times, but finally had to admit that, try as he might, he could not understand it at all.

Avicenna lived a turbulent existence and went through many vicissitudes, including imprisonment. Nevertheless he managed to settle and write many works on widely different subjects. He composed poetry; he wrote with authority on mathematics, physics, mineralogy and chemistry. He was a theologian of repute. When at last the meaning of Aristotle's *Metaphysics* began to dawn on him, he found his real vocation: the remaining years of his life were spent in studying philosophy.

His masterpiece is called *al-Quanun* (the *Canon*) and served as a textbook in the medical schools of the western world for a considerable period. It

The first truly important Arab author of original medical work was Rhazes, who assembled the corpus of Greek, Syriac and Arabian medical learning, to which he added his own clinical experience.

Avicenna's contribution was greater as a philosopher than as a doctor, although he was renowned in mediaeval Europe for his Canon *of medicine. This great work, in five volumes, attempted to relate the medical writings of Hippocrates and Galen and those in biology by Aristotle.*

Collection of writings of Galen translated into Arabic by Hunain ibn Ishaq (Mesue). The page shown has an autograph note by Avicenna. *Eleventh-century ms. Bibliotheque Nationale, Paris.*

Codex of Avicenna. *Fifteenth-century Hebrew manuscript. University Library, Bologna.*

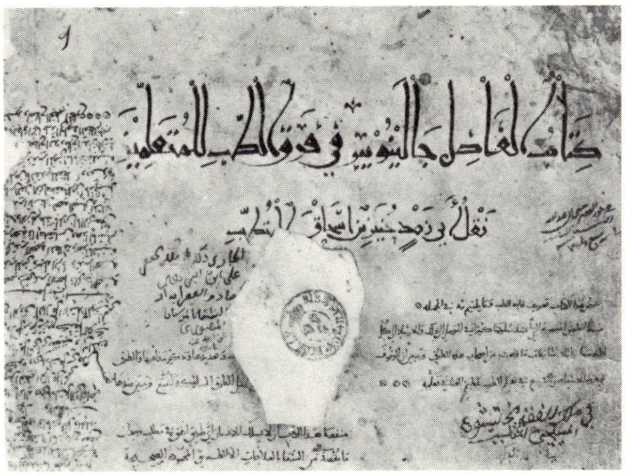

represented an attempt on the grand scale to coordinate the medical doctrines of Hippocrates and Galen and the biological ones of Aristotle. In the first of the five books of the *Canon,* Avicenna expounded the main doctrines of medicine, diseases and their symptoms, rules of health and hygiene, and also treatment. In the second book, largely based on Dioscorides, a series of medicaments are listed that were largely unknown to the Greeks. The third book dealt with pathology and contained recognizable accounts of pleurisy, jaundice, duodenal ulcer, pyloric stenosis and venereal diseases. The fourth book described the various contagious diseases, and included a treatise on surgery and a brief section on cosmetics, while the fifth book referred to the preparation of drugs and was the universally accepted text of materia medica up to the Renaissance.

The *Canon* was translated into Latin for the first time in the twelfth century by Gerard of Cremona. Together with the works of Galen, it dominated medical thinking in the Middle Ages; but in 1527 a copy was burned in public by Paracelsus, along with Avicenna's other works and those of Galen. The main drawback of the *Canon* was inadequate basic anatomical and physiological knowledge; at times it seemed as if Avicenna was indulging in a private joke, as when he enquired why the breasts did not grow on the abdomen, which would have been a more logical arrangement to his mind, or when he analysed the nature of love and concluded that it was a mental disorder.

The lasting success of the *Canon* is most probably related to ideology, for Avicenna's idea was to reconcile the biological and medical doctrines of Aristotle and Galen, just as in the thirteenth century Thomas Aquinas reconciled them with those of the Catholic church. The scholastic philosophy that was then elaborated by St Thomas to answer the attacks made on faith by reason recognized Avicenna and Averroes as masters who had transmitted the inheritance of Aristotle. This inheritance penetrated Spain and Sicily under the wing of Arab culture and thence to the rest of Europe, where Aristotle had been forgotten ever since the barbarians had severed the links with the eastern empire.

When Avicenna died at the age of 57, the school of Cordova was flourishing. In the tenth century, under the patronage of the great Caliph Abd al-Rahman III (912–961) of the Omayyad dynasty, the Spanish town became the leading cultural centre in Europe. The place was full of doctors, and the welfare of the million or so inhabitants was assured by the fact that there were 52 hospitals.

Among this host of Cordovan doctors appeared the greatest surgeon of Islam, Abu'l-Quasim, Albucasis in the Latinized form. Little is known about his life apart from the fact that he was born in 936 at El Zahra near Cordova. He left an encyclopaedic work entitled *al-Tasrif,* or the Method, translated into Latin by Gerard of Cremona, the most valuable part of which related to surgery. In fact, it contained observations which can be taken as revealing the hand of a highly skilled surgeon, and presented a mass of information on surgical practice at the time, with more than two hundred illustrations of the surgical instruments used by the Arabs.

Albucasis posed the question why Arabian surgery was so far behind and concluded that this was due to insufficient knowledge of anatomy and of Galen, whom he obviously regarded highly. On surgical practice, Albucasis told surgeons, 'God is watching you and knows if you are operating because surgery is really necessary or merely for love of money.' The indications for hernia operations and lithotomy make interesting reading for the modern surgeon. For bladder trouble he did away with the old bronze catheter and used a silver one instead. He recommended the use of false teeth

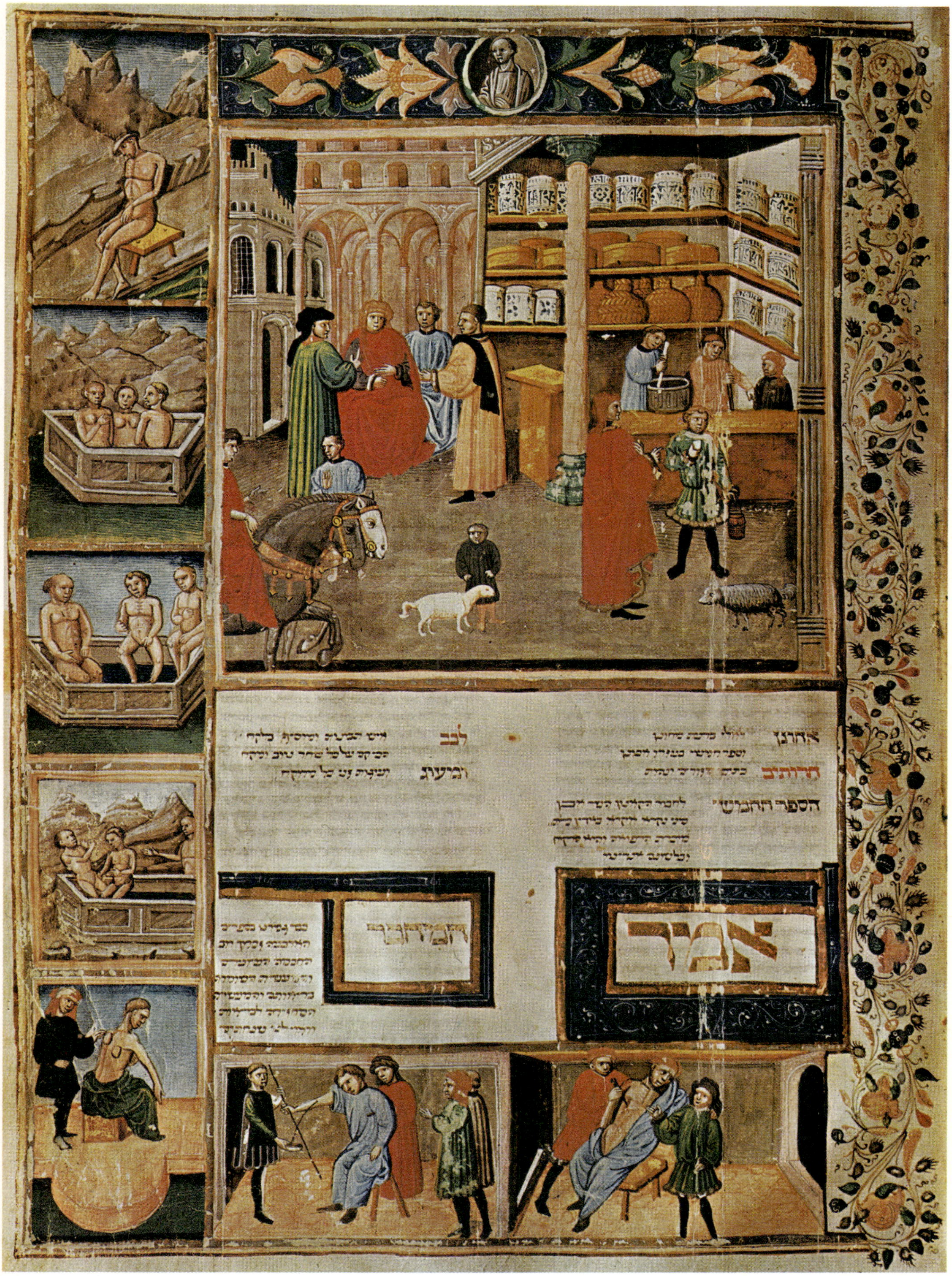

Oriental pharmacists still consult al-Tadhkira *(The Memorial), a medical lexicon by the last of the great doctors of the Arab school, Dawud al-Antaki. Another great Arab doctor was Abu'l-Quasim or Albucasis. His great work on surgery* al-Tasrif *(The Method) is evidence of his outstanding ability as a surgeon, and its illustrations give us an idea of mediaeval Arabic surgical instruments. Ibn Zuhr or Avenzoar, who lived in Seville and Cordova in the twelfth century, was a believer in practical medicine. Ibn Rushid or Averroes, who lived at the same time, was more a philosopher. He wrote the* Colliget *(Collection), a large work that was more concerned with the theory than the practice of medicine. Although a heretic to both Moslems and Christians, he was nevertheless influential. Arab learning declined after the*

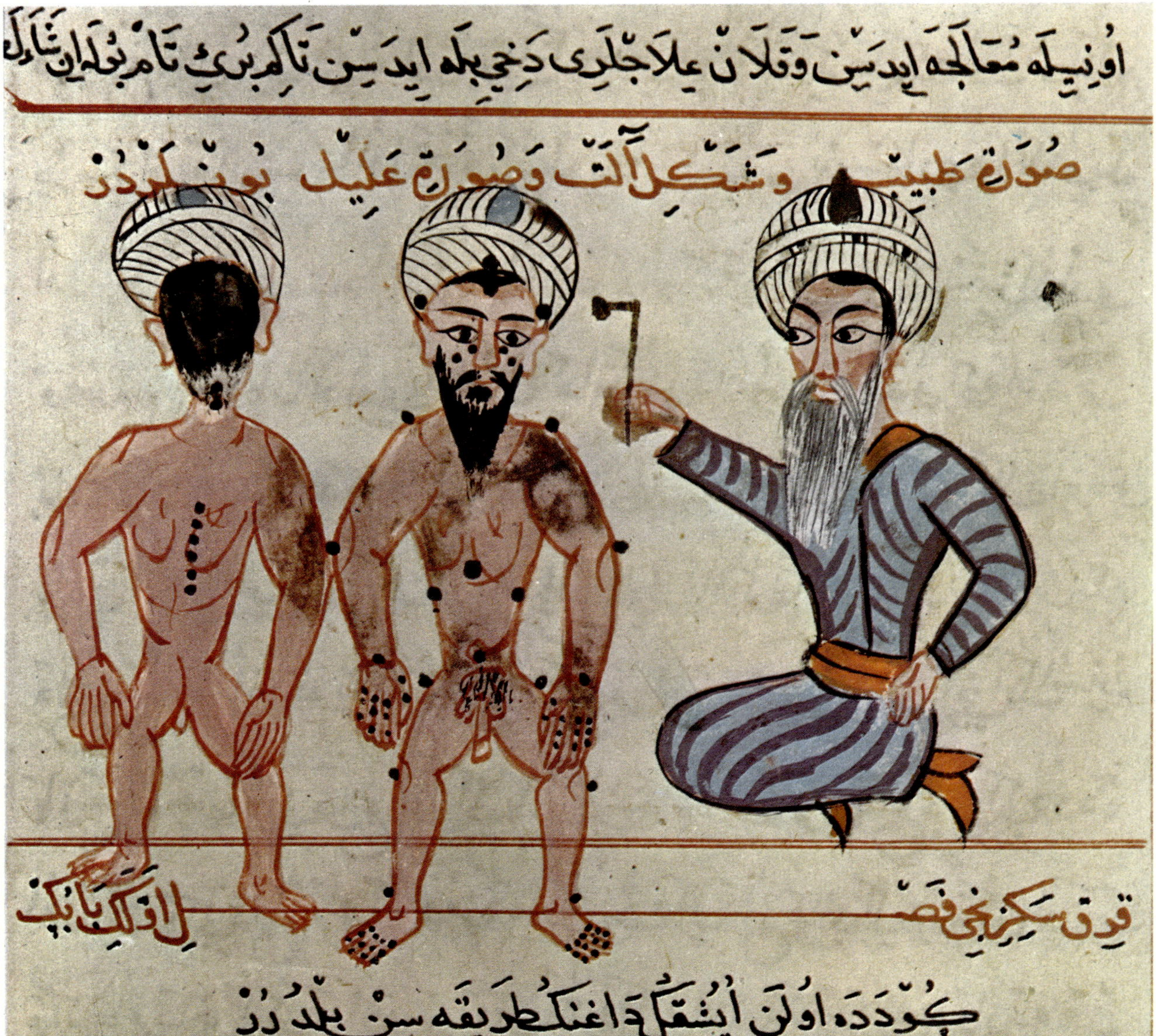

twelfth century, but it achieved considerable progress in chemistry and optics, as well as mathematics and mechanics, and the Arabs left important works on pharmacology and ophthalmology.

Finally, just as Arabian medicine collected and passed on the knowledge of the Greeks, so it itself was to be preserved in European medical thought, notably at the school of Salerno.

made from ox-bone, while for abdominal injuries he advised holding together the edges of the wound and applying large ants.

Avenzoar and Averroes

Under the Cordovan caliphate there lived at least one non-conformist who was courageous enough not to accept the doctrines of the great men of the past without first evaluating them: this was Avenzoar, in Arabic Ibn Zuhr. He was born in Seville about the beginning of the twelfth century, became a good practitioner and scholar, and died in 1162. As a doctor, he had no time for the metaphysical approach and placed great emphasis on practical experience. He therefore took, by and large, a negative view of the *Canon* of Avicenna, while not even Galen was spared from his critical approach.

Ibn Rushid, or Averroes, was better known as a philosopher than doctor. He was born in Cordova in 1126, and studied jurisprudence, philosophy and medicine; he became a magistrate in Seville and Cordova, and then governor of Andalucia. He died in Marrakesh in 1198, his heterodox teaching having been banned. He was the author of a commentary on Aristotle that was warmly praised by Dante. Averroes was accused of impiety as a result of his having denied the immortality of the soul. Following the teaching of Aristotle, he held that after death the soul re-entered universal nature. So to Moslems he was a heretic, while it goes without saying that his concept did not coincide with Christian doctrine of the immortality of the soul either. But that did not prevent Averroes from exerting a strong influence on the philosophy of the scholastics. His best known medical text is the *Colliget,* or Collection, an encyclopaedic work in the Galenic tradition, which however contains more theoretical discussions than practical observations.

Averroes' most celebrated pupil was Musa ibn Maimun, better known as Maimonides, who was not an Arab but a Jew. He in turn followed Aristotle in trying to reconcile faith and reason. He refuted part of the rabbinical tradition, thereby arousing the hostility of orthodox fellow-believers. Maimonides, like his master, became better known as a philosopher and religious scholar than as a doctor. Of special interest among his medical writings was the book of advice written for the depressive eldest son of the sultan Saladin, which

Cauterization of leprous lesions. *From Chirurgia imperiale (Imperial surgery), translated into Turkish from a treatise composed in Persia* c. *1300. Bibliotheque Nationale, Paris.*

Treatment of a fracture. *From Chirurgia imperiale.*

Blood-letting. *From a Persian ms. of the eighteenth century. Putti Collection, Rizzoli Institute, Bologna.*

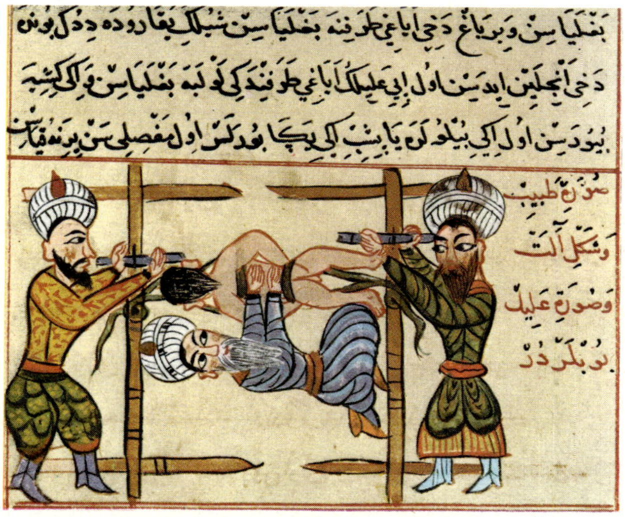

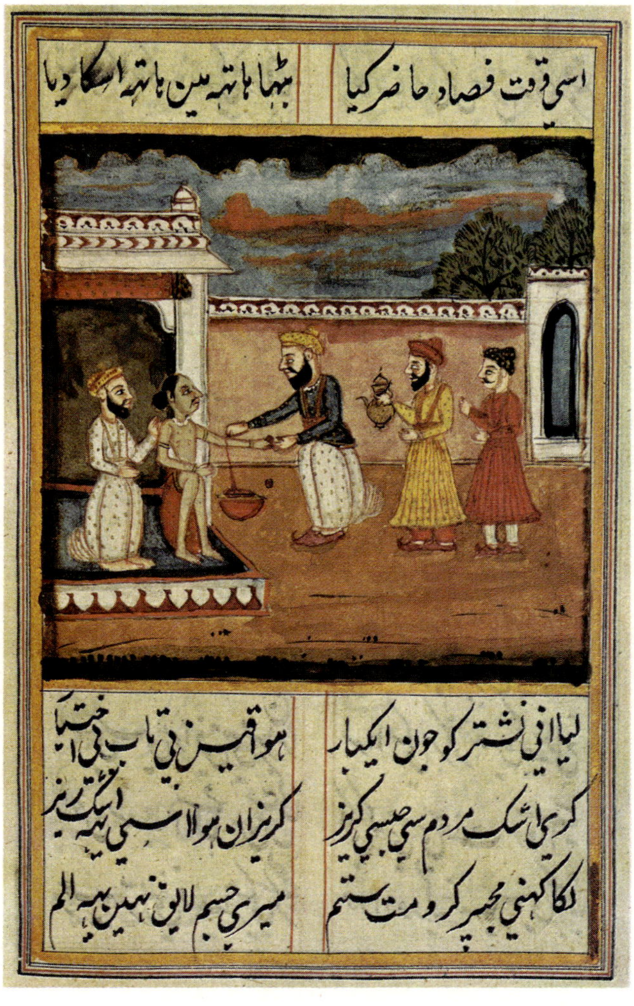

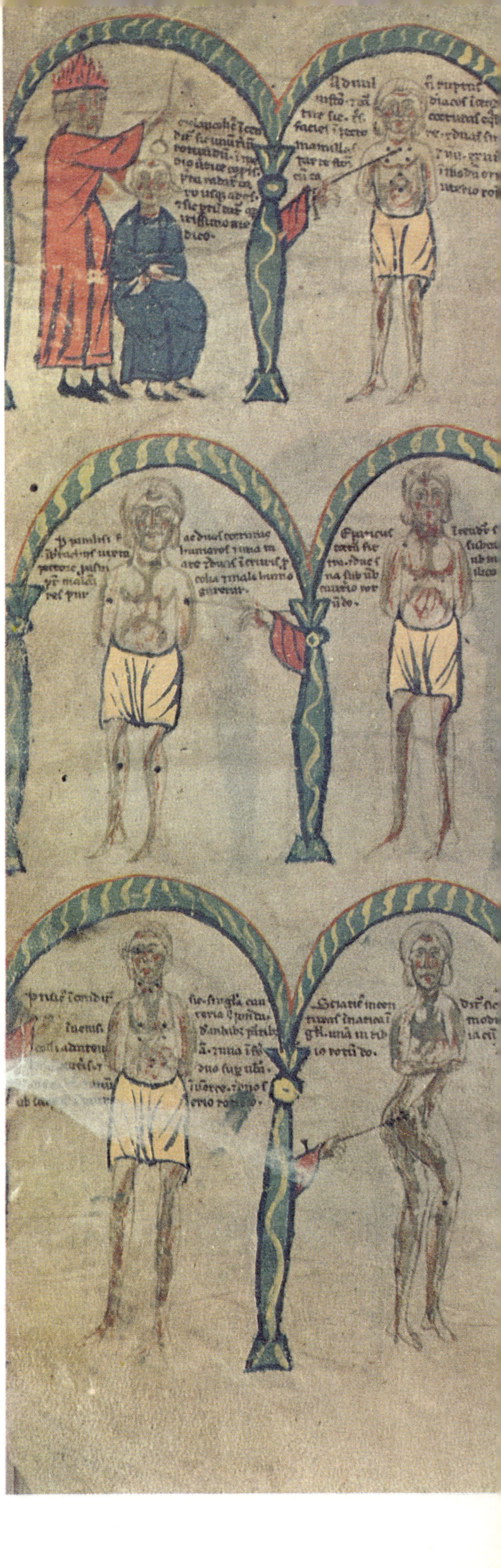

Page from the Chirurgia Magistri Rolandi. *Fourteenth-century codex. Casanatense Library, Rome.*

contained dietetic and hygienic rules and served as an example to Italian writers on health and hygiene from the thirteenth to the fifteenth centuries.

When Maimonides was thirteen, in 1148, the sect of Moslem fanatics called the Almohads displaced the Omayyads from Cordova, which then declined rapidly. The Almohads determined to expel all the Jews and all the Christians who had not been converted to Islam. Maimonides fled with his family, lost all his possessions in a shipwreck, and finally settled in Egypt, where he made a living from medicine, leaving aside philosophy and the study of the Talmud. As a physician he was so famous that Richard Coeur de Lion offered him the post of personal physician. Maimonides declined the offer as he was sick and tired of travelling. He died in Cairo in AD 1208; his tomb at Tiberias is still a place of pilgrimage.

Twenty-eight years after the death of Maimonides, Cordova was captured by Ferdinand II of Castile. Its culture had by then largely faded. The Moslems were gradually pushed back out of Europe; in 1258, the Mongols destroyed Baghdad, and so after five centuries the Arab empire lay in ruins, its way of life lingering only as a memory. In the field of science and philosophy, the Arab heritage was a precious one. Medicine is indebted to the enlightened caliphs and their physicians who salvaged and treasured Greek traditions and Greek texts, and to the chemists who laid a scientific basis for pharmacology, and the legislators who recognized the continuing existence of the figure of the lay medical practitioner.

The Arabs were creative as well as receptive, but to what extent is debatable. Some authorities, such as the Italian Puccinotti and the Frenchman Daremberg, denied that there was any value or originality in Arabic work. Castiglioni is more open-minded, conceding that some of their leading doctors achieved notable progress in the practice of medicine. 'Certainly', he wrote, 'they contributed no original or novel ideas to develop Hippocratic thought, but in a period of unrest they were preservers of tradition; they disseminated lay medical culture, they gave medical studies an honoured place in their civilization and they were in turn the intermediaries from whom the western world retrieved a precious heritage'.

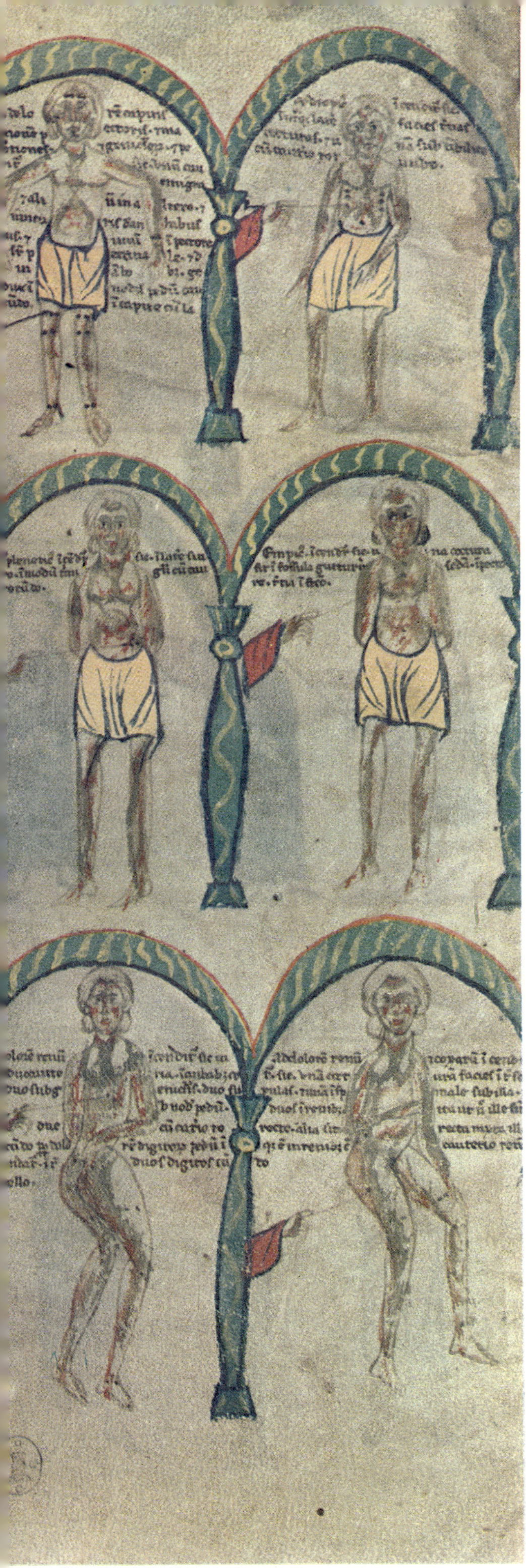

The school of Salerno

In the chaos which covered Europe, the heritage of one war after another, of epidemics and of famine, the welfare of the sick came within the sphere of interest of the religious orders. Nuns and monks were never involved in fighting, and so they were virtually the only people to enjoy the requisite detachment and peace to care for and comfort the sick, the wounded and the plague-stricken. During these centuries every possible setback retarded the advance of medical investigation, and monastic peace was perhaps the one remaining hope. But even the monks were only relatively isolated from the general situation, working and studying in the quiet spells between the recurring outbreaks of war.

This broken peace may be glimpsed in the history of the monastery of Montecassino, which was founded by St Benedict early in the sixth century. In the late sixth century it was pillaged and fired by the Longobards, and its inhabitants fled to Rome; in 720 they returned to Montecassino and set about the task of rebuilding their home. In the year 884 it was burnt down again, this time by the Saracens. Towards the middle of the eleventh century it was rebuilt once more by Pope Victor III. But Montecassino was not a happy choice of site on the part of the Benedictine community; in the second world war, it became a battle ground between the Allies and the Axis, and after heavy fighting only smoking piles of rubble remained where the monastery had stood.

St Benedict of Norcia had not created a nursing order by intent; chance circumstances were responsible for the progress of medicine, both in theory and in practice, in the hands of the Benedictine order. On the practical side, a number of monastic infirmaries were built. The best-known of these belonged to the Swiss monastery of St Gall, which had been founded in 720 by an Irish monk; Christianity had been taken to Ireland by St Patrick in the fifth century. The infirmary stood on the site of St Gall's own cell. Monastic hospitals were entirely autonomous; medicines were made up by the monks themselves from plants grown in the herb garden.

Help was always readily available for the sick who came to the doors of the monastery. In time, the monks who devoted themselves to medicine emerged from their retreats and started visiting the sick in their own homes. This infringed the rules

The art of replacing a missing part of the body by an artificial substitute, or prosthesis, is very ancient indeed; it was certainly known to the Etruscans, whose civilization was at its height in the sixth century BC. Over the centuries, development in this field was very slow. In the Middle Ages, artificial limbs were still primitive in execution, although some very ingenious aids were designed to deal with the mutilations resulting from the endless wars.

Surgical procedures. *From thirteenth-century French manuscript. Bibliotheque Nationale, Paris.*

Healing of cripples, showing various prostheses. *Detail from illustration in psalter of St Elizabeth. Archaeological Museum, Cividale del Friuli.*

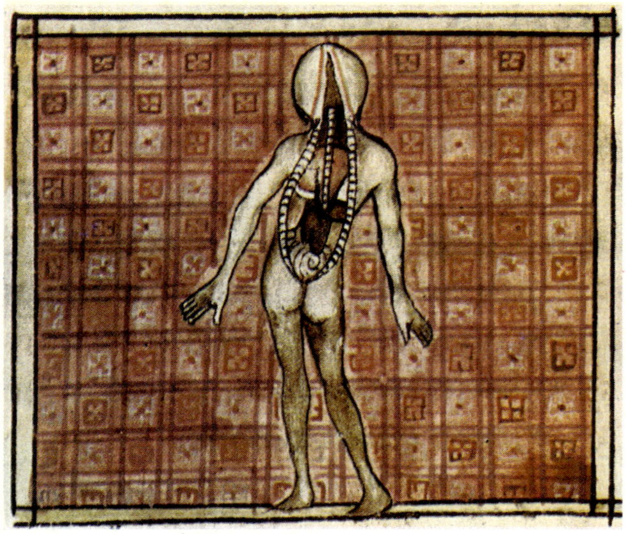

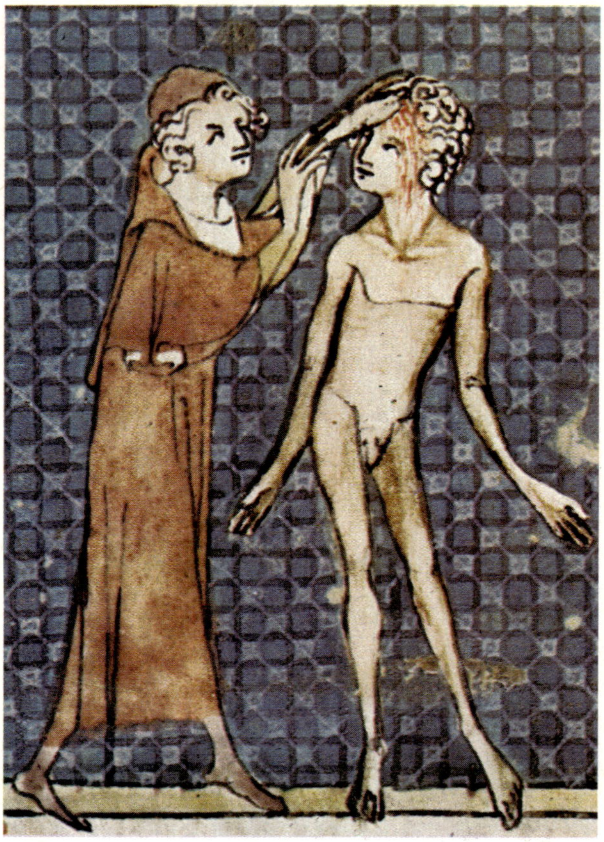

of the order by exposing the monks to the temptations of the world, and it became a hotly debated issue at ecclesiastical councils and synods. Eventually, monastic medicine was forbidden, but it was not easy for the church authorities to enforce this injunction. Many religious men had made a name for themselves as healers and were in great demand; and many sick people, especially those who professed the faith, preferred their services to those of the lay doctors, the leeches, who were sometimes perhaps not as competent as their clerical counterparts.

But lay medicine had not entirely disappeared, and after a long dormant period it came to the fore again and flourished in the famous school of Salerno. This town became a colony of Rome in AD 194 and had a long history as a health resort. In his work, *De virtutibus et vitiis,* St Thomas Aquinas called it a town of medicine. This was not because famous teachers worked there, but rather because excellent doctors were in practice and were highly regarded for their professional skill. No actual documentation or deed of foundation exists, but a doctor from Salerno is known to have been at the court of the French king in the year 904. Other doctors from Salerno looked after Alberon, Bishop of Verdun, while Desiderius, Abbot of Montecassino, went to Salerno for treatment in 1050.

As usually happens when an institution arises spontaneously and its origins are obscure, legend soon set to work. The tale of how the rabbi Helinus, the Greek master Pontus, the Saracen Adela and the Latin master Salernus all taught medicine at Salerno in their own tongues, may mean only that teaching was carried out in those languages and that the texts re-echoed the content of Greek, Latin and Arab works.

According to Busacchi, the formation of the school must remain conjectural, but two main sources are likely, lay and ecclesiastical. In the Christian period, Salerno, besides the salutary effects of its air and waters, offered an additional attraction, for it possessed the miraculous remains of St Matthew the evangelist, which were enshrined in a church. Doctors would be expected to congregate where there were many patients, and it would be logical for these doctors to take pupils and to organize and found a school. As the first of its kind

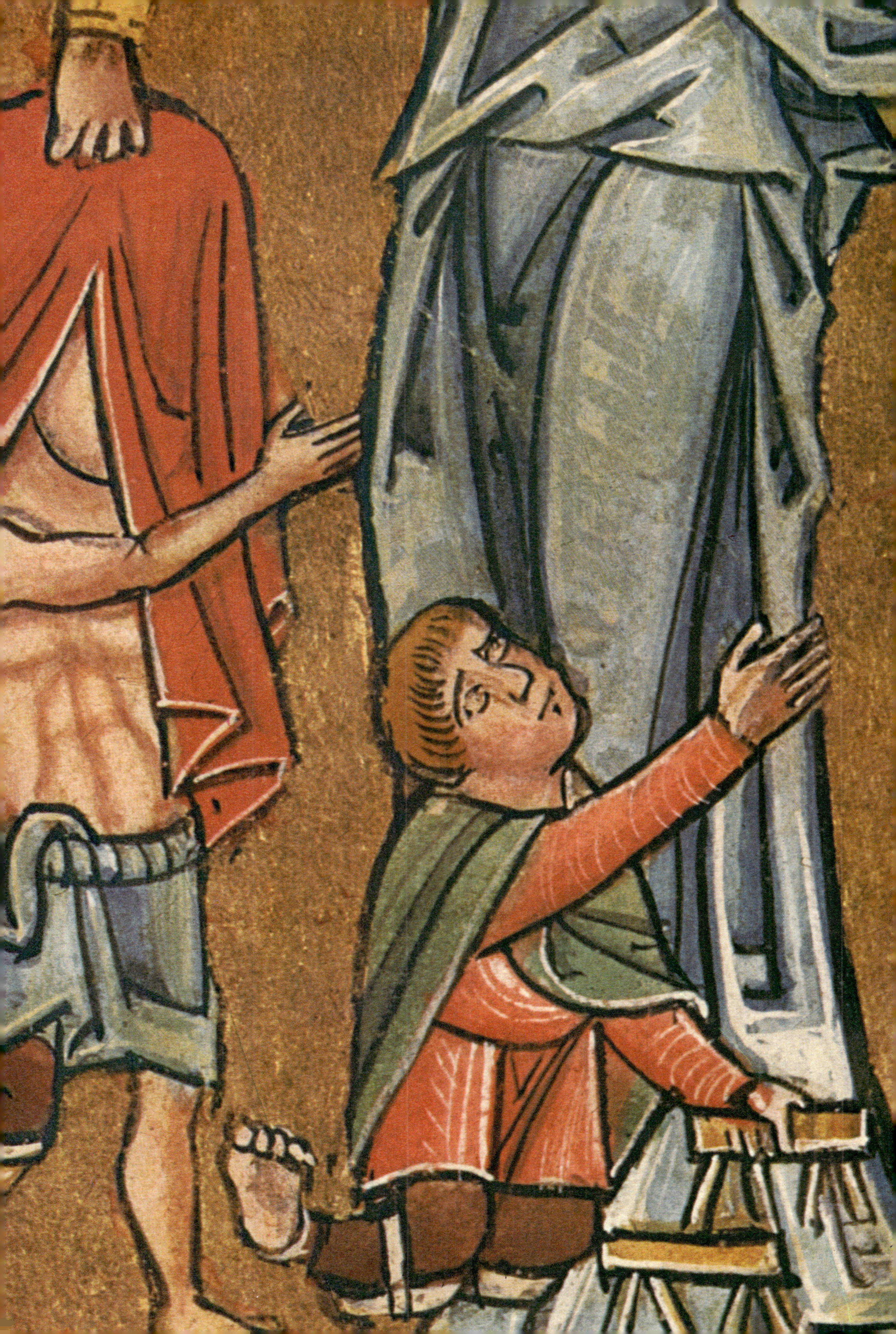

The unrest in Europe during the early Middle Ages caused scholars to seek peace in monasticism, and the practice of medicine came into the hands of monks and nuns. Infirmaries were built in the monasteries, and medicines were made from plants grown in the monastery grounds. The monks and nuns gave help to those who came to them, but eventually they went out to visit the sick in their homes, for their services were often preferred to those of the lay doctors. The bishops disapproved of this practice, since the orders were thus exposed to the temptations of the world, but found it difficult to enforce a ban because of the popularity built up by many individuals.

Lay medicine still existed, but remained dormant for a long period. In time, it began to flourish again, particularly in the town of Salerno in Italy. A school

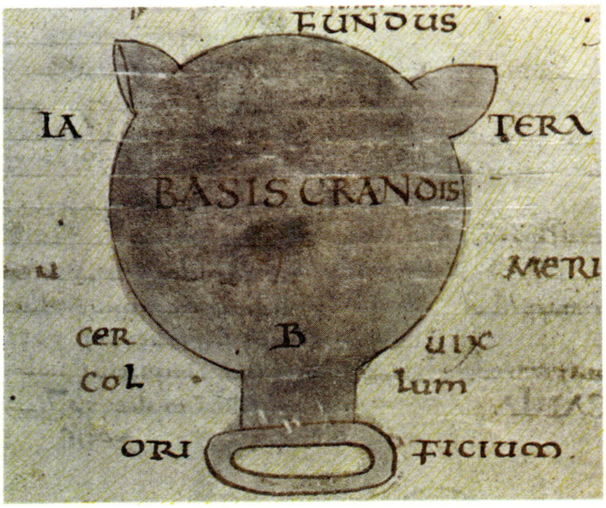

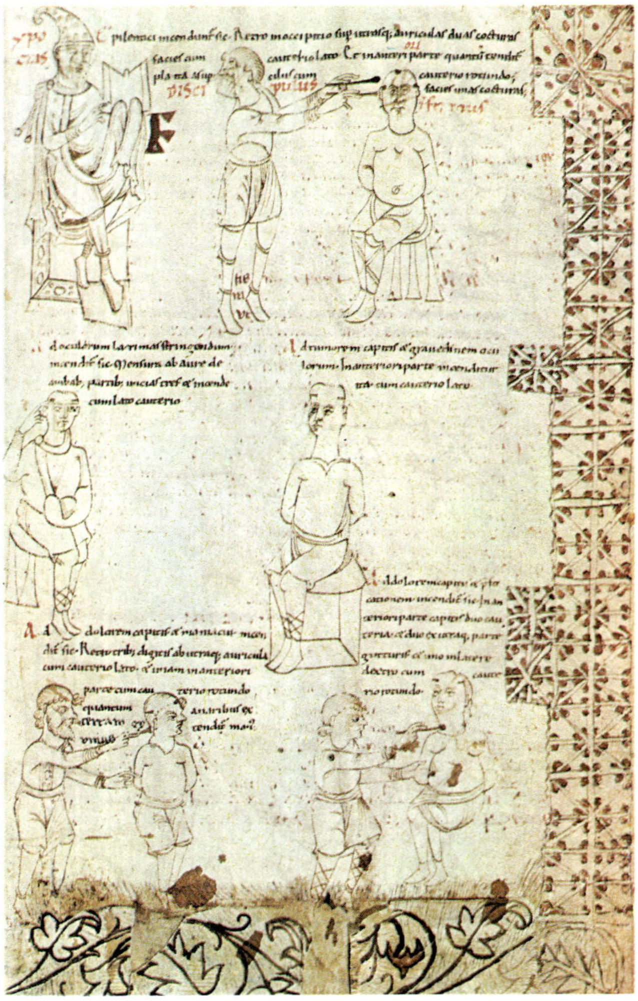

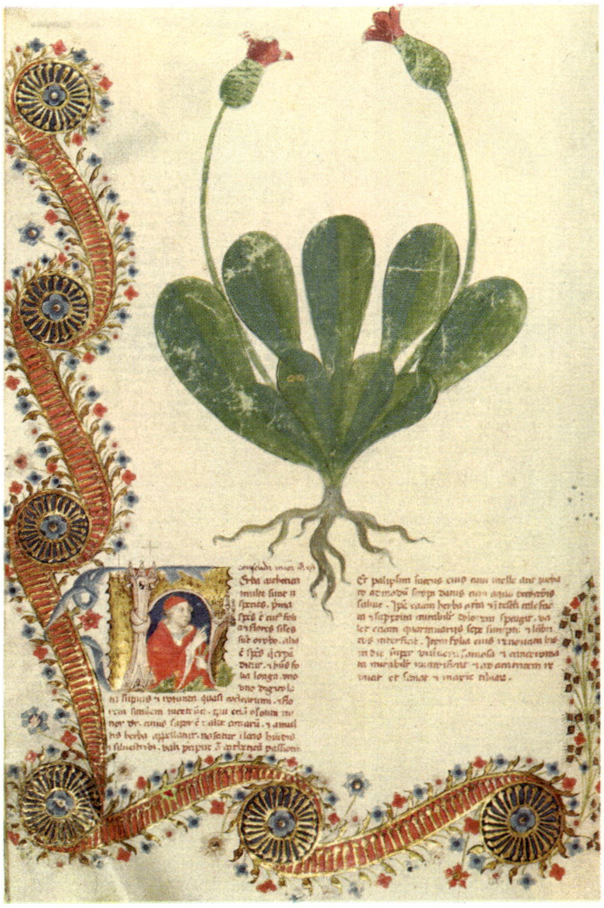

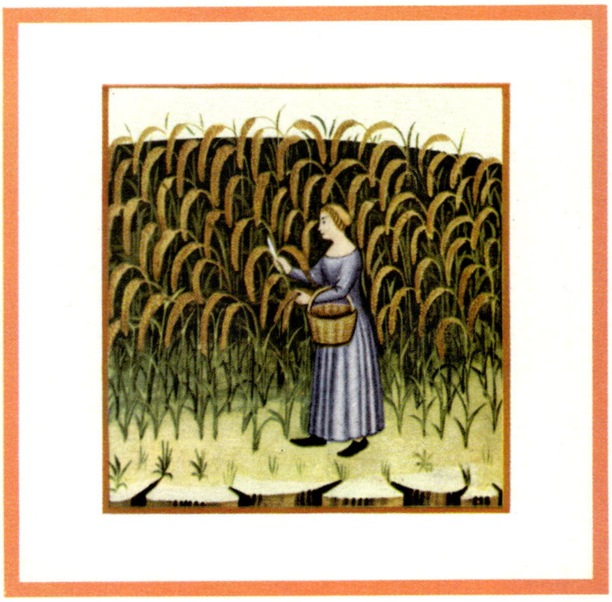

of medicine gradually came into being there in about the tenth century and reached its height in the late eleventh century. In 1240 Frederick II granted the school of Salerno the right to license doctors to practice their profession, and no one could work as a doctor unless he had been authorized. Permission was given after a five-year course of study and one year of practice under expert supervision.

Diagram of uterus. *From a sixteenth-century codex. Royal Library, Brussels.*

Surgical procedures. *From the Tacuinum sanitatis, a fourteenth-century codex.*

Medicinal plants. *From a fourteenth-century Lombard codex. Casanatense Library, Rome.*

Bathroom and bathers massaging themselves with leaves. *Miniature from a German ms. Sachsenspiegel, Heidelberg.*

in the Middle Ages, such a school would soon attract other pupils and masters.

Invaluable research on the history of Italian medicine by Salvatore de Renzi has brought to light the first real information about the school of Salerno which dates from the tenth century. The first manual for the use of students, containing the doctrines of Galen, Alexander of Tralles and Paul of Aegina, was written about 1050 by Gariopontus, who was the most famous teacher of his time. The work was entitled the *Passionarius,* and is of value today in giving the basis of modern medical terminology. Gariopontus latinized Greek terms and took words from common speech, for example, cicatrize and cauterize. Another broad compilation for students of the time was the *Practica* of Petroncellus. A noteworthy feature of both texts was a lack of quotation from Arab sources.

The knowledge of the school of Salerno was set down in the main in verse, much of which seems very amusing today. Many people knew a few lines: 'defecatio matutina bona tamque serotina' (defecation in the morning is as good as in the evening), for example. Another attractive feature of the school was the presence there of many women, often described in the writings as lively and imaginative. Some of the female students are mentioned by name: 'ut ferrum magnes, juvenes sic attrahit Agnes' (Agnes attracts the boys like iron to lodestone).

One of the Salerno women was Trotula, who wrote *De mulierum passionibus ante, in et post partum,* a useful treatise on obstetrics containing advice on what to do before, during and after childbirth, on the treatment of prolapse and polyps of the womb, and on the choice of a wet-nurse and her diet (excess of highly salted foods, as well as garlic, onion and pepper were strictly prohibited). In fact, the real identity of Trotula has not been ascertained; some authorities have suggested that she was not really a woman physician but merely a midwife, perhaps the wife of a famous doctor Johannes Platearius, and another theory is that Trotula was a nickname common to all Salernitan midwives. None of the works now bearing her name may be regarded as original, and much of it was written at a later period. Whatever its origin, the treatise continued to be cited as a standard text until the sixteenth century, and it was printed by Aldus in Venice in 1547. It is interesting to note that this Salerno character found popularity in early English literature under the name Dame Trot.

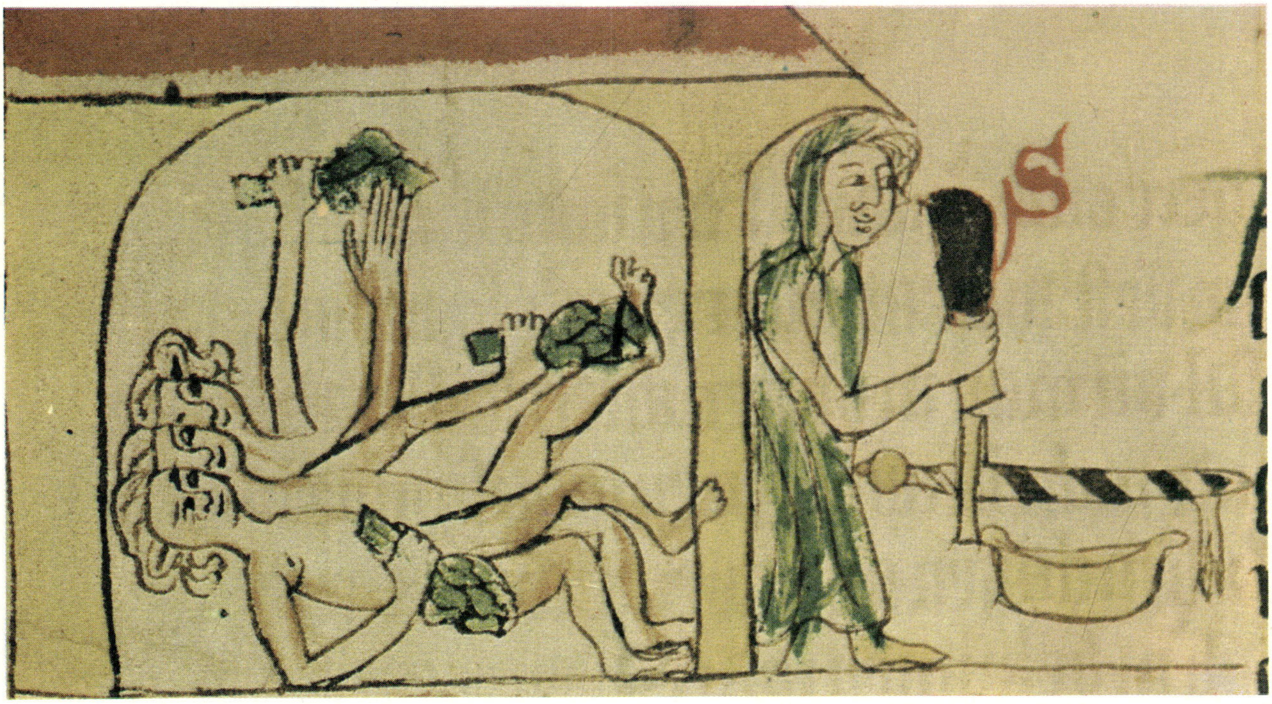

The first useful contribution to medicine from Salerno was the collection of its prescriptions in the celebrated Antidotarium, *the parent of subsequent pharmacopoeias. The Salernitan school specialized in diagnosis from examination of the urine, and in surgery. It was deeply indebted to Constantine Africanus, a scholar from Carthage and master of Oriental languages whose translations made Arabian medicine known in the West. He also translated Hippocrates' sayings and Galen's work* On the Art of Medicine. *After teaching for a while at Salerno he returned to Montecassino where he became a monk.*

The school of Salerno put its teachings into verse that could easily be remembered, and this populariza-

To the earlier period of the school belong also such works as the *Antidotarium,* a book of prescriptions on which subsequent pharmacopoeias were based, and the *Speculum hominis* (Mirror of man), which dealt with diseases in verse form.

The school of Salerno reached its zenith in the late eleventh century. Arabic literature became a source of influence through the work of Constantinus Africanus, a learned scholar famous for having bridged the gap between the culture of Islam and the Christian west. Constantinus was called Africanus because he was born in Carthage; he studied medicine and learned Oriental languages during long periods spent in Syria, Egypt and India. He was attracted to Salerno by the medical school and became secretary to the Norman duke Robert Guiscard after he occupied the town. Later Constantinus became a monk and retired to Montecassino, where he died in 1087. He was probably a plagiarist; allowing for the bitter enmity between Christians and Moslems, it is understandable that a Benedictine monk would not feel able to state in his translations the infidel names of the authors of the originals. His merit lay in that he made known the Greek concepts that the Arabs had worked on, a century before the more accurate translations of Gerard of Cremona.

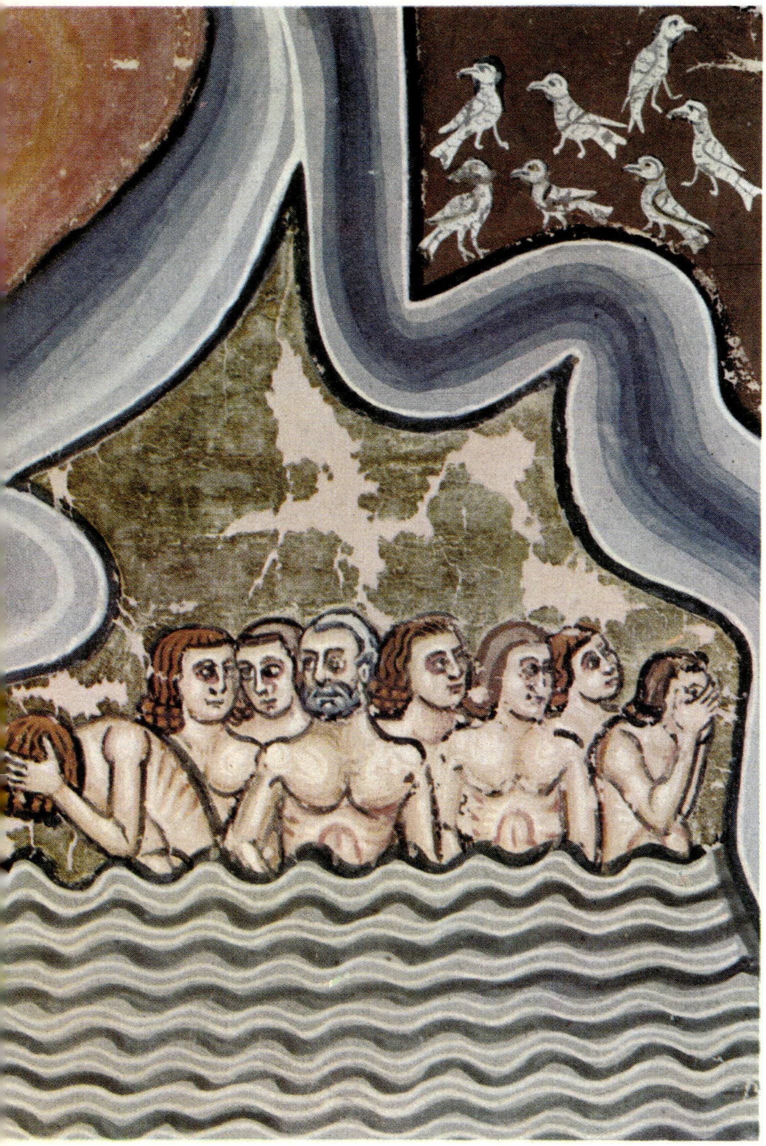

The writings of the Salerno school were mostly collaborations, although the names of some individuals stand out. Rogerius Frugardi was the author of a clear and concise text on surgery, which however often echoed ideas and methods used by Greek doctors. The chapters on cranial and abdominal wounds are of particular interest. Fractures of the head should be explored by palpation, and in the case of depressed fractures he advised trephining a series of perforations so that the damaged bone could be removed without damage to the membranes covering the brain. In abdominal injuries, if the intestine had protruded for long enough to have turned cold and hard, Rogerius suggested that before replacing the intestine it should be warmed and softened by placing over it the intestines of a newly-killed animal. Then it was to be cleaned with a sponge and replaced in the abdomen, the wound being left open as long as the damage remained visible, after which a drain was to be inserted and the wound dressed every day.

Salernitan anatomy was based predominantly on Galen. Doctors dissected animals, and especially pigs, believing that there was more resemblance between human and pig intestines than between those of man and other animals. At least they now recognized the importance of anatomy. A work by Copho belonging to the early period of the school was entitled *Anatomia porci* (Anatomy of the pig). Another anatomical treatise, produced in the twelfth century by Magister Maurus, was made famous by Gilles de Corbeil in a poem in Latin hexameters which summarized the medical thought of the period.

tion of medical knowledge was perhaps its greatest contribution. The best known work was the Regimen sanitatis salernitanum, *which dealt with hygiene ; its numerous verses were translated into other languages and became known throughout the civilized world.*

Among the sources recognizable in the Regimen *are many of the aphorisms of Hippocrates.*

Pierre Gilles de Corbeil, or Petrus Aegidius Corboliensis, was a Frenchman, born in 1140, who became a pupil of the school of Salerno and then a teacher in Paris. The section of his poem that dealt with urine remained the most widely known urological text for three centuries.

The Salernitan masters' idea of putting teaching matter into verse form was a happy inspiration. Their work, which was called the *Regimen sanitatis salernitanum* (The Salerno book of health), provided the basis of clinical medicine up to the end of the Middle Ages. The great contribution made by the school was its popularization of practical medical knowledge in the form of aphorisms, in verse and with a spice of humour, which had an appeal throughout the civilized world. But for the Salerno school, practical medical knowledge might have remained entirely esoteric, locked up in heavy volumes for the perusal of initiates, worthwhile enough but as difficult to study and interpret as Galen or Avicenna.

Grotto for thermal baths near Pozzuoli. *Miniature from De virtutis Balneorum Puteolanis by Pietro da Eboli. Angelica Library, Rome.*

De Thermis. *From the work of Rabanus Maurus of 1023. Codex from Montecassino.*

Drawings illustrating chemical experiments for the preparation of medicines. *From a fourteenth-century ms. University Library, Pavia.*

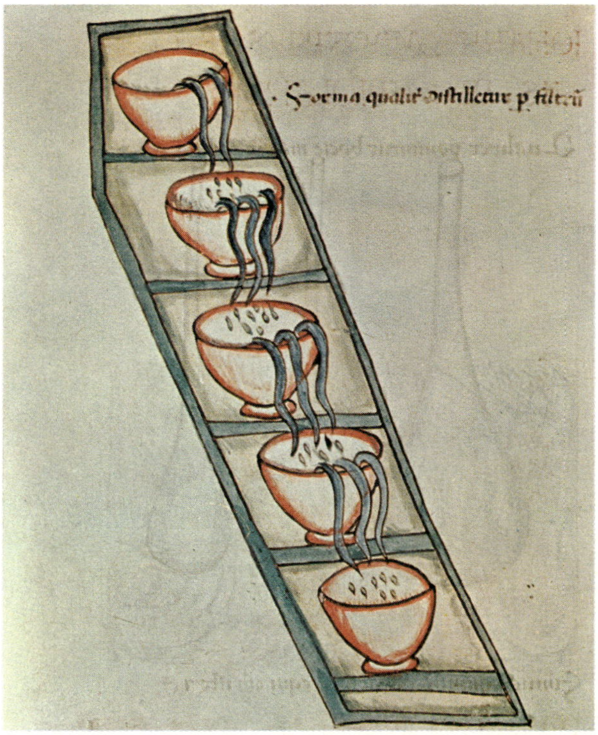

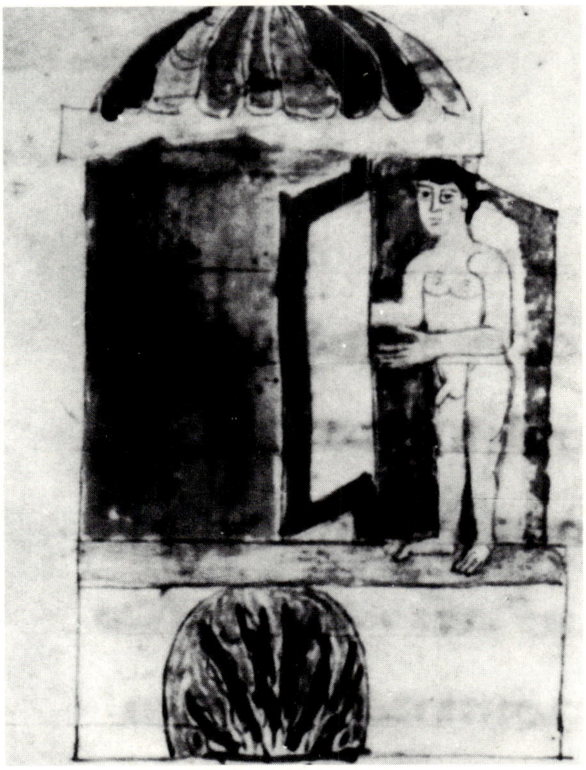

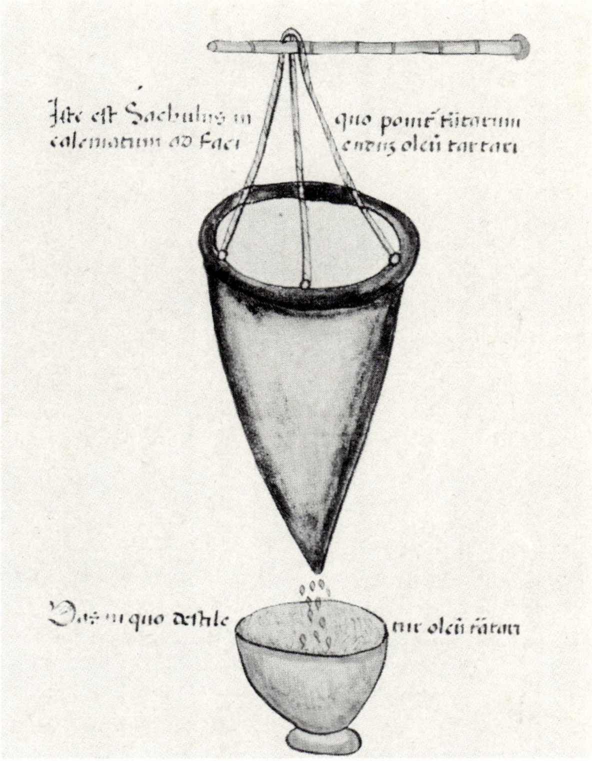

The Salernitan rules of health were based on common-sense: they advised washing the eyes and hands with pure, clean water in the morning, gentle exercise and brushing the teeth. 'When you come out of a hot bath, avoid the cold'. After lunch a short walk was indicated, but an afternoon sleep was not advised, for it caused headaches, lethargy and catarrh. A light supper was to be taken if a restless night was to be avoided. For indigestion and loss of appetite, purging was recommended before anything further was eaten. Wine was to be judged by its bouquet, taste, clarity, and colour. Bloodletting was beneficial, especially for acute illness and in the early spring; not too much blood was to be taken from old and young people. The Regimen sani-

The text was still in a phase of expansion when the first version was produced by Arnold of Villanova, who lived from 1235 to 1315. This was printed for the first time in 1480 and had 362 verses, though they increased with time; De Renzi discovered and published a version of 3,520 verses. The *Regimen* was dedicated to a king of England who has remained unidentified, in these well known lines which are typical of the spirit of the work:

Anglorum Regi scribit schola tota Salerni
Si vis incolumem, si vis te reddere sanum
Curas tolle graves, irasci crede prophanum.
Parce mero, coenato parum: non sit tibi vanum
Surgere post epulas, somnum fuge meridianum
Non mictum retine, nec comprime fortiter anum.
Haec bene si serves, tu longo tempore vives
Si tibi deficiant medici, medici tibi fiant
Haec tria: Mens hilaris, requies, moderata dieta.

Sir John Harington produced a translation of the text which was first published in 1607; he renders these lines:

The Salerno Schoole doth by these lines impart
All health to Englands King, and doth aduise
From care his head to keepe, from wrath his heart,
Drinke not much wine, sup light, and soone arise
When meate is gone, long sitting breedeth smart:
And after-noone still waking keep your eyes.
When mou'd you find your selfe to Natures Needs,
Forbeare them not, for that much danger breeds,
Use three Physicians still; first Doctor Quiet,
Next Doctor Merry-man, and Doctor Dyet.

This straightforward advice continues in the next three verses (which are quoted again in Harington's version):

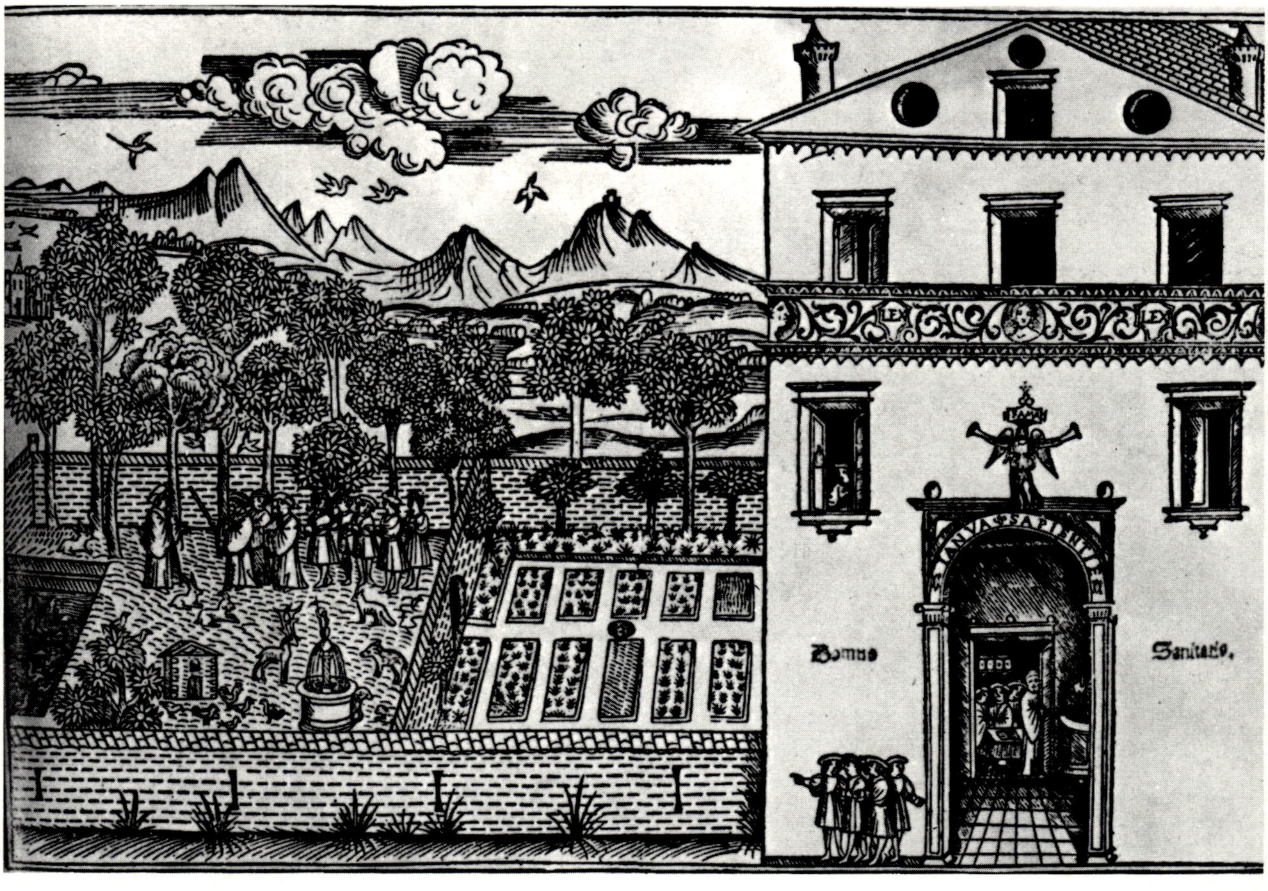

tatis salernitanum, *which contained these rules for health, remained the basis of clinical medicine up to the end of the Middle Ages. The school itself declined after the middle of the thirteenth century as universities sprung up in other places and culture, which had flourished for so long in Mediterranean lands, began to move to northern Europe.*

Domus sanitatis. *Sixteenth-century representation of the school of Salerno in Fabrica regiminis sanitatis, Pavia 1522.*

Surgery for haemorrhoids and nose polyps, and corneal incision. *From an eleventh-century ms. of the school of Salerno. British Museum, London.*

Following pages:
Miniatures illustrating the circulatory system and the muscles. *From Ashmole ms. of the thirteenth century. Bodleian Library, Oxford.*

Rise earely in the morne, and straight remember,
With water cold to wash your hands and eyes,
In gentle fashion retching euery member,
And to refresh your braine when as you rise,
In heat, in cold, in Iuly and December.
Both comb your head, and rub your teeth likewise:
If bled you haue, keep coole, if bath'd, keepe warme:
If din'd, to stand or walke will do no harme.

Some men there are that thinke a little nap breeds
no ill bloud:
But if you shall herein exceed too farre,
It hurts your health, it cannot be with stood:
Long sleepe at after-noones by stirring fumes,
Breeds Slouth, and Agues, Aking heads and
Rheumes:

To keepe good dyet, you should neuer feed
Untill you finde your stomacke cleane and void
Of former eaten meate, for they do breed
Repletion, and will cause you soone be cloid,
None other rule but appetite should need,
When from your mouth a moysture cleare doth
void.

This poem went all over the known world; it was a huge success and was translated many times – there were eleven versions in French, ten in German, and many in English and Italian. Official recognition for the school came in 1224, when an enactment of Frederick II made it incumbent upon anyone practising medicine in the kingdom of Naples to seek approval from the masters of Salerno. Subsequently, the school declined, for competition increased as universities sprung up in many other places. Culture, which had flourished on the shores of the Mediterranean, began to move northwards.

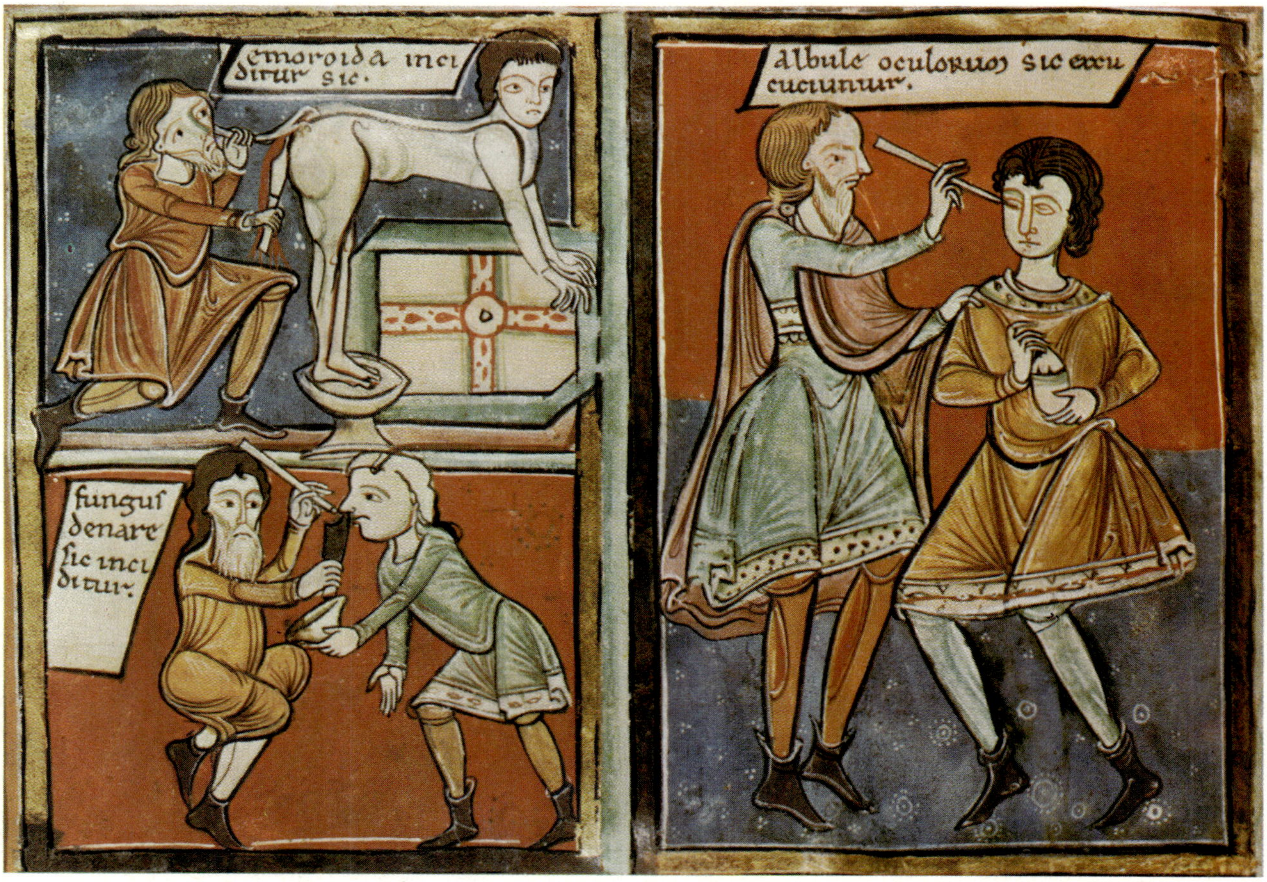

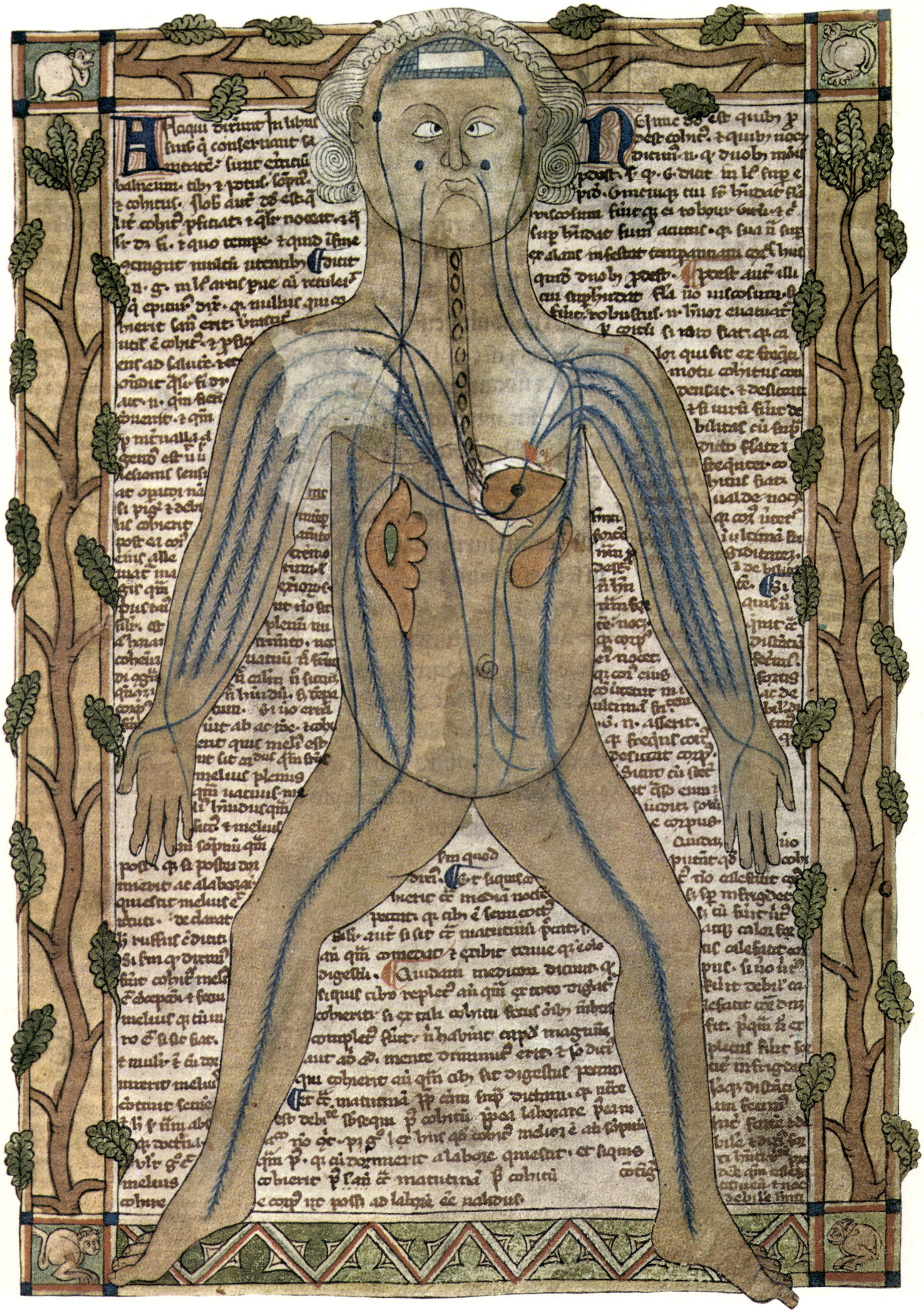

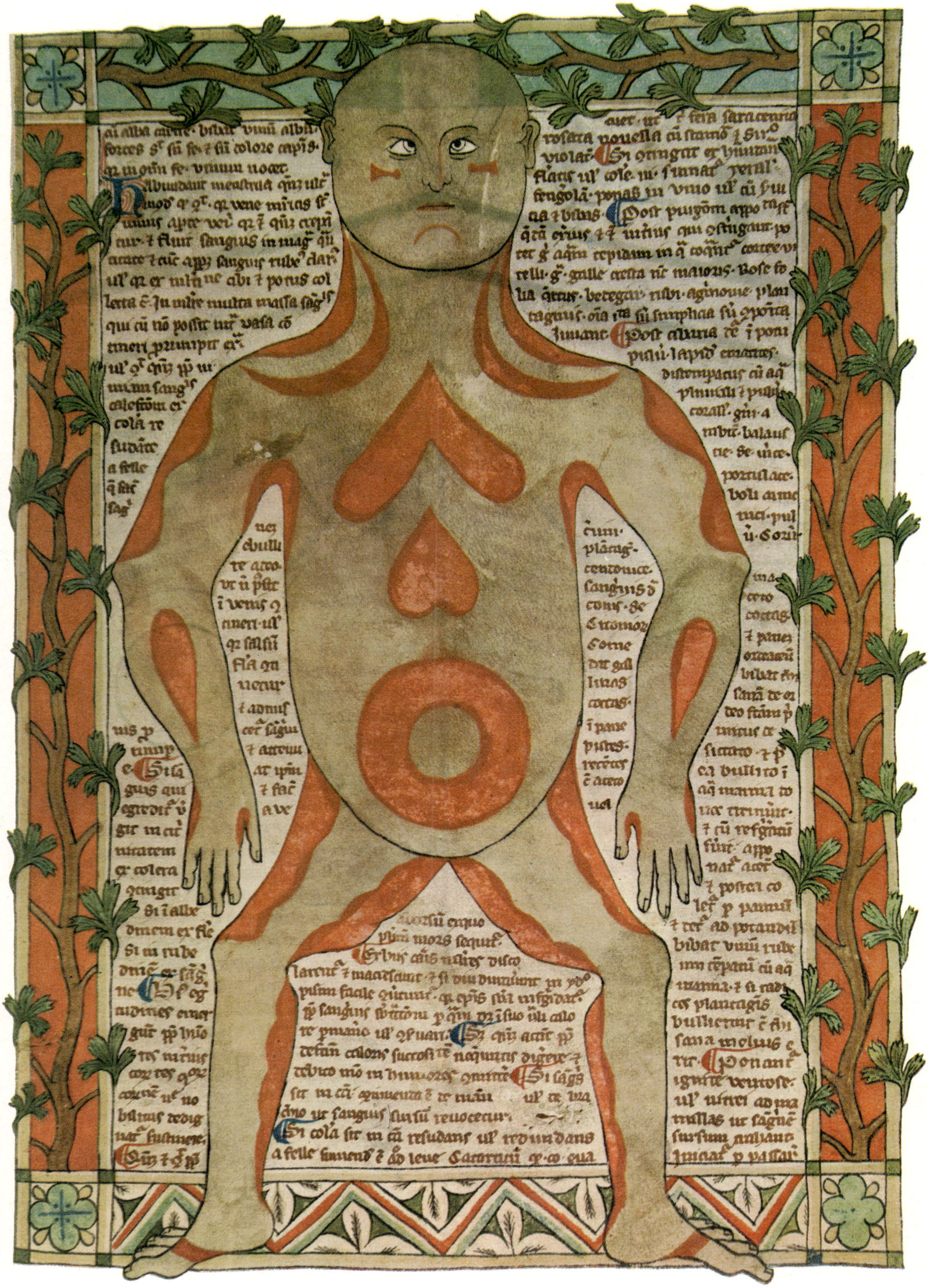

Foundation of the universities

The school of Salerno did not add instruction in other faculties to the teaching of medicine; it did not evolve into a *studium generale,* as the universities founded in western Europe at that time were called. The universities began to appear mainly in the twelfth and thirteenth centuries. Their foundation, one of the most important events in the history of civilization, was made possible by the growth and increasing wealth of mediaeval cities.

In the thirteenth century the secular movement, in conflict with the philosophy of Thomas Aquinas, tried deliberately to stand apart. This occurred within the framework of the universities, which had arisen at the instance of pupils or masters, usually with formal authorization by decree of emperor or pope or community. A discussion of the exact stage at which the corporations of students and of teachers got together to form the universities of Bologna, Montpellier, Naples, Salamanca, Paris, Oxford, Cambridge, Padua and Pisa is outside the scope of this book. The important point is that the rise of universities constituted the salient cultural feature of the early Middle Ages.

The greatest of the universities and perhaps the most ancient was Bologna, where a law school had been in existence since the eleventh century. It was run by the commune under democratic regulations, by which the students chose their professors and elected a rector, who had precedence over everyone, including cardinals, at official functions.

One of the first masters of medicine at this university of whom we have knowledge was a Florentine called Taddeo Alderotti (1223–1303), remembered because he is mentioned in the verses of Dante, who probably attended his lectures. In his native city he was held in low esteem, and was known as a poor man who sold candles to old women at church doors. In Bologna however he rapidly achieved success as professor of medicine, and his highly-priced professional services were in great demand. Taddeo also made translations of Aristotle and wrote a work, *Della conservazione della salute* (How to stay healthy), which was dedicated to a fellow-citizen Corso Donati, and in which he advised daily gymnastics. Another of his works, the *Consilia,* which described clinical cases in Italian rather than Latin, was an important presentation of practical observations.

The fame of Bologna as a school of surgery was linked to the names of Ugo and Theodoric, father

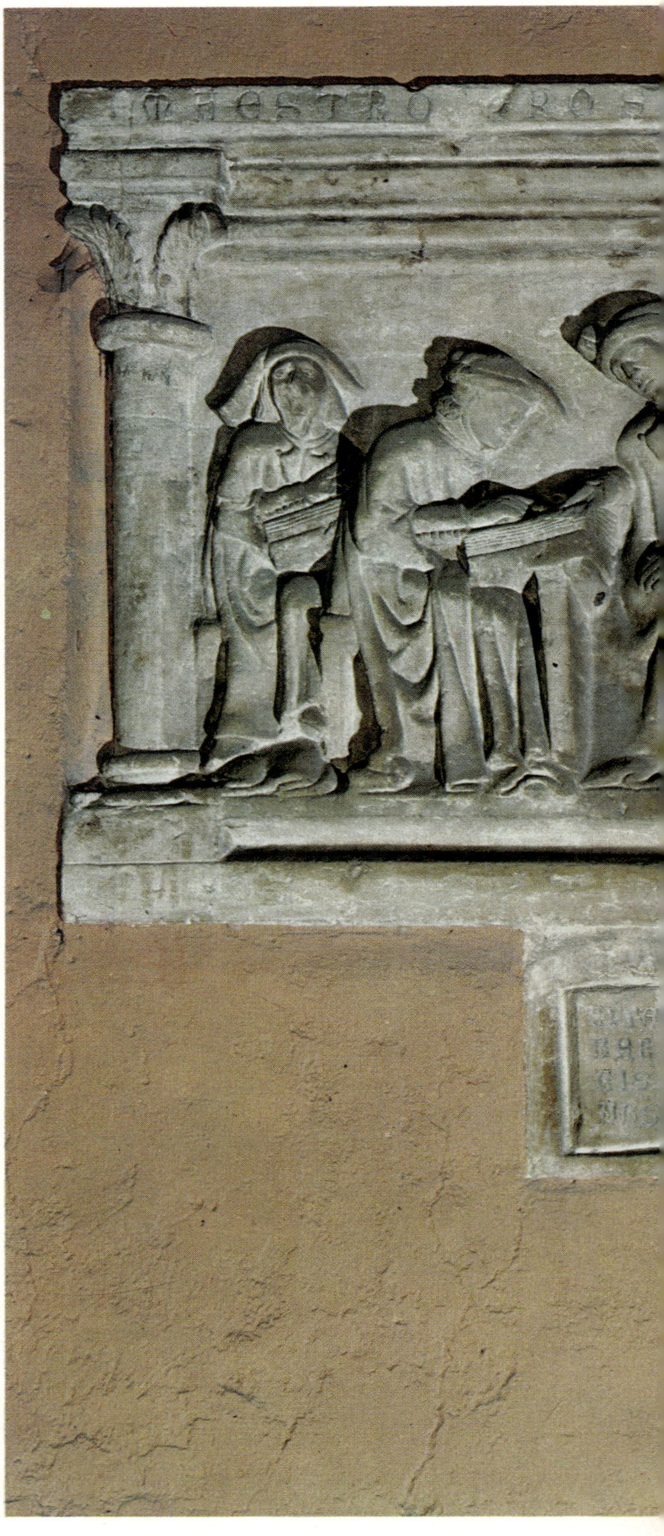

The greatest of the mediaeval universities was that at Bologna. Medicine was taught there, and Bologna became known particularly for its school of surgery and for the study of anatomy.

Mondino de Luzzi was the first distinguished anatomist of the Middle Ages. He performed the first dissections in 1315, and it was he who introduced the teaching of anatomy into the curriculum and drew to Bologna students from every corner of Europe. Although he practised systematic dissection of corpses, Mondino remained loyal to Galen's doctrines. His Anathomia, *written in about 1316, remained a textbook for nearly three centuries.*

Tombstone from the grave of Mondino de Luzzi, who is shown giving a lesson. *Church of S Francesco, Bologna.*

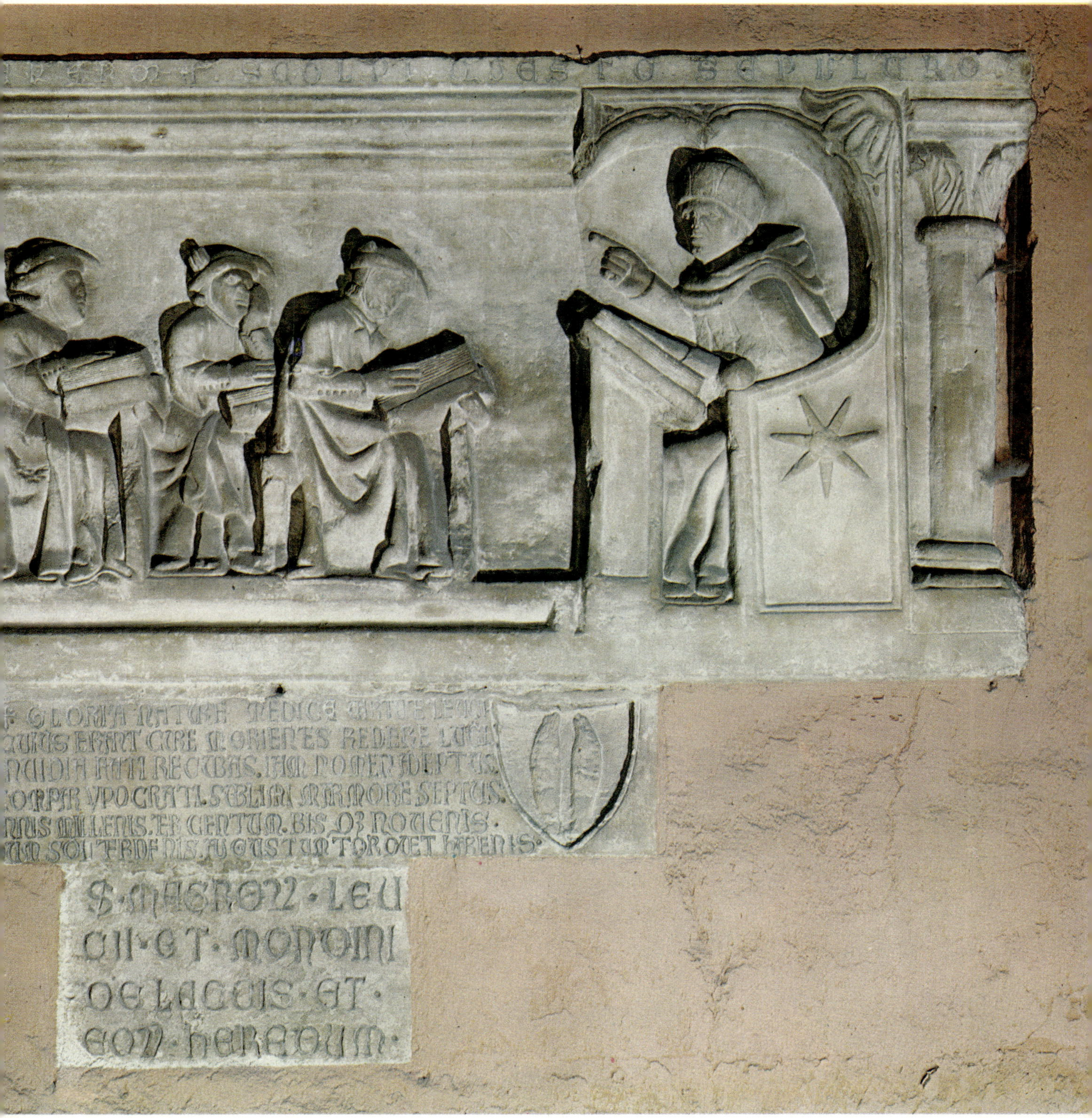

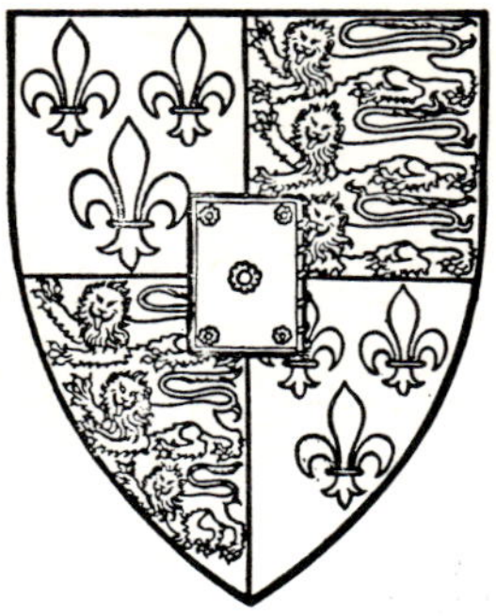

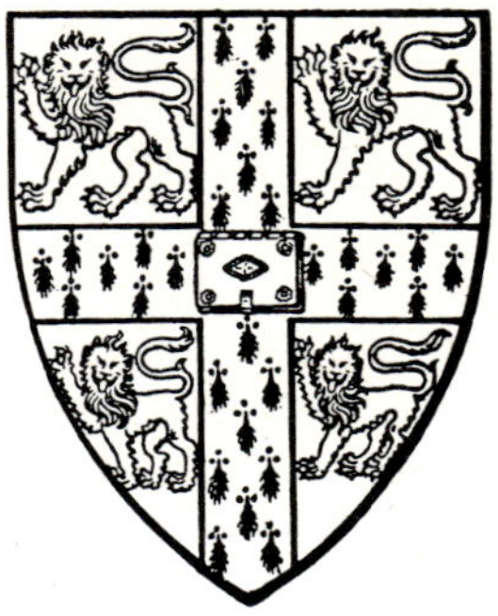

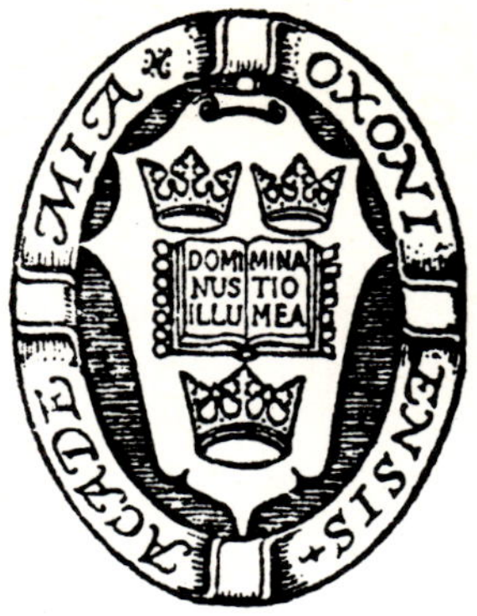

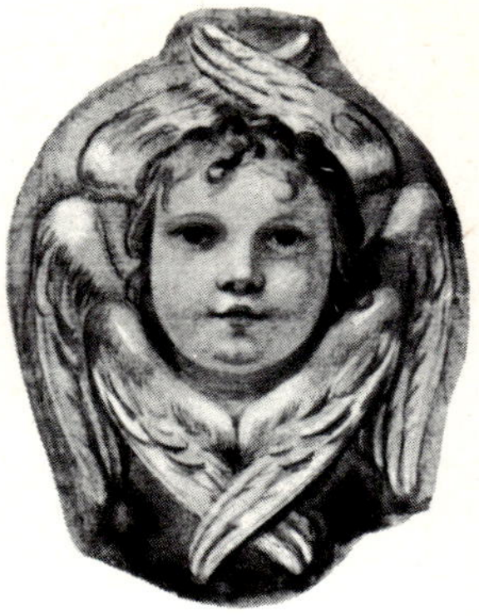

and son, of the Borgognoni family of Lucca. Ugo Borgognone is known to have died in 1252 although his birth-date is unknown; he learned surgery during the Crusades, when he saw service with the Bologna contingent. His son Theodoric (1205–1298) was a Dominican monk and had been bishop of Bitonto and Cervia before coming to Bologna. He collected his own and his father's experiences into a work called the *Cyrurgia* (Surgery). Theodoric made a valuable contribution to surgery by recommending the suturing of wounds to close them and prevent suppuration. This destroyed the old practice by which wounds were left open to the air, thus favouring the formation of pus.

The dissection of the dead is known to have been practised at Bologna at this date, initially under orders from the magistrature. In 1302, a nobleman called Azzolini met his death in suspicious circumstances. Doctor Bartolomeo da Varignana was instructed to examine the corpse and find out if death had been due to posioning. He performed the autopsy with the assistance of a colleague and three surgeons. The report he wrote excluded the possibility of poisoning and is of importance in suggesting considerable practical knowledge of anatomy. Again, from the anatomy taught to his pupils by William of Saliceto (1210–1277), it is likely that this surgeon was not merely repeating information obtained from ancient authorities but must also have known about human dissection.

Mondino

Anatomy took on a new lease of life in the hands of Remondino de Luzzi, known as Mondino. He was born in Bologna about the year 1270, studied medicine and philosophy and taught at Bologna for a decade from 1314, and was also a diplomat and politician. Mondino practised systematic dissection and although his knowledge was bounded by Galen he wrote a work of fundamental importance called the *Anathomia*. He explained that the way to begin a dissection was to open up the abdomen by a vertical incision, followed by a horizontal one slightly above the umbilicus; dissections could then be performed, region by region, with careful display of the organs. For three centuries, anatomy lecturers were required by medical schools to use Mondino's text in their teaching.

In Bologna anatomy was taught by surgeons until Aranzio occupied the chair of anatomy in the sixteenth century and anatomy became an independent study. Mondino's great contributions were that he collected anatomical ideas together into one work, and that he taught anatomy from the human cadaver. But much of his information was sketchy; on the size of the heart, Mondino wrote, 'it is not big and it is not small'. There was an air of finality in his work, a legacy of Aristotle and Galen; this led him to say that men were not provided with tails so that they could sit down.

Some teachers of medicine were heretics. One of these taught at Montpellier university, where the school of medicine was among the most ancient, dating from the end of the tenth century. His name was Arnold of Villanova, and he was probably Catalan or Provençal; he lived from about 1235 to 1316. He wrote in one of his works that he was doctor of theology, jurisprudence, philosophy and medicine, and that he knew Arabic, Greek and Hebrew as well as Latin. He adopted the new lines of thought contributed by the Arabs to chemistry; he had a high opinion of the rules of diet and hygiene of the school of Salerno, editing as we have seen a version of the *Regimen sanitatis salernitanum*. He indulged in alchemy and magic, and sought a universal remedy, the elixir of immortality, in experiment after experiment. He was argumentative and since Galen and Avicenna went for little with him, he was under constant surveillance by the Inquisition. He was accused of heresy and it was only the intervention of Pope Boniface VIII (whom Arnold had treated for kidney stones) that saved him from death. But his works were burned and now all knowledge of the fourteen heresies of which he was accused has been lost.

An Englishman at Montpellier, dean in the year he died, was Gilbertus Anglicus (1180-1250), who became well known as the author of a *Compendium medicinae,* also known as the *Rosa Anglicana,* which contained extracts from the doctrines of Salernitan and Arabic doctors. He suggested as a 'safe' treatment for goitre: 'take a frog when neither the sun nor the moon is shining in the sky; cut off its legs and wrap them in a deerskin; apply the right leg of the frog to the left foot of the patient, and the left leg to the right foot'. But he is remembered for his excellent descriptions of leprosy and smallpox, the

Shield and symbols of the universities of: Cambridge, old shield; Cambridge, 1573; Oxford; Pisa.

Shield of the Sorbonne in Paris.

First document of foundation of the Ticino studium in the year 825 by enactment of the Emperor Lotharius.

University of Salamanca.

Anatomical theatre of Fabrizio. *From Gymnasium Patavini by Tomasini, Udine 1654. Civic Museum, Padua.*

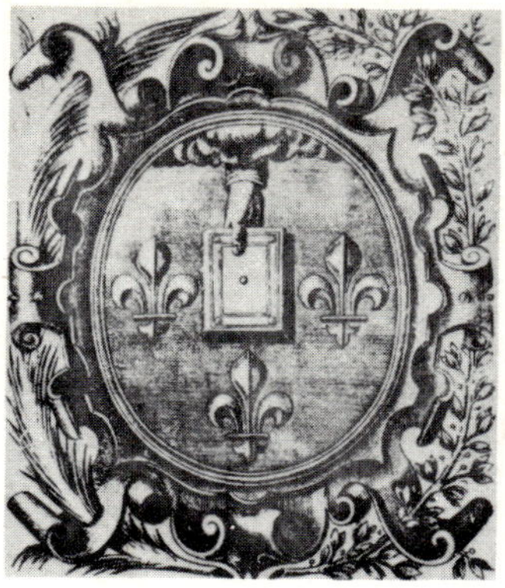

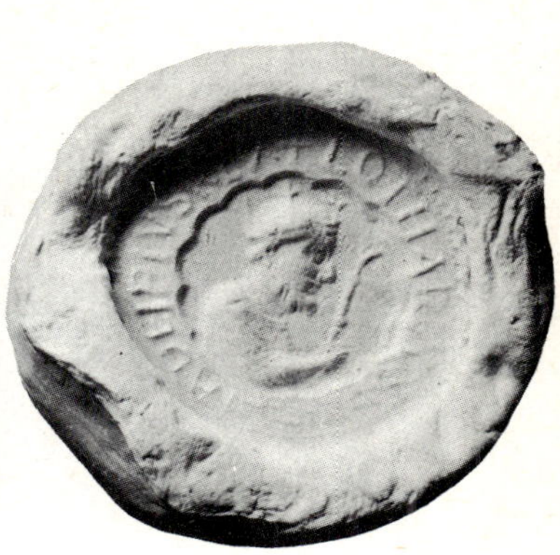

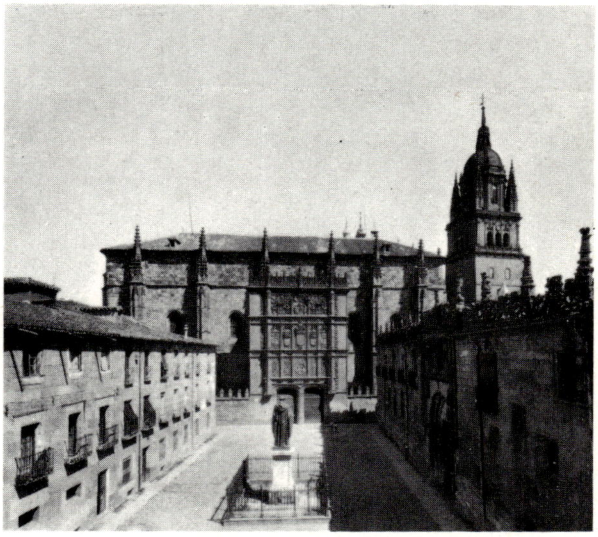

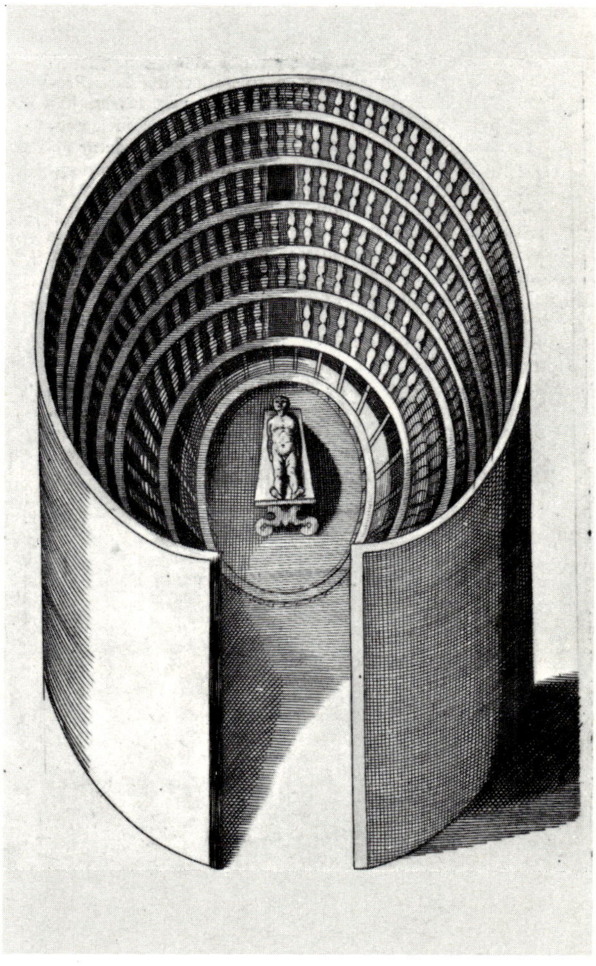

contagious nature of which he was one of the first to recognize.

Pietro d'Abano (1250–1315) was another heretic, and the first distinguished representative of the great medical school of the university of Padua. A disciple of Averroes, he wrote a work called *Conciliator controversiarum quae inter philosophos et medicos versantur,* which attempted to reconcile points of dispute between Arab medical doctrine and Catholic philosphy. He too was accused by the Inquisition but was taken ill and died during his trial. He was condemned posthumously to the stake and the sentence was ordered to be carried out on his dead body; but the corpse was carefully concealed by a loyal servant, and the judges had to be content with burning an effigy.

Dante may well have been a pupil of Pietro d'Abano for a time; some think that Dante was a doctor, for in 1300 he was elected prior of the guild of doctors and apothecaries in Florence. Most experts on Dante do not hold this view, though he possibly studied medicine at Bologna and Padua, and his *Divine Comedy* shows obvious first-hand knowledge of a number of diseases.

The Paris school of surgery

Surgery was beginning to make progress in France. The head of the surgery school at Paris was a pupil of William of Saliceto, a Milanese called Guido Lanfranchi, who was born in the first half of the thirteenth century. Although he was in holy orders, Lanfranchi may have married at some stage for he had a son who practised medicine at Montpellier. Obliged to leave Milan for political reasons, he went to Lyons and wrote the *Cyrurgia parva* (The little book of surgery). In 1295 he was summoned to Paris to lecture on surgery and was very successful there. He finished writing the *Cyrurgia magna* (The big book of surgery) in 1296 and died early in the fourteenth century.

Lanfranchi restored surgery to an honoured place in France. One of the reasons why it was practised largely by itinerant barbers was that physicians thought it beneath their dignity to get blood on their hands. Lanfranchi established the principle that no good doctor could ignore surgery and conversely that a surgeon was duty-bound to acquire some knowledge of medicine. Lanfranchi's

The study of anatomy, based on the dissection of human corpses, advanced the scope of surgery. Many physicians of the thirteenth century would not perform operations, believing it to be beneath their dignity to get blood on their hands, and surgery was largely carried out by barbers. In the fourteenth century, the principle that doctors should have a knowledge of surgery became established. Guy de Chauliac, the best known of mediaeval surgeons, stressed the importance of a knowledge of anatomy to his art.

Dissection in the Middle Ages. *Thirteenth-century Anglo-saxon ms. Bodleian Library, Oxford.*

Dissections. *From the Anathomia of Guido da Vigevano. Condé Museum, Chantilly.*

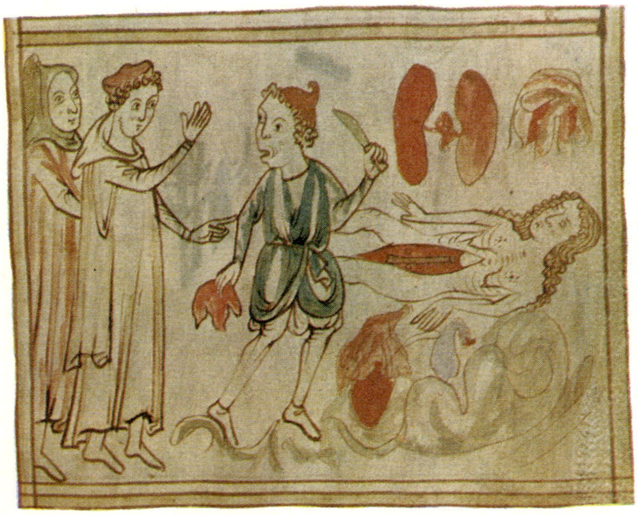

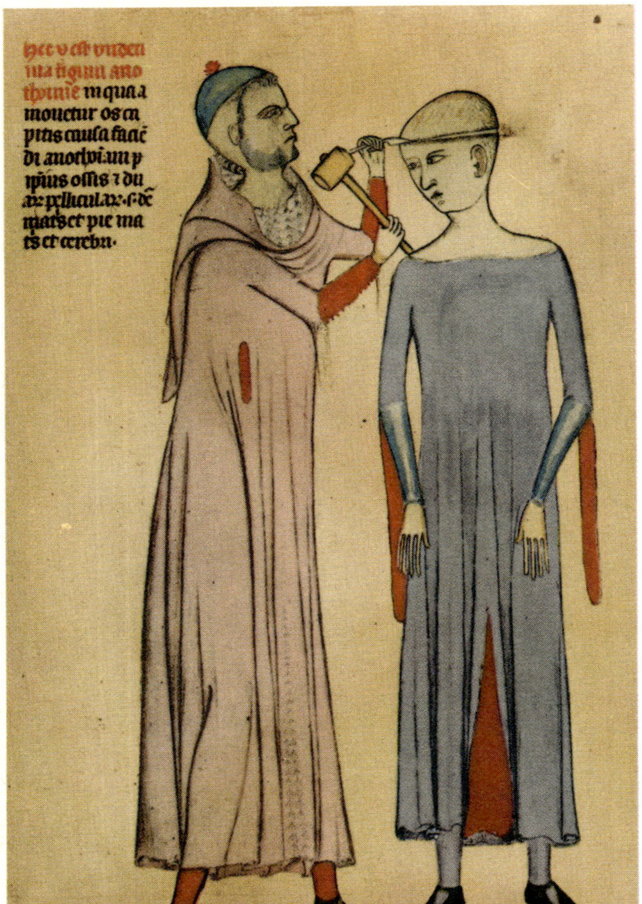

work was based both on contemporary Italian practice and on his own experience.

The first specifically French work on surgery was written by a colleague of Lanfranchi, Henri de Mondeville, who lived from about 1260 to 1320. He studied medicine at Paris, Montpellier and Bologna, where he was a pupil of Theodoric, following the latter in the practice of suturing wounds to prevent the formation of pus. Henri's skill brought him the post of physician to Philip the Fair and Louis X, and he also saw active service.

In the introductory part of the *Cyrurgia,* written at the insistence of his colleague Bernard de Gordon, a famous master of the university of Montpellier, Henri documented customs of the time in an entertaining manner. He dealt frankly with the question of fees, advising brother surgeons always to ask more than doctors did, and putting them on their guard against rich patients who appeared in rags in order to be let off lightly.

Another celebrated French surgeon of the same period was Guy de Chauliac (1300–1368), who studied at Bologna and Paris and took his degree at Montpellier. He was probably the most famous surgeon of the Middle Ages. In his *Chirurgia,* Guy scorned the approach of Theodoric but stressed the importance of anatomical knowledge, following what he had been taught at Bologna by Bertuccio, pupil of Mondino. He took holy orders and went to Lyons, where he continued to practise as a surgeon, was summoned to Avignon and became personal physician to Pope Clement VI and later to Innocent VI and Urban V.

Guy de Chauliac seems to have been a disagreeable man. At Avignon he so moved Petrarch to wrath that the poet wrote the Pope a long letter about the bad behaviour of doctors. The letter began, 'As always and most especially in the circumstances, brevity becomes the man who wishes to address His Holiness, so I will say my say in brief, speaking my mind with sincerity and a devout heart. I know that your bedside is besieged by the doctors. This is the very mainspring of my fears. They never agree among themselves, judging it blameworthy to contribute nothing new or merely to follow in another's footsteps. There is no doubt that they all trade in our lives, as Pliny put it, while hoping for fame as a result of new discoveries. It is a singular privilege of their calling that a man need

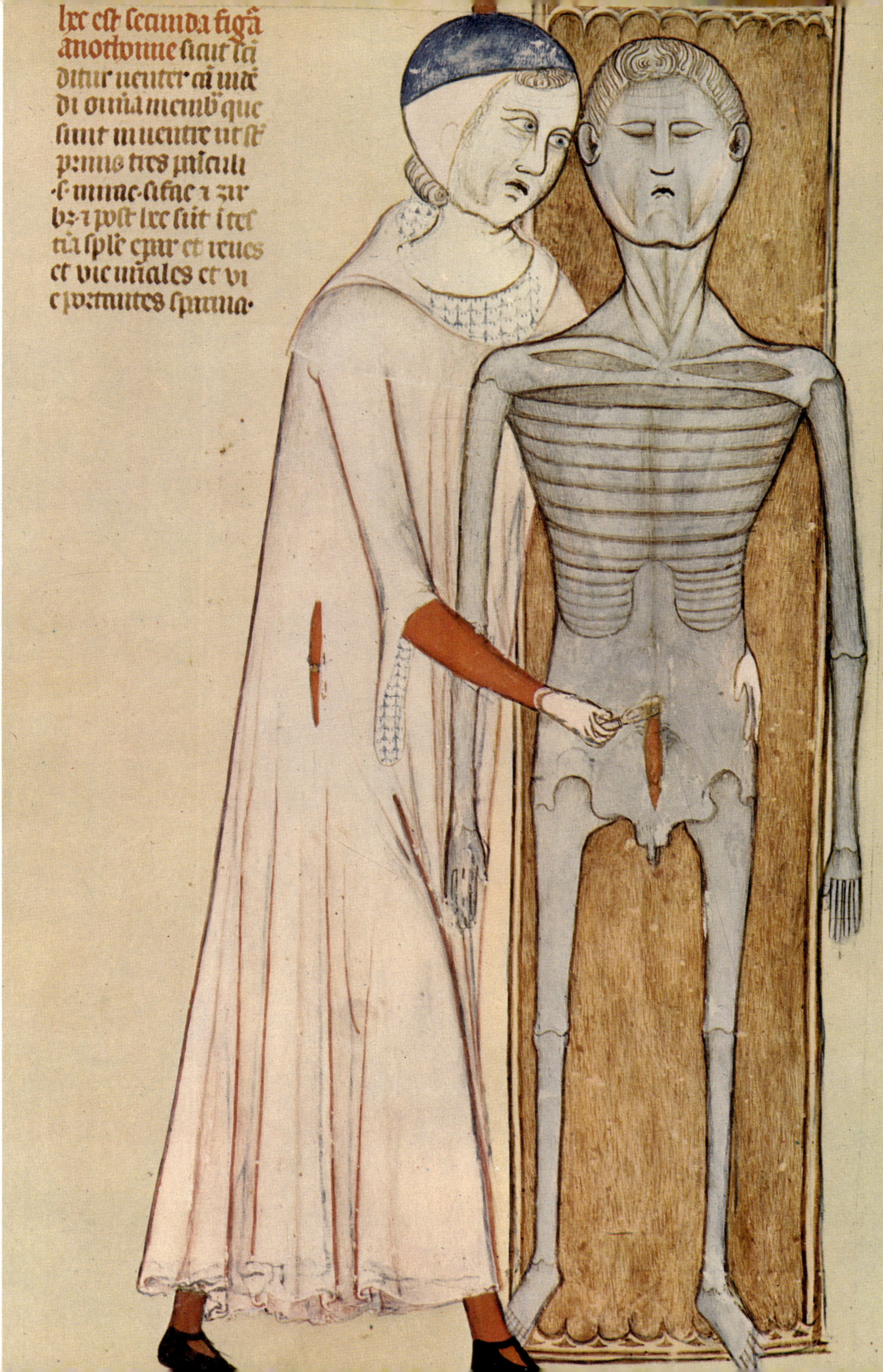
hec est secunda figura
anothomie sicut sci
ditur venter cum vide
di omnia membra que
sunt in ventre ut sunt
primo tres panniculi
scilicet mirac sifac et zir
bus et post hec sunt intes
tina splen epar et renes
et vie urinales et vi
e portantes sperma.

Anatomy started to flourish in the thirteenth century. We have records of an autopsy carried out at Bologna in 1302 that must have required a considerable knowledge of anatomy, presumably gained from the dissection of corpses. The subject advanced in the early fourteenth century under Mondino de Luzzi, but anatomy did not become an independent study in the universities until the sixteenth century. During the Middle Ages, dissections were often carried out in public and were sometimes spectacular occasions.

Mondino de Luzzi directing dissection. *Woodcut frontispiece from Mondino's Anathomia, 1493. Putti Collection, Rizzoli Institute, Bologna.*

Mondino in the chair at a dissection. *Engraving from Fasciculus medicinae by Johannes de Ketham, 1493. Putti Collection, Rizzoli Institute, Bologna.*

only say he is a doctor for people to put blind trust in him. Yet falsehood is more dangerous in this art than in any other. Beware: anyone may be deceived, so great is the power of hope. There is no law punishing homicidal ignorance and no punitive precedent. They learn and it is we who foot the bill; they become expert as they kill. Only a doctor can commit murder and get away with it. Most merciful Father, think of that band as of enemy forces. Let the memory of the man who chose this for his epitaph bear witness, "I died of a surfeit of doctors". The elder Cato's prophecy seems at last to have come true, with ruin following on the heels

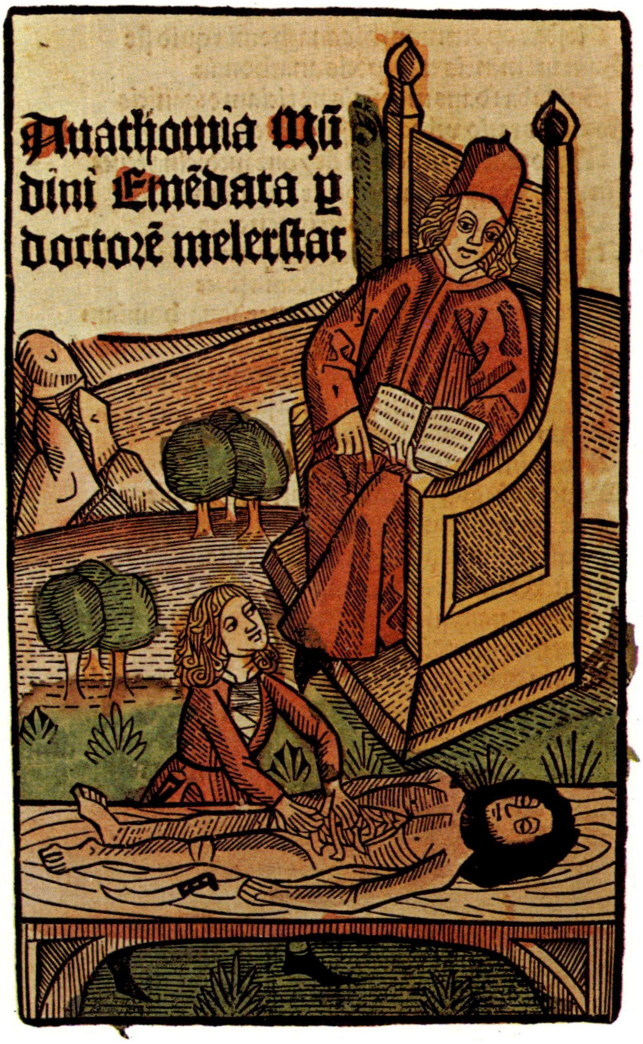

of the Greeks and their learning, especially their medical men. Having got to the stage when men dare not do without doctors, although countless nations manage without them as well and better than we do, and in good health. . . . then find yourself a single one who is worthy, not on account of his manners, but on account of his knowledge and integrity.

'Their art is almost forgotten ... as if their business were not with ill-health but to bring people round to their point of view. They crowd the sick-beds of the unfortunate, high-flown phrases flowing from their lips. A poor sick man dies and all they do is discourse of Hippocratic this and Ciceronian that, trying to turn all occasions – however tragic – to their own advantage. . . . . In conclusion, let me say that from a doctor intent on his eloquence and not on advice, you must guard your life as you would from an assassin or sly poisoner. Plautus was right, in the *Aulularia,* when the cook was told, "Be off with you! I pay you as a cook not as a chatter-box!" For the rest, take care of your health, doing what is good and needful to that end. Be of good cheer and hopeful if you wish yourself, and the Church and us – suffering with you – to be well again. And may God keep you.'

It is a moving letter, its only fault being that so good a poet should have known people so poorly; for he should have realized that the Pope had already joined the ranks of those for whom 'so great (was) the power of hope' that they 'dare not do without doctors'. Clement V promptly showed the letter to Guy de Chauliac, who later issued a counter-attack. Other writers of the time had portrayed the doctor as a figure of fun: he was said to be so intent on showing off his fine new clothes, that he thought he had done quite enough when the urine was examined and the most propitious hour and day for blood-letting decided on. It would have been all to the good if Guy de Chauliac's conduct had been such as to save doctors from being satirized by Petrarch.

The most promising pupil of Lanfranchi's Paris school was a Fleming, Jan Yperman, whose work helped to promote the cause of medicine in the Low Countries. The Paris school was in fact greatly influenced by the teachings of the German Dominican Albert von Bollstaedt (1193–1280), famous as St Albertus Magnus, who recognized the work of Aristotle as the basis of knowledge.

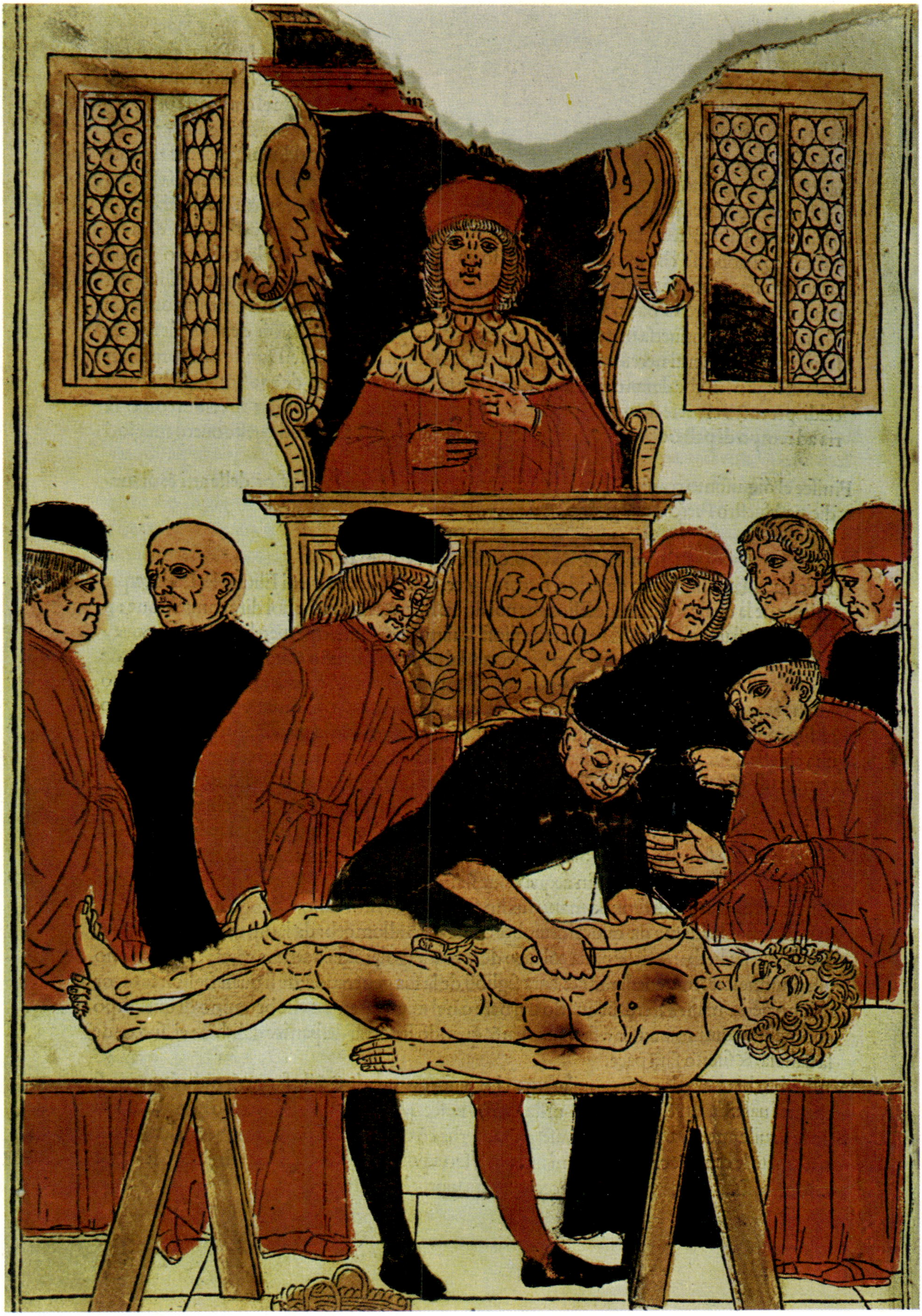

In the Middle Ages, the practice of medicine was often linked with the Church. This was particularly true of mediaeval England – the earliest doctors learned their craft in Church schools on the Continent, and afterwards remained in the Church. Subsequently only clerics could enter the training schools, and they studied under the direction of the Church. Surgery and gynaecology were not thought to be suitable for clerics to undertake, and cases needing such treatment were the province of the barber-surgeons and midwives.

The stultifying effect of the Church prevented any great advances being made in medicine; study was concerned with theory rather than practice and there was a great shortage of working doctors. A consequence of this was the popularization of medical know-

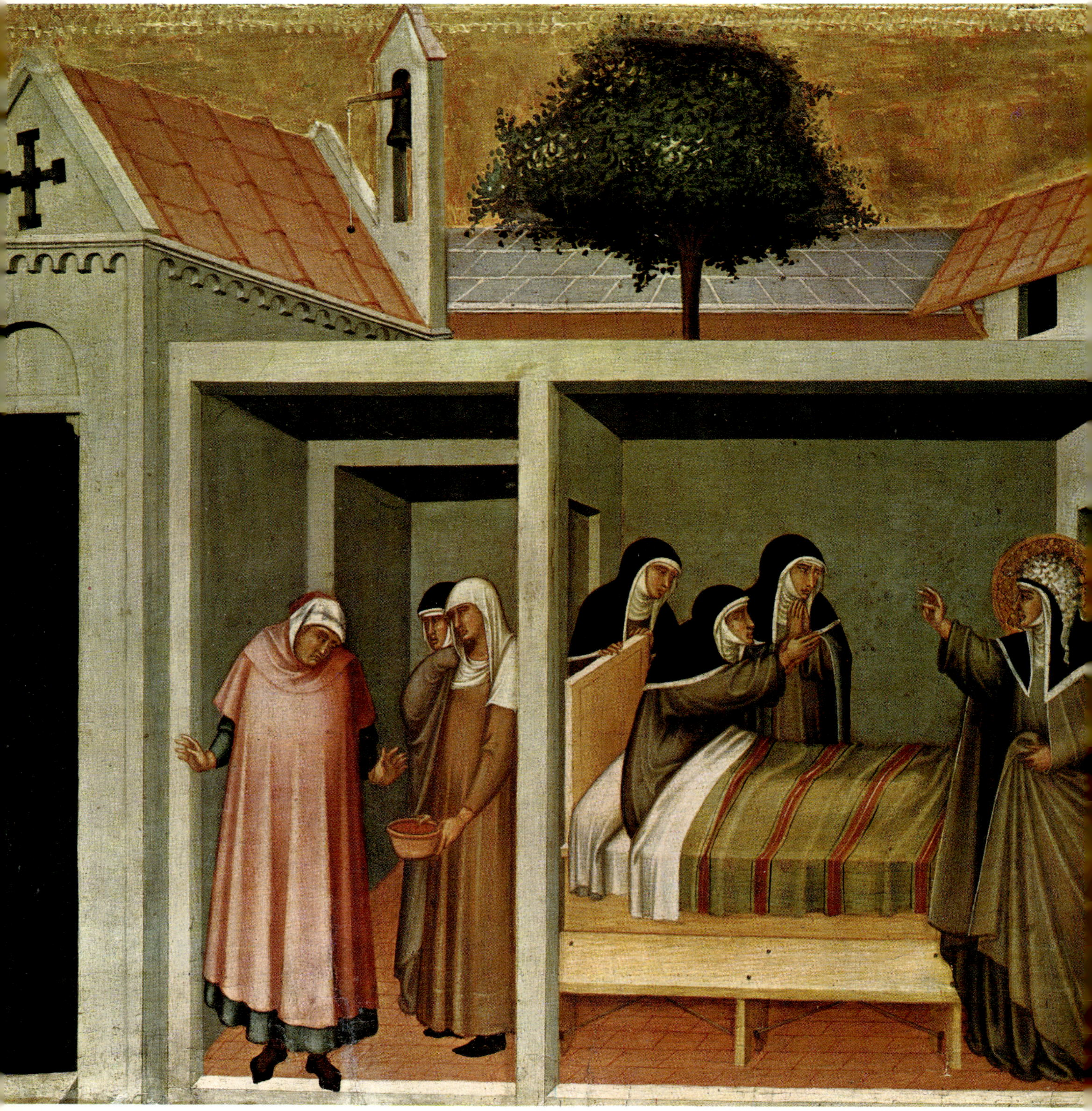

ledge for wide consumption, as happened with the school of Salerno.

The best-known mediaeval English physician was John of Gaddesden. His work, Rosa anglica, *helped to make the medicine of the Arabs better known in England. It is possible that Gaddesden was the model for the character of the learned doctor in the* Canterbury Tales *by Chaucer.*

The doctor gives up treatment on account of the seriousness of the illness. *From Pietro Lorenzetti, Storie della Beata Umilte, detail from a predella. Pinakothek, Berlin.*

Mediaeval England

In mediaeval England, medicine came strongly under the influence of the Church; the earliest well-known physicians, products of cathedral or monastic schools on the Continent, remained clerics. Even subsequently, when students went to the French universities, they still studied under ecclesiastical direction and since none but clerics could be admitted for training, the English and French medical professions were officially celibate. Degrees and university appointments in England could only be obtained by married men at the end of the fourteenth century, and since surgical and gynaecological cases were regarded as unsuitable for clerics to treat, they could not be dealt with by physicians. Barber-surgeons and midwives thus exercised their skills independently, and in addition the latter had to act as intermediaries when a woman patient was to be treated by a doctor. The basic uniformity of medical education prevented any really new works being written; at the same time study was far more theoretical than practical, with emphasis being placed on scholastic rather than clinical ability. There were several important consequences of this trend. The first was a great shortage of practising doctors; villages and small towns had to continue to use the services of the folk healers or leeches, who had a vast lore of herbal and other remedies. Another was that medical works on every imaginable subject were translated from Latin into English. A third effect, also to do with the popularization of this knowledge, was the incorporation of medical facts into the poetry of such writers as Chaucer and Lydgate, something that paralleled the Salernitan school and its *Regimen*.

A number of English physicians of the Middle Ages are known to us today through their own writings and through those of others. The most famous of these was John of Gaddesden, who lived from 1280 to 1361. A fellow of Merton College, Oxford and prebendary of St Paul's in London, he became physician to Edward II. He wrote a medical work called the *Rosa anglica* (the English rose–not to be confused with the work by Gilbertus Anglicus), of which he said rather confidently, 'As the rose excelleth all other flowers, so this book excelleth all other'.

John of Gaddesden helped to make Arabic medicine better known in England, for the *Rosa anglica* contained many quotations from Arab as well as Greek sources. Geoffrey Chaucer (1340–1400) may well have used Gaddesden in the *Canterbury Tales* as the model of his learned doctor who knew the work of Arab writers on medicine. Both Chaucer and Gaddesden were in the service of the Crown, and so were probably acquainted. In the Prologue to the *Canterbury Tales*, which describes, in the style of the *Decameron*, pilgrims passing the time by taking it in turns to tell a tale as they journeyed to the saint's shrine at Canterbury, the learning of the Man of Phisik was described thus:

With us ther was a Doctour of Phisik,
In al this world ne was ther noon him lik
To speke of phisik and of surgerye;
For he was grounded in astronomye.

Wel knew he th' olde Esculapius,
And Deiscorides and eek Rufus,
Old Ypocras, Haly and Galien;
Serapion, Razis and Avicen;
Averrois, Damascien and Constantyn,
Bernard and Gatesden and Gilbertyn.

A great influence on thought in thirteenth-century England was the Franciscan Roger Bacon (1214–1292), who was known as Doctor Mirabilis. Unlike Albertus Magnus, who upheld the Aristotelian approach, Roger Bacon saw this as a grave danger to knowledge, on the ground that the best way to know was to find out by experience. Roger Bacon taught in Paris, and many stories about him tell of his invention of the magnetic compass and of gunpowder, though both these had in fact been invented earlier. He returned to England where, because of attacks on the Franciscans and Dominicans, he was imprisoned and released only shortly before he died.

In spite of the real advances made, many of the medical writers of this period were highly superstitious, and many of these believed in astrology. What went on in each part of the body was supposed to be determined by the influence of a particular planet or constellation of the Zodiac; the sun ruled the right side of the body and the heart, the moon ruled the left side and stomach, Venus ruled the neck and abdomen, Jupiter the lungs, liver, hands and feet, and so on.

The Black Death

When the terrible epidemic known as the Black Death arrived in Europe, astrologers rapidly reached agreement over its cause, stating that it was the result of the conjunction of Saturn, Jupiter and Mars. The Franciscan monk Michele di Piazza wrote that the plague was spread 'propter infectionem hanelitus' (by infection of the breath). This statement is significant in using the term infection for the first time, though in too generic a sense to have a specific implication.

The Christian Era has witnessed three pandemics of plague. The first spread through Europe from the East during the reign of Justinian in 542 and 543; the second, the Black Death, reached England in 1348; while the third, which began in 1894, resulted in very few cases in the British Isles.

All these plagues were characterized by enormously high death-rates. There is little documentary evidence to give a reliable figure for the casualties of the first, but it has been estimated that a quarter of the population of Europe, or twenty-five million people, died in the Black Death; in some parts the population was reduced by three-quarters in the first pestilence. The nineteenth-century pandemic started in China and on reaching Hong Kong in May, 1894 spread rapidly throughout most parts of the world; in Europe and America deaths were comparatively few, but in the ten years following its arrival in India it claimed nearly ten million victims.

Like the first pandemic, the Black Death came from the East. It is thought that the first Europeans to be affected were the Italian merchants who traded in central Asia and fled from the Tartans to Caffa (now Feodosiya) in the Crimea, which was a Genoese trading port. Caffa was besieged for three years, during which time the plague broke out among the Tartars. Dead bodies were catapulted inside the walls, and after the Tartars had dispersed, those of the Italians that survived returned home in a ship, apparently healthy but in fact carriers of the deadly pestilence which immediately broke out in Genoa.

From Genoa the plague spread throughout Italy; the start of its progress was described by Fra Michele di Piazza, the author of *Historia Sicula ab anno* 1337 *ad annum* 1361 (History of Sicily 1337–1361):

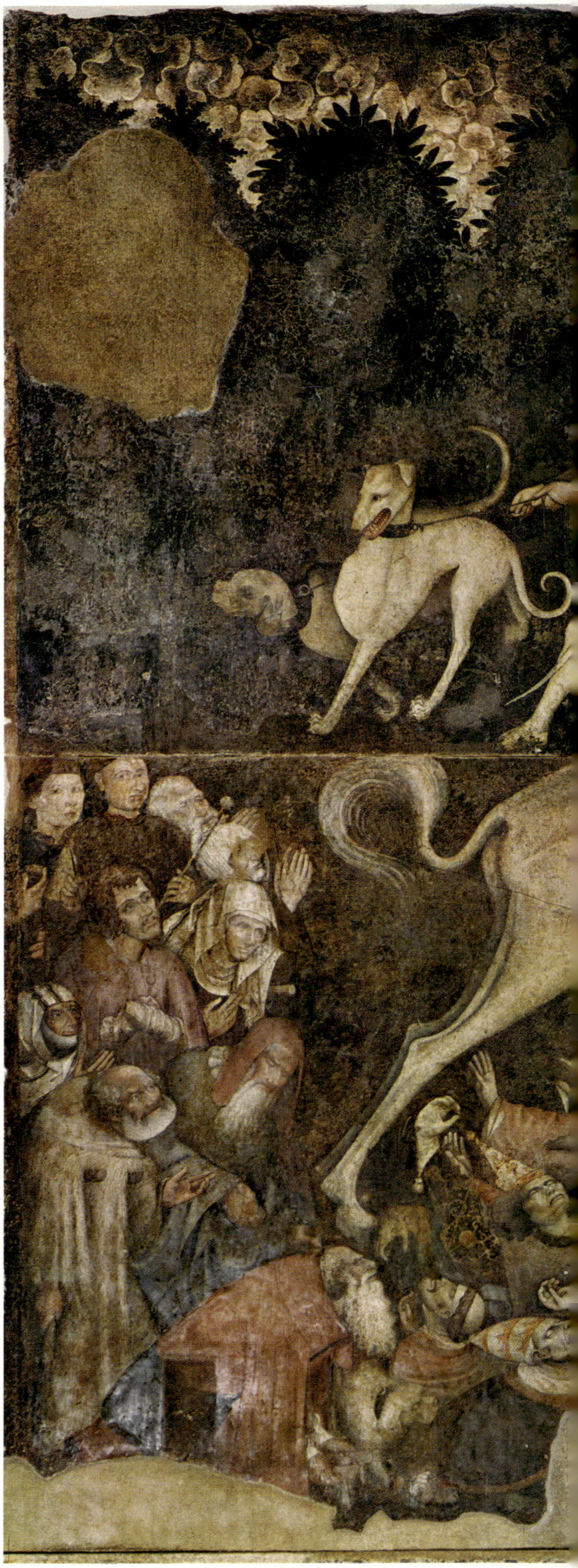

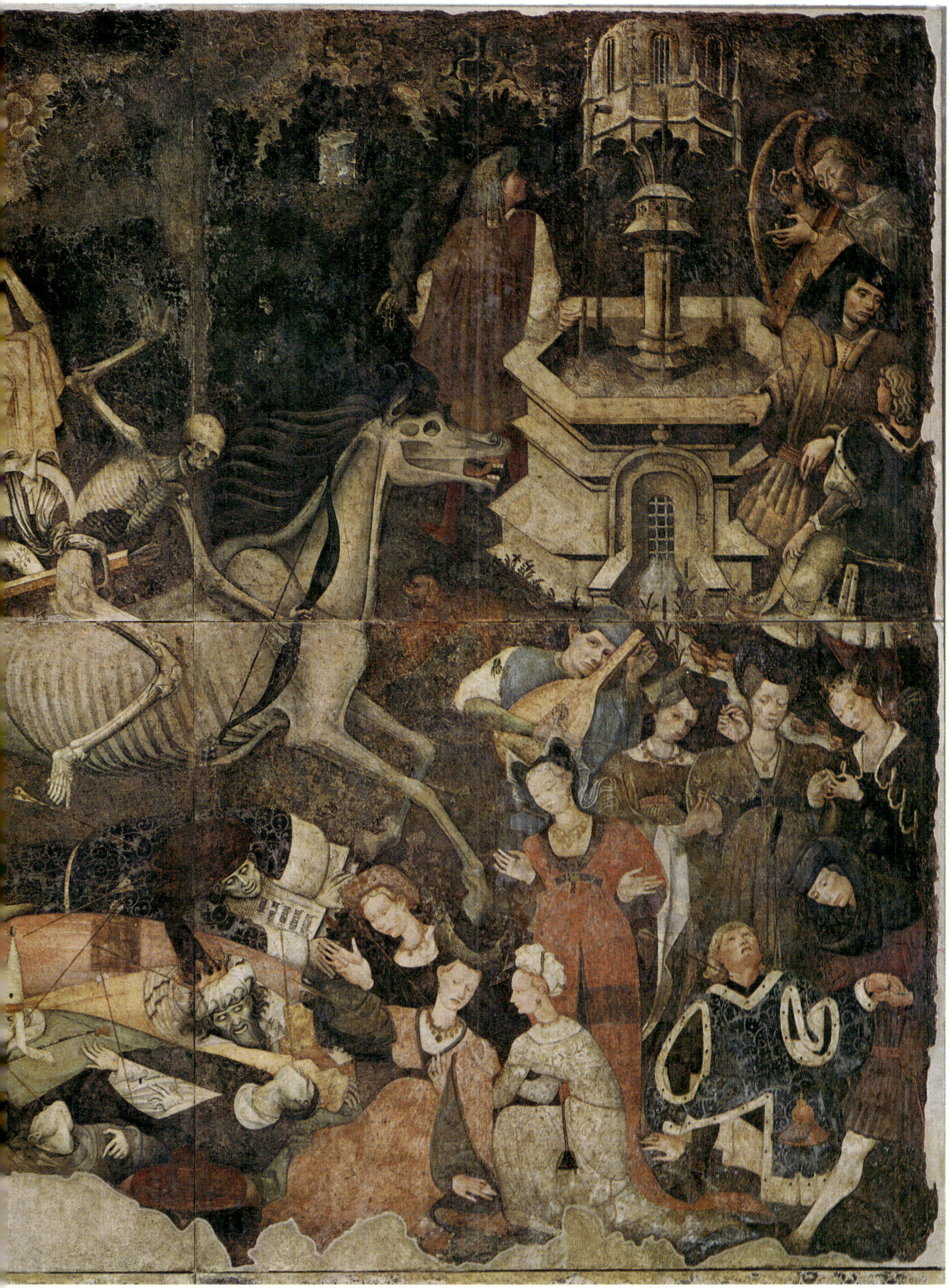

Previous pages:
The triumph of Death. *Fresco of the Catalan school, fifteenth century. National Museum, Palermo.*

This page:
The plague in 1348 at Florence, described by Boccaccio. *From the Parisian-Italian codex of the Decameron,* c. *1380.*

The plague at Tournai in 1349. *Gilles le Muisit, ms. Royal Library, Brussels.*

Three terrible plagues have spread through the world since the time of Christ. The first came from the East and spread through Europe in 542 and 543. The second was the infamous Black Death, which came from the East and reached Europe in 1347. This plague is estimated to have killed about 25 million people in Europe, or a quarter of the population. The

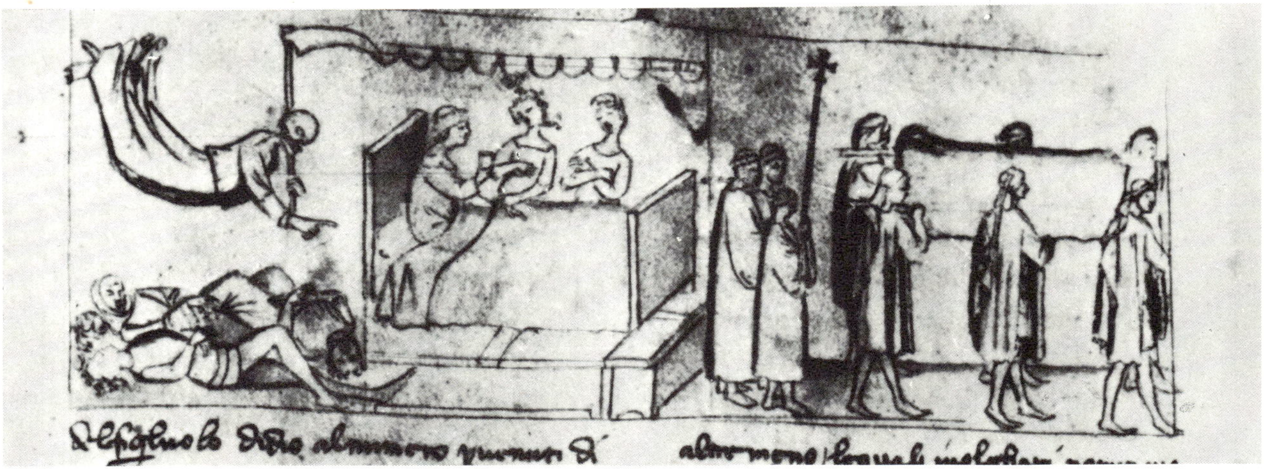

'In the first days of October 1347, the year of the Incarnation of the Son of God, twelve Genoese galleys fleeing before the wrath of our Lord over their wicked deeds, entered the port of Messina. The sailors brought in their bones a disease so violent that whoever spoke a word to them was infected and could in no way save himself from death. Those to whom the disease was transmitted by infection of the breath were stricken with pains all over the body and felt a terrible lassitude. Then there appeared, on a thigh or an arm, a pustule like a lentil bean. From this the infection penetrated

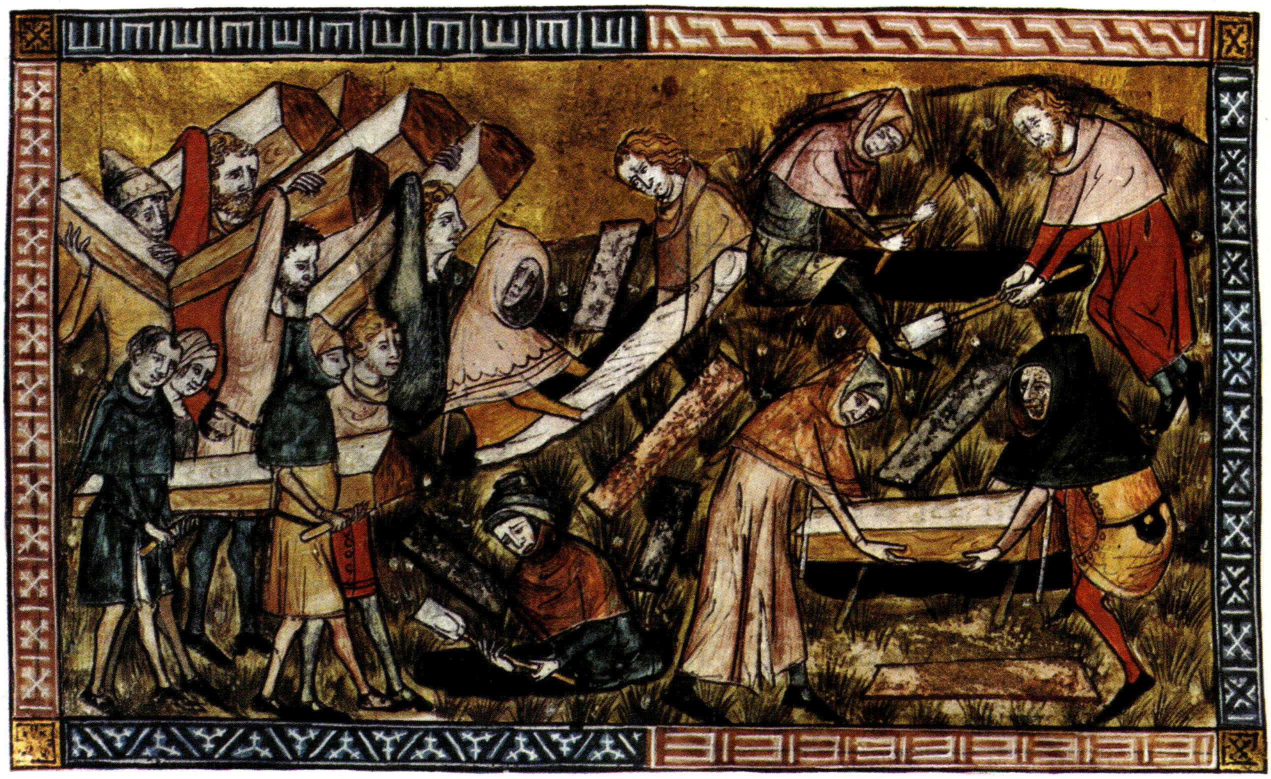

third plague began in China in 1894, and spread rapidly through most parts of the world.

The despair caused by the Black Death had several manifestations. One was the rise in Italy of bands of people calling themselves Flagellants. These fanatics travelled about the country flogging themselves with whips, imagining that their suffering would move the Lord to take away the plague. Another was the killing of Jews and lepers (meaning almost anyone with a skin disease) as scapegoats. After the plague, an outbreak of dancing mania or St. Vitus' dance occurred in Germany. It was a kind of communal hysteria of epidemic proportions, and spread to France and the Low Countries.

the body and violent bloody vomiting began. It lasted for a period of three days and there was no way of preventing its ending in death'.

The Genoese ships were subsequently expelled from the port but the infection remained, depopulating the town.

Plague reached Florence in 1348. Giovanni Boccaccio wrote about it and its deleterious effect on morale: '... heavy drinking, debauchery, singing and trivial amusements, and sating the appetite with anything that was fancied became the normal way of life, Whatever happened was received with laughing and joking, a certain remedy for so great a curse. People truly exerted themselves to this end, day and night, calling now at this tavern, now at that, drinking anything and in great quantity, and doing the same in their houses, behaving in a way that was agreeable to them and for their own enjoyment'.

Boccaccio confirmed what Michele di Piazza had written: 'This trouble struck such terrible fear into the hearts of men and women that brothers deserted each other, an uncle left his nephew and a sister left her brother; women often abandoned their husbands and worse, incredible though it is, fathers and mothers acted towards their children as if they were not their own, by refusing to see them or look after them'.

The first English town to be affected by the plague, in August 1348, was Weymouth, and from here the Black Death spread through the West Country and reached Bristol in a few weeks. Spread eastwards occurred rapidly, and London was attacked three months after the arrival of the disease. East Anglia and the North were affected in the following spring and summer. By the end of 1349 the Black Death was over, but it had had the devastating effects of reducing the English population by perhaps a third, and of establishing epidemic plague, which persisted for a period of three hundred years.

We know, from many contemporary accounts, of the grave demoralizing effect of this terrible pestilence on superstitious people ignorant of its nature. This extract from the chronicle of an Irish friar conveys the sense of desolation and despair of the times:

'I, Friar John Clyn, of the Order of Friars Minor, and of the convent of Kilkenny, wrote in this book those notable things which happened in my time, which I saw with my eyes, or which I learned from persons worthy of credit. And lest things worthy of remembrance should perish with time, and fall away from the memory of those who are to come after us, I, seeing these many evils, and the whole world lying, as it were, in the wicked one, among the dead waiting for death till it came—as I have truly heard and examined, so have I reduced these things to writing; and lest the writing should perish with the writer, and the work fail together with the workman, I leave parchment for continuing the work, if haply any man survive and any of the race of Adam escape this pestilence and continue the work I have commenced'.

Demoralization resulted in disturbances of collective behaviour. Thus, among other grotesque developments, there arose the confraternity of the Flagellants. In dark cloaks, with a scarlet cross on their breasts, these fanatics passed in procession through the towns and countryside, flogging themselves with three-tailed lashes in the belief that the Lord would be moved to compassion by their suffering and would remit the plague. Wherever they went, the Flagellants made converts and these frenetic bands themselves became a plague, committing vandalism, looting, arson and rape. On reaching Avignon, they were threatened with excommunication by Pope Clement V.

The Flagellant movement was of Franciscan origin and came from Umbria, from where it spread to various places. It is of interest that the Flagellants founded hospitals, including one at Bologna, in 1260, and at Imola, Ferrara and Treviso, among others.

Preventive measures in the years when the plague was devastating Europe were on a very small scale, as might be expected with populations so resigned to their fates. In some towns the authorities attempted to isolate the plague-stricken away from any dwellings, and to isolate for ten days anyone who had treated those infected by the contagion. Milan and Venice refused access to any suspect persons or goods. Strict quarantine regulations (that is forty-day isolation) were introduced in the tiny Dalmatian republic of Ragusa (Dubrovnik) somewhat later, in 1377. Doctors, for their own protection, had adopted a mode of dress that made them look rather like great birds of prey; the

Apart from the Black Death and its aftereffects, several other epidemics hit Europe in the Middle Ages. On a small scale, epidemics of ergotism, known as St Anthony's Fire, occurred when a certain fungus infected the crops. An unusual epidemic took place in England after the victory of Henry VII at Bosworth Field in 1485. It was caused by a fatal disease known as 'sweating sickness'; Henry's coronation was delayed because several important councillors died. A serious epidemic of syphilis broke out in Naples in 1495 and slowly spread through Europe.

Physicians were powerless to treat these infectious diseases, and people turned to superstition. Scrofula, tuberculous enlargement of lymph glands in the neck, was known as 'king's evil' and was treated in England and France by the king's touch. According to English

effect was heightened by a beak-like facepiece that was in reality a sponge soaked in vinegar and aromatic substances held in front of the nose.

'Leprosy' and other epidemics

As the imagined aides of the devil, who was assumed to be the cause of the plague, Jews and lepers became scapegoats. Thus in many parts of Europe, but especially Switzerland and Alsace, Jews were massacred together with those lepers who had escaped the plague.

Just as 'plague' was used as a generic term for any epidemic, so in the Middle Ages 'leprosy' was the name given to a large number of skin diseases, doubtless including non-infectious conditions such as eczema and psoriasis, as well as diseases like smallpox and syphilis. It is very likely that few of the green-gowned 'lepers' of mediaeval England, who were excluded from public places and made to wear wooden clappers on the ends of their sleeves to warn of their approach, were suffering from the ravages of *Mycobacterium leprae* (the tuberculosis-like organism discovered by Hansen in 1871). Leprosy is in fact contagious, but is spread only with difficulty. The evidence for its existence in this country in the Middle Ages lies chiefly in the description of Gilbertus Anglicus:

'The eyebrows falling bare and getting knotted with uneven tuberosities, the nose and other features becoming thick, coarse and lumpy, the face losing its mobility or play of expression, the raucous voice, the loss of sensibility in the hands, and the ultimate break-up of the leprous growths into foul running sores'.

It seems that in this country true leprosy died out completely by the fifteenth century. Certainly, some of the accounts of 'venereal leprosy' in the reign of Edward III resemble nothing so much as secondary syphilis.

After the plague a new epidemic broke out in Germany; this was the dancing mania. It spread hysterically, at first to people in places where there were victims of St Vitus' dance. It raged through the Low Countries and northern France; the priesthood tried exorcism, convinced it was caused by collective possession by devils.

Another epidemic disease which was widespread and much feared during the Middle Ages was the holy fire or St Anthony's fire (ergotism). This manifested itself as progressive gangrene of the limbs and ended in serious mutilation and death. It was first mentioned in the middle of the ninth century, and there were at least six outbreaks up to 1129. The name 'St Anthony's fire' was given during the Middle Ages when some sufferers were miraculously cured while praying at the tomb of St Anthony, at a church in the French Dauphiné. It was then realized that the epidemic broke out in years when rye ripened badly; the condition has almost disappeared now, thanks to advances in the processing of flour and the discovery of the causative agent, *Claviceps purpurea,* a fungus which infects the grain and produces a toxic substance.

Towards the middle of the fifteenth century, a serious epidemic disease broke out in England; this was 'sudor anglicus' or the 'English sweating sickness'. The first outbreak took place among the victorious forces of Henry VII after Bosworth in 1485. It spread rapidly all over England, affecting the young and fit, and the devastation was so great that, as Holinshead wrote, 'scarce one amongst an hundred that sickened did escape with life; for all in manner as soone as the sweate tooke them or in a short time after yielded up the ghost'. It recurred in 1507 and 1517, with a tendency to spread to Calais, and, most virulent of all, in 1529, when Europe as far as Vienna, together with the Turkish army besieging it, was devastated. The last outbreak took place in 1551 and remained confined to England.

John Caius, president of the Royal College of Physicians of London, wrote in 1552 an account of the sickness which was in fact the first English monograph on any disease; the symptoms were high fever, shivering, pains in the hands and feet, delirium, profuse sweating, coma and death; some accounts also mention a rash. The cessation of sweating was a very bad sign. The disease remains unidentified, but some authorities have suggested that it may have been a mild form of typhus.

Medicine and suggestion

As is plain, the Middle Ages were exceptionally troubled times. Medicine had little to offer. Pathology was still based on the doctrine of the humours, and so diagnosis rested on examination of the blood, urine and sputum. Consequently treatment *sources, the first king to cure this condition was Edward the Confessor (1002–1066), but the French say that it was Clovis in the year 496, when he was crowned king of the Franks. The practice continued for centuries and was still in vogue in the eighteenth century. William of Orange is said to have touched only one victim, saying 'may God give you better health and more sense'.*

Edward the Confessor curing the scrofulous. *Thirteenth-century English miniature.*

Plague. *Plate by Hans Weiditz for De Remediis of Petrarch, 1520.*

consisted of blood-letting, purging, emetics, enemas and blistering – all debilitating procedures liable to turn the scales against the sick patient. Magic and suggestion were major therapeutic tools, and at a time when impotence, loss of memory, hysteria and other complaints were attributable to possession by the devil or to witchcraft, it was natural that exorcism should come within the sphere of therapeutic practice.

At this time the 'king's touch' began to be used to cure scrofula (tuberculous enlargement of the lymph nodes in the neck) and the custom continued up to modern times. In France, the practice went back to King Clovis, who in the year 496 – according to St Thomas Aquinas – laid hands, at the prompting of an angel, upon the neck of his favourite page, who had been sick for some time, and cured him by pronouncing the words 'I touch you, God heals you'. The formula was used thereafter by all the kings of France. In England, the practice of healing scrofula by the royal touch was introduced by Edward the Confessor, who reigned from 1042 to 1066. Some cures may have resulted, for the practice continued for over a thousand

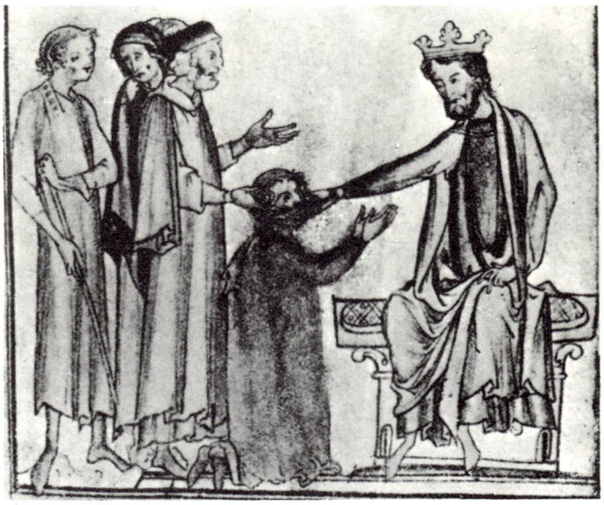

years. John of Gaddesden's writings on scrofula (in the *Rosa anglica*) support the effectiveness of the custom, for after giving advice on drugs and diet, he says, 'If this does not suffice, go to the King that he may touch and bless you; because this disease is called the royal disease and the touch

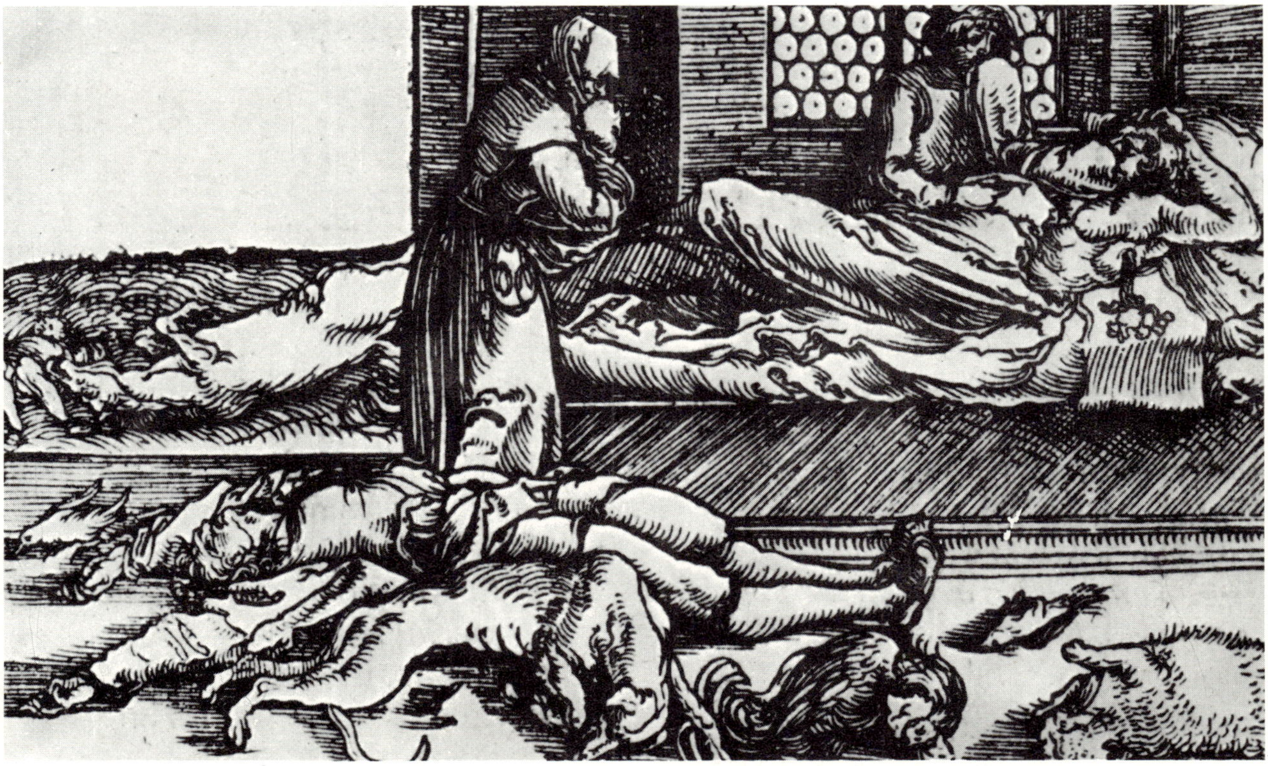

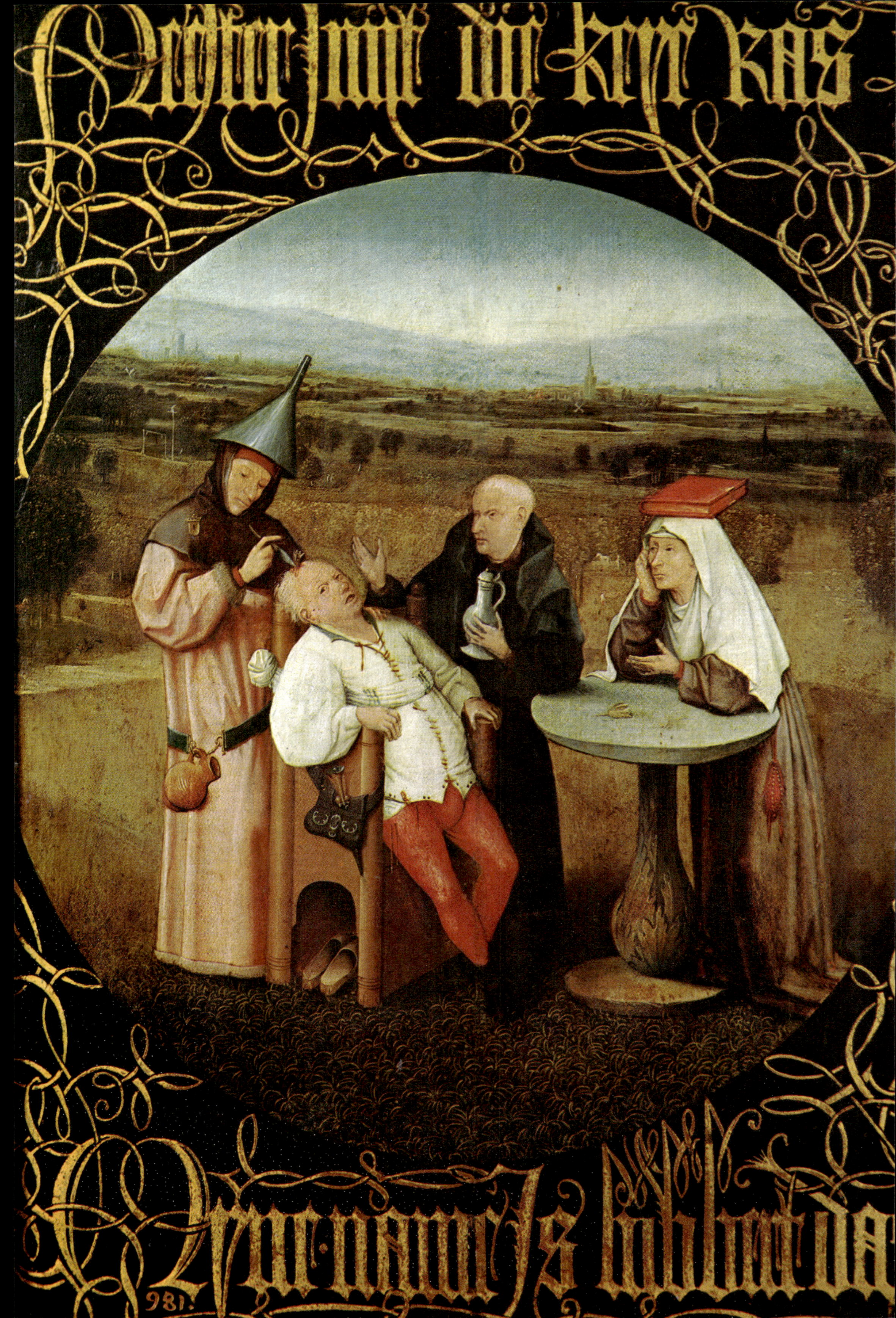

The widespread despair caused by the seemingly endless epidemics of the Middle Ages was fertile ground for the growth of all types of quackery. Some of the strangest of the itinerant charlatans were the stone-cutters, who claimed to cure madness and all mental disorders by removing stones from the head of the sufferer. They would make a small incision in the scalp then by sleight of hand pretend to take out a stone, which was thrown noisily into a basket. It is interesting that as late as the seventeenth century the mentally ill were still described as having 'a stone in the head'.

Removal of the stone of folly. *By Hieronymus Bosch. Prado Museum, Madrid.*

St Vitus' dance. *By Brueghel the Elder, 1564. Albertina Collection, Vienna.*

of the Most Serene King of the English is valuable for it'. He added that if this treatment failed, a surgeon could take over treatment, provided that he took every care not to sever arteries and veins.

The tradition of this healing power as a divine (and therefore a royal) attribute can be traced back to much earlier times. For example, in some representations of Aesculapius, as that in the temple at Athens, the Greek god of medicine is portrayed in the act of placing his hands on a patient. The Roman historian Pliny records that Pyrrhus cured diseases of the spleen by touch, while Tacitus states that Vespasian cured the blind and another emperor, Hadrian, relieved sufferers of dropsy, both by their imperial touch. The Christian tradition of the laying on of hands sprang from these more ancient practices.

Edward the Confessor undoubtedly treated a great number of people for scrofula: the king's household accounts record, for example, 288 subjects touched at Easter, 1277. But after Richard II the practice is not mentioned in the English chronicles until 1462, when it was revived by Henry VI, who also instituted elaborate rituals to accompany the touching, including the distribution of a specially minted gold coin, called the gold Angel, as a touchpiece. In *Macbeth* (IV, 3) written in the reign of James I, Malcolm describes the disease and the treatment:

'Tis called the evil:
A most miraculous work in this good king;
Which often, since my here-remain in England,
I have seen him do. How he solicits heaven,
Himself best knows: but strangely visited people,
All swoll'n and ulcerous, pitiful to the eye,
The mere despair of surgery, he cures;
Hanging a golden stamp about their necks,
Put on with holy prayers: and 'tis spoken,
To the succeeding royalty he leaves
The healing benediction.

Shakespeare records here that the power to heal was said to pass down from reign to reign; it was in fact thought to come to the monarch after his consecration with the holy oil.

Richard Wiseman, the skilled and famous surgeon of the time of Charles II, wrote a classic account of the Evil in which he testifies to the healing power of the king's touch. The ceremony, together with the golden Angels, and later with medals issued as admission tickets, continued through all the reigns up to that of William of Orange, who is said to have touched only one victim, saying cynically: 'May God give you better health and more sense'. Queen Anne later revived the tradition, touching, among others, Dr Johnson – but without success.

The King's Touch had a longer career in France. Louis XVI touched no less than 2,400 sufferers at the time of his coronation in 1775, and the practice was actually revived when Charles X was crowned in 1824, when 121 patients were presented by the two great physicians Alibert and Dupuytren.

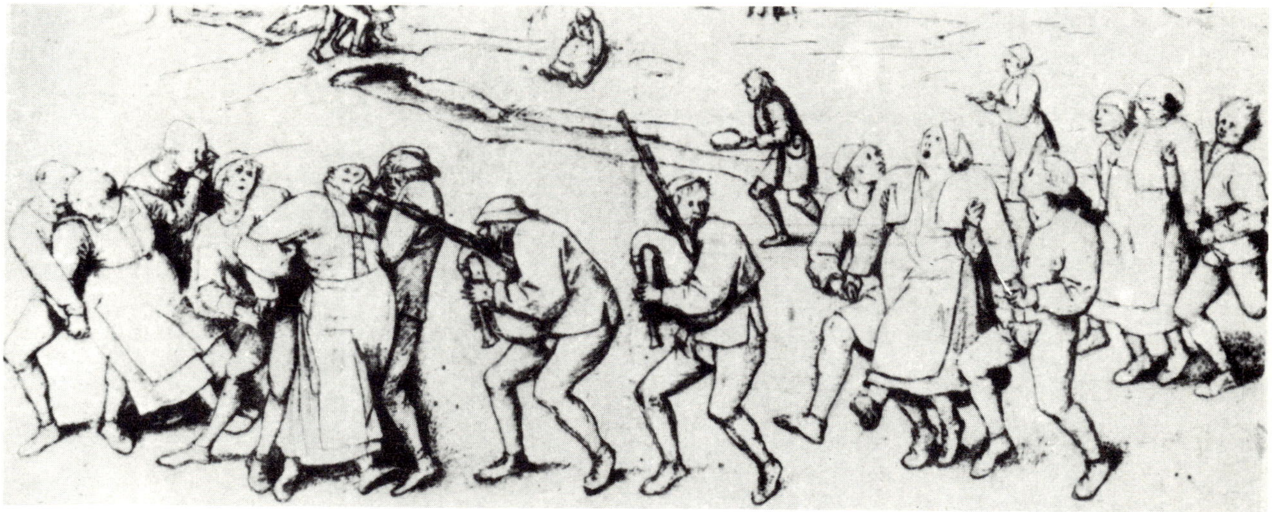

Guilds, pharmacies and hospitals

By the late centuries of the Middle Ages, medicine, still developing along the lines of the school of Salerno, passed entirely into the hands of the laity: Pope Honorius III had in fact forbidden the clergy to practise. The physicians began to organize themselves into professional bodies, with rights protected by the law of the land. This was the period which saw the formation of the guilds, which had strict regulations ensuring that no one could practise a profession without having completed the required course of study and attained the necessary degree of knowledge.

The status of physicians in society improved, but in practice, little had changed. Pathology was still based on the theory of humours, while diagnosis, except in the case of a few rare physicians who made their deductions from their own positive observations at the bedside, was usually based on interpretation of the colour, density and smell of the blood, of the smell and colour of the sputum, and above all on examination of the urine. There were innumerable systems, each explaining how detailed diagnosis of all types of diseases could be determined not only from the colour and odour of the urine, but from the layers of sediment formed in the collecting flask. The diagnosis was often optimistically simple: cloudiness in the upper layer indicated that the seat of the disease was in the head, in the lower layer conditions of the bladder or genital organs.

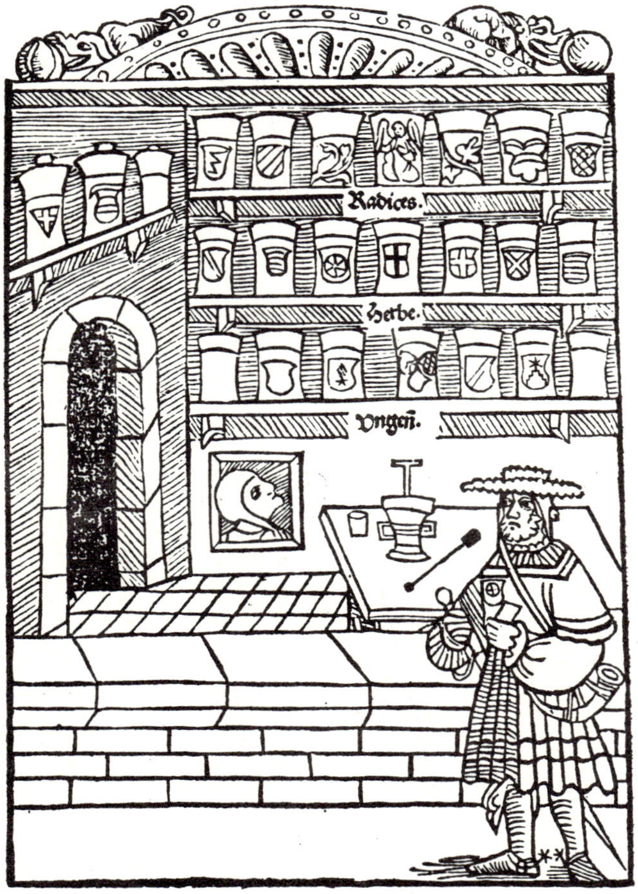

Therapy was still based on the theory of opposites (contraria contrariis), as it had been in Galen's day, so that for diseases thought to be caused by 'fullness' (plethora), blood-letting was the main treatment. This procedure was supposed to deflect the material causing the illness and make it pass from one organ to another. When blood was taken from the side of the body opposite that where the disease was situated it was revulsive, but when taken from the same side as the disease, derivative, tending to relieve the patient's plethora and pain. The most detailed directions were given regarding the most favourable days and hours for blood-letting, the correct veins to be tapped, also the amount of blood to be taken and the number of bleedings.

Blood-letting was often performed at public baths, which were themselves a popular form of therapy, especially in the Germanic countries. The baths were enormous tanks in which the bathers stood or sat, and some were steam-baths, in which the patients were covered to the neck with a cloth while steam was introduced from below. Bathing was often mixed, and was also often made the occasion for feasting and drinking, so that in time it was commonly associated with debauchery. In the early sixteenth century, increasing knowledge of the nature of contagion led to regulations suppressing mixed bathing, and in time the use of common bath tanks died out completely until re-introduced in modern times.

Mention has already been made of the barbers, who performed many of the functions of the doctor, including blood-letting, purging and tooth-drawing, and who were important figures in medicine right up to the seventeenth and even eighteenth century. They had probably begun to gain their importance around 1100, when monks went to barbers for their tonsure and also for

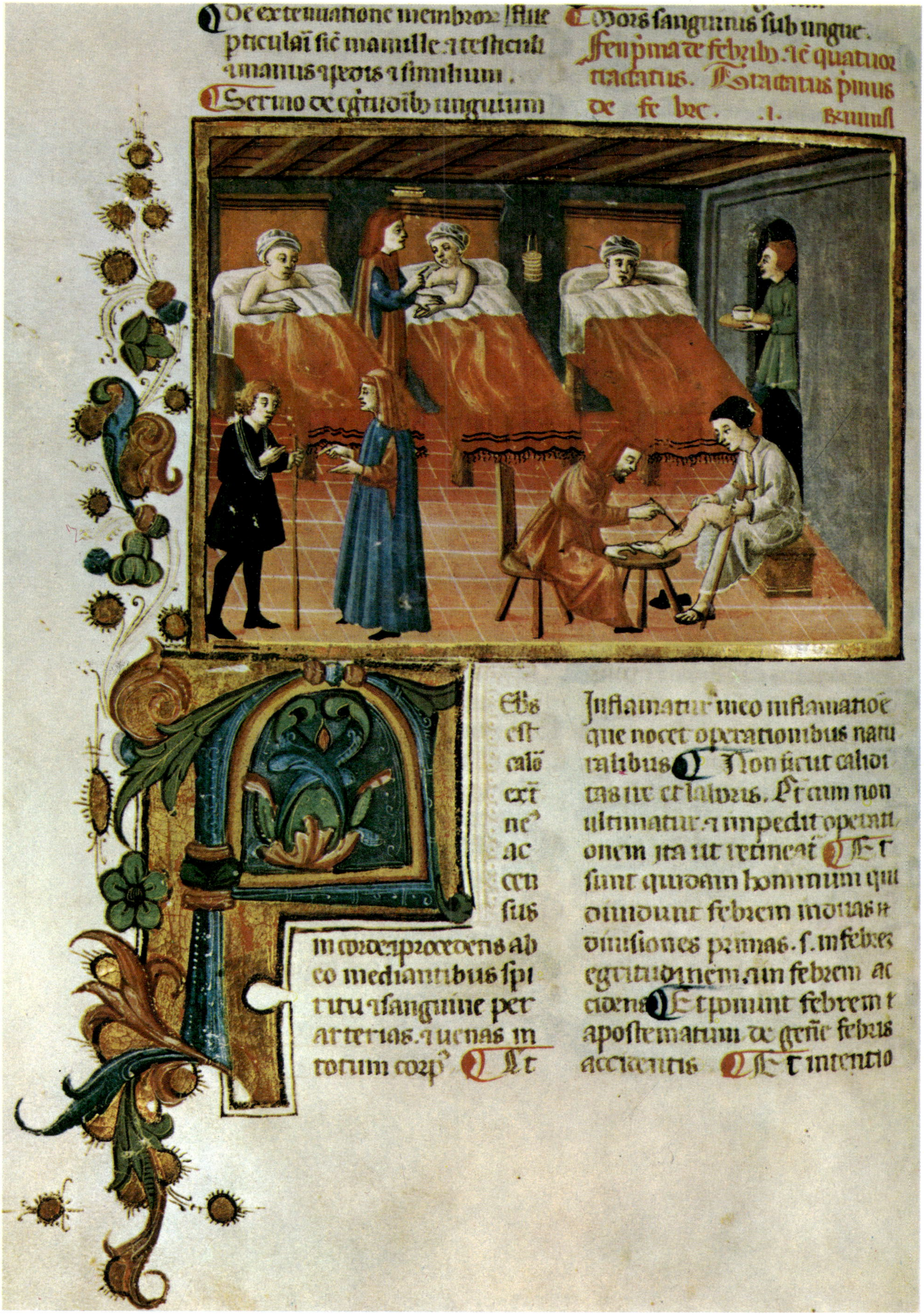

Previous pages:
German pharmacy of the sixteenth century. *From Bossler, Dialogus des Appostolicums, 1521. Bertarelli Collection, Milan.*

Italian hospital of the sixteenth century. *Squarcialupi codex. Laurentian Library, Florence.*

These pages:
Child in swaddling-bands. *Majolica by Andrea della Robbia. Ospedale degli Innocenti, Florence.*

The birth. *From the Story of Griselda by an unknown painter of the fifteenth century. Sforza Castle Museum, Milan.*

By the late Middle Ages, three institutions were established which were to be the foundations for the practice of medicine in Europe for centuries to come, and which, in one form or another, exist to this day. These were the guilds–the forerunners of modern medical associations–pharmacies and hospitals.

The pharmacies, which had their own guilds, first appeared towards the end of the thirteenth century,

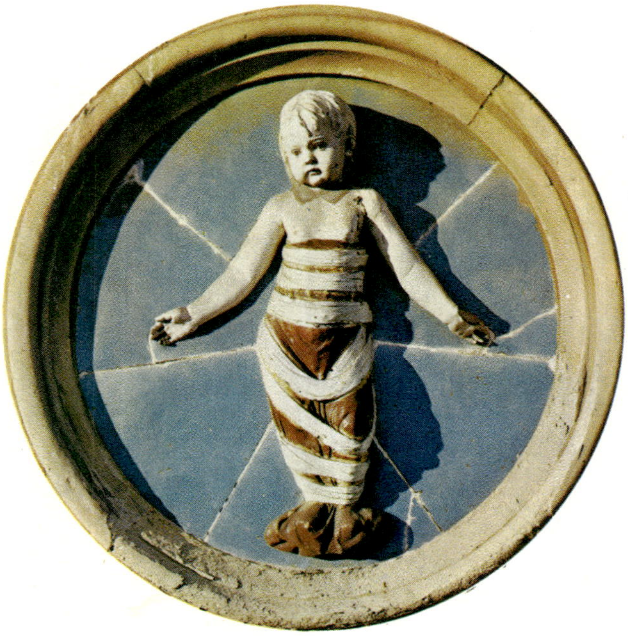

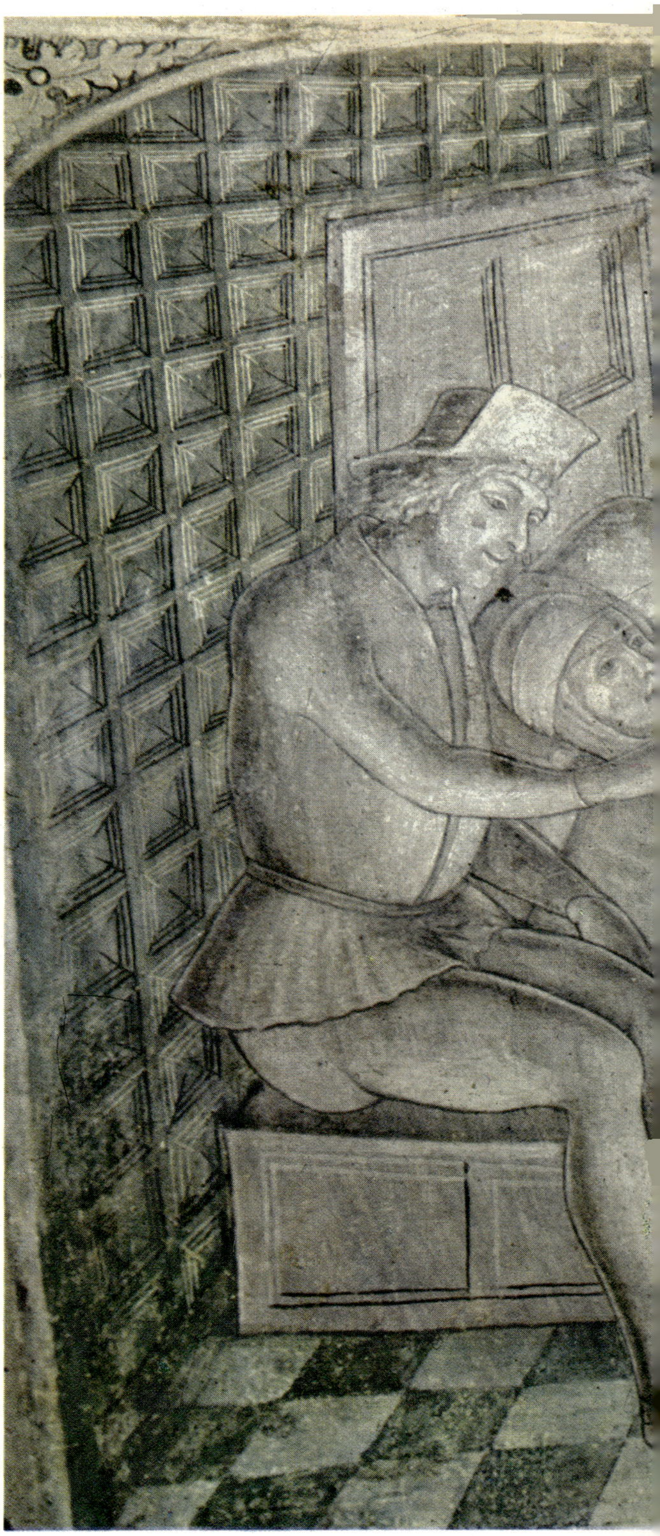

bleeding, which they were required to undergo regularly by church law. By the end of the Middle Ages the barber-surgeons were well established, and in 1505 the faculty of medicine in Paris instituted a course for barbers, to spite the surgeons proper, of whom it was jealous; in time the barbers became more closely associated with the physicians. In England, in 1462, the large and prosperous Guild of Barbers became the Company of Barbers, while the surgeons obtained a special charter in 1492. Under Henry VIII, in 1540, the Barber Company was joined with the small and exclusive Guild of Surgeons to become the United Barber-Surgeon Company.

Italy, towards the end of the thirteenth century, saw the establishment of the first public pharmacies; the statute of the Venetian Guild of Physicians and Pharmacists dates from 1258. Based on the Arabian model, the pharmacies developed originally in the monasteries and courts of rulers, later to become private shops where physicians came not only to buy drugs but also to confer with colleagues and even to see patients. The pharmacist himself was often an astrologer or alchemist who became the centre of a sort of scientific circle.

The drugs used in treatment were drawn from

and were based on the Arabic model. A typical feature was a great number of jars and pots, often of rare and beautiful design, full of various drugs and potions. Each pharmacy also had its special sign, a great wooden counter, and often a wall-niche containing a bust or statue of Aesculapius or Hygiea. Doctors went to pharmacies not only to buy drugs, pointing out the jars with a stick, but often to see their patients. They also went to consult the pharmacist himself, who was often an alchemist or astrologer and a man of some learning.

Physicians also visited the hospitals, which were now quite highly organized, or saw patients in their homes. Women usually had their children at home, but were attended by the midwife rather than by a doctor.

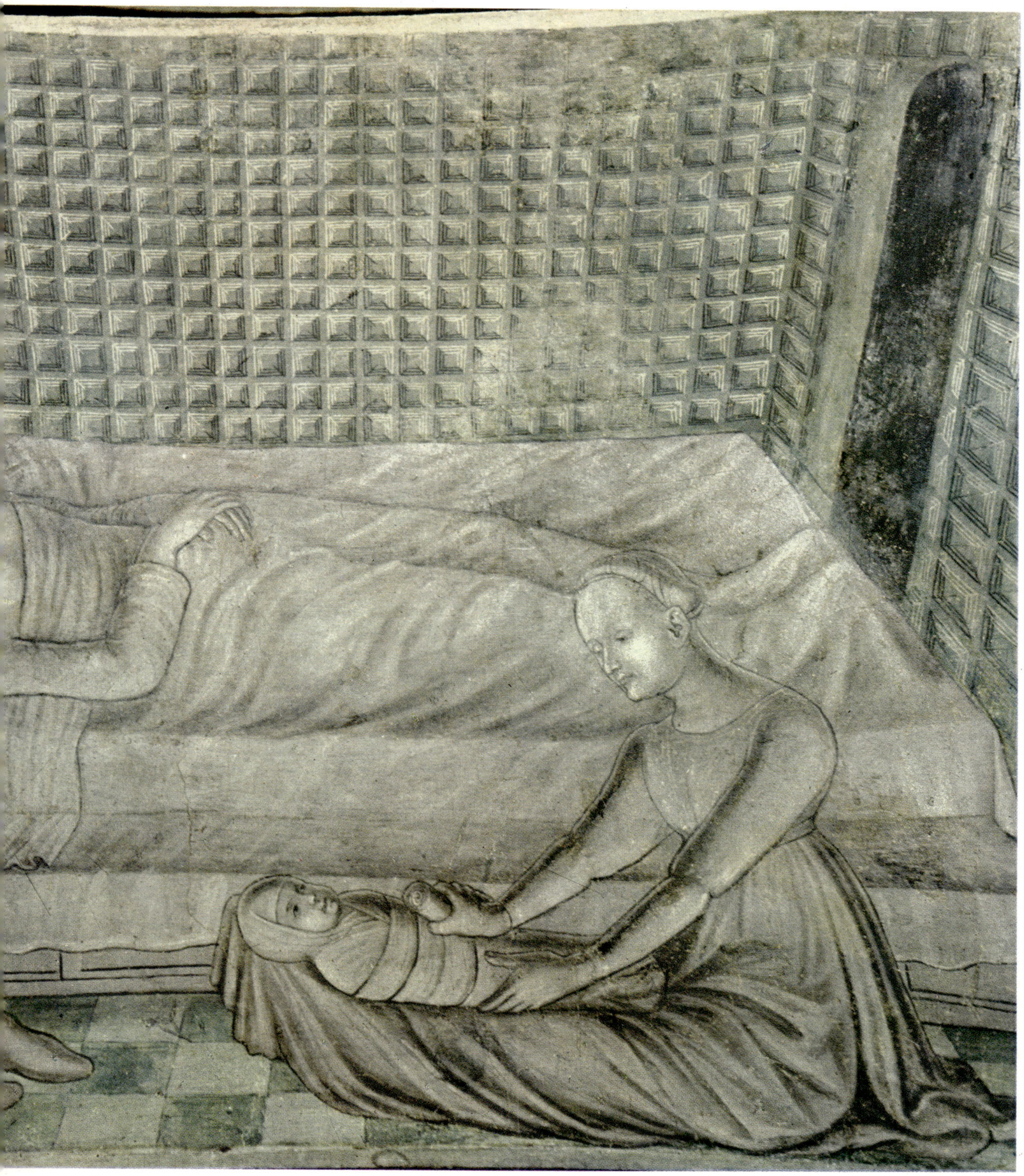

The great hospitals built during the late Middle Ages were the proud achievements of the flourishing cities of Europe, and considerable thought was given to their construction. In Italy, the finest architects were often commissioned to design them, while they were also decorated by some of the outstanding artists of the day. Famous examples are the Ospedale del Ceppo at Pistoia and the Ospedale degli Innocenti at Florence, which have magnificent bas-reliefs in coloured, glazed ceramics by Giovanni and Andrea della Robbia. Although the hospitals had now largely passed out of the hands of the church, the subjects of these works, like the names of the institutions themselves, reveal the profound influence of the Christian spirit; such nursing as existed at this time was invariably carried out by various religious orders.

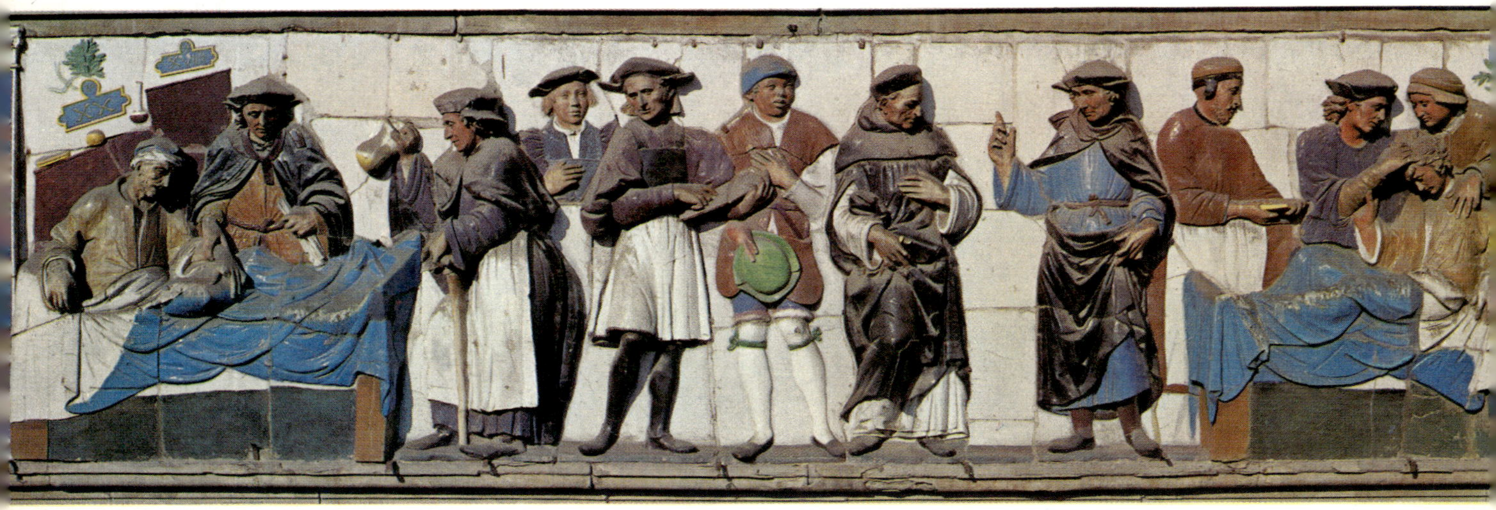

all sources, especially from plants, and many preparations with genuine pharmacological properties were known. At the same time, there was widespread use of various complicated prescriptions containing innumerable constituents from precious stones to vipers' flesh, which had to be compounded according to the most rigid and nonsensical instructions; the most fashionable was 'theriacum', said to have been invented by Nero's physician, which contained fifty-seven substances. Many of the drugs were imported from the Orient, and as they formed light and compact cargoes they became one of the most important factors in the growth of trade and the opening up of new sea-routes.

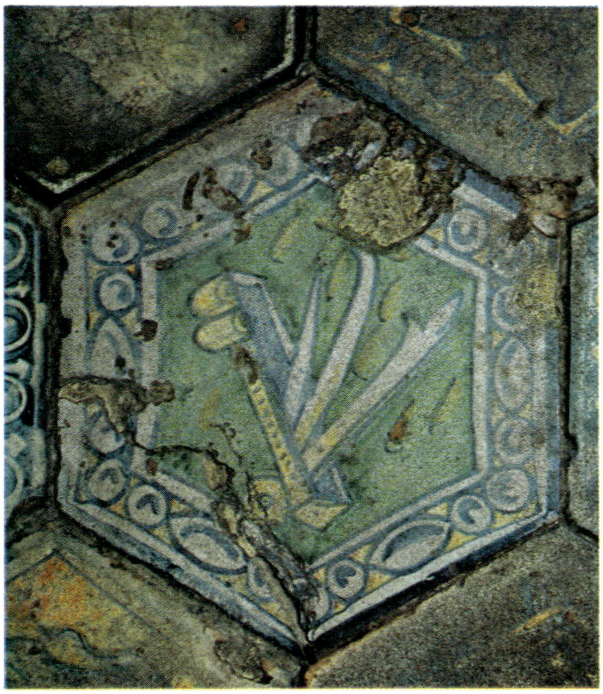

Hospitals can be traced back in one form or another as far as the sanctuaries of Aesculapius in ancient Greece, but the institution as we know it today was probably a product of the Christian principle of charity. The Middle Ages saw the founding of hundreds of hospitals all over Europe and in the lands visited by the Crusades. One of the most important developments was the widespread foundation of leper hospitals; at the height of the epidemic era there were over two hundred in England and Scotland and about two thousand in France.

About the beginning of the thirteenth century, the hospitals began to pass from the hands of the church to those of the civic authorities. This was the period which saw the founding of the great city hospitals, like the Hôtel-Dieu in Paris, the Santo Spirito in Rome and St Bartholomew's and St Thomas' in London. Cities lavished great wealth on these buildings, particularly in Italy, where many of the great architects and artists of the day were commissioned to design them. This inspired patronage formed the foundations of an association between medicine and the arts which was to bear rich fruit in the glorious age of the Renaissance.

Apart from the drugs used, some of which were probably effective but most not, therapy still rested heavily on hygienic measures like bathing, on diet, and on blood-letting, which was thought to relieve 'fullness.' Blood was usually taken by opening a vein with a lancet, but sometimes by blood-sucking leeches or using cupping vessels. Most of these techniques were not without dangers for the very ill.

Visiting the sick. *Majolica by Giovanni della Robbia. Ospedale del Ceppo, Pistoia.*

Lancet for blood-letting, arms of the Manfredi family, Dukes of Faenza. *Majolica of the sixteenth century. Church of S Petronio, Bologna.*

Healing the sick. *Majolica. Ospedale del Ceppo, Pistoia.*

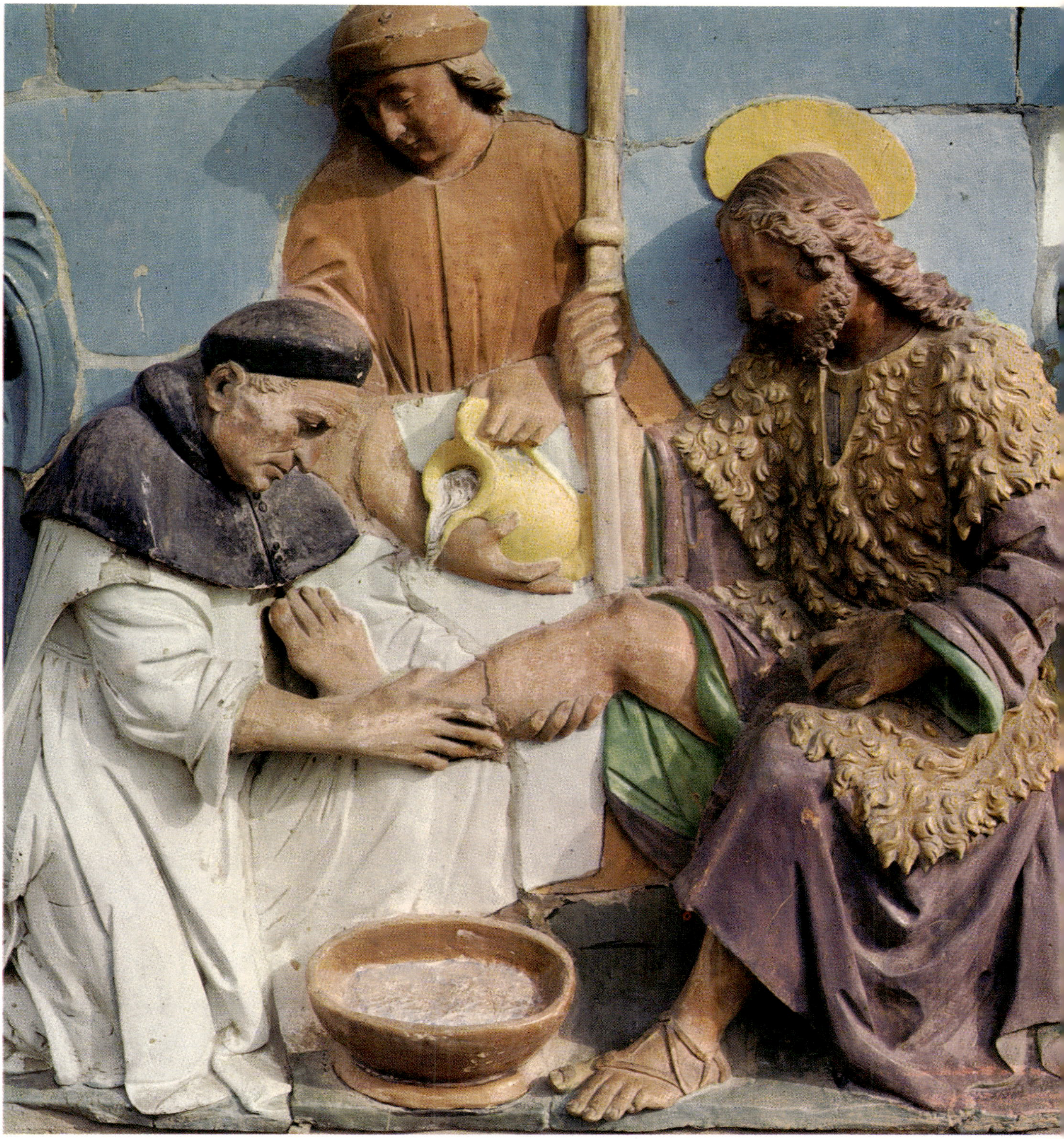

THE RENAISSANCE
Medicine and humanism

With the end of the Middle Ages began a cultural movement characterized by the re-awakening of ancient learning through direct knowledge of Greek and Roman authors. This movement was not confined to the arts and resulted in a new general outlook, with emphasis on knowledge of nature and the view of man as nature's masterpiece. This was the beginning of Humanism, within the wider framework of what is known as the Renaissance.

The movement originated in Italy, from where it spread to other countries. Interest in classical antiquity was cultivated, while metaphysical speculations ceased and the fetters on learning imposed by the mediaeval attitude to religion fell away. There were repercussions in all aspects of life, but especially in politics, in the arts and in science, which prospered in consequence of direct observation of nature. In the fifteenth century observation of phenomena replaced theoretical procedures; science advanced from the dark into new territories. The same held true of medicine.

Many simultaneous events contributed to this revival of learning. The finite world of the Middle Ages disappeared for ever with the discovery of America, the great voyages of da Gama and Magellan and with Copernicus placing the sun at the centre of the universe. Ancient Greek culture and the open-minded rationality of Plato and Hippocrates came to Italy with the scholars fleeing from Constantinople after its fall to the Turks in 1453. Perhaps the most powerful single factor in the spread of knowledge was the invention of printing by Laurens Janszoon Coster of Haarlem and Johann Gutenberg of Mainz. After the sack of Mainz in 1462 the German printers became scattered all over Europe, and presses were set up in many cities, producing books as beautiful as manuscripts but much more cheaply. Medical learning advanced from the dissemination of the ancient knowledge, soon copiously to be printed in superb editions, and from the humanists of the Renaissance, who sought to reconcile all fields of knowledge with medicine and so were equally at home with classical texts and with the sick patient.

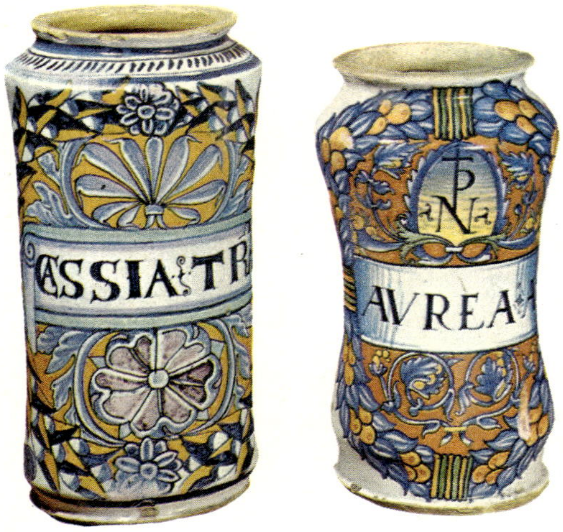

The great physicians of the period, like Niccolo Leoniceno, were humanists and men of letters, and certainly many Renaissance doctors were very different from their mediaeval predecessors. Although astrology was used, and diagnosis and treatment depended on examination of the urine and on blood-letting, and although quacks of every description still flourished, nevertheless the best doctors were held in the highest esteem. For during the Renaissance the physician became a true scholar, the student of natural philosophy who had been freed from Aristotelian dialectics. He was the friend and adviser of princes and the patron of printers and painters.

Doctors were of the wealthier classes. They were educated at the universities, and those of Italy, the cradle of the Renaissance, were at this time at their zenith. Padua in particular received very many foreign students, who were organized into 'nations' (English–later including William Harvey–German, Polish, Hungarian, and others) and strongly influenced academic life. Ferrara and Bologna were other universities with especial attraction for the student from abroad. In these, as at others throughout Italy, great power was placed by the constitution in the hands of the students, who elected their officials and directed the course of studies. This took place at a time when much of Europe was being laid waste by religious wars. In 1565 Pope Pius IV decreed that the doctorate of medicine could be conferred only on Catholics; such ecclesiastical interference with learning could not be tolerated by the independent, and the Venetian Senate, which earlier had granted admission to Padua University to Jews and Protestants, appointed a procurator to confer degrees regardless of

The Renaissance, the great revival of learning which flowered in Italy towards the end of the fifteenth century, was one of the most important events in the history of our civilization. It overthrew much of the dogmatic teaching and metaphysical speculation which had held back learning in the Middle Ages, restoring the rational attitudes of ancient Greek culture. Strongly aided by the invention of printing, which facilitated the spread and cross-fertilization of ideas, it saw huge advances in the sciences, in medicine, and in the arts, producing some of the greatest writers, scholars and artists who have ever lived.

Fifteenth-century pharmacy jars. *Sforza Castle, Milan.*

The healing of the deacon Justinian by Saints Cosmas and Damian. *By Beato Angelico. S Marco, Florence.*

the faith of the candidate. This was in the spirit of the Renaissance, and fifty years later the Venetian Republic broke completely from the Church and founded its own college, conferring state diplomas.

Medical teaching in the Renaissance remained, on the surface, like that of the Middle Ages. Many teachers continued to express conservative views, and Galen and Avicenna were still the standard authors. Nevertheless new attitudes began to make themselves evident. Public dissections were practised in ever-increasing numbers, and although the old custom persisted of reading from the pages of Galen while a dissector displayed the organs, ignoring the discrepancies between text and fact, the anatomical knowledge made available to the medical student increased little by little. More and more teachers carried out dissections themselves, and towards the end of the sixteenth century anatomy theatres began to be built by the universities. Until the end of the century anatomy was always taught together with surgery, and it was only in 1570 that the first separate chairs for the two subjects were created.

Anatomy, the study of which is necessary for a rational approach to medicine, was to be reborn in the sixteenth century with the work of Leonardo and Vesalius, but from the time of Mondino many crude attempts at depicting the organs of the body had begun to appear in print. These sketches might be taken as the first tentative gropings of anatomists in the light of science, but it has been shown that none of the illustrations in books printed between 1478 and 1539 represented original observations or research, and that for the most part they were copies of old manuscript drawings. In the Middle Ages anatomy was usually shown in five schematic pic-

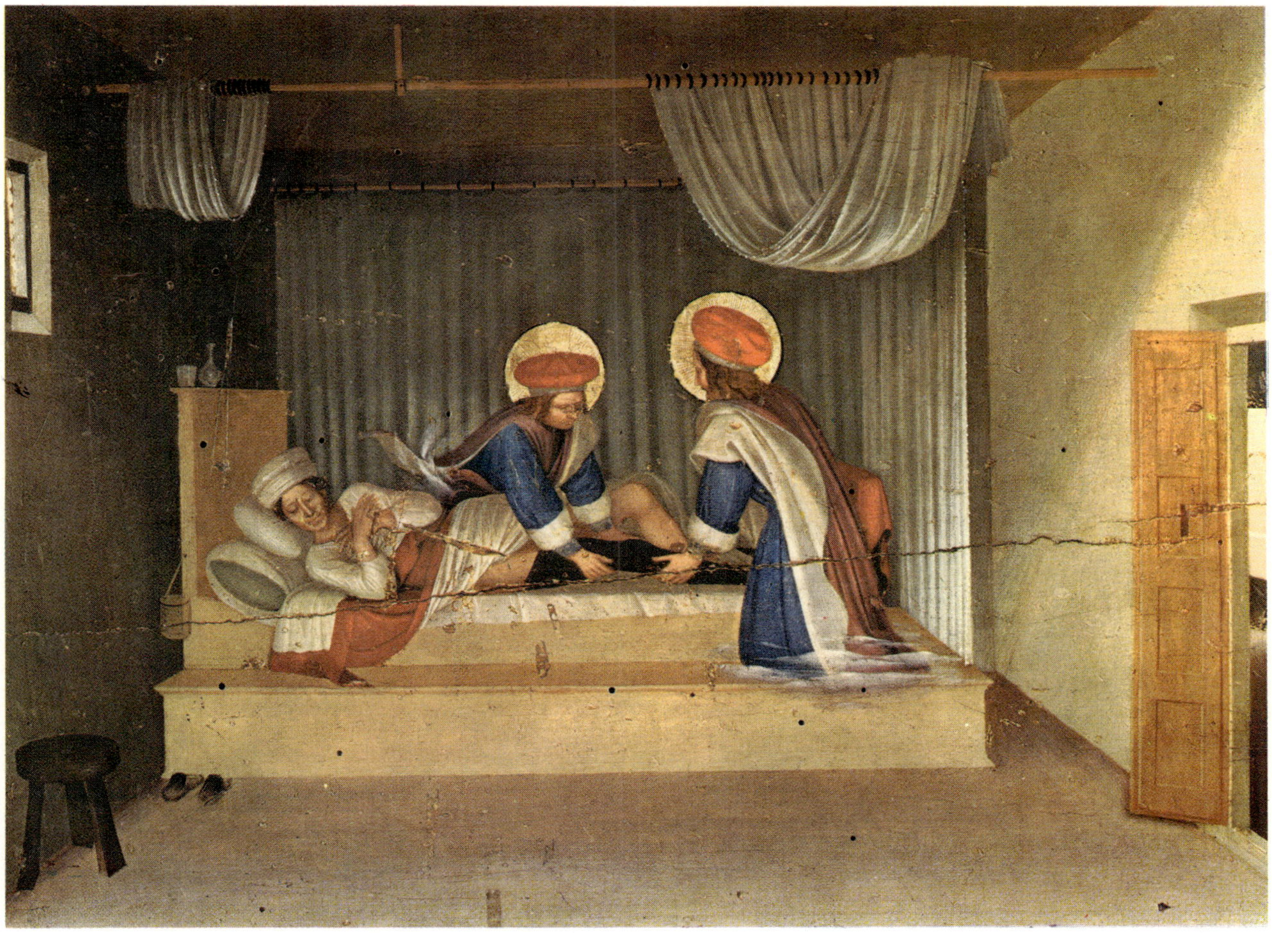

Although medical teaching in the Renaissance retained much of the Galenic tradition of the Middle Ages, there were outstanding advances in knowledge of two subjects–anatomy and physiology–which in time were to have profound effects on the practice of medicine and surgery. Interest in anatomy was shared by doctors with the painters and sculptors of the Renaissance, many of whom were themselves skilled in dissection. In addition, the painters bought their paint pigments from the apothecaries, which thus brought them into close contact with the physicians.

A sick woman in her room. *From Miracles of S Vicenzo Ferrer by Ercole de Roberti. Vatican Gallery, Rome.*

Infants in swaddling-bands. *Detail from The Madonna protecting the Innocents. School of F Carracci. Ospedale degli Innocenti, Florence.*

tures, illustrating the skeleton and nervous, muscular, arterial and venous systems, with the body in a frog-like, half-crouching position. The scheme is found in Persian as well as French and German drawings, while the characteristic position is seen on Chinese acupuncture illustrations as well. Such mediaeval drawings were diagrammatic memory aids, and contained medical folk-lore as well as fanciful ideas. The traditional pictures of the foetus in utero found in works up to the end of the fifteenth century were a thousand years old, while other didactic pictures, such as the zodiacal pictures representing diseases and wounds, were produced unchanged over hundreds of years.

In contrast to these crude and inaccurate drawings produced for, and presumably by, doctors, the portrayal of human anatomy by the great Florentine painters of the fifteenth century had reached a state of high perfection. Perspective, geometry and human proportions were studied assiduously, and an interest in dissection came about through the fact that the painters formed part of the Florentine Guild of Physicians and Apothecaries, an association which Masaccio joined, first as an apothecary and two years later as a painter. Artists bought their pigments from the apothecaries and so came into close contact with the physicians. In this way dissection, strictly regulated by statutes of the university, became a desired means for artists to acquire anatomical knowledge, and perhaps the painters were helped by the doctors. At one end of the time-scale is Giotto's assistant Stefano, who was so successful that physicians would learn where to let blood by studying the veins painted on his canvases; at the other end of this quest for truth stands Leonardo da Vinci.

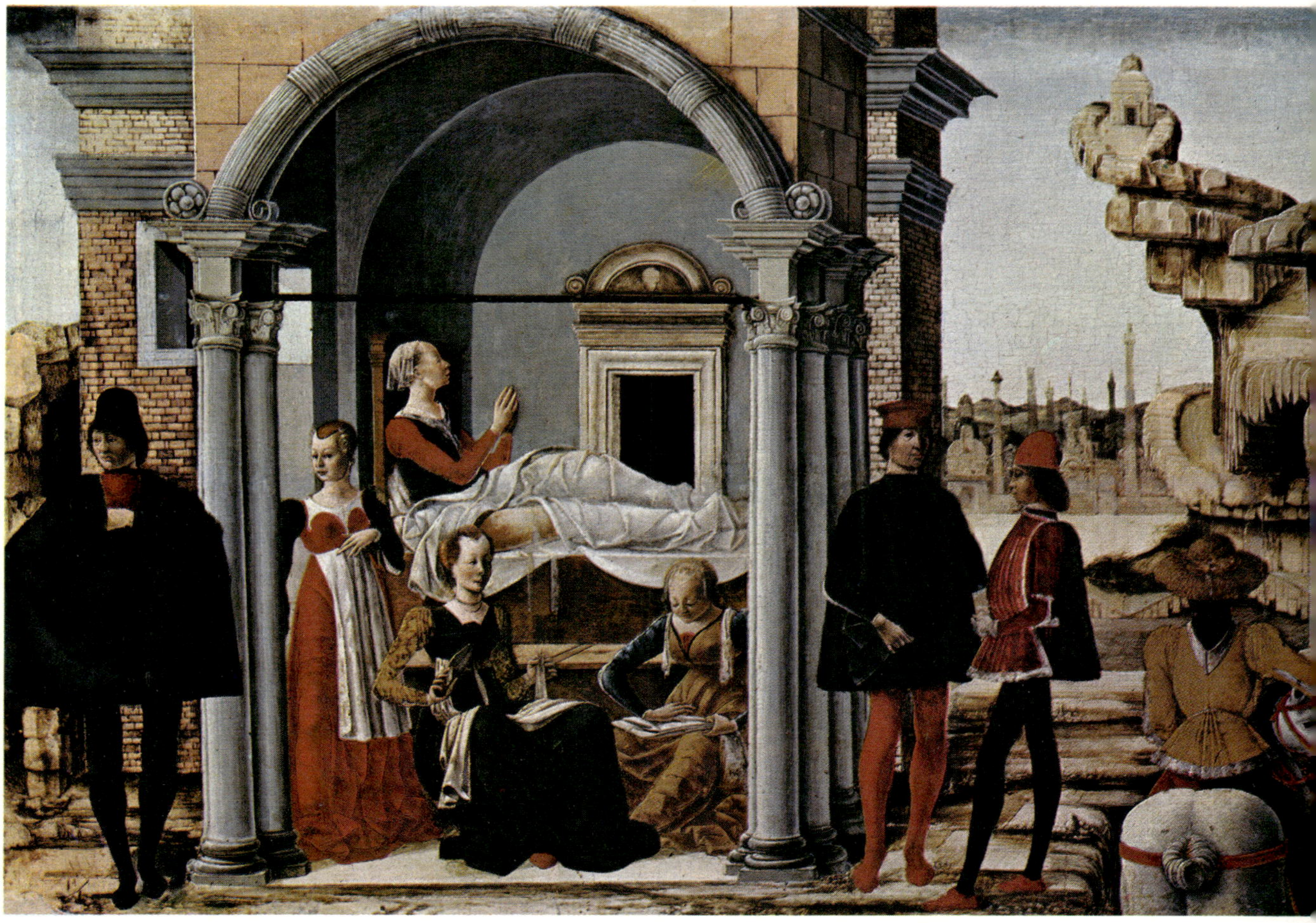

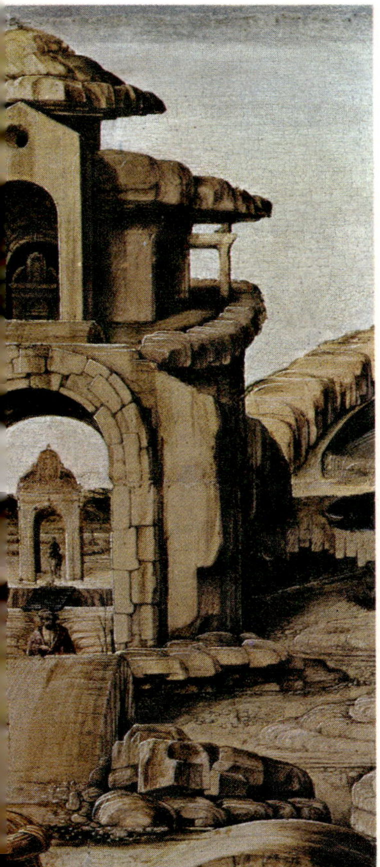

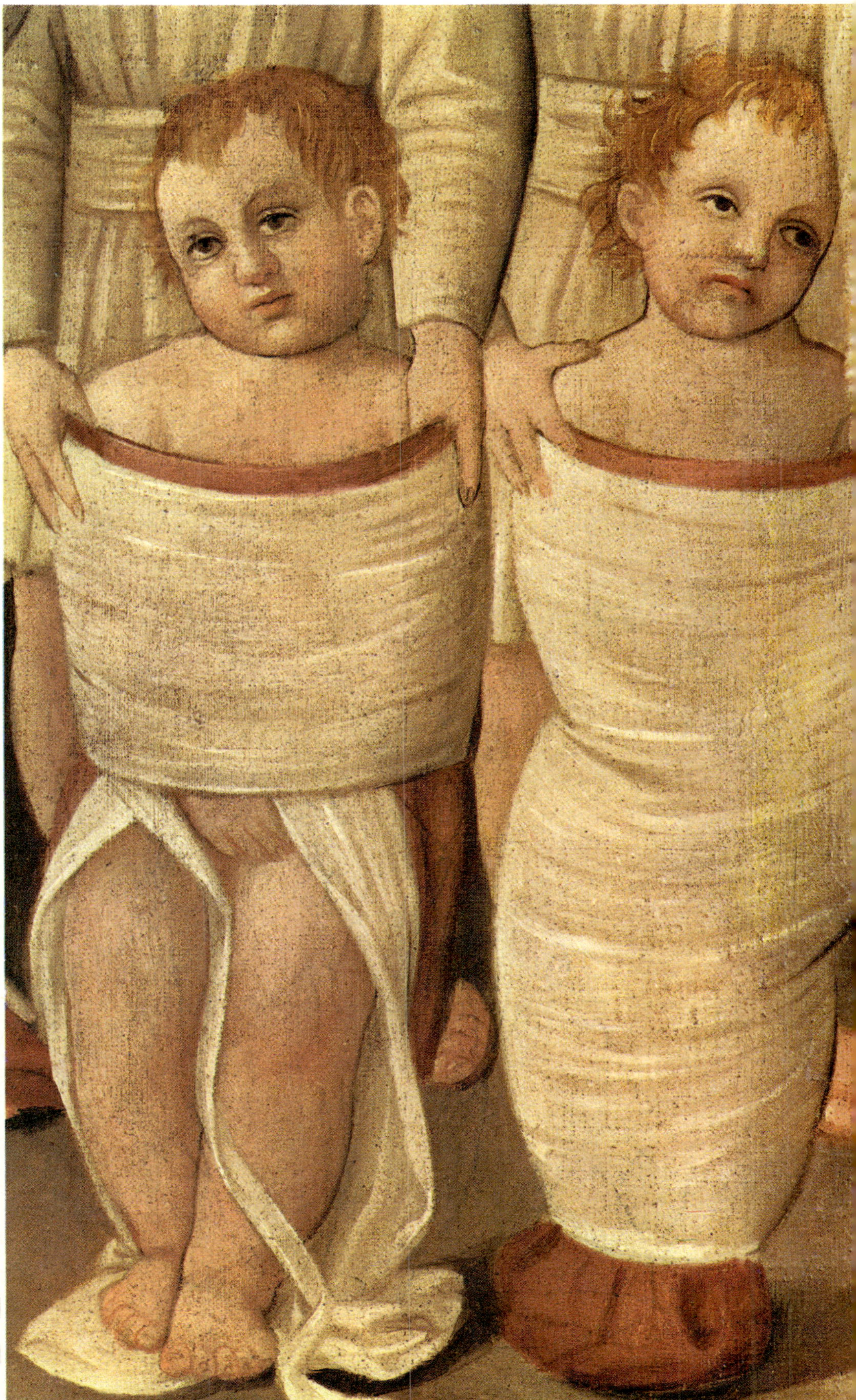

Surgical instruments made in the sixteenth century to designs by Ambrose Paré. *Putti Collection, Rizzoli Institute, Bologna.*
Table of anatomical instruments used by Vesalius. *From de humani corporis fabrica, Basle, 1543.*
Fifteenth-century bistoury. *Putti Collection, Rizzoli Institute, Bologna.*

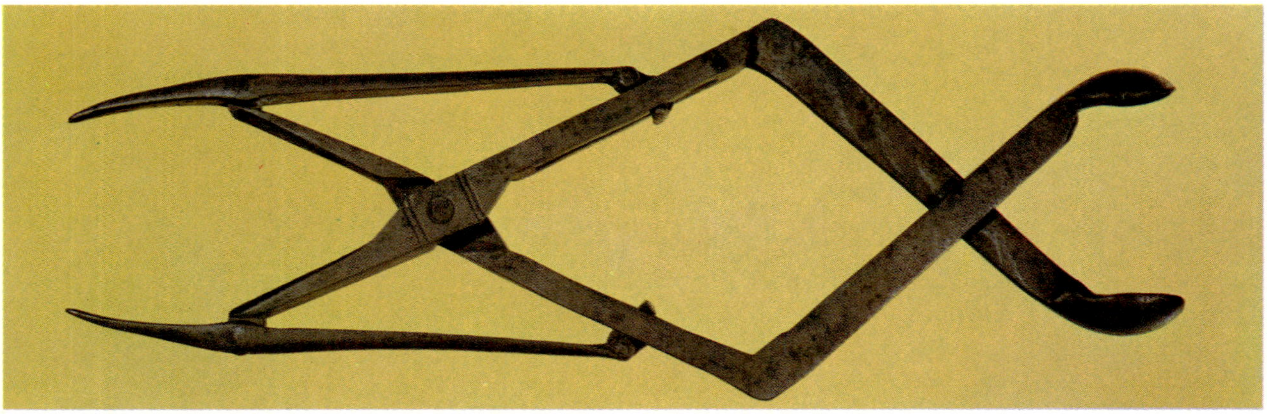

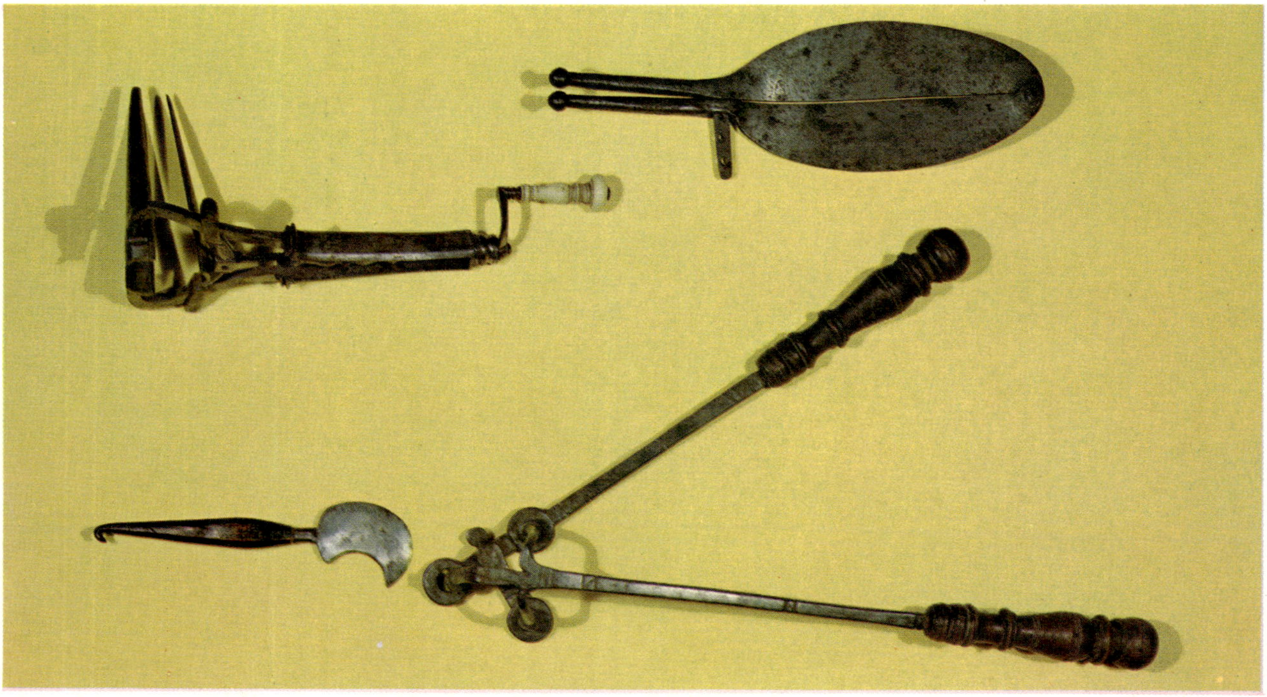

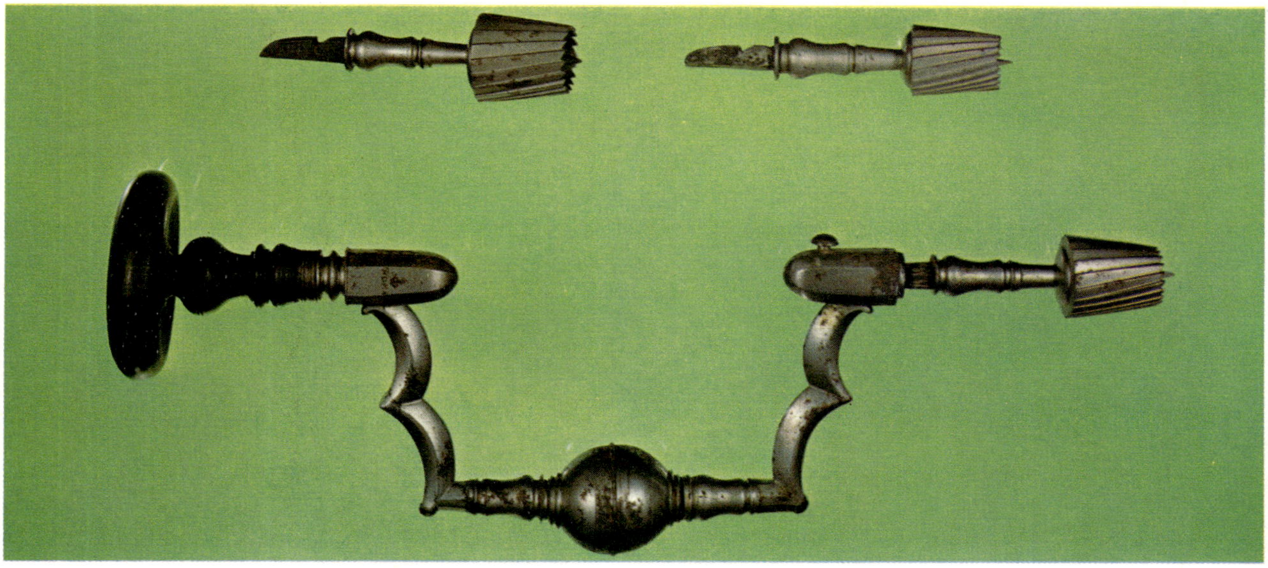

Art and anatomy

Leonardo was a genius who excelled in both the arts and the sciences, and approached anatomy without the preconceptions of others, preconceptions derived from Galen and Mondino, placing trust only in direct observation and experiment. When he was in the service of the Borgia family in Rome he dissected more than thirty bodies by candle-light in the mortuary of the Santo Spirito, producing a thousand drawings of his dissections. One anatomical technique he devised is still employed; he injected liquid wax into the body cavities to reveal their exact structure. By this method he proceeded to study the heart, lungs and womb. He was the first man to attempt to trace the course of the cranial nerves and to dissect the foetal membranes.

Leonardo analysed the muscular system and recognized the specific action of each muscle; he gave attentive study to the valves of the veins which he clearly understood to prevent the back-flow of blood. He also made incomparable drawings of the coronary arteries and their course, but did not grasp correctly the place of the septum dividing the right and left parts of the heart; had he done so he might have discovered the circulation of the blood.

Leonardo da Vinci was recognized in his lifetime as a genius for his artistic masterpieces and for his work as architect, engineer, scientist and inventor. He might also have been regarded as the father of anatomy, had his remarkable notebooks not lain undiscovered for two centuries. From the drawings and notes in them it seems that he intended to write a major treatise on anatomy, in collaboration with Marc Antonio della Torre of Verona, to whom Vasari attributed the attempt to break new ground

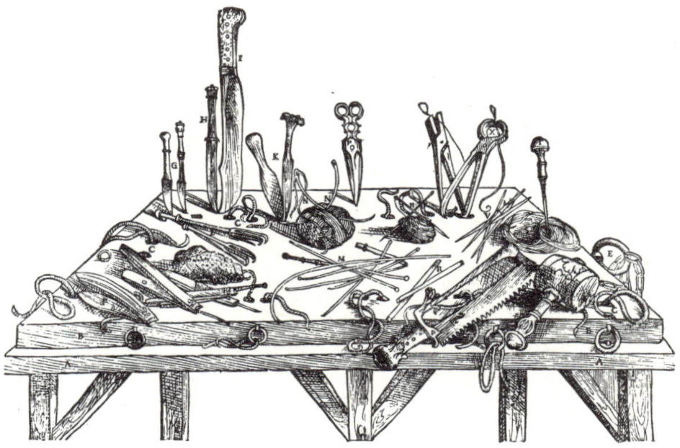

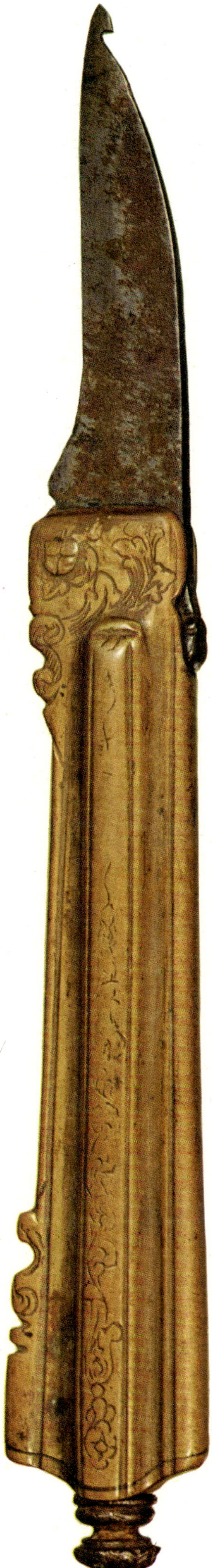

Anatomical drawings by Leonardo da Vinci. *Royal Library, Windsor Castle.*

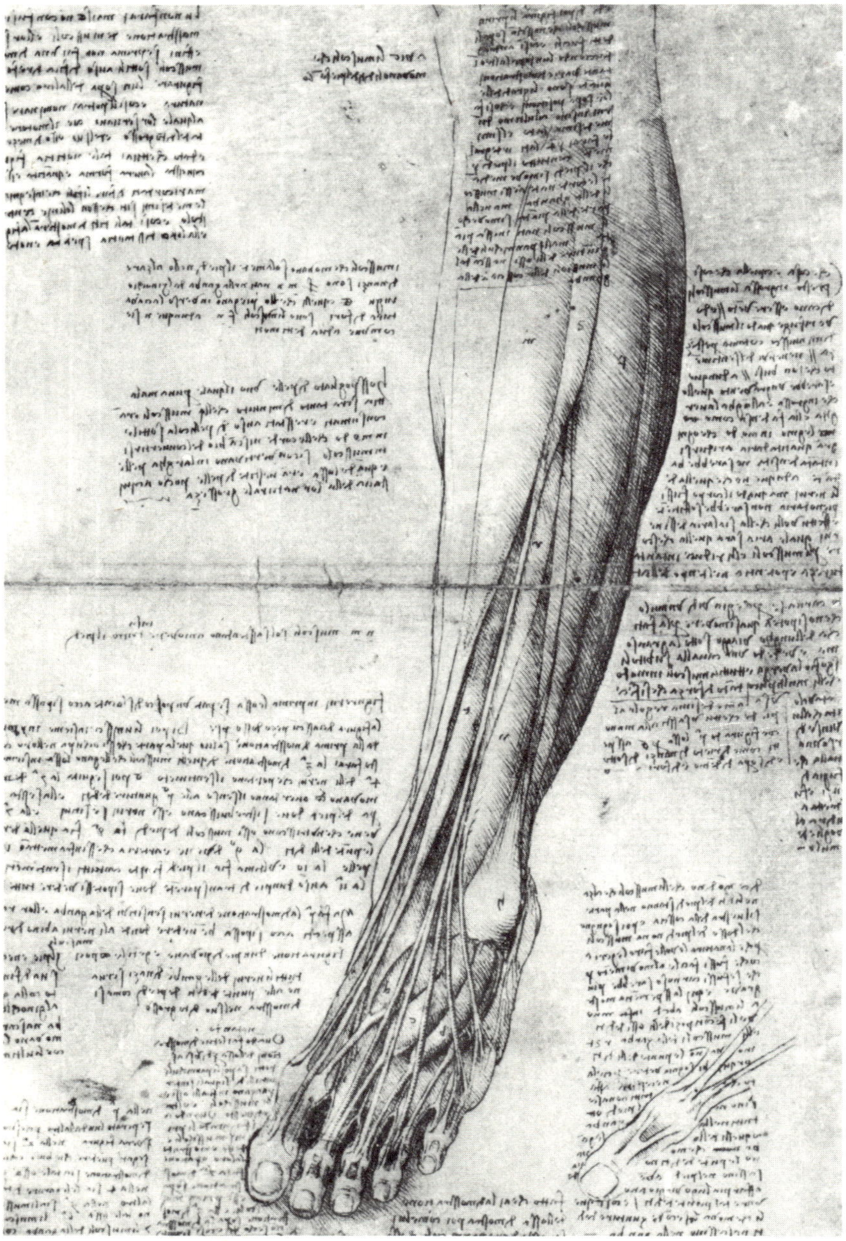

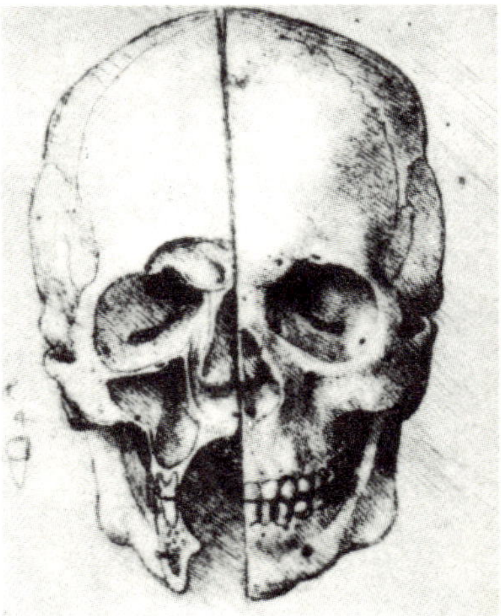

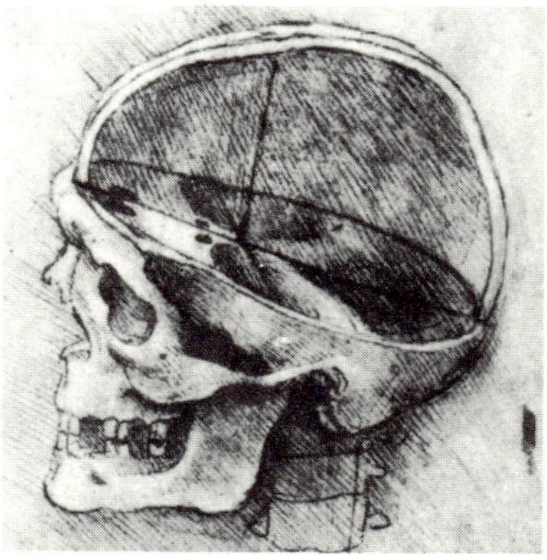

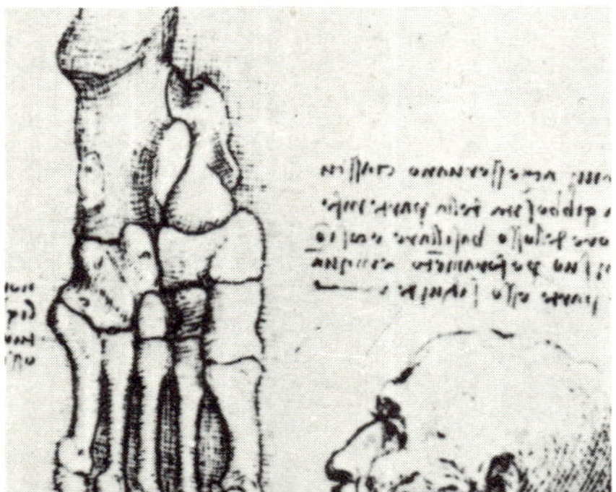

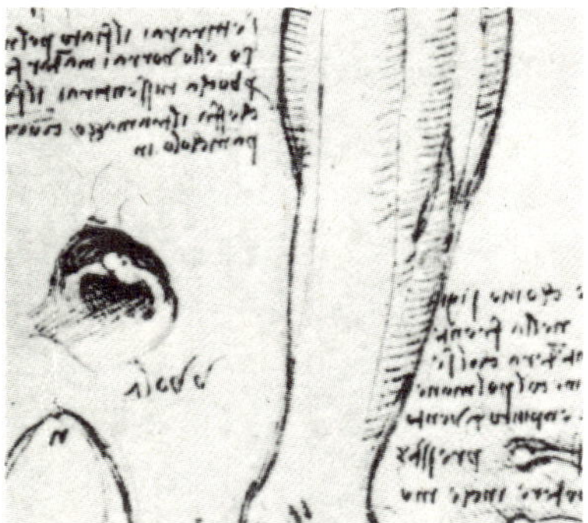

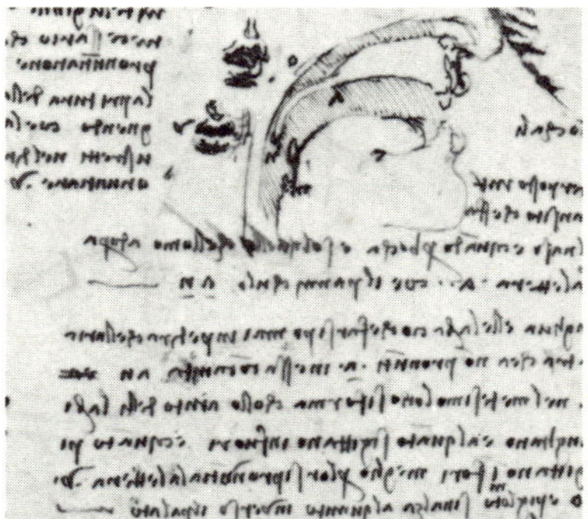

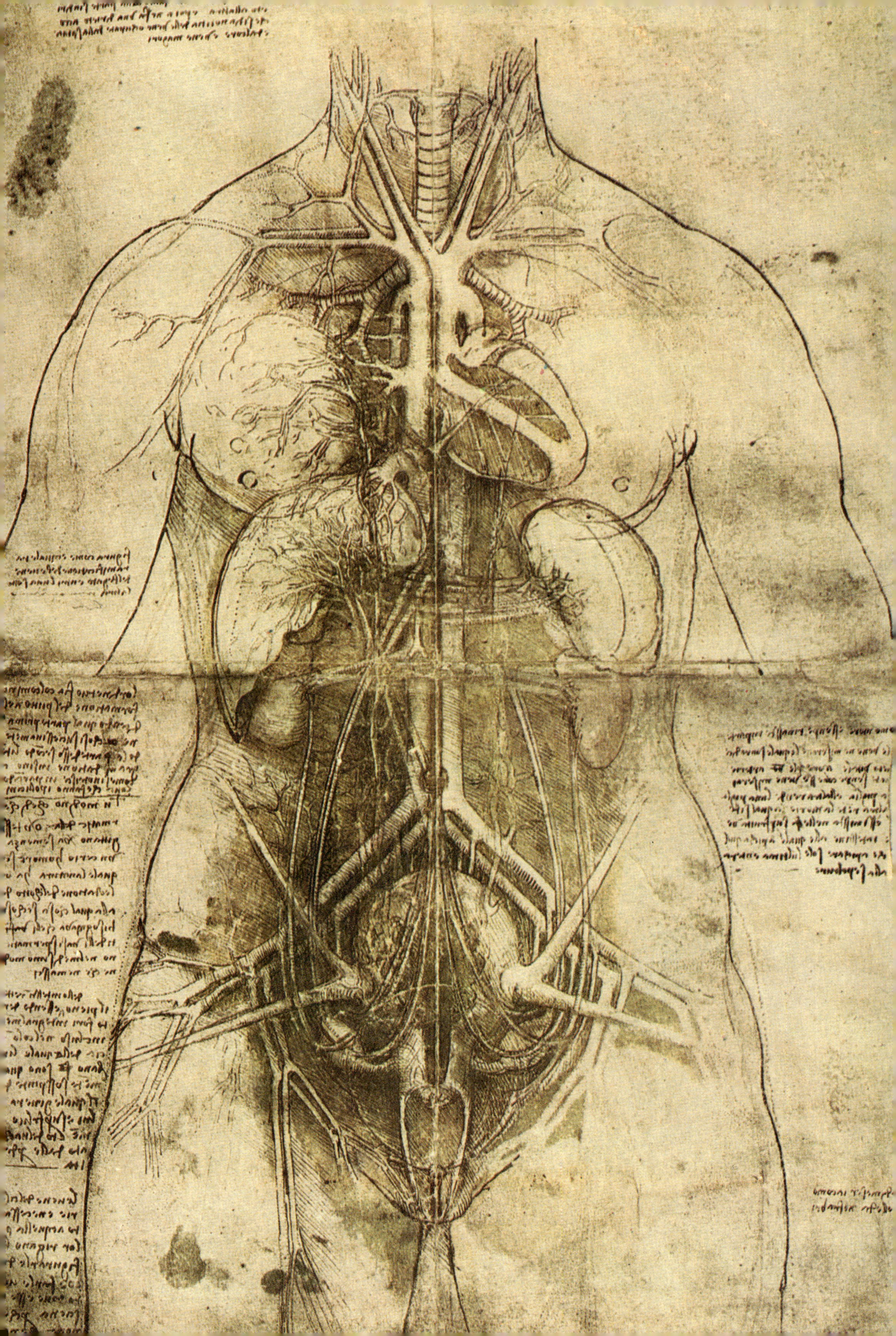

Leonardo da Vinci – the genius who excelled as a painter and engineer and in countless other fields – dissected more than thirty bodies, made many discoveries and produced hundreds of superb anatomical drawings. His investigations even took him some way towards discovering the circulation of the blood. Medicine was yet to benefit directly from the new knowledge; blood-letting was to be a popular treatment for centuries to come. But one artist made use of his anatomical studies: Durer once sent his doctor a now-famous sketch to indicate where he had a pain.

Dürer's sketch of himself indicating his spleen. (The artist sent it to his doctor, with the message 'Where the yellow patch is with the finger pointing, that is where it hurts me'.) *National Museum, Nuremberg.*

Diagram showing veins for blood-letting. *From Regime contre la pestilence par les Médecins de Basle, Lyons, 1519.*

in the teaching of anatomy. The idea for the joint work may have come from della Torre but he died in 1506 when barely thirty-three. When Leonardo died at Amboise in the year 1519, at the age of sixty-seven, while in the service of King Francis I of France, his notebooks went to his friend Francesco Melzi; subsequently they were in part donated to the Ambrosian Library in Milan and part dispersed as a result of war. An outstanding collection of drawings by Leonardo now belongs to the Queen, and is kept in the Royal Library at Windsor Castle.

These drawings show the artist to be the creator both of medical illustration and of anatomy in relation to physiology, and his scientific objectivity, powers of independent observation and stupendous technical skill make him, historically speaking, the father of anatomy. The following passage from his notebooks contains his justification of anatomical illustration, and by stressing the need for presenting collected facts in an easily comprehensible and unequivocal form he shows himself to be the true scientist and in a way anticipates the scientific journals and standard technical vocabulary of later centuries.

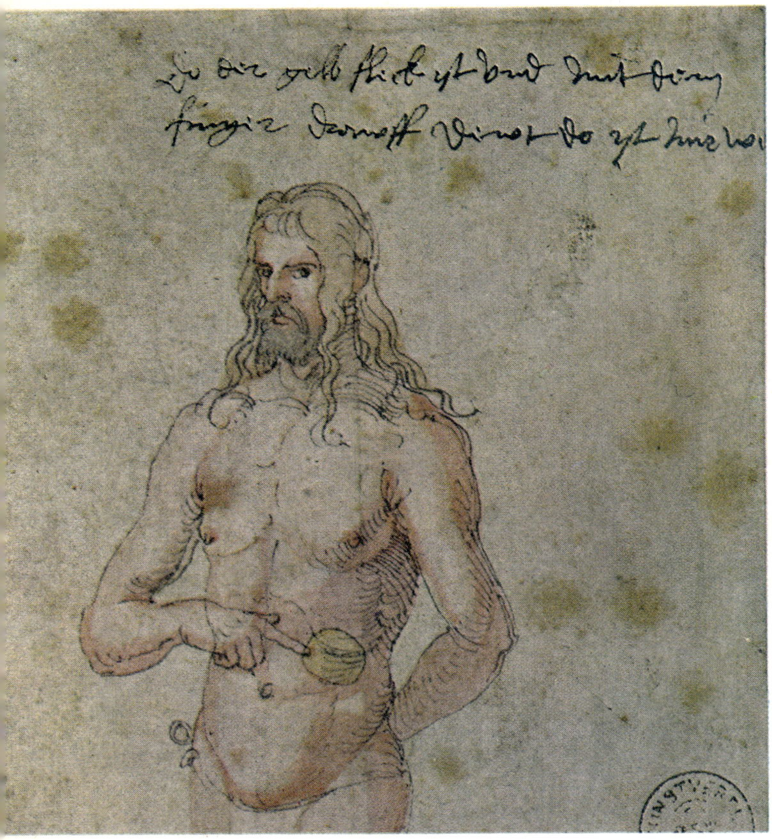

'You who say that it is better to watch an anatomical demonstration than to see these drawings, you would be right if it were possible to observe all the details shown in such drawings in a single figure, in which with all your cleverness you will not see or acquire knowledge of more than some few veins, while in order to obtain a true and complete knowledge of these, I have dissected more than ten human bodies, destroying all the various members and removing the minutest particles of flesh which surrounded these veins, without causing any effusion of blood other than the imperceptible bleeding of the capillary veins. And as one single body did not suffice for so long a time, it was necessary to proceed by stages with so many bodies as would render my knowledge complete; this I repeated twice in order to discover the differences. And though you should have love for such things you may perhaps be deterred by natural repugnance, and if this does not prevent you, you may perhaps be deterred by fear of passing the night hours in the company of these corpses, quartered and flayed and horrible to behold; and if this does not deter you, then perhaps you may lack the skill in drawing, essential for such representation; and if you had the skill in drawing, it may not be combined with a knowledge of perspective; and if it is so combined you may not understand the methods of geometrical demonstration and the methods of estimating the force and strength of muscles; or perhaps you may be wanting in patience so that you will not be diligent.

'Concerning which things, whether or no they have all been found in me, the hundred and twenty books which I have composed will give the verdict "yes" or "no". In these I have not been hindered either by avarice or negligence, but only by want of time. Farewell.'

It could be said that now the study of anatomy, and with it medical knowledge, was at last on the right road. Not only medical students, but every great artist learned anatomy and some, especially of course Leonardo himself, were skilled anatomists: Donatello and Verocchio were experts in this field, and Vasari wrote of Pollaiuolo that he 'cut up many men to see how they were made and was the first to show how to find the muscles'.

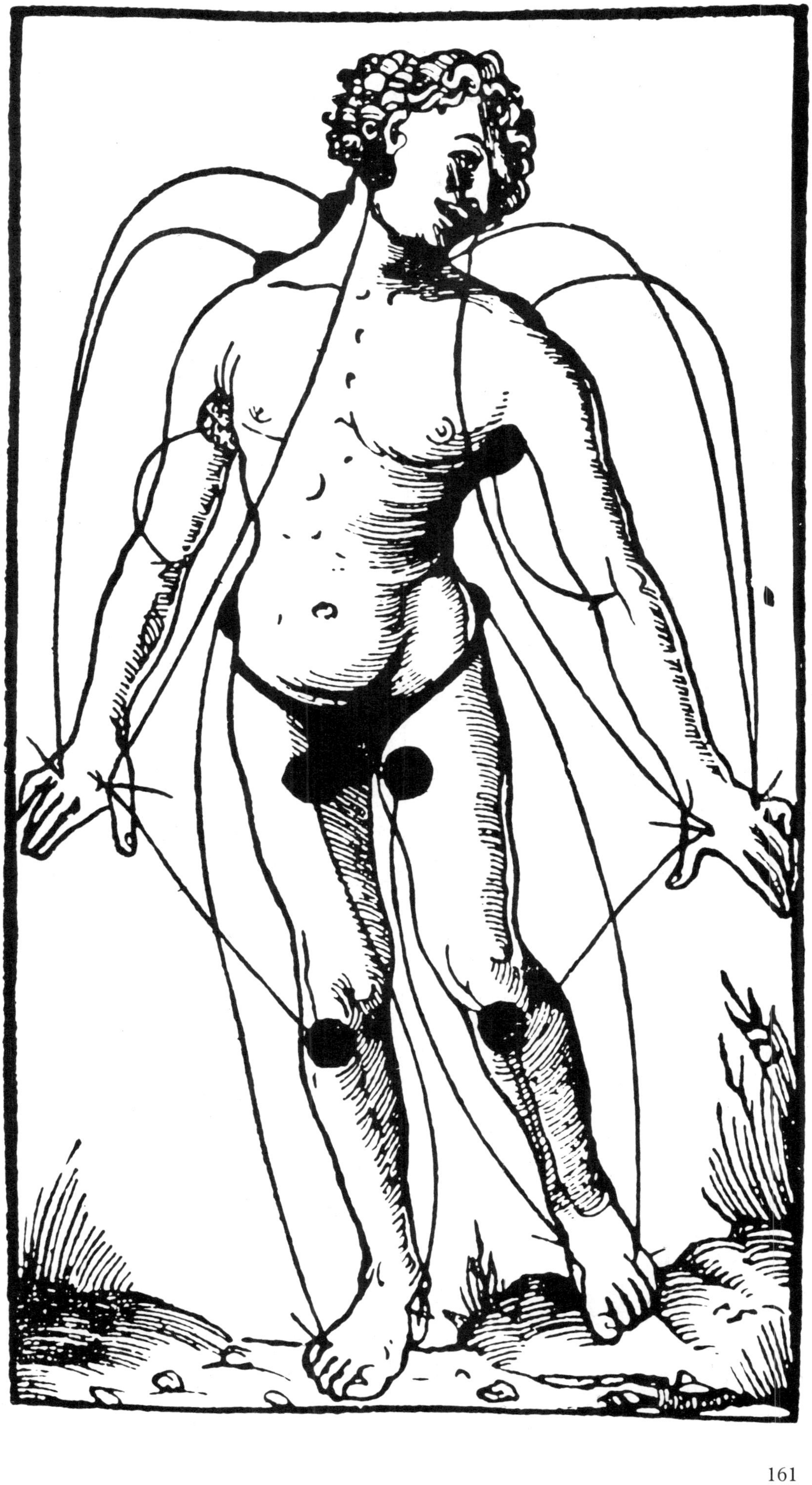

Vesalius and the end of Galenism

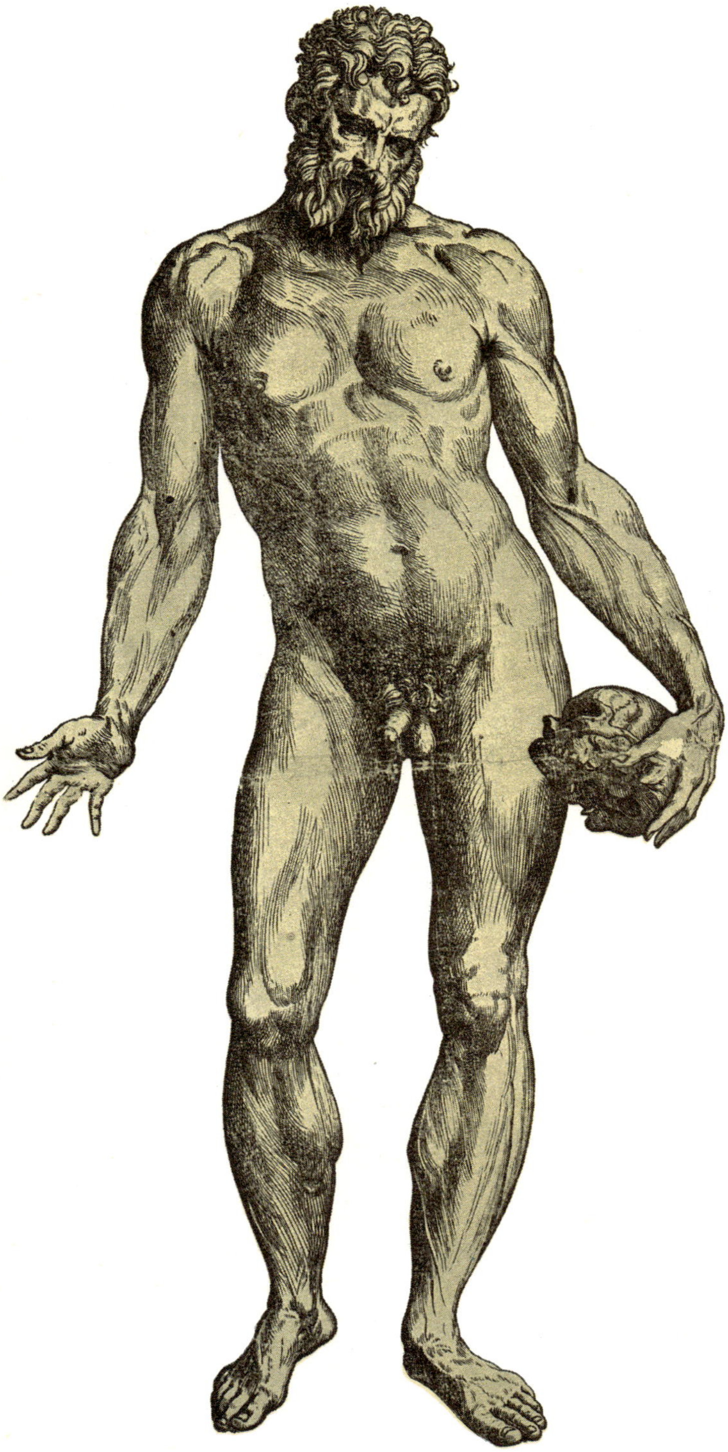

The man who is celebrated as the father of anatomy was not Leonardo da Vinci, but a Fleming called Andreas Vesalius, who was born in Brussels in 1514, the son of an apothecary from Wesel on the Rhine, whence he took his name. He began his studies at Louvain, continued them at Montpellier and then at Paris, where his master was Jacques Dubois, also known as Jacobus Silvius or Silvio. Silvius unfortunately held that nothing new could be added to the anatomy of Galen. From Paris Vesalius went back to Louvain for a short while; in 1537 he left for Padua where he joined a compatriot, Johan Stephen Kalker, who was studying painting at the school of Titian. Under the name of Stephen Calcar, this artist made superb illustrations for Vesalius' works, thereby contributing a good deal to the fame of the anatomist himself.

In the same year Vesalius took a degree and was then appointed to the chair of medicine and anatomy. In 1538 his work *Tabulae anatomicae sex* (Six anatomical tables) was published, with both text and illustrations containing age-old errors of Galen. But over the next five years Vesalius displayed his brilliance as an experimenter and observer. Slowly, perhaps without being fully aware of the processes at work, he discarded the anatomical dogma of Galen; this was made possible by the freedom of investigation then permitted at Padua, which was enjoying its heyday.

In 1543, when he was just twenty-eight, Vesalius finished his monumental work, *De humani corporis fabrica libri septem* (Seven books on the structure of the human body), which was printed at Basle. It caused an unprecedented uproar; most of the dons of the university were Galenists and they sided against him, violently denying the truth of Vesalius' statements. Even his former teacher, Silvius, maligned him. But Vesalius' conscience was clear; he had worked hard for five years to portray the human body faithfully – not on the lines of outworn doctrines, but solely on the basis of his own observations.

Vesalius showed where Silvius had erred, but he had no wish to triumph for personal reasons. The sea of ignorance facing him was vast, and there was also the ill-will of his accusers to contend with. Unable to withstand them, irritated by his colleagues and threatened by the church, he gathered together his unpublished work and burned it all. Then he left Padua to become the highly-paid physician of

De humani corporis fabrica libri septem, *Vesalius' monumental work on anatomy, superbly illustrated by Stephen Calcar, has been described as the greatest medical book ever written. It presented a very complete investigation of the structure of the human body, including many original discoveries, and refuted many of the concepts of Galen. For this reason it had a very hostile reception from the established staff of the universities. Vesalius himself, who completed the work at the age of twenty-eight, soon turned to medical practice, forsaking forever his original studies, to die in comparative obscurity before the age of fifty.*

Male and female figures. *From the Epitome by Vesalius, Basle, 1543.*

Emperor Charles V, and subsequently of Philip II of Spain, from 1556. A brilliant scientific career was over. Vesalius made no more original observations, although he followed the work of his successors in the study of anatomy. He died in 1563 on the island of Xante, on the return journey from a pilgrimage to Jerusalem, in circumstances which have never been made fully clear.

Some little time passed before other scholars began to appreciate his work at its true value. The revelation of Galen's fundamental errors was a tremendous shock. The worst of the errors was related to the anatomy of liver, bile duct, upper jaw and uterus. What upset the Galenists most of all was Vesalius' denial of the existence of the pores in the septum through which blood was supposed to flow from the right to the left ventricle of the heart. It is strange that Galen, who after all made numerous dissections, should have erred also in the description of such parts of the skeleton as the sternum, sacrum and articular cartilages of the knee. Naturally, Vesalius' work itself was not entirely free of errors. He had not fathomed the mechanism of circulation; he placed the lens in the centre of the eyeball; he believed the vena cava came from the liver; that there was a muscle inside the nose and seven (not twelve) cranial nerves. These and other faults did not however stop the new work done by this great anatomist from producing positive long-term results, and *De humani corporis fabrica* must be regarded as one of the most important books ever published, and the foundation of modern medicine.

Many anatomists at this time were accused of practising vivisection on humans, and this charge was brought against Vesalius; there was indeed a chapter in *De humani corporis* dealing with vivisection, but this referred to animals. The charge must be viewed with due caution as it emanated from his bitterest enemies in France, the Galenists Dulaurent and Riolan, who cited only one instance, that of a Spanish nobleman who was dissected in the belief that he was already dead. It seems improbable that a man of Vesalius' stature would have been capable of committing an error of this kind.

The publication of the work of Vesalius in the magnificent Basle edition had one curious consequence: it smothered a treatise on anatomy planned on a vast scale by Giovanni Battista Canano of Ferrara (1515–1579). This was to be regretted

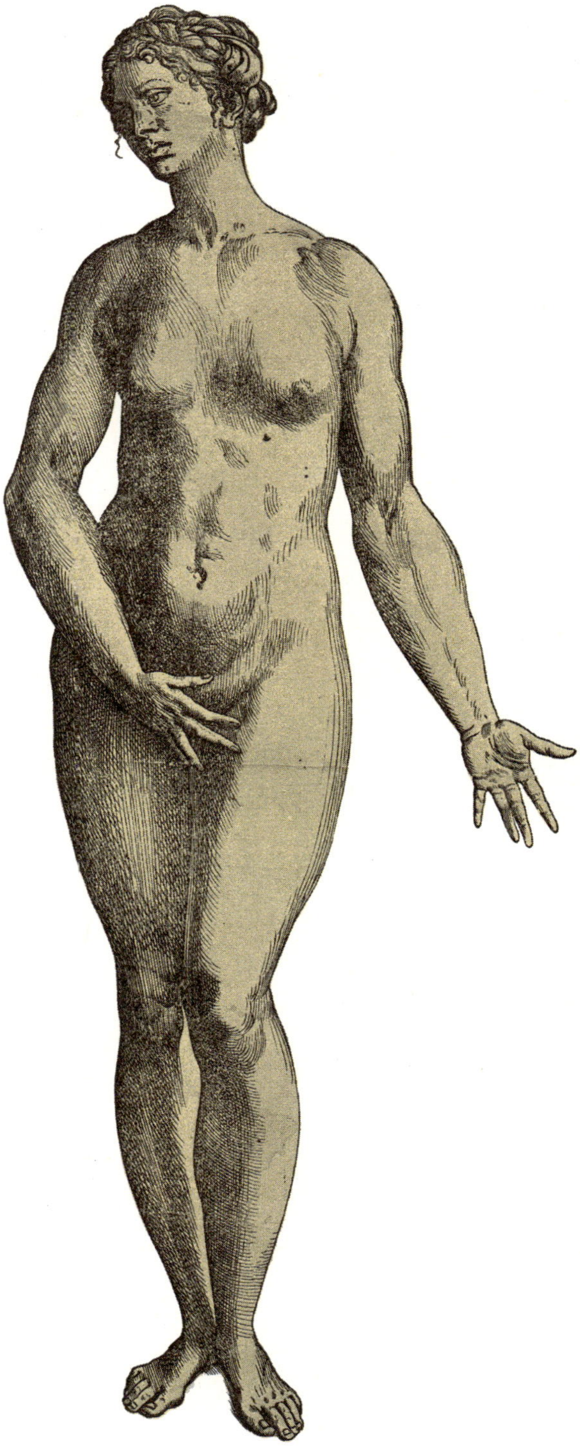

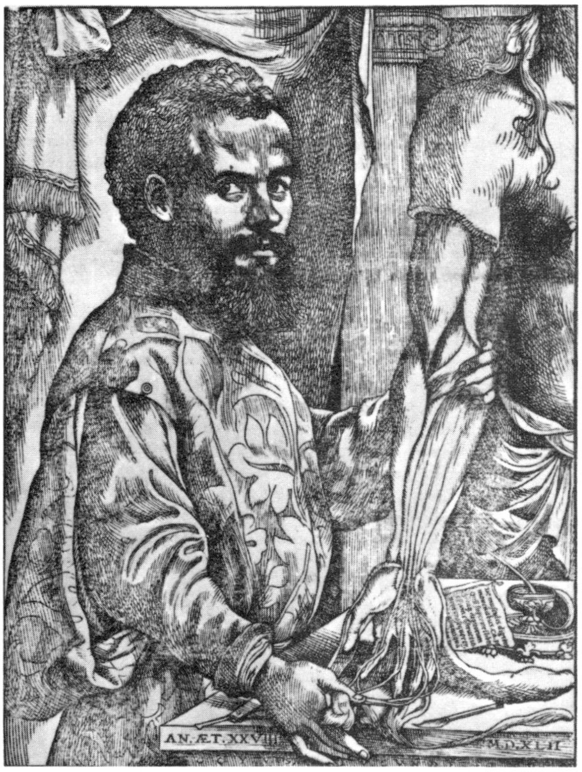

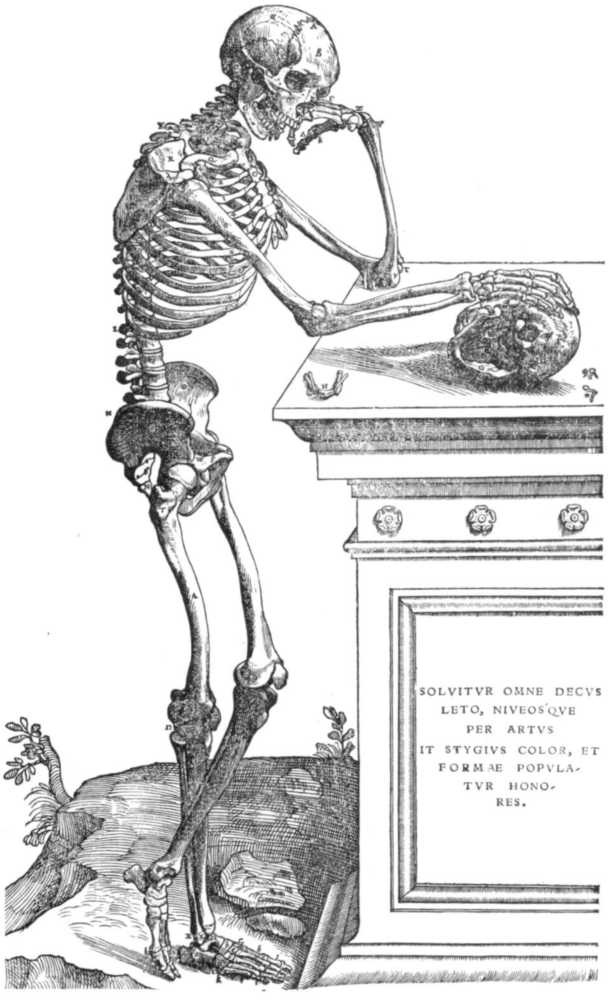

Portrait of Vesalius at the age of 28. *From De humani corporis fabrica, Basle, 1543.*

Skeleton. *From De humani corporis fabrica by Vesalius, Basle, 1543.*

Anatomical dissection. *Frontispiece from De humani corporis fabrica, Basle, 1543.*

because the first part, entitled *Musculorum humani corporis picturata dissectio* (Illustrated dissection of the muscles of the human body), published in Ferrara in 1541, two years prior to the completion of Vesalius' *Fabrica,* showed considerable understanding and observation. It has been maintained that Canano failed to publish the rest of the book because he lost heart on seeing Vesalius' work, which he said was unsurpassable. It is probable that he was modest enough to prefer not to compete with a brilliant colleague, but however modest it is unlikely he had no idea of his own worth or thought the *Fabrica* was perfect. It was Canano who first discovered the valves in veins and communicated the discovery to Vesalius, whose greatness, after all, was not generally admitted until later.

Although he was a superb observer and undoubtedly a man of great learning, as an innovator Vesalius was not so very far ahead of some of his colleagues, for example Jacopo Berengario da Carpi. Born in 1470, the son of a famous surgeon and a pupil of Aldus Manutius, creator of the famous press in Venice and its Aldine type-fount, Berengario took his degree in medicine at Bologna, taught at Pavia and Bologna and practised in Rome and in Ferrara, where he died in the early sixteenth century. His heirs inherited his considerable wealth, obtained largely from treatment of patients with syphilis; he was among the first to popularize the use of mercurial ointments in the treatment of this disease.

It seems that Berengario was an unscrupulous man. Benvenuto Cellini, who knew him well and had been under his care, did not speak favourably of him, and he was criticized by many others besides. But Berengario was a resilient character and survived such attacks. And above all he was a very accurate anatomist. In 1518 he published *De fractura calvariae sive cranii* (On fracture of the cranium), which was followed in 1521 by *Commentaria super anatomia Mundini* (Commentary on the anatomy of Mondino), a broadly-based and most original work. The *Isagogae,* an anatomical compendium, appeared in 1522 and featured some magnificent illustrations of the heart.

According to the French medical historian Daremberg, the finest original work in anatomy was done not by Vesalius but by Gabriele Fallopio (1523–1562). Fallopio belonged to the Ferrara school and taught for a long time at Pisa, ending

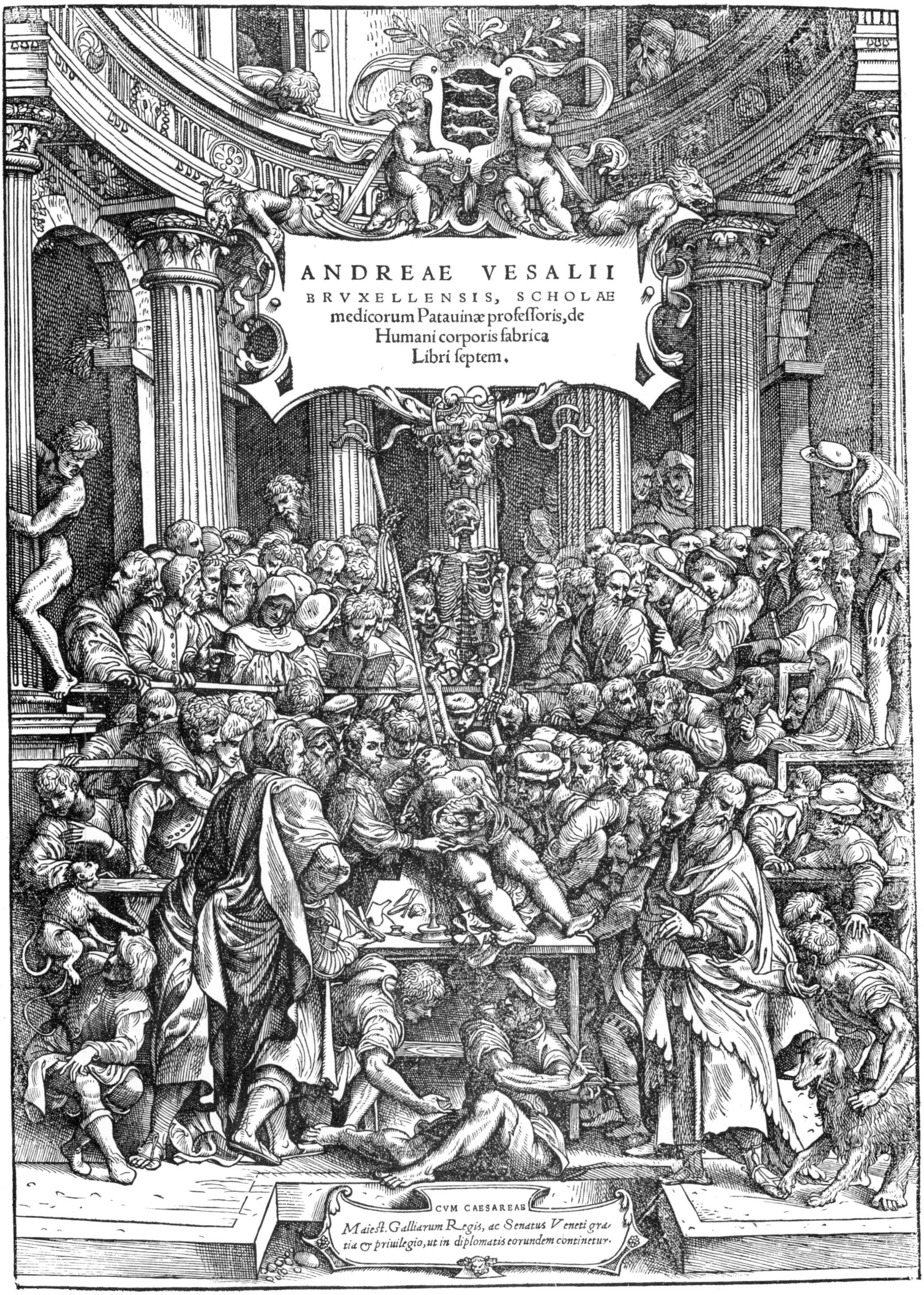
ANDREAE VESALII
BRVXELLENSIS, SCHOLÆ
medicorum Patauinæ professoris, de
Humani corporis fabrica
Libri septem.
CVM CAESAREAE
Maiest. Galliarum Regis, ac Senatus Veneti gratia & priuilegio, ut in diplomatis eorundem continetur.

In spite of the liberal intellectual climate of the Renaissance, the study of the human body was not without problems. The investigations of almost all the anatomists of the time, including Vesalius, gave rise to accusations that they performed dissections on living people. Perhaps the lifelike poses of the figures in anatomical illustrations of the period had something to do with the charges, which were apparently unfounded, although animal vivisection was practised. But most anatomists were also surgeons, and it is likely that people confused their operations with vivisections.

Flayed man. *Statue by Ludovico Cardi (Il Cicogli), apparently made from anatomical plates by Vesalius. Bargello Museum, Florence.*

Judgement of Cambises. *By Gerard David, detail from panel.*

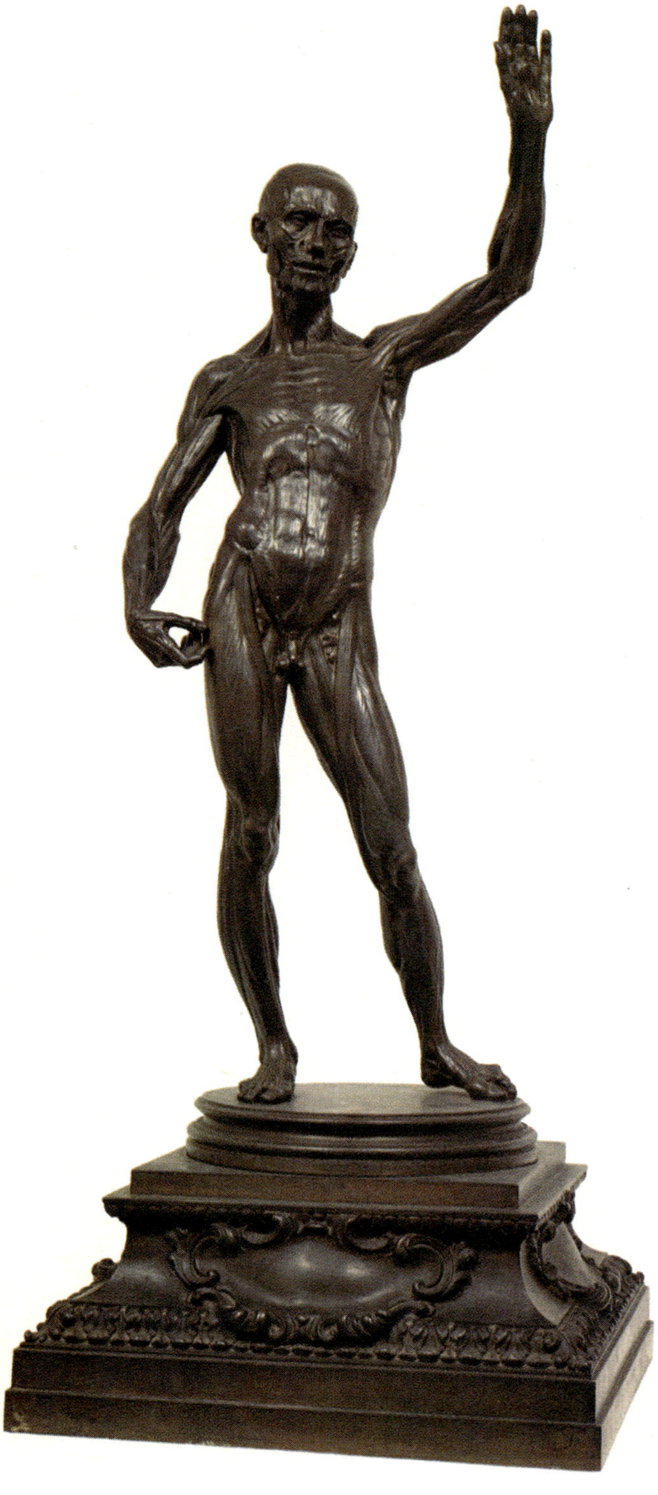

his career in the chair of anatomy at Padua left vacant by Realdo Colombo, Vesalius' successor. Colombo was a good scholar but had shown weakness by siding with the opponents of his master Vesalius. After the storm had passed, he was ready enough to point out certain errors in Galen. Colombo discovered the pulmonary circulation, and described with more accuracy than his predecessors the pleura, peritoneum and mediastinum; he also located the lens correctly. His work, *De re anatomica,* was published posthumously.

Gabriele Fallopio was estimable as a scholar and as a person. His behaviour towards his colleagues was exemplary. He spoke of Berengario as 'without doubt the restorer of the art of anatomy, which Vesalius then perfected'. Of the *Fabrica,* he said that it was Vesalius' divine monument and would last for ever. Then, having praised it, he began correcting the errors in the work: he described the ear and cerebral arteries, which Vesalius confused with the sinuses, and the clitoris and the (Fallopian) tubes that still bear his name. He was the first to describe the circular folds of the small intestine, the inguinal ligament, the chorda tympani, the semicircular canals and the lacrimal duct. In addition he wrote an excellent account of the eye muscles and of the cerebral nerves, and because of his contribution to the study of tissues he has been regarded as the precursor of Malpighi and Bichat (Castiglioni). Fallopio's most important book was the *Observationes anatomicae,* first published in Venice in 1561; his *Opera omnia* appeared there in 1584, over twenty years after his death. He died in 1562 at the early age of thirty-nine.

Fallopio studied and taught at Ferrara, Pisa and finally at Padua, where he was succeeded by his pupil Gerolamo Fabrizio d'Acquapendente (c. 1533–1619), called Fabricius. Famous in his day as a surgeon, Fabricius was also a great anatomist and physiologist. He was the first to give a good description of the valves of the veins, although he thought that the blood in the veins flowed away from the heart. His best work was done on reproduction, childbirth and the anatomy and physiology of the foetus; it is interesting that the discoverer of the circulation, William Harvey, who was one of Fabricius' pupils, also wrote on embryology. It was in the time of Fabricius that the famous anatomy theatre at Padua was built, as a model of its kind.

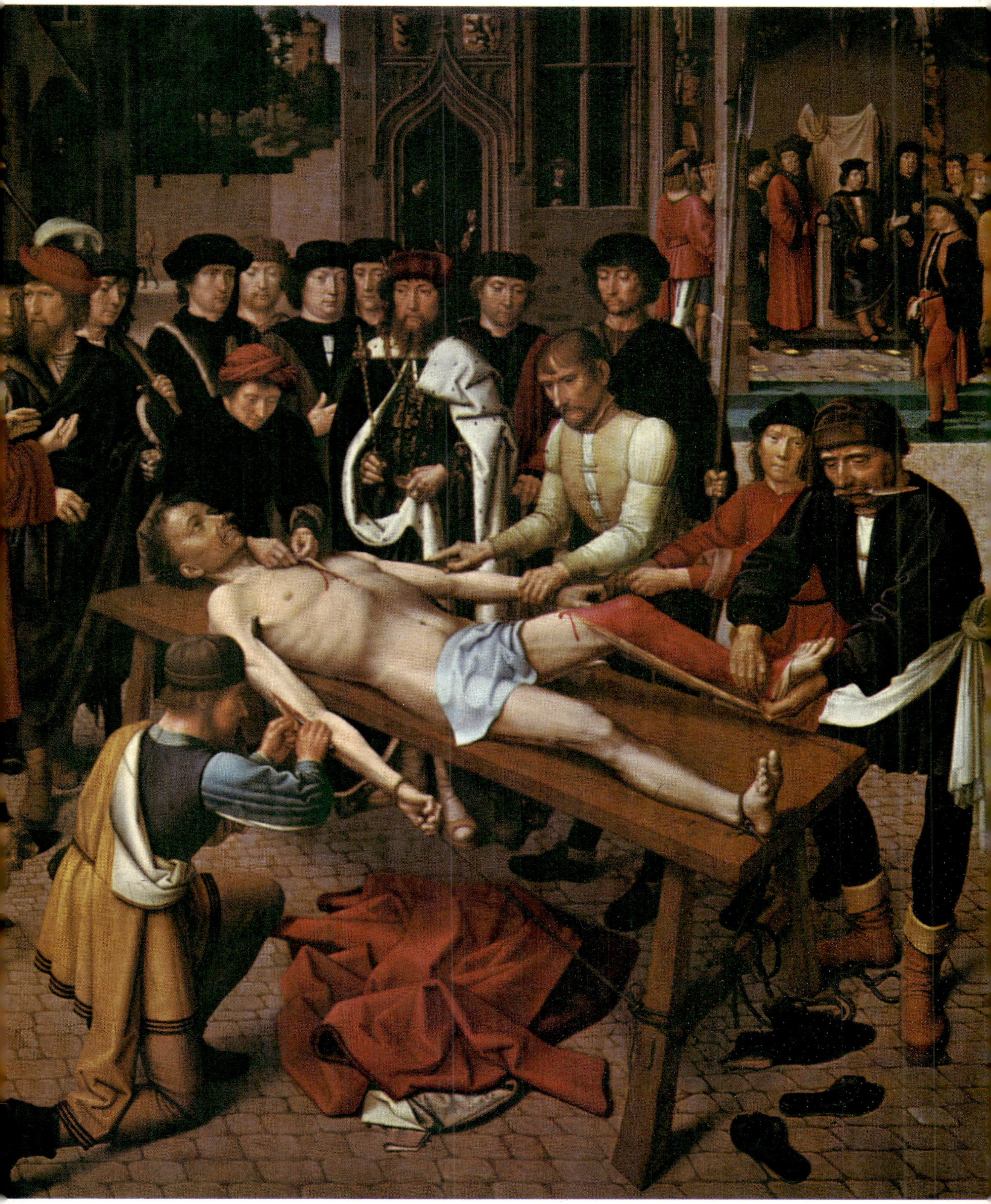

Syphilis and early theories of infection

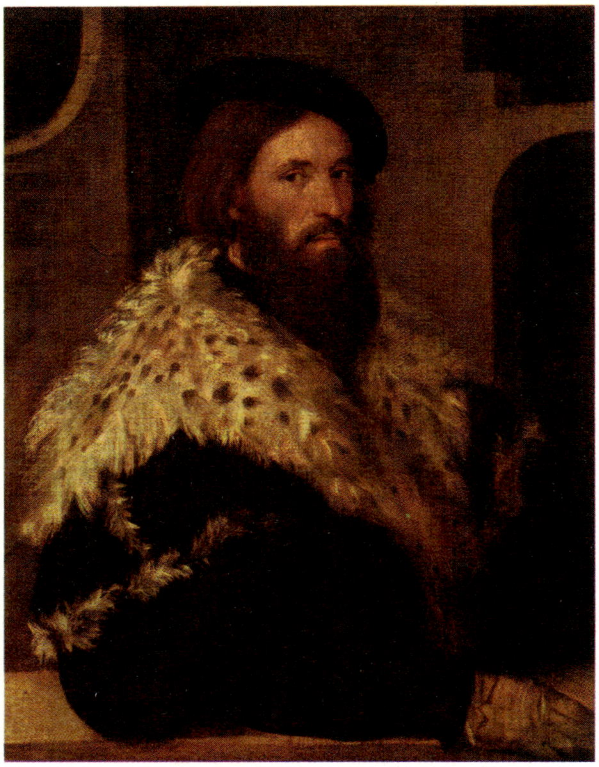

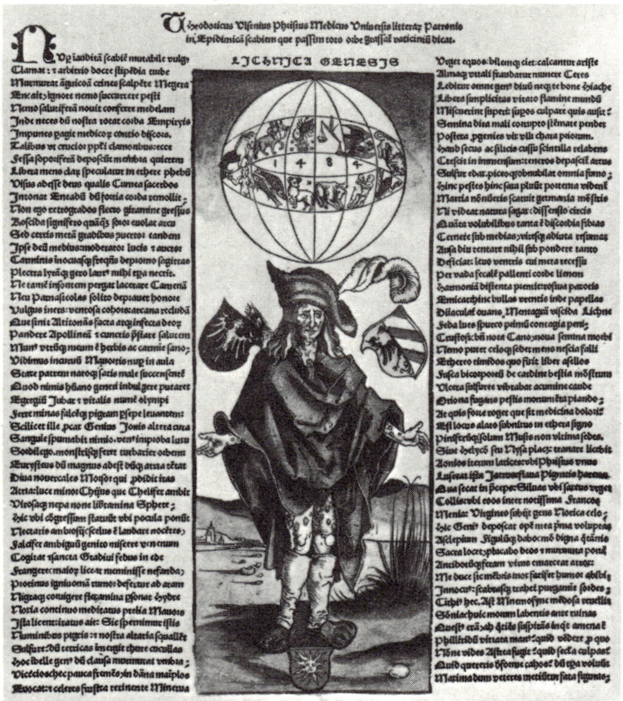

In the last years of the fifteenth century, a terrible new epidemic appeared, a lethal infection which produced repulsive rashes and ulcers and was spread by sexual contact. It became rife when the army of Charles VIII of France invaded Italy and was first known as the Neapolitan disease, for a major outbreak occurred among the troops when Naples surrendered without a siege; many desertions followed, and surviving mercenaries returned home, bringing the name and the disease with them. Morbus Gallicus became the term in general use until Girolamo Fracastoro (1478–1553) published in 1530 his poem dedicated to Pietro Bembo, entitled *Syphilis sive morbus gallicus* (Syphilis or the French disease), in which a young shepherd, Syphilus, insults Apollo; in revenge the god causes the flesh to fall from the young man's limbs, revealing his bones, his teeth to rot, his breath to stink and his voice to fail.

Fracastoro noted that the disease appeared simultaneously in many countries, and he doubted the popular theory that it came from America with Columbus' sailors. This doubt we must share today. It is likely that syphilis has always existed in the Old World, and that the causative organism *Treponema pallidum* underwent a world-wide mutation at the close of the fifteenth century, attacking previously resistant hosts in the Orient as well as in Europe. Mediaeval medical writings refer to cases of venereal leprosy, probably cutaneous syphilis, which was treated with mercury then as in the 1500s. Besides, there are a few undoubted descriptions of the disease in tracts written before 1492.

Perhaps commercial factors had something to do with the encouragement of the idea that syphilis had come from America. It is a common primitive belief that a disease and its cure exist side by side; guaiac, the 'holy wood', was used by the natives of the New World and was brought by Spanish mariners to Europe, where, in the form of infusions, its remarkable efficacy against the new disease was reported. Fracastoro and the German knight Ulrich von Hutten (who died miserably of syphilis) were enthusiastic about the new treatment, which was in fact quite useless. Guaiac was particularly popular in Germany, and one of the Baltic trading companies largely controlled its import; continued belief in the worth of this New World 'cure' sustained and was sustained by trade.

Conditions then prevalent in Europe were all

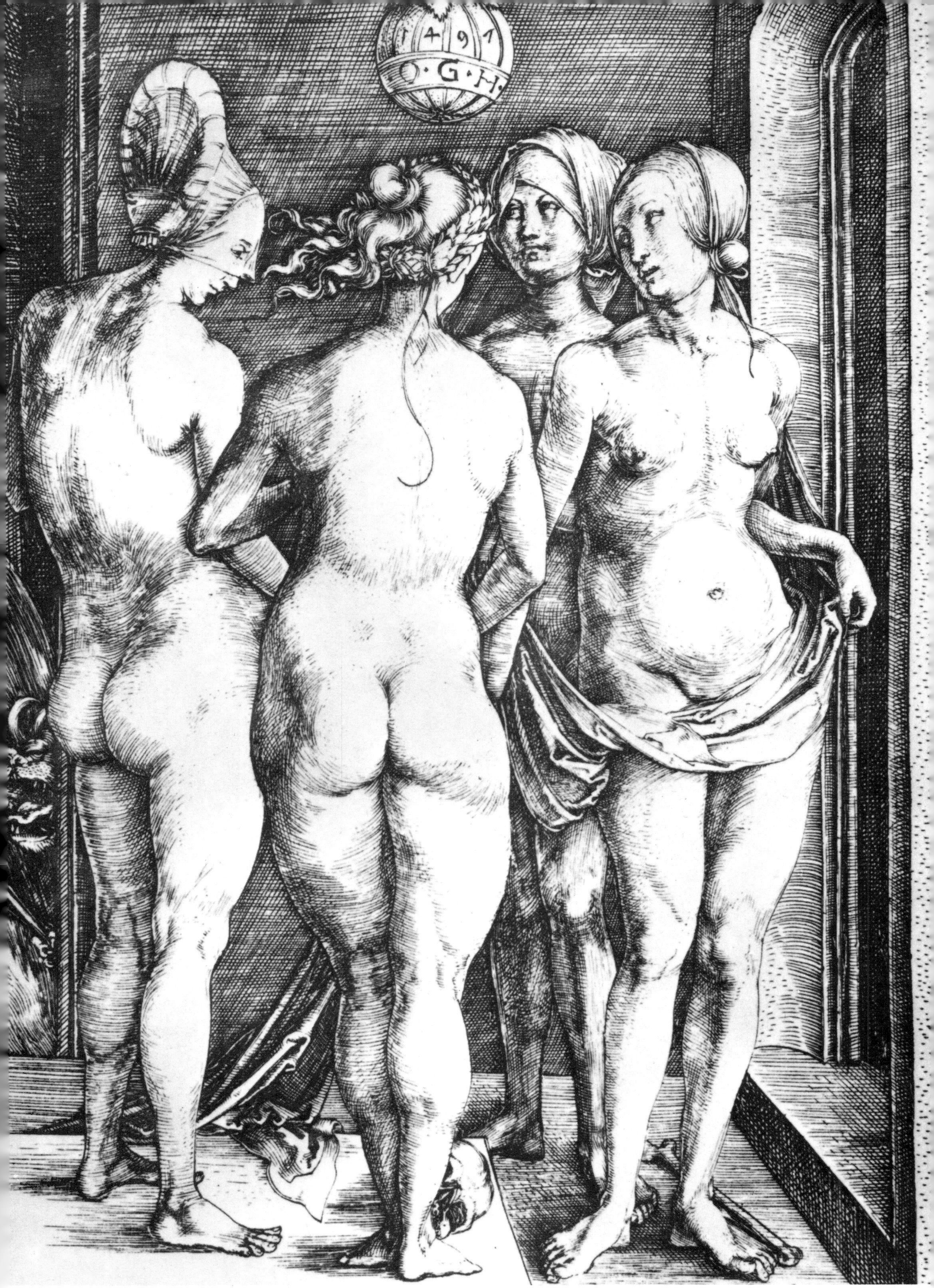
1497
O·G·H·

Previous pages:
Girolamo Fracastoro. *Portrait attributed to Il Torbido. National Gallery, London.*

A man suffering from syphilis, with text describing the disease. *By Albrecht Dürer. Museums, Berlin.*

The four witches. *Engraving by Dürer. Museums, Berlin.*

These pages:
Louèche baths in the Valais. *By Hans Boch. Basle Museum.*

A disease which reached epidemic proportions in Europe during the late Middle Ages and the Renaissance was syphilis. It was recognized by physicians as a contagious infection spread by sexual contact, so that it was realized that it was aggravated by the widespread immorality of the period, when the cities contained thousands of prostitutes, male and female. But other means of contagion were postulated; when

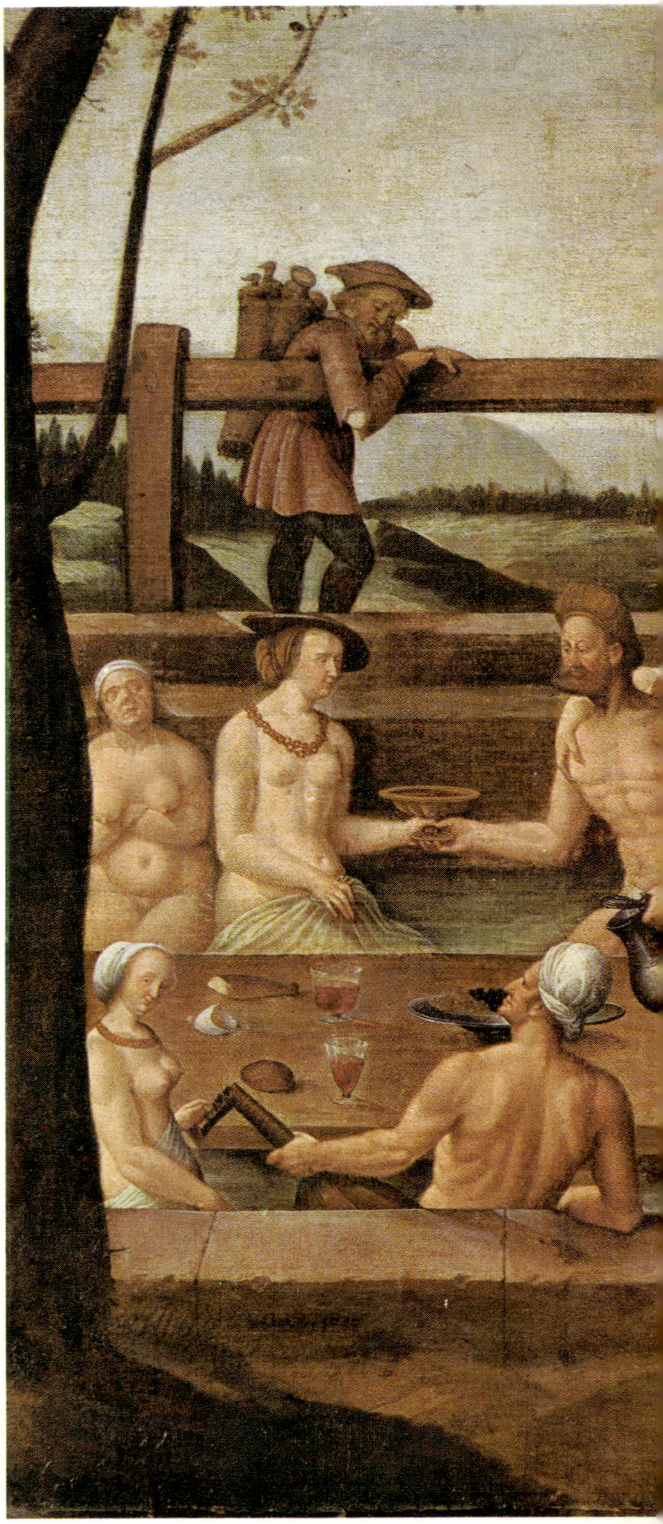

too suitable for the spread of syphilis. In Rome, during the period when America was being discovered, the town treasury collected over thirty thousand scudos a year from brothels. The historian Marino Sanudo gave a figure of twelve thousand prostitutes for Venice, when then had a population of three hundred thousand.

If it is true that prostitution facilitated the spread of the disease, it is also true that medicine in the fifteen-hundreds – in comparison with previous centuries – approached this plague quite differently. In particular, various prophylactic measures, effective to a certain extent, were adopted. The times were gone when an unknown disease appeared and a corner had to be found for it in the theory of the humours, and interminable debates centred on the nature of the humoral imbalance at the root of it. Old theories had been discarded and doctors tried to build up a picture of the disease grounded solely on their own experience and observation.

In Paris in 1497 the civic authorities issued an order under which all syphilitics not habitually resident in Paris were to leave. Residents were isolated in the Faubourg St Germain. The Scots were among the first to become aware that the contagion spread through sexual contact. In fact, a regulation made by the town council of Aberdeen stated that to protect citizens against the disease that had come over from France, women of ill-fame were to stop working on pain of being branded.

Nicolo Leoniceno described syphilis accurately as early as 1497, while Antonio Benivieni (1440–1502) observed that the infection could be transmitted from mother to foetus. Fracastoro was the first to suggest that invisible germs, which he called 'seminaria', caused contagious disease, distinguishing between poison (like snake bites) and 'live contagion' and noting the need to destroy the germs. 'Were it possible to destroy them with caustics,' he wrote in reference to tuberculosis, which he defined as contagious, 'there could be no better remedy; but as these substances cannot be used without endangering the lung, treatment can be tried through neighbouring organs.' Fracastoro recognized three kinds of contagion: one by simple contact; another by means of some carrier (fomites) such as clothing, bed linen, personal belongings; and a third kind at a distance, as when germs propagated in the air and chose the most suitable spot to fasten on.

Cardinal Wolsey fell from power he was accused among other things of having infected Henry VIII by whispering in his ear. Civic authorities (which often had a considerable income from town brothels) attempted to curb the disease by restricting the activities of those who were known to be sufferers.

One regulation prohibited mixed bathing in public baths, which in many places were a very popular treatment for ill-health. The bath was sometimes accompanied by other procedures such as blood-letting or the application of medicaments, and it was often also made an occasion for feasting, drinking and other entertainments. As knowledge about contagion increased, the practice of bathing in common tanks died out almost completely; by the eighteenth century bathing itself had become a luxury.

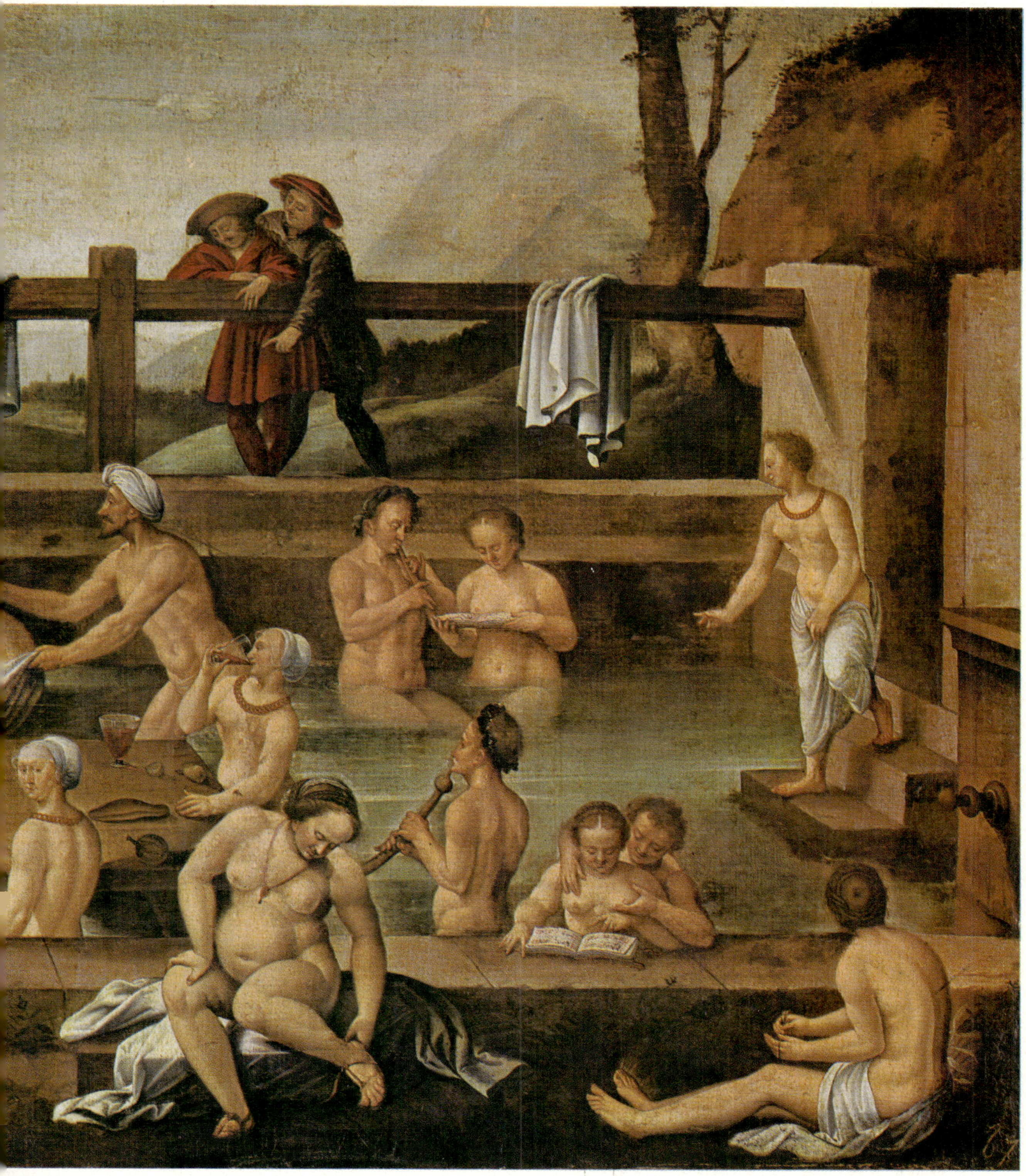

Paracelsus

The Renaissance was above all an Italian phenomenon; its spirit gradually permeated to France and eventually to the Teutonic countries where universities, of later date, were still not numerous. The two most ancient were at Prague and Heidelberg, founded in 1347 and 1386 respectively. In 1500 no German faculty of medicine as yet had more than two professors. The Silesian Johannes Lange (1485–1565) studied and then took his degree in medicine at Pisa; on his return to Germany he described the position of medicine and 'ignorant and over-weening' medical men in his own land as pitiful.

The great English medical humanist was Thomas Linacre (1460–1524), the founder of the Royal College of Physicians of London and physician to Henry VII and Henry VIII. He studied in Italy and gained medical degrees at Padua and later at Oxford. Apart from his Latin translations of a number of Galen's works and his foundation of medical lectures at Oxford and Cambridge he wrote books on grammar, and on account of his broad-based humanism he was called by Fuller the 'restorer of learning' in England. His translations, accurate and clear, were widely read throughout Europe and superseded the garbled versions previously in circulation.

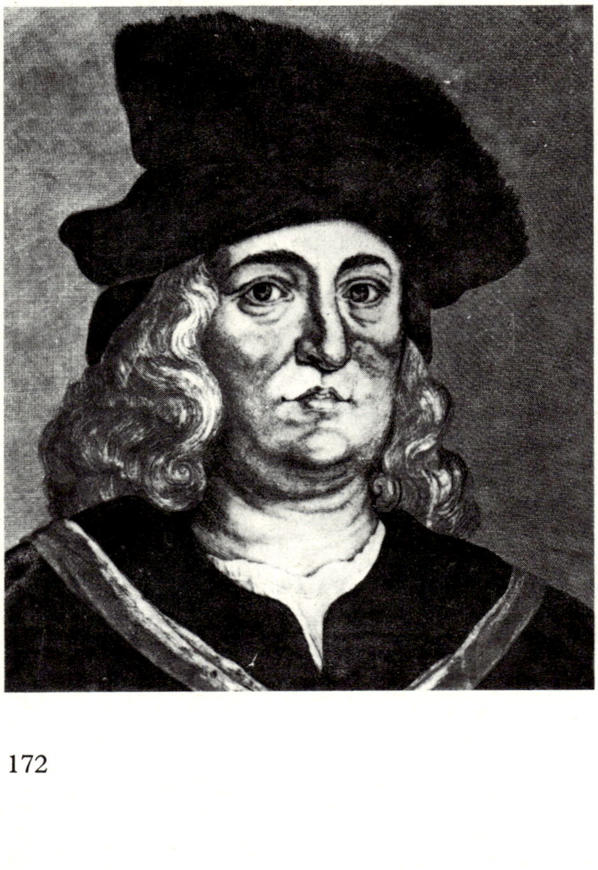

In France, a typical Renaissance figure was François Rabelais (c. 1495–1553), like Linacre a priest as well as a doctor, who studied medicine at the famous university of Montpellier and became physician to the hospital at Lyons. He also produced one of the first Latin translations of Hippocrates' *Aphorisms*, but it is as the author of the cruelly satirical *Gargantua* and *Pantagruel* that Rabelais has gone down in history. Certainly, his own profession did not escape his scorn: 'Stercus et urina, medici sunt prandia prima' (faeces and urine, a doctor's dinner) says his Doctor Rondibilis.

The most notable German-speaking reformer of medicine of the Renaissance was, beyond doubt, Philippus Aureolus Theophrastus Bombastus von Hohenheim, or Paracelsus. A brilliant man, he collected as many admirers as critics during his life-time; the fact that he was so controversial a figure was his own doing: his works were written in involved and sometimes obscure language, containing many precise ideas often overlaid with extravagant concepts. Perhaps Paracelsus never decided whether his main interest was natural science or magic, cabalistic knowledge and alchemy. He was well aware that medicine must forsake the teaching of Galen and start afresh, but he erred in his theory of the composition of matter from sulphur, mercury and salt. In the alchemical concept of Paracelsus these three elements were the outcome of distillation: the vapour condensing in the alembic was called sulphur, mercury was the scanty dense liquid remaining, while salt was the dry residue.

But the man who called himself Paracelsus was beyond question a great medical practitioner, and an innovator who spoilt a good deal of his work by not being able to keep his violent and mystical traits within bounds.

He was born in 1493 in the devout atmosphere of Einsiedeln in Switzerland, which had a Benedictine monastery and a shrine of Our Lady which was an object of pilgrimage. There is little reliable information about the life of this bizarre character: it is known that he was an only son, and that his father was a doctor who went to the Tyrol when Theophrastus was nine years old. It is also known that in Austria Theophrastus started studying minerals and metals and that he was initiated into the secrets of alchemy and astrology by Abbot det donec totú includat deinceps ad Zoná ferat, ab eaq3 ad colé at q3 inde rurs' ad Zoná, nouissime testiculos ãplexa in Zoná demittatur.

Idem ex fascia scissa ac Zona.

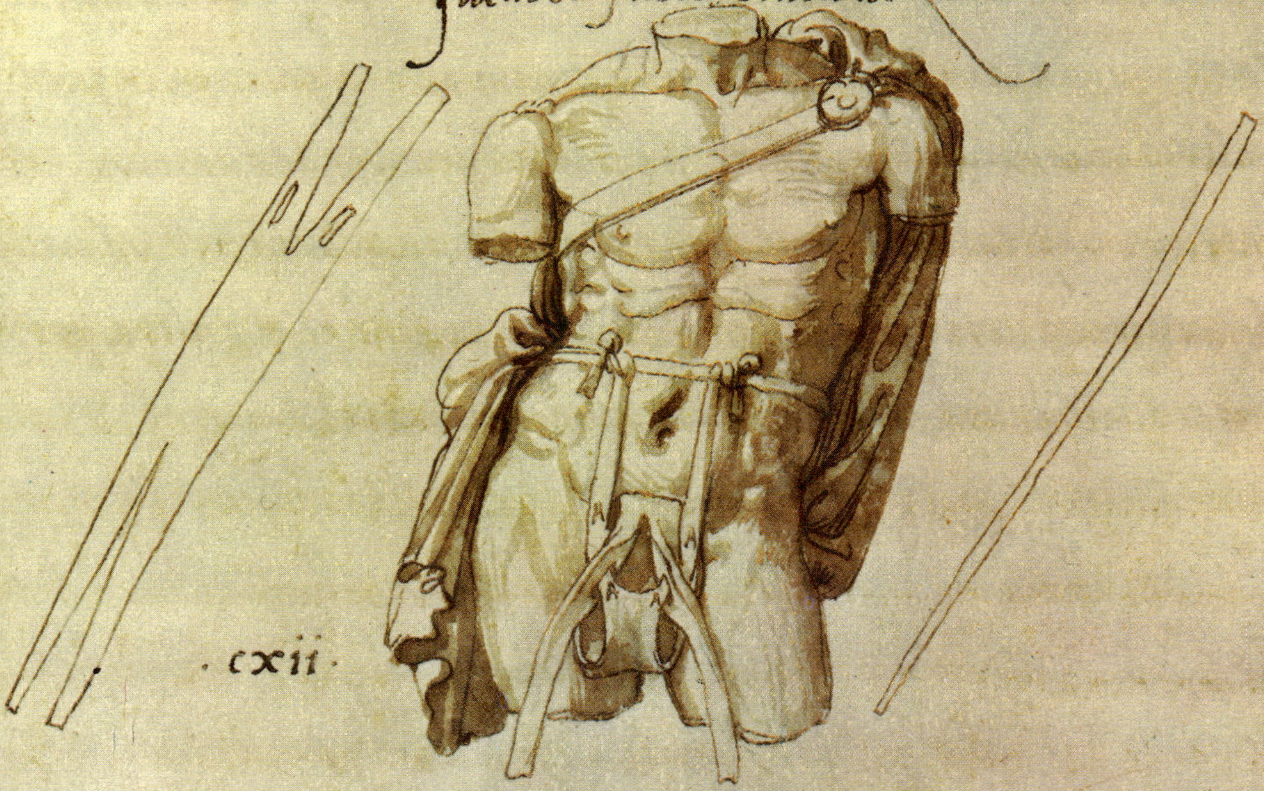

cxii

Linteú iustæ magnitudinis scindito in ptes quatuor sic ut mediú integrum relinquatur quo colé excipito tú ab altero capite scissas ptes i uicinia colis fidito, in eaq3 fissa alteri' capitis ptes cõijcito, ciguloq3 inserito et nodo alligato. Iinculú ad alter, ingué qđ nónulli Cancrú pigue dixerut. Ad utrúq3 inguen

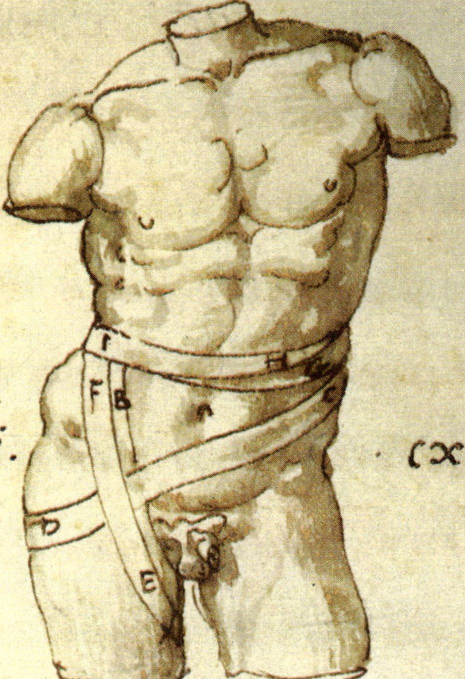

cxiii.

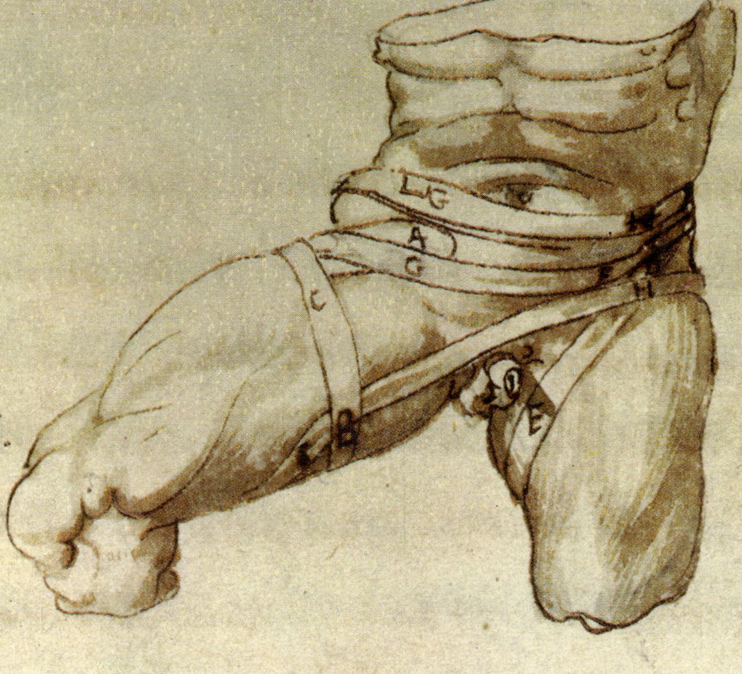

cxiiii.

Previous pages :
Paracelsus. *Engraving by W. Hollar after Rubens. Impression in the Wellcome Historical Medical Museum.*

Bandages. *Drawings attributed to Primaticcio. From Chirurgia by Guido Guidi. Bibliothèque Nationale, Paris.*

These pages :
Reduction of dislocations. *Drawings by Primaticcio (?) from Guidi's Chirurgia.*

Ward at the hospital of S Matteo, Florence. *By Jacopo Pontormo. Accademia Gallery, Florence.*

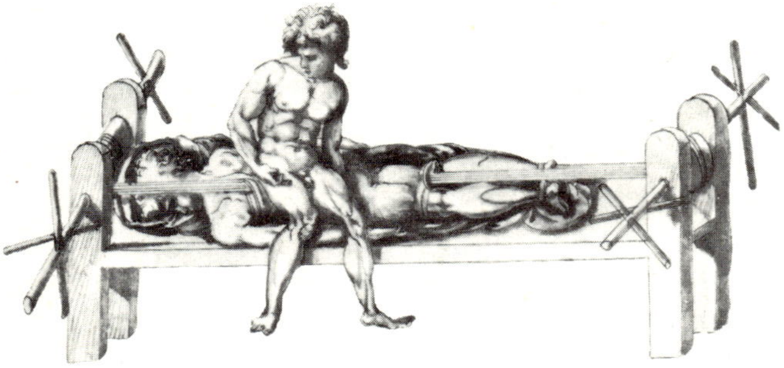

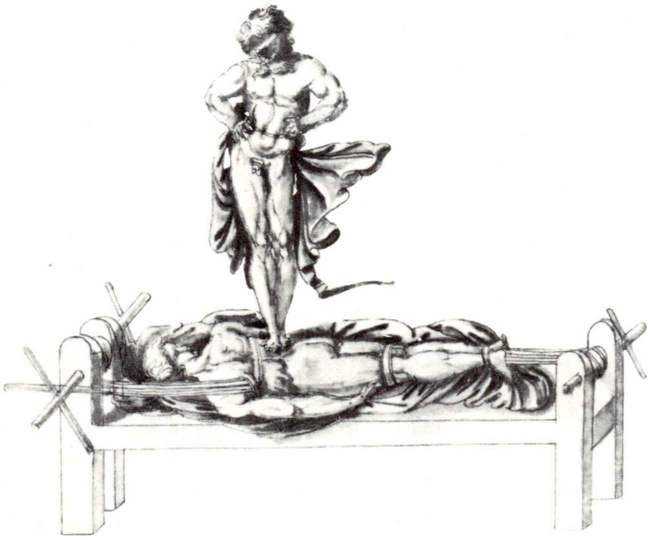

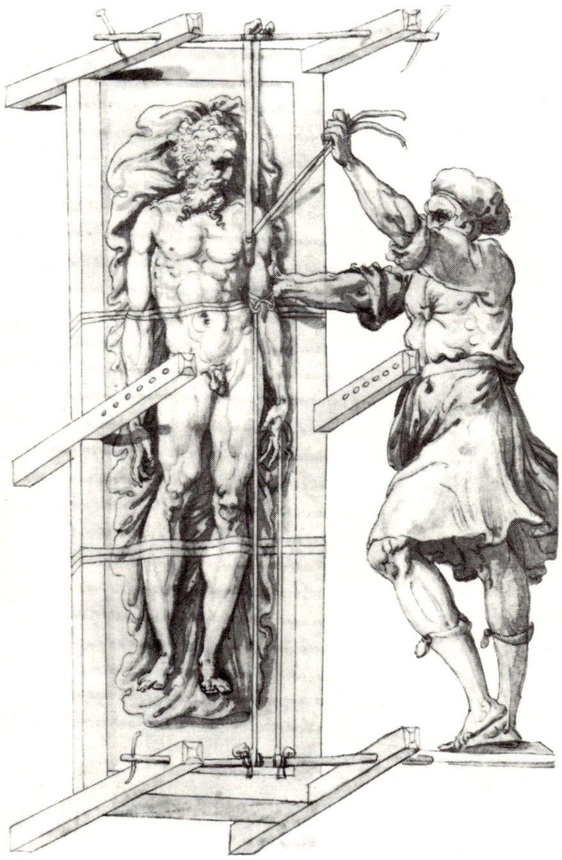

Tritheim of Wurzburg. He travelled from 1517 to 1526, studying for brief intervals at Vienna, Cologne, Paris and Montpellier. He himself said he took his medical degree at Ferrara in 1519, where his master was Leonicenus, author of the treatise on syphilis previously mentioned and of a work on Pliny's errors in botany and anatomy, but the documentary evidence for this statement is lacking. From his own writings it would appear that he had visited the Iberian peninsula, Pomerania, Poland, Lithuania, Russia, had been to the tin mines of Cornwall and Sweden, and had served as an army surgeon with the Dutch and the Venetians. Surprise was often expressed that he could have written so great a number of works despite this incessant travelling from one country to another. In answer to those who wondered about the sources of the extraordinary information of all kinds contained in his books, he wrote, 'I went in search of my art, often hazarding my life. I have not been ashamed to learn from tramps, butchers and barbers things which seemed of use to me'.

In 1526 his restless way of life changed. In that year Johannes Froben, or Frobenius, the Basle humanist and publisher, who had long been suffering from leg trouble, was advised by his doctors to have his leg amputated if he wished to save his life. Frobenius put himself in Paracelsus' care, and in a short time he recovered. Soon afterwards Erasmus of Rotterdam, a great friend of Frobenius, wrote to Paracelsus describing his illness and asking advice. The doctor prescribed treatment and Erasmus got better. It was probably on account of the reputation from these and other cures that Paracelsus was offered appointment to a university chair and as municipal doctor to the town council of Basle. This was an unexpected and welcome reward for a man who had identified with mercenaries and vagabonds, and had often been considered undesirable by the authorities in places which he had visited.

The speech with which Paracelsus made his debut at the university was characteristic and must have amazed his colleagues, who followed Galen assiduously and had never dreamed of prescribing commonsense treatment from their own experience. Paracelsus remarked: 'Thanks to the post offered me by the Basle authorities, which is an honour, I can proceed to teach students my methods, expounding for a two-hour period every day my precepts of treatment with the utmost diligence for the

The greatest physician of the Renaissance outside Italy was the Swiss-born Paracelsus, whose resounding full name was Philippus Aureolus Theophrastus Bombastus von Hohenheim. It seems that this remarkable character gave himself the name Paracelsus because he rated himself above Celsus, although it has also been suggested that he was given it because of his weakness for the prefix 'para', which appears in the titles of many of his works. Although involved with alchemy and mysticism, Paracelsus upheld Hippocrates' view that the place of the doctor was by the sickbed, and he contributed widely to the medicine of his day. When appointed as professor at Basle, he caused a furore firstly by lecturing in German, then by burning in public the works of Galen and Avicenna to demonstrate his revolt against unquestioning acceptance of medical dogma.

utmost benefit of my audience'. He then broke with tradition by lecturing in German instead of the customary Latin. He did worse: he burnt in public the works of Galen and Avicenna, condemning the pusillanimity that for so many centuries had held back progress in medicine. To this act of revolt he added invective against his new colleagues, accusing them of propagating falsehood and thereby feeding the troubles of the world. After having held his post for only two years, as might be expected, Paracelsus felt it necessary to leave Basle and revert to his life as a wandering physician.

It is unfortunate that in his iconoclastic fury Paracelsus rejected the good things in the works of the ancient authors. Yet he upheld the Hippocratic principle that the place of the doctor was by the patient's sickbed. Paracelsus was a clinician in the best sense of the word; he said, 'The doctor's character can influence the patient's recovery more than any medicine'.

During his journeys he collected a great deal of useful observation and experience. He was a chemical pathologist and a vitalist; according to the Paracelsian concept, the body's manifestations were subject to chemical and vital laws. He introduced the concept of metabolic disease and concerned himself with questions of hygiene. His admirable practical knowledge was shown in his works on surgery and his observations on syphilis and its treatment (mercury effective, guaiac useless). Through Paracelsus chemical remedies were introduced into medicine, and pharmacology began to make use of many new products. Paracelsus wrote a treatise on the diseases of miners, which may be considered the first work on occupational disease. He discussed 'diseases that deprive man of reason', and he recognized the connection between cretinism and goitre. He also wrote on epilepsy and the dancing mania, which was very widespread at the period. He died in 1541 at Salzburg when he was only forty-eight.

The greatest contemporary of Paracelsus was Jean Fernel (1497–1558), a native of Amiens who became professor of medicine in Paris, and, while

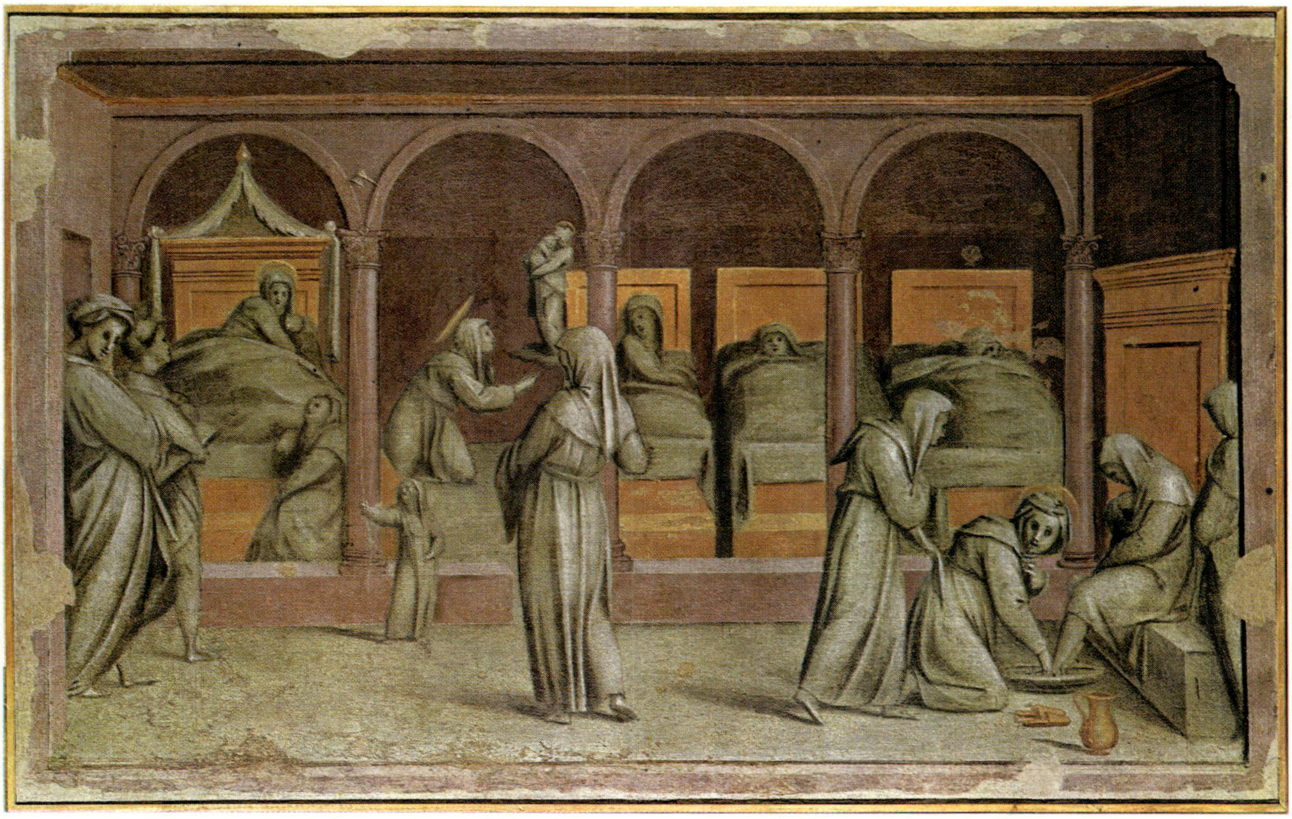

Paracelsus was a humanist, a man who travelled widely and studied many subjects, and his attitudes and beliefs were shared by several of the great figures of the Renaissance. This movement had arisen in Italy, but in time it spread throughout the continent of Europe and to the British Isles. Most countries produced men of medicine who were also well versed in other fields of inquiry, both in the sciences and in what we would now call the humanities. Often, the physician might also be an ordained priest, like the Englishman Thomas Linacre, founder of the Royal College of Physicians in London, and the Frenchman François Rabelais, creator of Gargantua *and* Pantagruel. *In his famous books, Rabelais ridiculed the mediaeval practice of forcing a diet of dogmatic teaching on the young student, praising instead the Greek ideal of*

very much a man of his time, was instrumental in loosening the hold of Galen on medical thought and added much to medical progress. He invented the terms physiology and pathology, and his writings, collected as *Universa medica,* remained the standard text for two centuries. Fernel was the first to give a clear description of appendicitis and to suggest a syphilitic origin of aortic aneurysms, and he saw something that Vesalius missed, namely that the spinal cord is hollow (perhaps this was in fact a description of syringomyelia, a disease where there is an abnormally large cavity, as the central canal of the cord is normally invisible to the unaided eye).

Girolamo Cardano was a man of great brilliance whose life was also very disturbed. He was born in Pavia in 1501 and was maltreated in childhood by both his parents. His father Fazio was a jurist and public lecturer in geometry in Milan, and a friend of Leonardo da Vinci. Girolamo attended the university of Pavia and then went to Padua, where in 1525 he was elected rector and a year later he took his degree in medicine. Because of his illegitimacy, he was refused admission to the Milan college of physicians.

Cardano lived wretchedly and for a while he was obliged to accept lodging in an almshouse with his wife and son. But circumstances improved when he made his name with the publication of *Practica arithmeticae et mensurandi singularis* in 1539. In 1545, he composed the *Ars magna,* the most important algebraic work of the Renaissance, which contained the solution of the cubic equation (still wrongly called Cardano's formula) and resulted in a bitter altercation with Nicolo Tartaglia, the mathematician from Brescia; Tartaglia was in

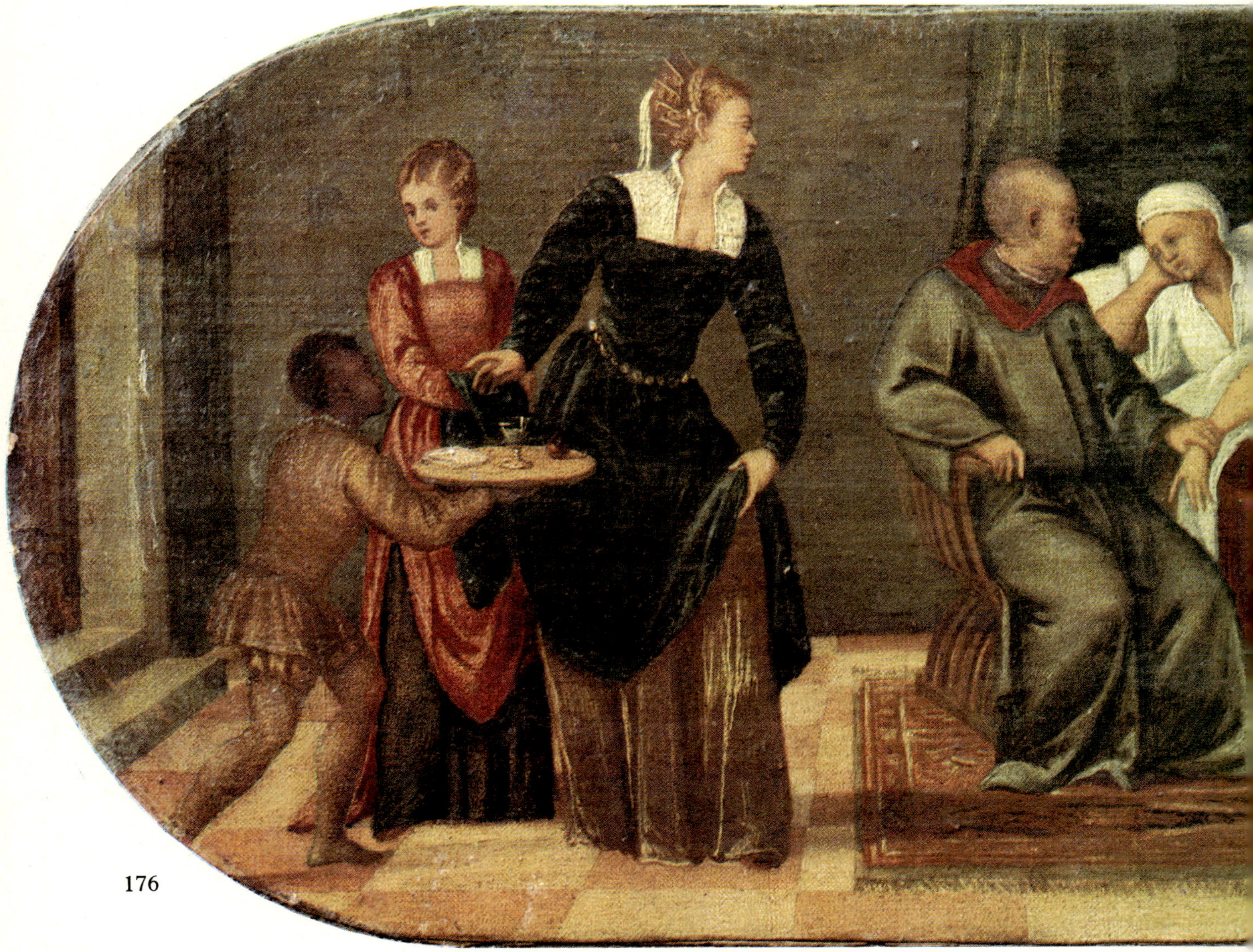

education in which the master drew out the pupil's innate faculties, intellectual, physical and social.

Jean Fernel was the greatest French physician of the Renaissance. He also studied philosophy and mathematics, but his greatest passion was astronomy, to which he devoted much of his life. A fascination with the mystical, as in astonomy and alchemy, marked many Renaissance scholars.

possession of the method and had confided it to Cardano, who swore to keep it secret.

Although involved with mathematics and philosophy, Cardano was also a great doctor. In 1552 he was invited to Edinburgh to treat the archbishop of Scotland, John Hamilton, who was thought to be suffering from a tubercular condition. After six weeks' observation, Cardano diagnosed asthma and recommended that the archbishop sleep between sheets of raw silk and without feather pillows. John Hamilton recovered; it may be supposed that he was allergic to feathers.

Tragedy darkened Cardano's life: his son poisoned his wife, was sentenced to death and beheaded. Cardano wrote *De utilitate ex adversis capienda,* in which he described the psychopathic trait. He stated it was 'nothing but a disorder of the mind, a malignant doltishness, which does not show the signs of complete insanity, for those suffering from it are able to exercise some choice'.

He was nominated professor at Bologna in 1563, imprisoned for impiety in 1571 and died in misery in Rome at the age of seventy-five. At the end of his life he was a superstitious man, dedicated to astrology and chiromancy.

Felix Platter of Basle (1563–1614) earned distinction as the first man to try to distinguish between various mental disorders: mentis imbecillitas (mental deficiency), mentis consternatio (loss of consciousness, as in epilepsy and in some strokes), mentis alienatio (psychosis) and mentis defatigatio (anxiety state). Platter studied medicine at Basle, Montpellier and Paris and was a follower of Vesalius in anatomy, although he held such traditional views as to believe melancholia to be the work of the devil.

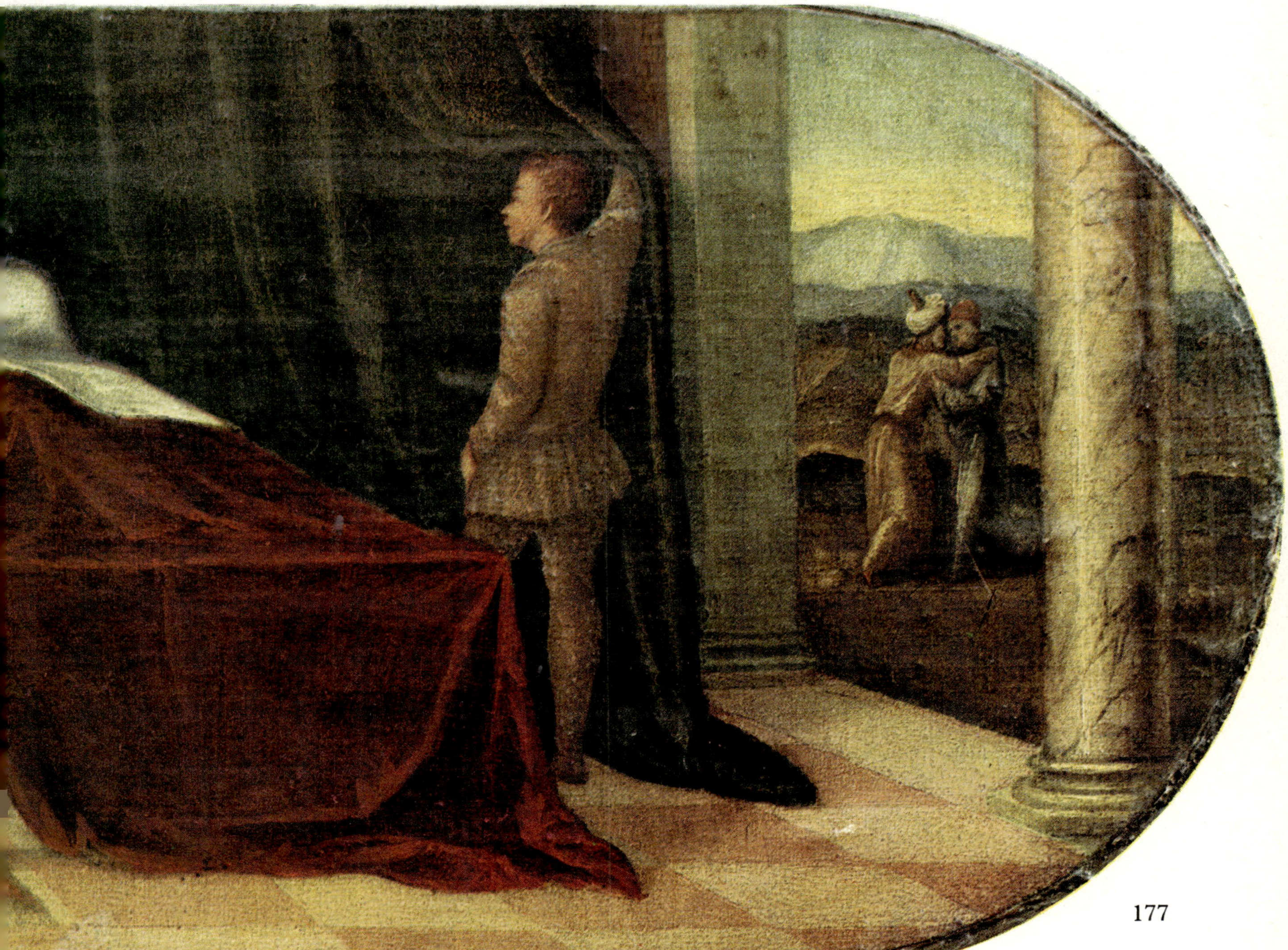

The doctor's visit. *By Bonifacio de' Pitati. Poldi Pezzoli Museum, Milan.*

Paré and sixteenth-century surgery

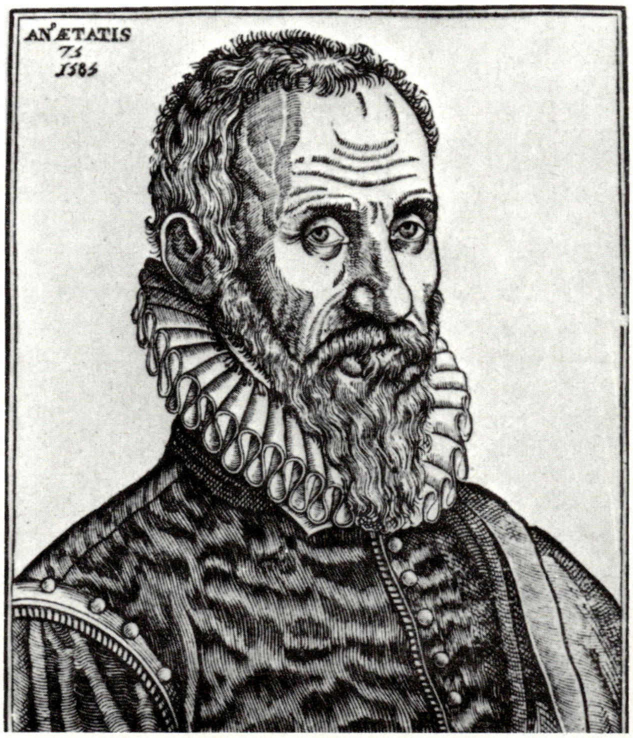

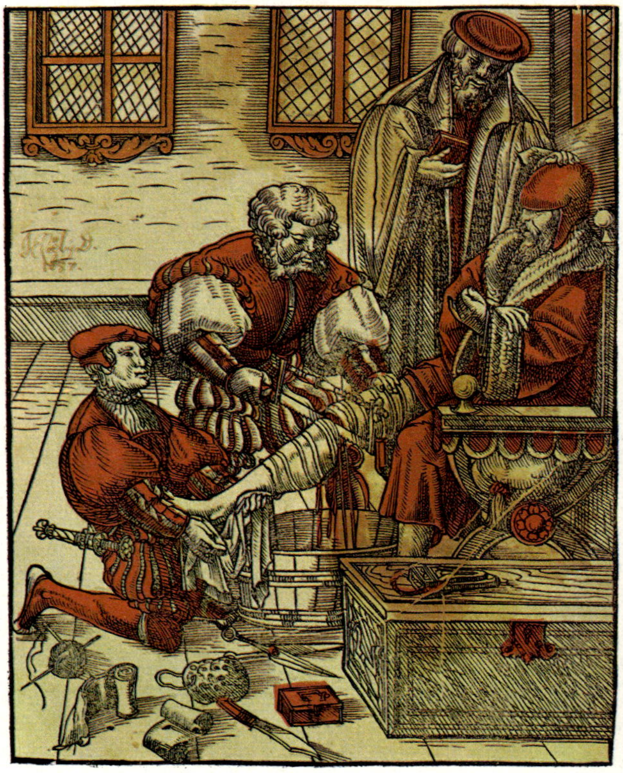

'In the year 1536, Francis the King of France sent a great expeditionary force to Piedmont to conquer Turin and recapture cities and castles ... The soldiers of the fort, seeing our forces launching an all-out attack, did their best to defend themselves and killed and wounded many with all types of weapons but chiefly gunshot, so that the surgeons had a great deal of work on their hands. At that time, to tell the truth, I was still a beginner, never having seen gunshot wounds treated. True, I had read in the eighth chapter of the first book of Giovanni da Vigo's *Delle ferite in generale* that wounds caused by firearms were poisonous because of the gunpowder and that the best treatment was to cauterize them with boiling oil of elder mixed with treacle.

Knowing that boiling oil was sure to cause the wounded terrible pain, before applying it I asked what the other surgeons used for the first dressing. It was only when I learned that they poured the oil as hot as possible into the wound that I summoned up courage to do likewise. But then I ran out of oil and was obliged to apply a mixture of egg yolk, oil of roses and turpentine. That night I was unable to sleep thinking I was going to find that my wounded patients had died because I had not performed the cauterization with boiling oil. So I got up before daybreak and went to have a look at them. What I found was beyond my wildest hope, for those to whom I had given my mixture felt little pain and their wounds were not inflamed. On the other hand, I discovered that all those to whom I had adminstered the boiling oil were in dreadful pain and with the injured part inflamed. At this I decided that never again would I burn so cruelly the poor men who had been wounded by arquebus shots.'

Thus is was a novice who put an end to the atrocious practice of burning wounds with hot iron or boiling oil. This beginner was Ambroise Paré, maistre barbier chirurgien, the leading surgeon of the Renaissance. The passage quoted reveals the honest professional, full of compassion for the suffering of others, intelligent, endowed with acute powers of observation and also lacking in knowledge in some respects. In fact, the treatise on gunshot wounds was written in French; 'I do not wish', he said, 'to be able to boast of having read Galen, in the Greek or in the Latin; God was not pleased to be so kind to me in my youth as to

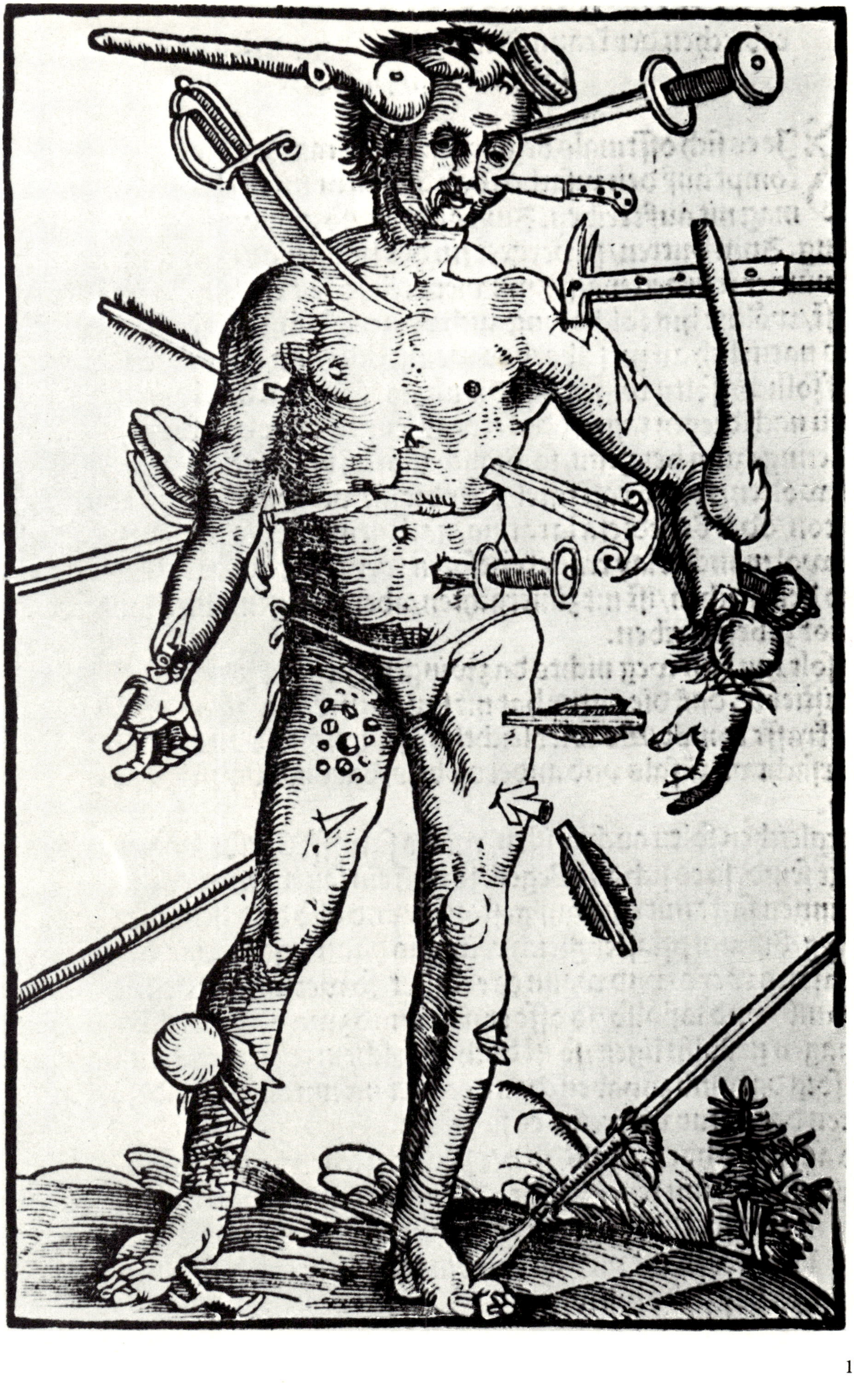

Previous pages :
Ambroise Paré at the age of 73. *Portrait from Opera omnia, 1585.*

Amputation of a leg. *Colour plate from Die grosse Chirurgei by Walter Ryff, 1545. Putti Collection, Rizzoli Institute, Bologna.*

The wound man. *Plate from the Grosse Wundartzney by Paracelsus, 1536.*

These pages :
Rhinoplasty. *From Chirurgia curtorum per insitionem by Tagliacozzi, Venice, 1597.*

Portrait of Tagliacozzi with his books. *Attributed to T Passarotti. Putti Collection, Rizzoli Institute, Bologna.*

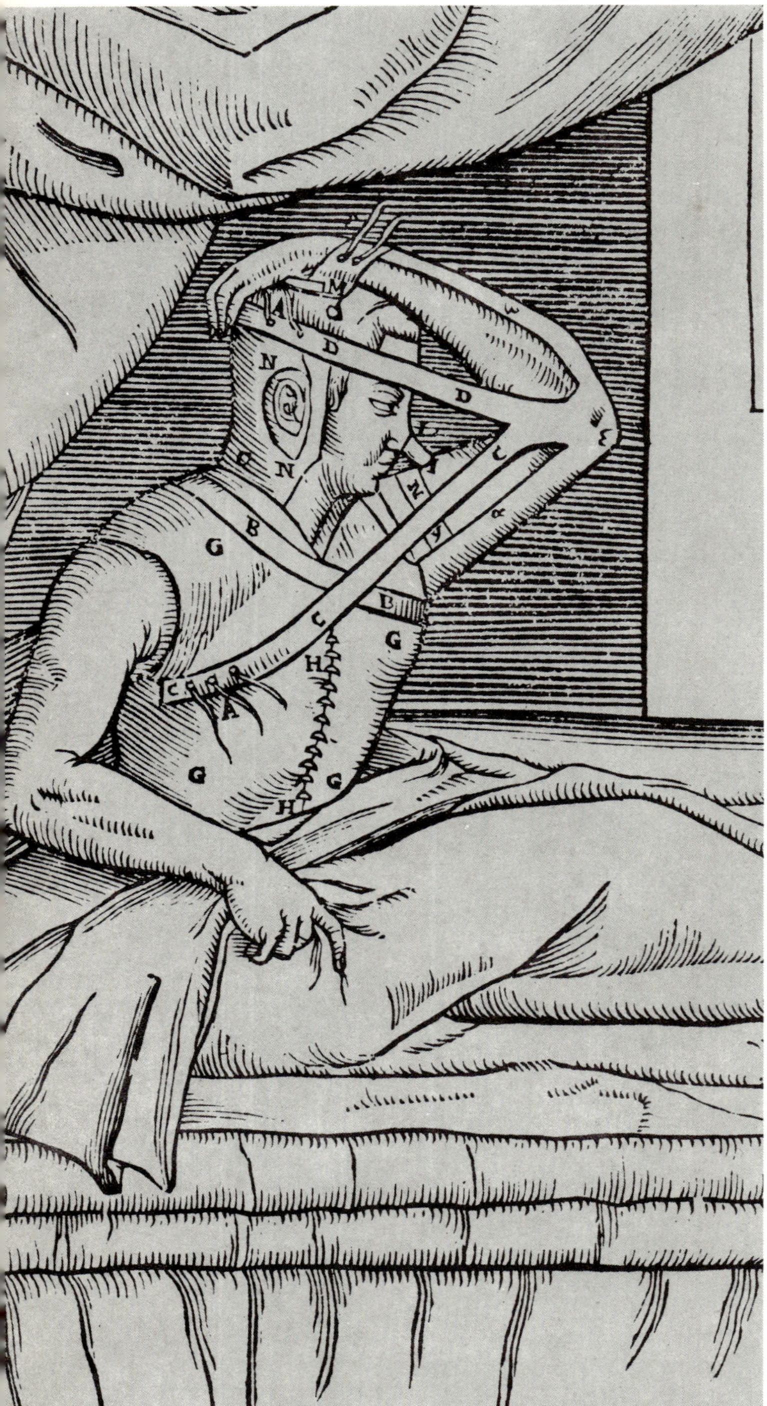

provide for my instruction in the one or the other of these languages'.

Ambroise Paré was born in 1517, at Bourg-Hersent near Laval in Mayenne. His father and a paternal uncle were barber surgeons, representing the lowest grade in the medical hierarchy. Surgeons formed the confraternity of St Cosmas and concerned themselves with the treatment of wounds, cauterization, the lancing of abscesses and the application of ointments and plasters. Major operations were entrusted to these modest practitioners, who besides shaving their customers used to let blood by application of leeches or cupping vessels. The ambition of Paré, who had had little schooling, was ignorant of Latin and Greek and so unable to enter the university, was to become a barber surgeon.

A deficient education became an asset, for Paré learned the art from first-hand experience, initially with a relative who was a barber surgeon in Paris, then as house surgeon at the Hôtel Dieu, an old hospital which had been founded by monks in the Middle Ages, and then as an army surgeon. His career progressed with his mind unburdened by the weighty heritage of Galen and Albucasis but without his neglecting recent anatomical advances. It was through his intelligence as well as his lack of reverence for the old masters that he was able to abolish overnight the cauterization of wounds. In the tenth century Albucasis was apologetic about the use of the cautery, which he advised only as a last resort, but it had subsequently come into indiscriminate use. Because of his opposition to barbarous systems practised by surgeons on the battlefield, Paré became the idol of the army.

He also made systematic use of procedures devised by other people but seldom adopted, for example control of haemorrhage by ligation of arteries, and operation for hare-lip. He devised new surgical instruments, including haemostatic forceps. He was interested in the problem of cripples, for whom he devised ingenious artificial aids. He also wrote on obstetrics and the procedure of podalic version for abnormal presentation of the foetus. The humble barber surgeon rose to become a councillor of state and surgeon to four kings of France, Henri II, Francis II, Charles IX and Henri III. He died in 1590.

That Parè eventually decided to take up the pen himself and start writing was due to the inaccurate statements committed to paper by a traditionalist,

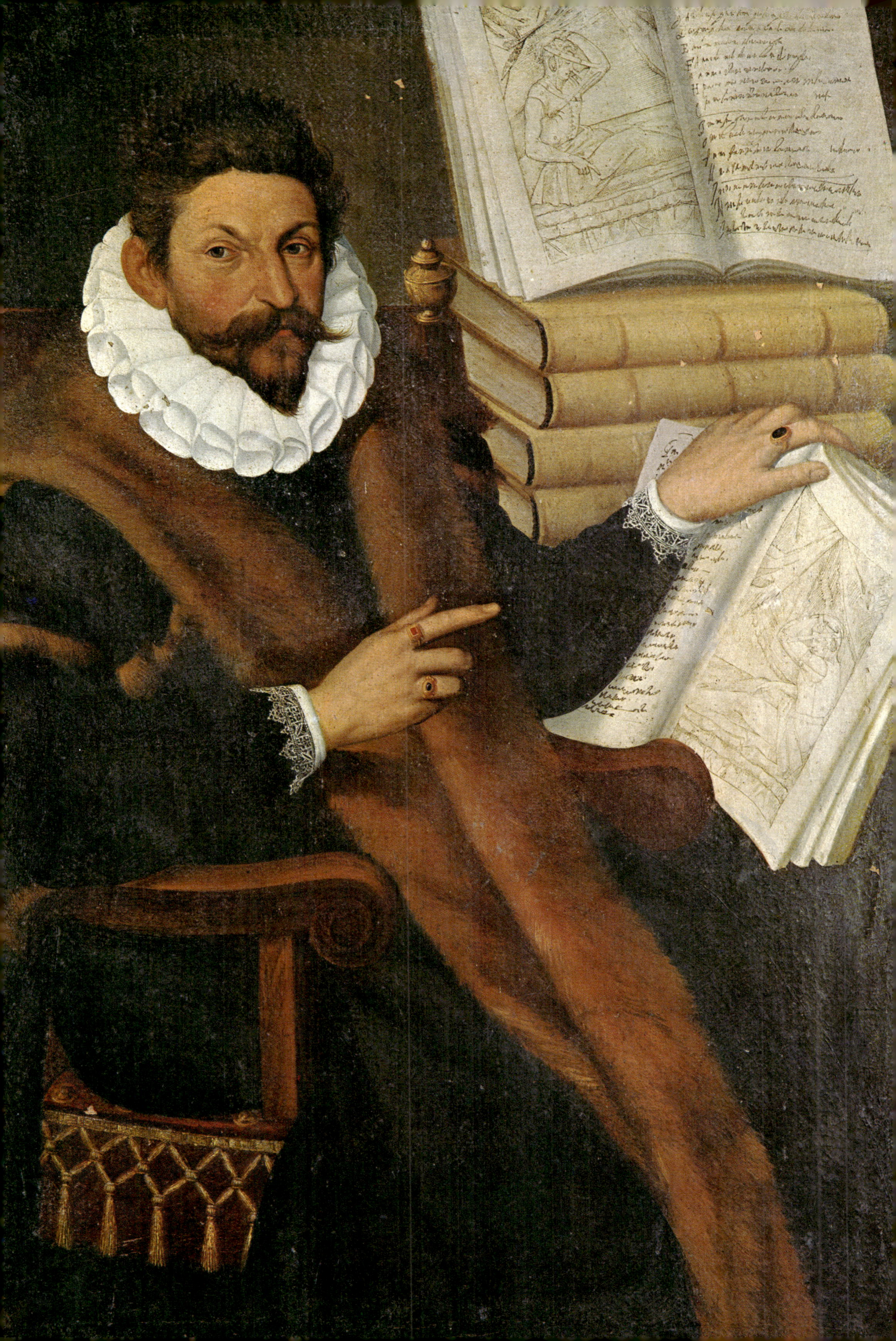

The reforming, original spirit of the Renaissance, together with the big advances in anatomy and physiology, in time had a stimulating effect on the practice of surgery. The greatest surgeon of his day was the Frenchman Ambroise Paré, who won enormous popularity with the army because he rejected the custom of burning wounds with hot iron or boiling oil. He also designed many surgical instruments and introduced new operative techniques, such as the ligation of arteries (which had been developed earlier but not adopted). Paré devised numerous prostheses for cripples, including an ingenious artificial hand; the writings of Hippocrates had described methods of reducing hip dislocations and for making orthopaedic shoes, but generally progress in this field was very slow until the eighteenth century.

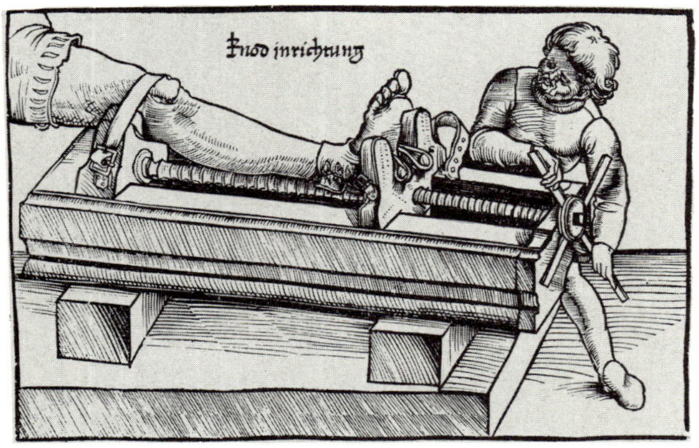

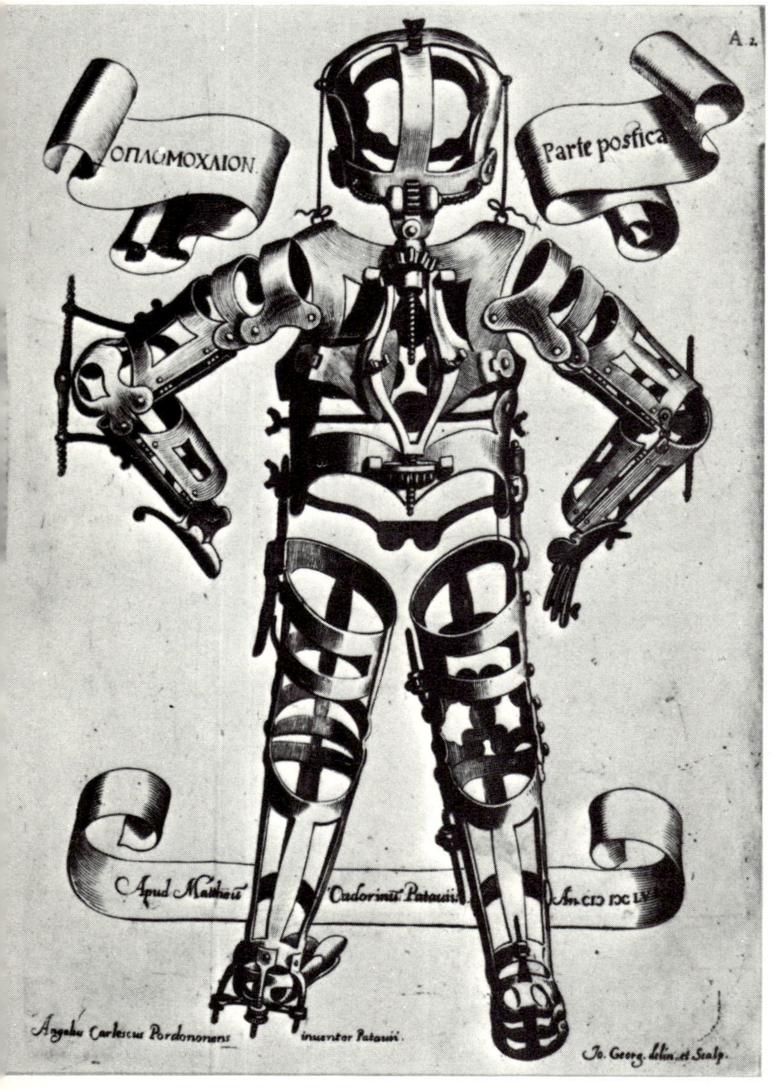

Etienne Gourmelen, who attacked Paré in a long diatribe, criticizing in particular arterial ligation. 'How dare you teach me surgery', Paré replied, 'you who have done nothing all your life but look at books! Surgery is learnt with the hand and eye. And you – mon petit maître – all you know is how to talk your head off, sitting comfortably in your chair'. He was already famous when he began writing, and he found pleasure in giving a full account of his experiences as a surgeon and in war. The completed text was entitled *Oeuvres de M. Ambroise Paré, conseiller, et premier chirurgien du Roy,* and was published in 1575 at Paris, in a magnificent volume of nearly a thousand pages.

In the first engagement during the Piedmont campaign, a badly wounded officer named Le Rat was brought to Paré. The young surgeon saved his life; when asked how, he replied, 'I treated him, God healed him'. This phrase, which was engraved on his tombstone, was more than an impromptu answer from a humble and devout man; it was his expression of faith in natural healing power, and it recurs in Paré's diaries, especially apropos of desperate cases.

One of these cases is illuminating, for it leaves no doubt about the great surgeon's belief in the healing mechanism. It was a patient who was such a problem that nothing his own doctors could do for him was any help. Paré, who retired from the army in 1559 and bought a house near the Pont St Michel in Paris, was invited by the king to treat the Marquis d'Aurel. The patient's condition had steadily deteriorated over a seven-month period since his femur had been fractured by a bullet. Paré began his account of the case by describing a man suffering from an infection. 'The young marquis had a high temperature, his eyes were sunken in their sockets, his face yellowish, his tongue dry and spotted, his body wasted away and his voice feeble as that of a dying man'.

The wound was suppurating and the sick man lay in incredible filth. The sheets had plainly not been changed for months. 'I carried out an examination with a silver probe', he wrote, 'and found one deep cavity in the middle of the thigh and others round the joint, with many bone fragments, some separate and others not. He had extensive bedsores, got no rest by day or night, had no appetite and was thirsty. Noting these serious complications and the weakening of the life force, I was sorry I had seen him for it

Another notable surgeon of the sixteenth century was the Italian Gaspare Tagliacozzi, who developed an effective rhinoplasty operation. He transplanted onto the nose a strip of skin from the patient's arm, the strip being only partly detached and the patient strapped up in such a way that the graft continued to be fed by its blood supply until it had taken on the new site.

looked as if there was little hope of avoiding death. All the same, to give him hope and strength, I told him he would be on his feet again with the help of God and his physician and surgeons'.

Paré was shocked to discover, in the course of the consultation, that the bone fragments had not been removed and he asked the doctors concerned why this had not been done. He also asked why they had not drained and dressed the wound, and why they had never had the linen changed on the sick man's bed. 'They replied that the sick man would never have agreed to the operation; nearly two months had gone by since they changed the sheets because his sufferings were so dreadful that they could hardly contrive to smooth down the bed, let alone to make it'. Paré won the young man's confidence and was able to make the incisions to drain the wound and remove the bone fragments. Then he ordered his patient to be given a good wash and laid in a clean bed, with a cushion to relieve the discomfort from the bedsores; he also had a rudimentary sort of shower fixed up in the room – the drops of water, falling into a large basin, made a sound like rain and the patient was lulled to sleep, soon getting four hours' rest at a time. The Marquis d'Aurel lived to tell the tale; during his convalescence, Paré encouraged the household to keep his spirits up and they enlisted the help of a strolling player and the songs and dances of the local peasants.

Ambroise Paré lived during the long wars of Francis I with Charles V and Philip II and the wars of the Reformation. He was young when the reform movement, initiated by Luther and Calvin, bore its first fruits. Some authorities say that the surgeon was a Huguenot but this is unlikely. Certainly he was a devout Christian, a doctor in the service of a Catholic king who also treated the leader of the Huguenots, Admiral Coligny, during the Huguenot wars. When the massacre of St Bartholomew took place, his life was spared only by the king's intervention.

Giovanni da Vigo (1460–1525), whose works had been studied by Paré, was a native of Rapallo, surgeon to Pope Julius II and one of the most famous Italian surgeons of his time. His *Practica copiosa in arte chirurgica* (1514) went through more than forty editions and was translated into English and German as well as the Romance languages. It was composed of nine books, the first of which con-

Traction of a leg. *From Feldtbuch der Wundartzney by Hans Gersdorff, Strasburg, 1517. Putti Collection, Rizzoli Institute, Bologna.*

Artificial limbs with various structures in metal and leather. *From Opera chirurgica by Fabrizio d'Acquapendente, Paris, 1613.*

Artificial hand designed by Ambroise Paré, 1551. *National Library, Vienna.*

Trephining the skull. *From Feldtbuch der Wundartzney by Hans Gersdorff, Strasburg, 1517.*

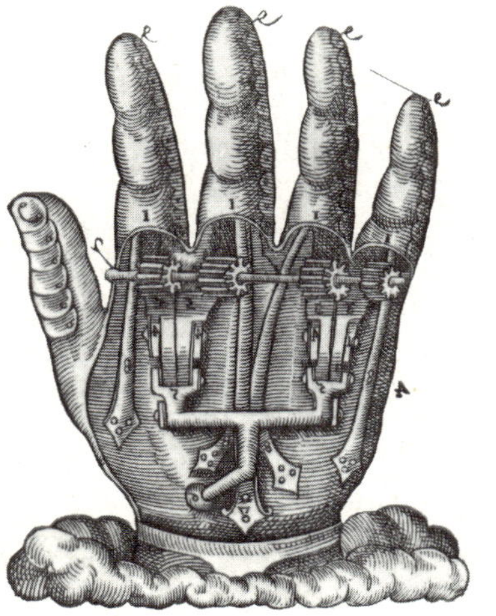

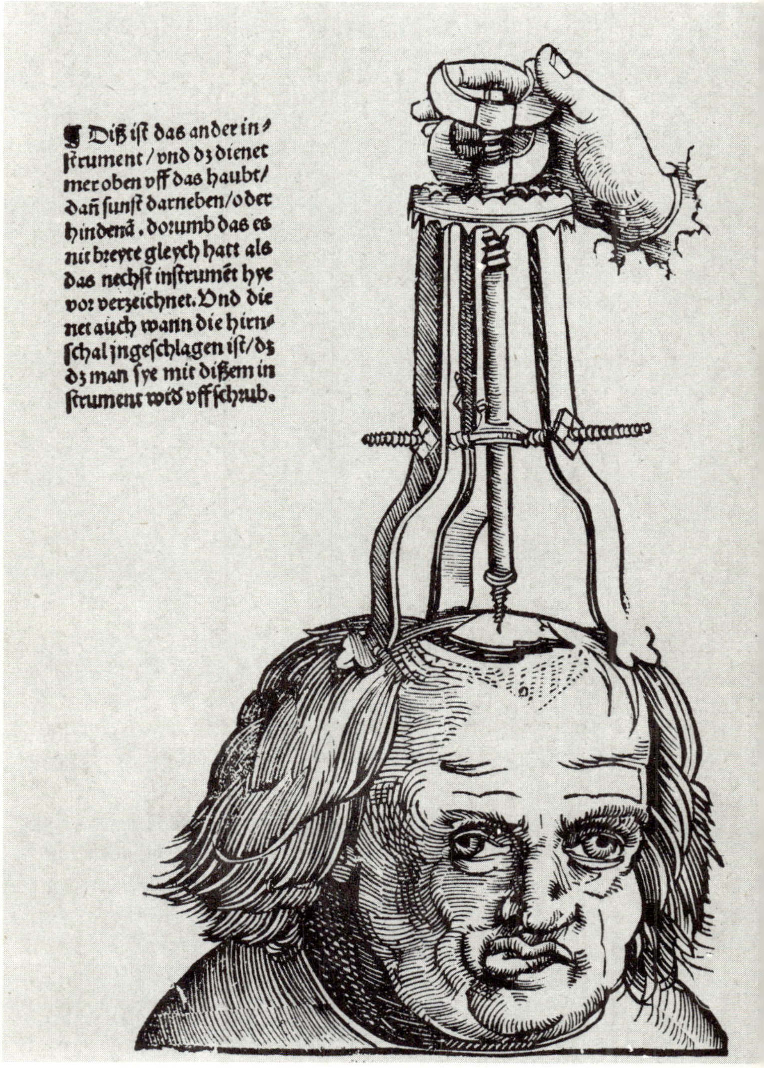

The anatomy of the eye; an eye operation; device to correct squints. *Illustrations from Ophthalmodouleia by G Bartisch, Dresden, 1583. Putti Collection, Rizzoli Institute, Bologna.*

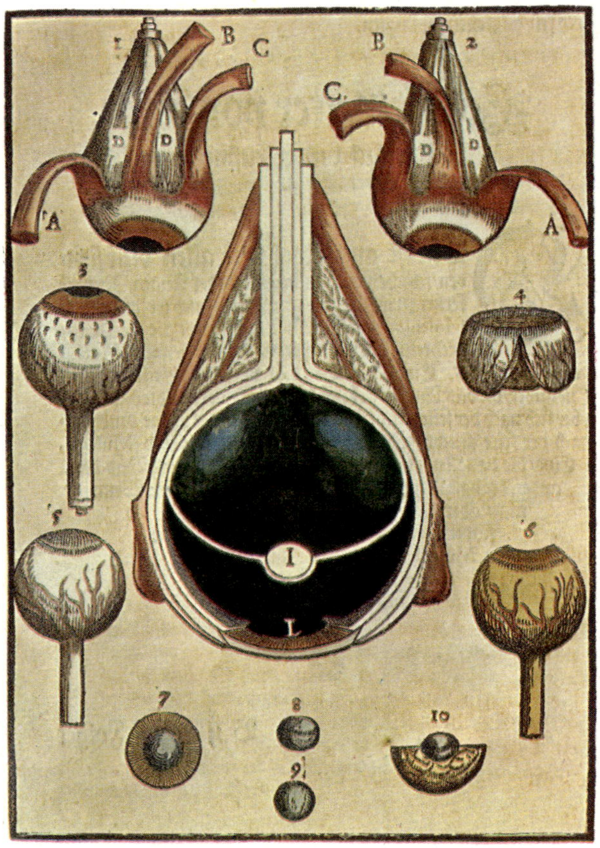

tained the necessary anatomical knowledge as a preliminary for surgery, while the others dealt with a range of surgical disorders and their treatment. A noteworthy feature in Vigo's work was his advocacy of the practice, long disused, of ligating blood vessels by introducing the needle below and tying the thread from above. In the belief that wounds were poisoned, he recommended treatment by cautery and also by a plaster containing pulverized frogs, worms and vipers.

Among the surgeons of the later Renaissance mention should be made of Gaspare Tagliacozzi (1546–1599), professor of medicine at Bologna, who made considerable advances in plastic surgery, using his great knowledge of anatomy. Plastic surgery had been practised in Sicily in the fourteen-hundreds by members of the Branca family and also in Calabria by members of the Vianeo di Maida and Boiano di Tropea families; they all regarded rhinoplasty as a family secret. Tagliacozzi gave his technique wide publicity: it consisted in restoring the nose with a strip of skin from the arm of the patient, who was strapped up so that the graft did not have to be removed completely until it had taken. He met opposition from the ecclesiastical authorities, who charged him with impiety and prohibited his operation, which was revived only in 1822.

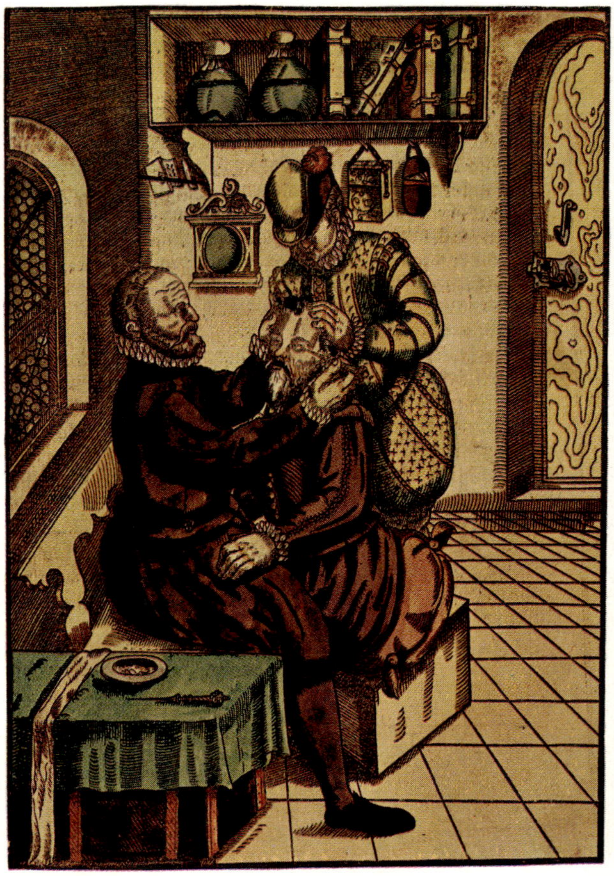

During this period the German-speaking lands produced, among other notable figures, Georg Bartisch (1535–1607), the author of the first book on eye surgery, *Ophthalmodouleia,* published at Dresden in 1583, and also fflilhelm Fabry or Fabricius Hildanus (1560–1624), who was born at Hilden near Düsseldorf. Hildanus practised in Berne, having studied medicine in Italy and France. He carried out amputations with a red-hot knife; according to him this horrifying system had the advantage of reducing haemorrhage to a considerable extent.

Hildanus was also the first to amputate above, rather than through, a gangrenous part, and to amputate through the thigh, but he advocated a curiously archaic magical practice in dealing with wounds–the application of weapon-salve to the causative knife or sword.

Another famous German surgeon of the period was Felix Wurtz (1518–74), a native of Zurich and

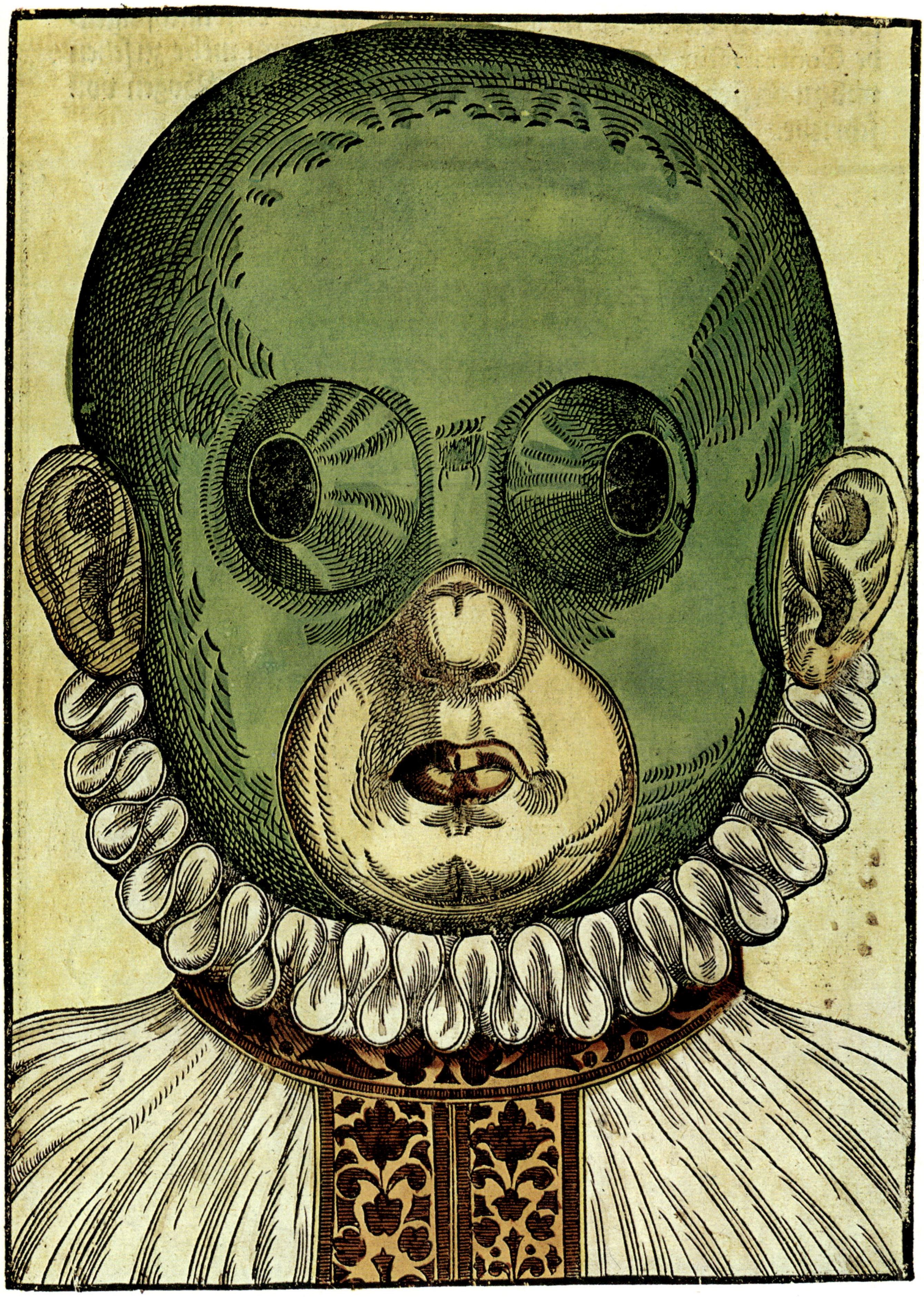

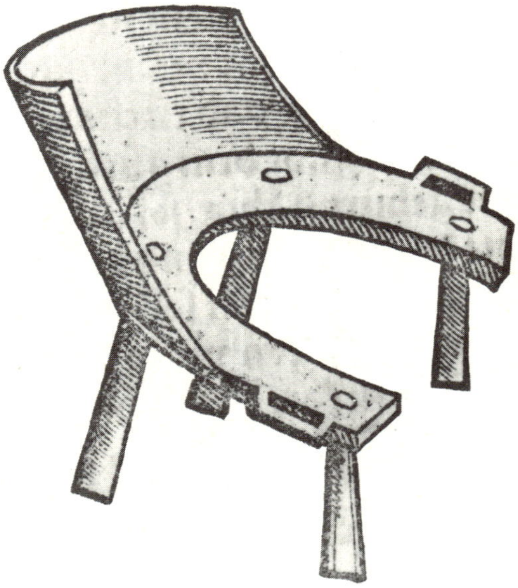

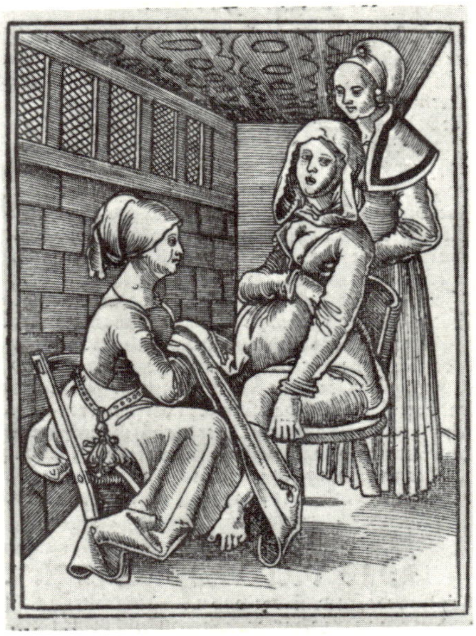

Der frawen Rosegarten

¶ Wo aber das kind sich in müter leib nit wolt vmbwen
den damit das das haupt [illegible]dersich keme/so soll die heb-
am den andern füß auch zü der geburt schicken, ond dem
kind vßh.ffen/doch allwegen das die arm vnd hend ne-
ben seiner seiten hinab gestreckt seyent/als obstat.

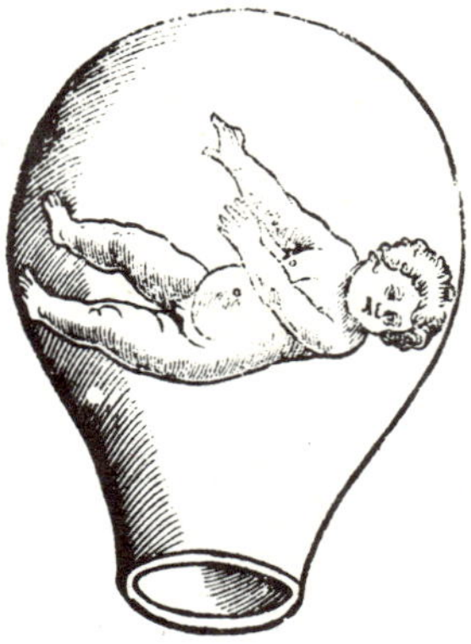

¶ Wo aber das kind ke-
me mit einer seitē an die
geburt/So soll aber die
hebam̄ das kind schickē/
richten vnd wysen vber-
sich/wie es vorhin in mü
ter leib gesessen ist vñ im
darnach zü bequēlichem
vßgang helffen.

¶ So aber das kind kem mit ge
teiltē füessen/ So soll die heb-
am̄ die füß züsamen thün/vnnd
darnach vßfüren/als obstadt.
Doch soll sie allzeit fleiß anke-
rē das die hend des kindes neb-
seiner seiten hinab gestreckt sey-
ent/als dick gemelt ist.

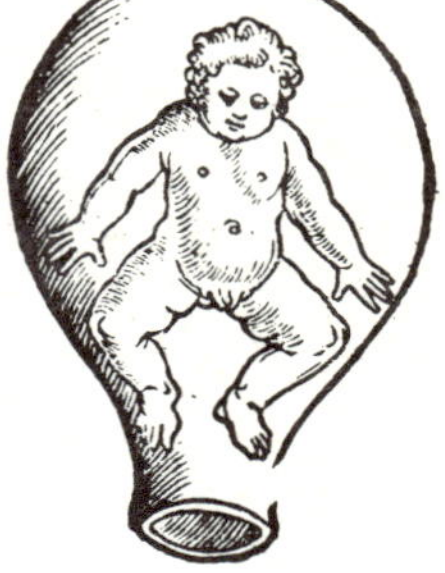

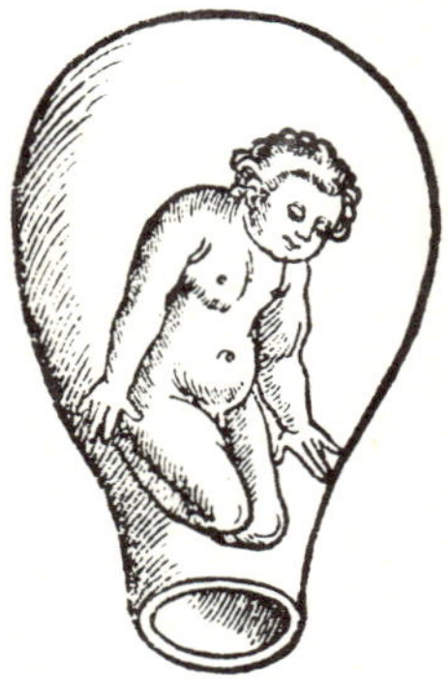

¶ Vnd so das kind sich mit
den knüwen erzeugt/od̉ mit
einē knü kem an die geburt
So soll die hebam̄ dz kind
vbersich heben vnd die füeß
begriffen/vñ wie obgeschri-
ben ist dem kind zü vßgang
helffen

¶ Itē ob das kind ein hand
erzeugte/So sol die hebam̄
das kind nit empfahē/ sond̉
sie soll mit yngelaßner hād
die schultern des kindes be-
greiffen vnd hindersich k:bē
vnd die hand neben des kin-
des seyten hynab streckē/dz
haupt begreiffen/ vñ im zü
vßgāg helffen. Wo aber sō
lich wysen vnd schicken der
hend nit ein fürgāg wolt ha
ben So ist aber not dz man
die fraw an ruckē lege/ vnd
mit dē haupt nider vnd mit
dē hindern hoch/damit das
das kind hindersich fall/ vñ
als dan wider sitzē/vñ dem
kind zü vßgang helffen.

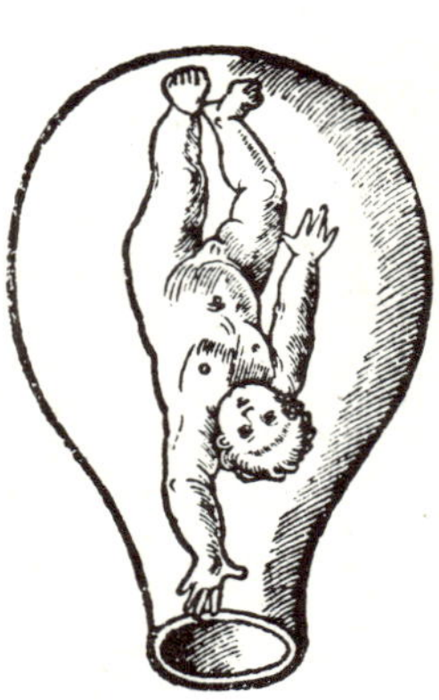

Many of the books published during the Renaissance were written in the vernacular, rather than Latin. Some of the most popular books of the period were on the subjects of obstetrics and paediatrics, and of these many went into hundreds of translations and editions and were standard texts until centuries later. Obstetrics gained richly at this time from the work of the anatomists and surgeons, notably Ambroise Paré.

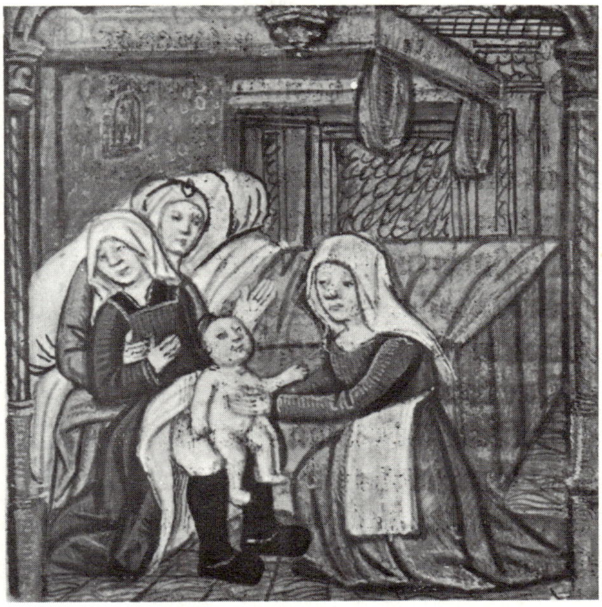

a friend of Paracelsus, who adopted some of his methods in the treatment of wounds. He must have had little practical anatomical knowledge, for his work on the practice of traumatic surgery deals exclusively with fractures, dislocations and the dressing of wounds, for which purpose he used cautery, ointments and plasters.

During the Renaissance numerous books appeared on the subject of obstetrics, many of them written in the vernacular. In 1513 the most successful of these was published at Strasburg, *Der Swangern Frawen und Hebammen Rosengarten* (The rose-garden of pregnant women and midwives), written by Eucharius Roesslin (d. 1526), a physician who practised at Worms and later at Frankfurt. The *Rosengarten* was essentially a collection of Greek and Latin works on obstetrics, but rendered in German and illustrated with twenty woodcuts by Conrad Merkel, a friend of Dürer. The use of the common language and the inclusion of illustrations probably account for the enormous success of Roesslin's work; it was translated into several languages in numerous editions until as late as the eighteenth century. An English version by Richard Jonas, called the *Byrthe of Mankind,* was published in 1540.

One of the best-known of all Renaissance

Obstetric stool; childbirth; positions of foetus in the uterus. *Illustrations from the Rosengarten by E Roesslin, Worms, 1513.*

Delivery standing up. *Illustration from Passetemps de tout homme, by Guillaume Alexis, Paris, 1505.*

Ivory statuette of pregnant woman, with removable parts designed to show internal organs. *Probably sixteenth-century German. Putti Collection, Rizzoli Institute, Bologna.*

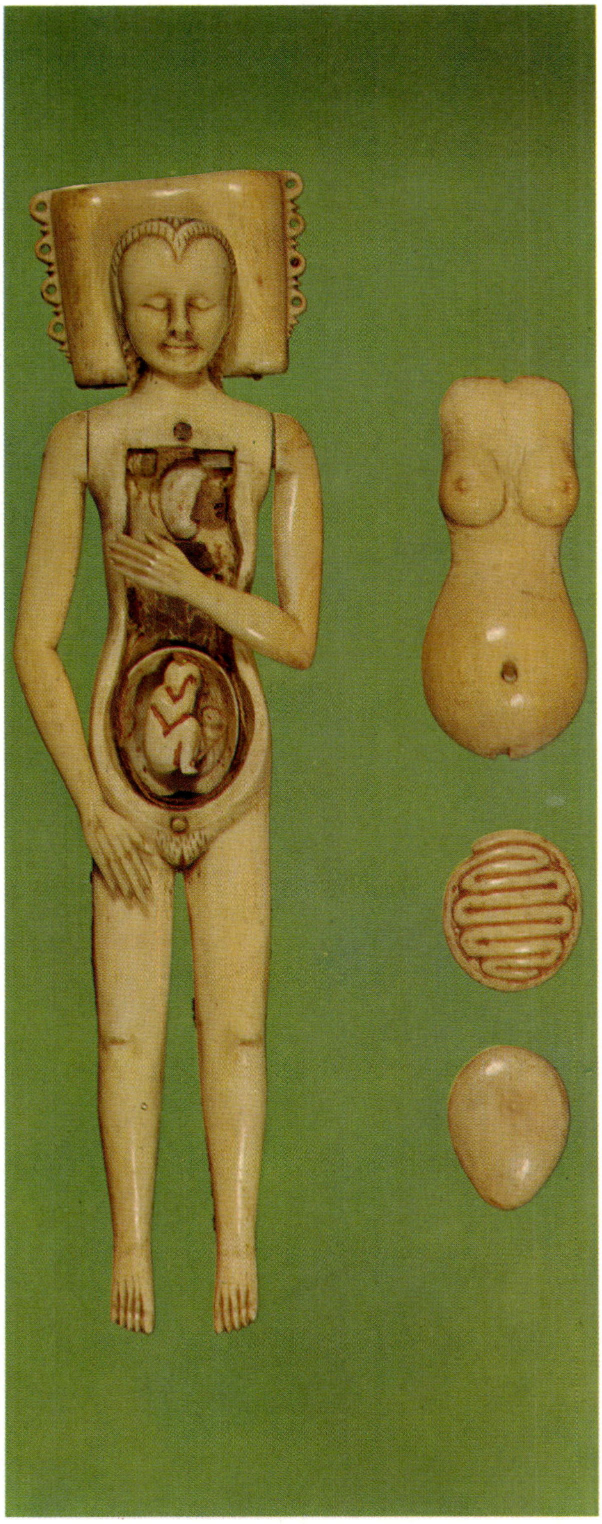

Birth of the Virgin. *By Boccaccio Boccaccino. From the Cathedral, Cremona.*

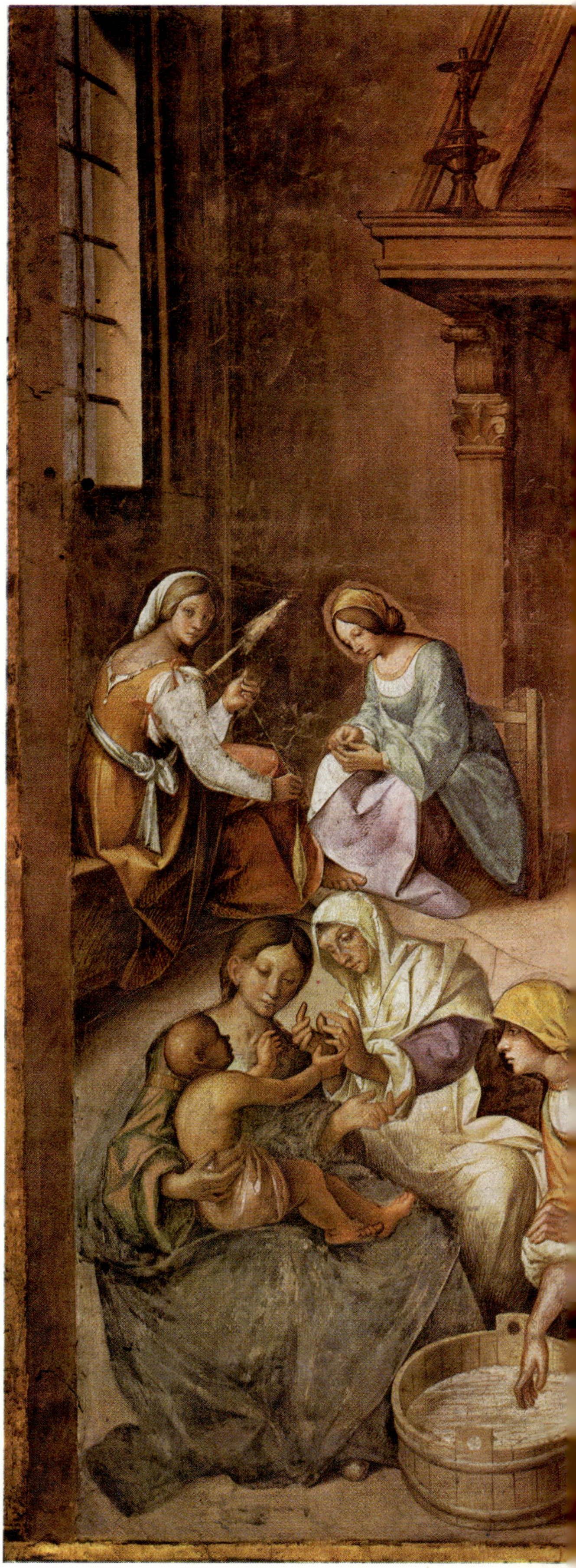

medical works, and one which like the *Rosengarten* was republished in innumerable editions until well into the eighteenth century, was an Italian book on obstetrics, *La comare o raccoglitrice* (The midwife) by Scipio Mercurio, first published in 1595, the year of his death; it is notable for containing one of the earliest statements that Caesarean section should be performed in the case of contracted pelvis.

Advances in anatomy and surgery in the sixteenth century had an important influence on the practice of obstetrics. Vesalius and all the other great figures of the time paid attention to the various deformities that may occur in the structure of the pelvis and studied the mechanics of childbirth. Paré is regarded as one of the founders of modern obstetrics; his *De la génération de l'homme* (Paris, 1573) combines Hippocratic principles with Paré's own original observations and modifications, and recommends podalic version, a procedure which Paré was probably the first to put into successful practice. Another book advocating this method was *L'heureux accouchement des femmes* (Paris, 1609), written by Jacques Guillemeau (1550–1613), a surgeon and obstetrician who was a pupil of Paré.

The publication of practical books on obstetrics was matched during the Renaissance by the growing number of works on the subject of paediatrics, many of them written in the vernacular. The first English contribution was the *Boke of children* by Thomas Phayre (d. 1560), published in 1545 as part of his *Regiment of life,* a version of the Salernitan *Regimen sanitatis,* while the first one in French was Simon de Vallambert's *De la manière de gouverner les enfants dès leur naissance* (Poitiers, 1565).

An Italian work was *De morbis puerorum* (On the diseases of children, Venice, 1583) by Gerolamo Mercuriale (1530–1606), who was also the author of a famous book on medical gymnastics, *De arte gymnastica* (1573), and of the first systematic treatise on skin diseases, *De morbis cutaneis* (Venice, 1572). Mercuriale also attempted to explain certain psychiatric conditions, stating for example that the increase in melancholia which he observed was caused by the life of pleasure and excessive luxury that more and more people were leading, tracing its origin to a disturbance of the imaginative faculties.

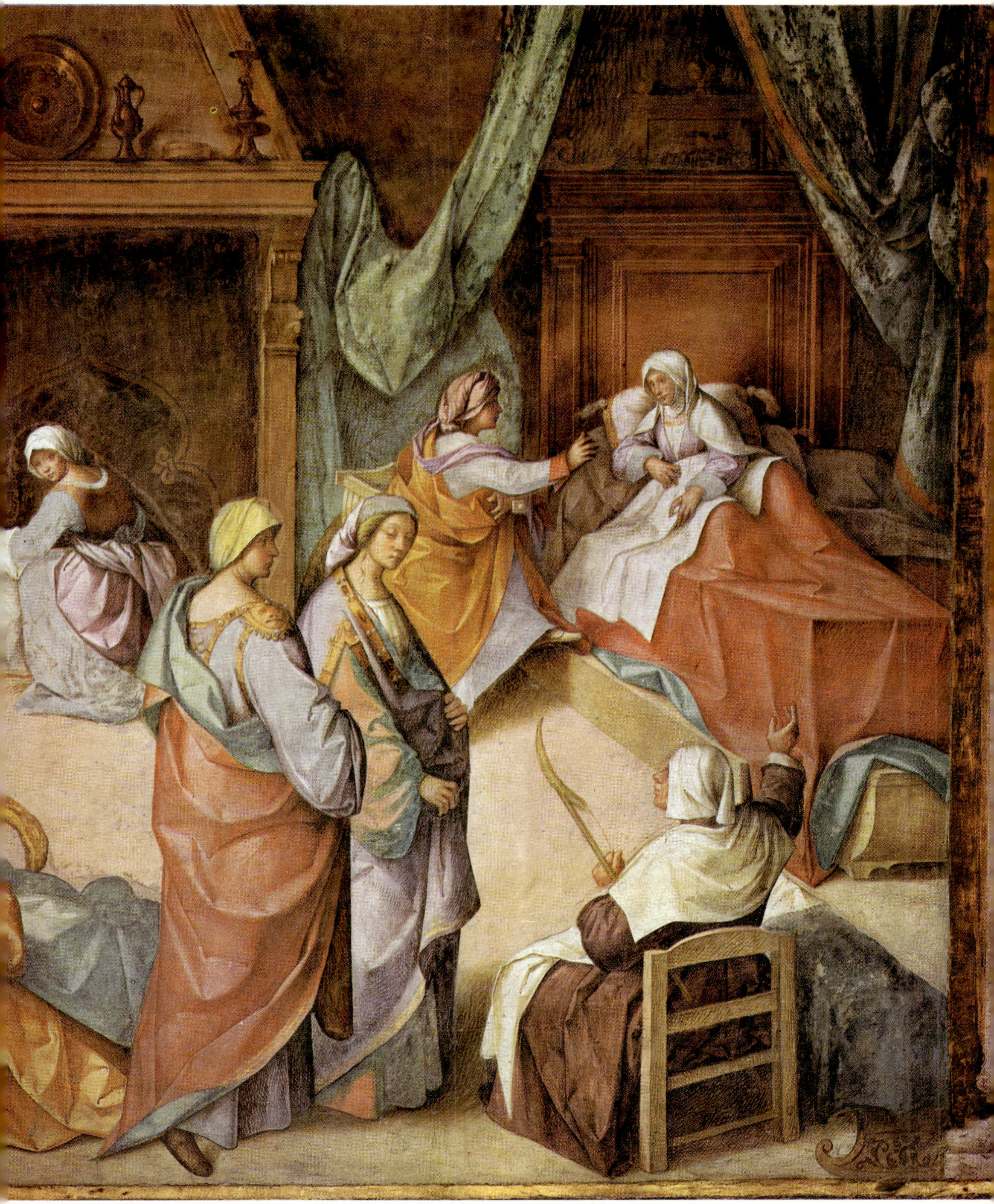

SEVENTEENTH CENTURY

A golden age of science

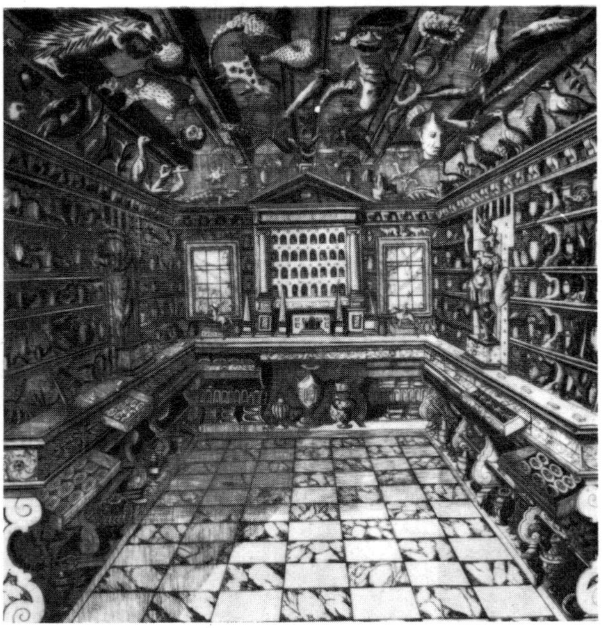

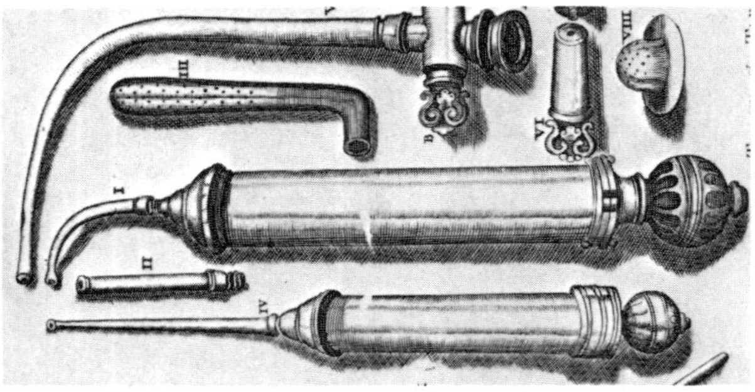

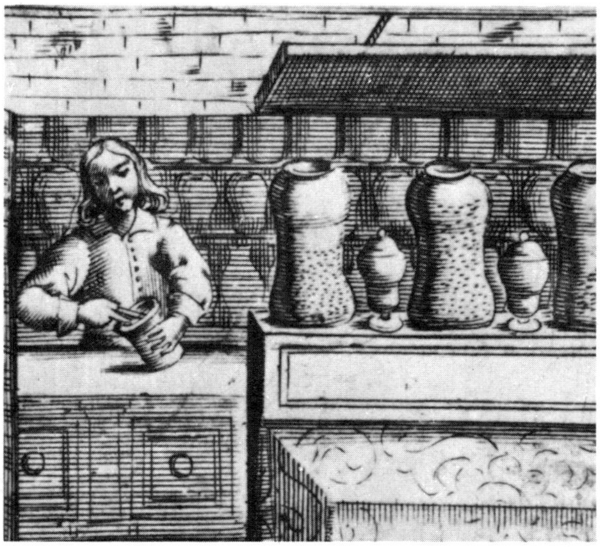

In the seventeenth century the gulf between medical practice and advances in research was wider than at any time before or since. Medical practitioners were for the most part poorly trained and loth to keep abreast of developments; they continued to prescribe, whatever the disease, the same old remedies – enemas, blood-letting and purging. Thus in Molière's *Malade Imaginaire* Doctor Dyafoirus remarks about his son Thomas that 'the good thing about him, which pleases me most of all, and in which he follows my example, is that he adopts blindly the opinion of our ancient doctors and has never wished to understand or hear the why and wherefore of the pretended discoveries of our century concerning the circulation of the blood and other opinions of the same mark'. Molière made fun of doctors and their presumptuous ignorance in five of his comedies; among the reasons for his anti-medical prejudice was his conviction that his only son had died from antimony prescribed by the physicians.

When a new drug becomes popular, even today, it is often used enthusiastically and without every note being taken of side effects and specific indications for its use. This happened 350 years ago with antimony. Lesage, in *Gil Blas*, pilloried 'the wretches who go by the name of doctors, hitching their unworthy persons to the triumphal car of antimony or at the very least tagging along behind'. Although as a drug antimony was known in the time of Paracelsus, by the name of stibium, its fortunes only prospered after the publication in 1604 of the book *The Triumphal Chariot of Antimony* by Johann Thölde, an alchemist, the author attributing it to a mythical friar, Basil Valentine. Thölde had observed pigs growing fat on a diet rich in antimony, and he applied this knowledge to treat a group of undernourished monks. Unfortunately the monks died. Over the next century violent controversy arose over whether this substance was a useful drug or a poison. The argument abated when Louis XIV was cured of typhus after a dose of antimony. No one considered if the king would also have recovered without it, and so the substance became a universal panacea; it might be said that doctors of that time were no better than the physicians of an earlier age who based diagnosis and treatment entirely on experience gained from individual cases; naturally with such a case as Louis XIV the course and outcome of the illness

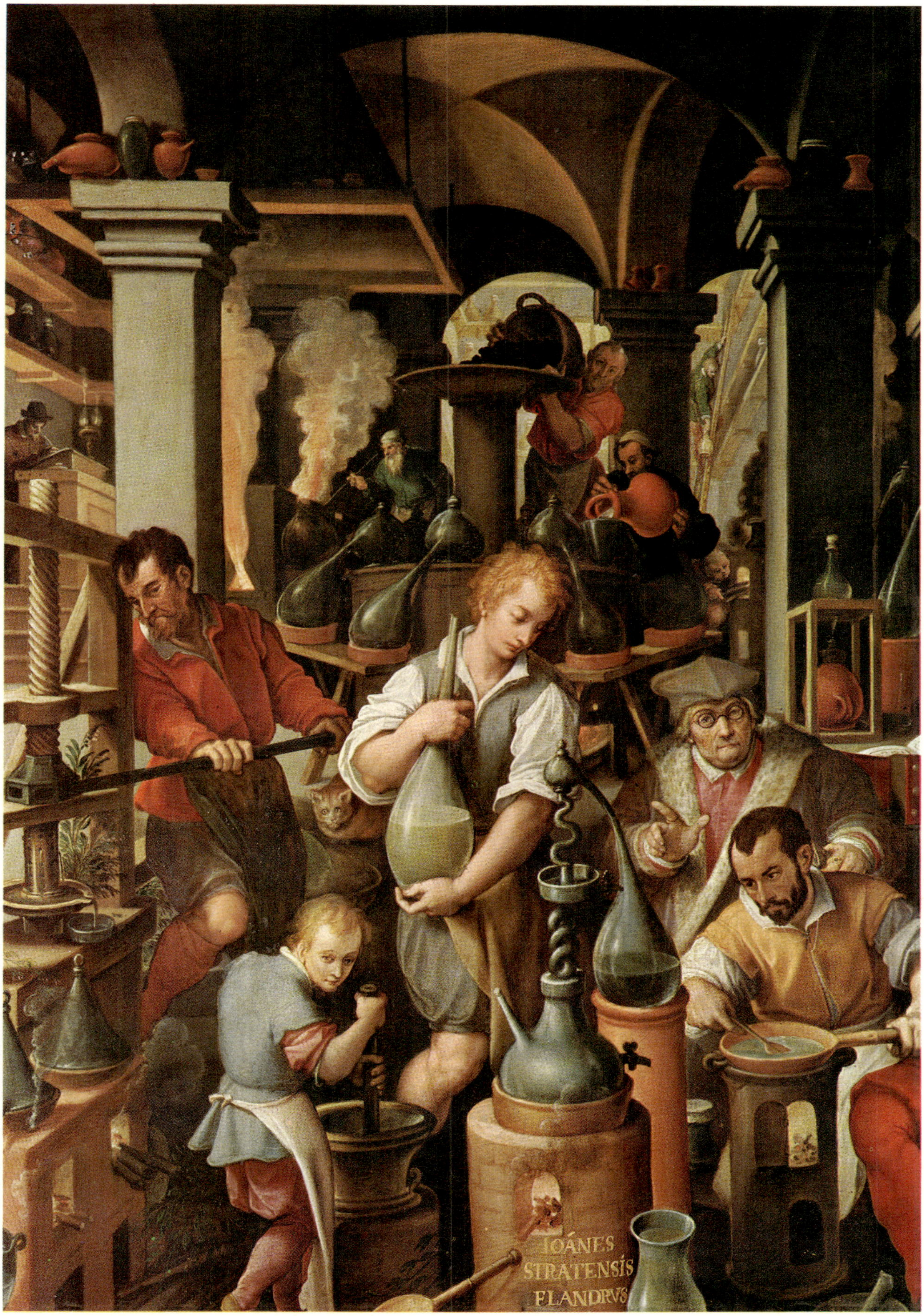
IOÁNES
STRATENSIS
FLANDRUS

Previous pages :
Natural history museum. *Plate from Museum Franc. Calceolarium Veronensis a Benedicto Ceruto Medico incaeptum. By Andrea Chiocco, Verona, 1622. Bertarelli Collection, Milan.*

Surgical instruments. *Plate from Armamentarium Chirurgicum by Johann Schultes (Scultetus), Venice, 1665.*

Pharmacy. *Seventeenth-century engraving. Bertarelli Collection, Milan.*

The alchemist. *By Giovanni Stradano. Palazzo Vecchio, Florence.*

These pages :
Dissection (frontispiece) and other plates from Armamentarium Chirurgicum. *By Johann Schultes, Venice, 1665.*

dictated the law. Another drug that was welcomed indiscriminately was quinine, introduced into Europe in 1632 under the name of Jesuit's bark, because it had cured the malaria of a missionary in Peru. The Inca medicine-man who administered it would not reveal the ingredients, and the Jesuit decided to find out the truth for himself; after a long search, he discovered that the remedy was the bark of a plant. The Jesuits held the export monopoly to Europe, earning great rewards from the acceptance of quinine as the cure that had been created alongside the disease. Others, like the Englishman Robert Talbot, an apothecary's apprentice, also turned it to advantage. Talbot made up a prescription based on rose petals, lemon juice, water and quinine, which cured malarial fever in a few days, and became famous, eventually being summoned to the French court at Versailles where he cured the King and the dukes of Burgundy and Anjou.

Soon after its introduction quinine started fierce arguments, because doctors were over-prescribing it in their ignorance of its toxic side effects, such as disturbances of hearing. Nevertheless its therapeutic worth was inescapable, and it had one other important effect, for it may well have played a leading part in the overthrow of Galenism. The Galenists held that the effective treatment of many diseases involved purgation, and while they could argue that the success obtained in treating syphilis with mercury was due to salivation being really only another way of expelling toxic material, there

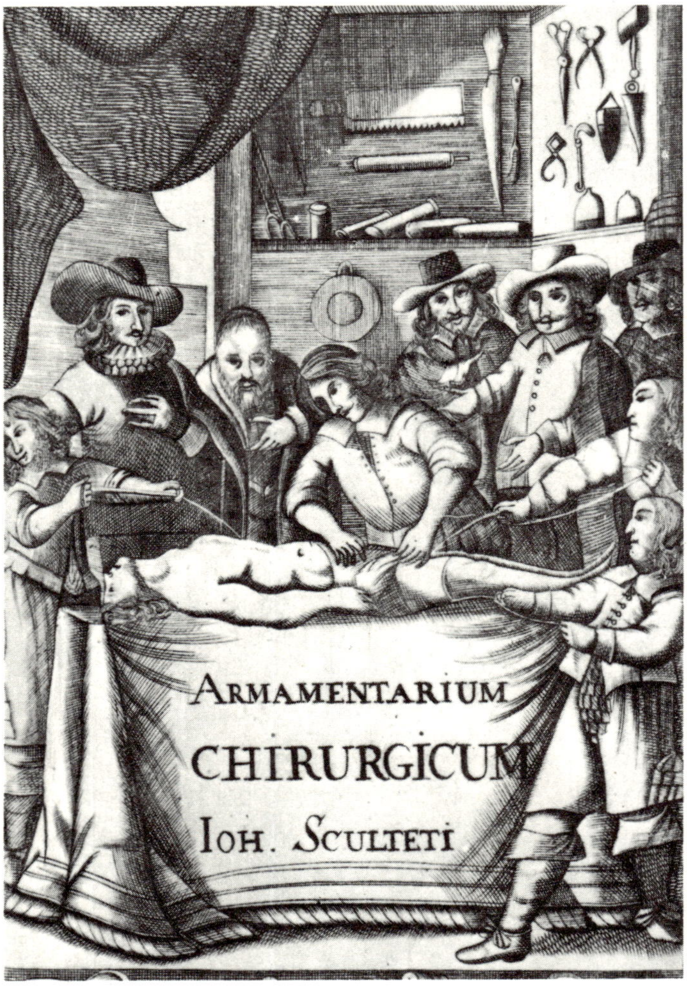

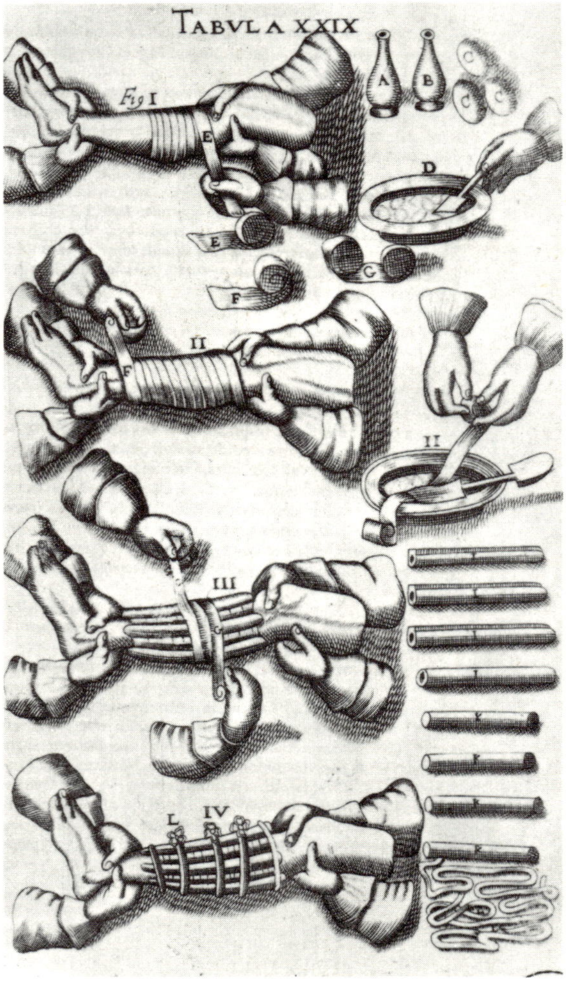

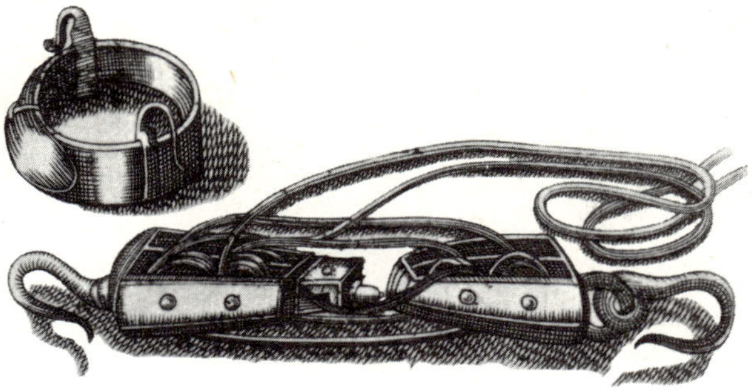

The seventeenth century presented a paradoxical situation in which the natural sciences were developing broadly and swiftly but medicine seemed to be if anything retreating into a more dogmatic attitude than it had adopted during the Renaissance. Alchemy and the sale of panaceas flourished, while surgery seemed to benefit little from the great advances of the previous century.

was no hope of explaining the effects of quinine in the same way. Bernardino Ramazzini (1633–1714), founder of the pathology of occupational disease, compared the medical revolution brought about by quinine with the effect on the art of war of the introduction of firearms.

Quinine was the great pharmacological advance in an era which clung by and large to the medicaments of an earlier age. Pharmacopoeias of the period included many recipes containing ingredients with magical properties–worms, foxes' lungs, lozenges of dried vipers, oil of wolves, moss from the skull of a victim of violent death, and crabs' eyes, to list but a few–and such treatments were prescribed by the leading physicians of the day. In addition many proprietary preparations earned fortunes for private individuals. Garrison describes these in fascinating detail. One of the best known of these was Scot's Pills, a mixture of aloes, jalap, gamboge and anise, introduced in 1635 and still on sale in 1875. Baffy's Elixir was made up to the beginning of the present century. The formula of Goddard's Drops, prescribed by Sydenham and said to be made from raw silk, was bought by Charles II for more than £5,000.

These recipes and many others, some complex and some of the simplest formulation, formed the basis of treatment for a wide variety of diseases. Prices were often high, and apothecaries' bills were a source of dissatisfaction to patient and physician alike. Overcharging sometimes got out of hand: in 1633 George Buller asked for thirty shillings per

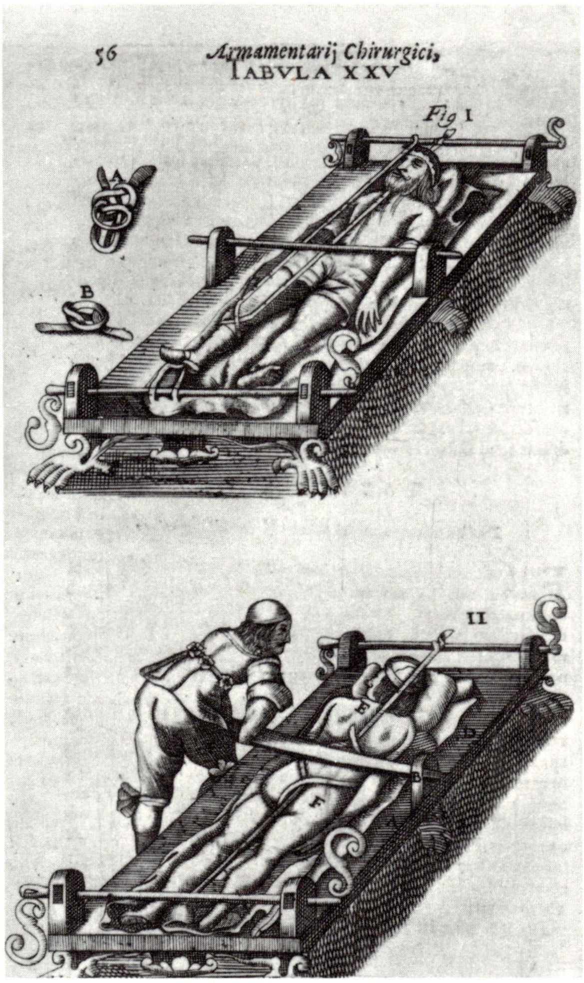

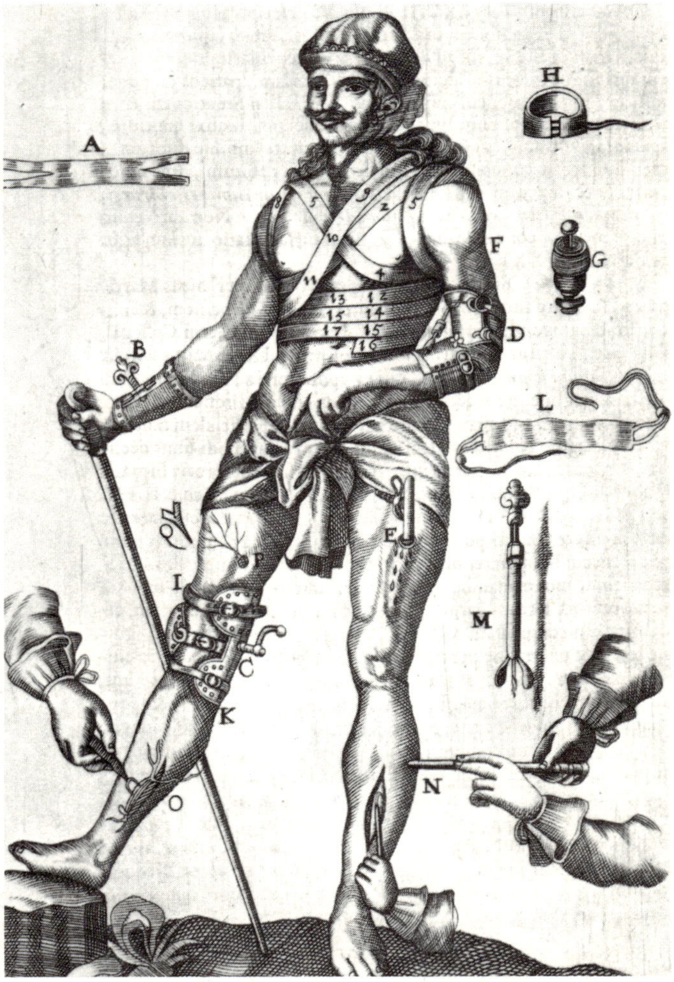

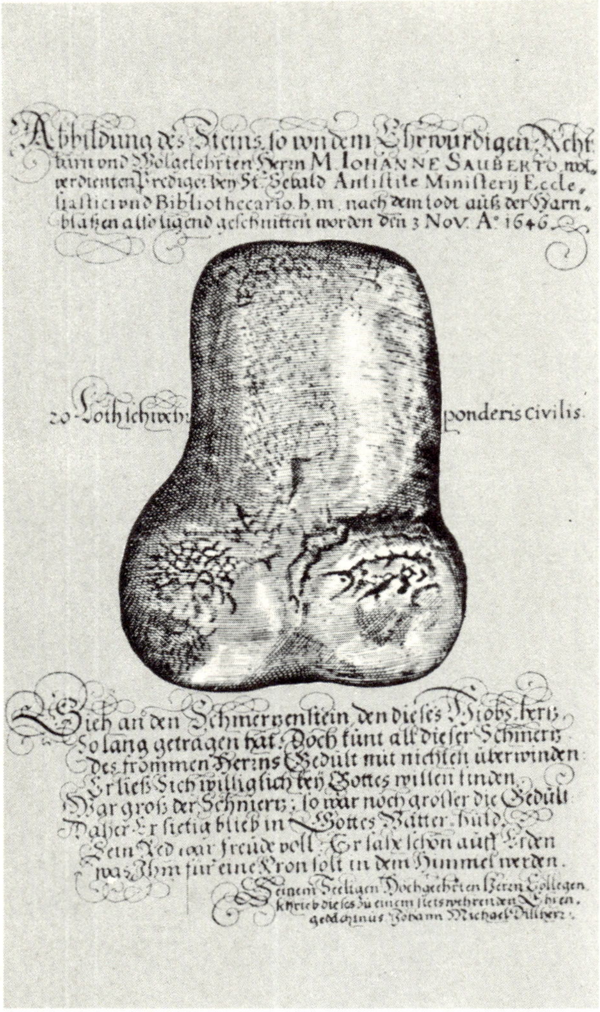

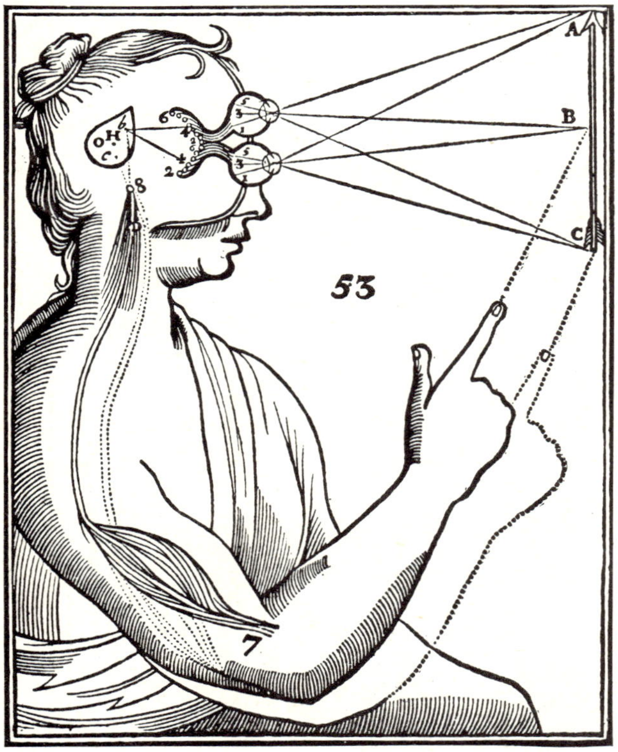

Kidney stone. *Engraving of 1644. German Museum, Nuremberg.*

Vision. *From De homine by René Descartes, 1644.*

The tooth-drawer. *Seventeenth-century engraving. Bertarelli Collection, Milan.*

pill, while a few years earlier the Royal College of Physicians prosecuted Dr Tenant for charging £6 for a pill and a decoction.

The great progress made in anatomy in the latter half of the sixteenth century had surprisingly little effect on surgery in the seventeenth. Despite academic conservatism and the slow diffusion of the new knowledge it might be expected that surgeons would seize on the facts revealed by Vesalius and his successors and put them to practical use. However the surgeons, with the barbers, were still an underprivileged subclass, lacking a scientific education and far below the physicians in status. In England the company of Barber-Surgeons, incorporated in 1540, was allowed to perform dissections in its own hall, but not elsewhere. In France, the surgeon was regarded rather more highly and a gain in status led to his assuming the pompous airs and bombast of the successful physician; but he was still an inferior being. Guy Patin (1601–1672), the dean of the medical faculty in Paris, showed his hate of his upstart surgical colleagues in words which might have been applied to his fellow physicians by Molière: 'Mere booted lackeys–a race of extravagant coxcombs who wear moustaches and flourish razors'.

The positions of surgeons, in France at least, was improved not by learning but by an event in 1686 which the historian Michelet considered 'more important than the work of Paré'. This was the treatment of Louis XIV's chronic anal fistula by the surgeon Felix, with marvellous results. The happy surgeon was rewarded with an estate, a title, and a fee of 300,000 livres, three times that paid to the royal physician. Thus at one stroke surgery was shown to be a noble and a profitable calling. Felix was followed by Mareschal, who continued to improve the social standing of the surgeon in the following century.

The seventeenth century saw a great advance in obstetrics with the introduction of the forceps by the Chamberlen family. The first practical instrument to assist childbirth was designed in 1561 by Pierre Franco, but in 1647 Pierre Chamberlen produced a pair of curved forceps similar to those in use today. The family kept its invention a closely guarded secret, and with the forceps several members acquired highly successful practices in London, earning great sums of money. Hugh Chamberlen tried to sell the secret in Paris, but

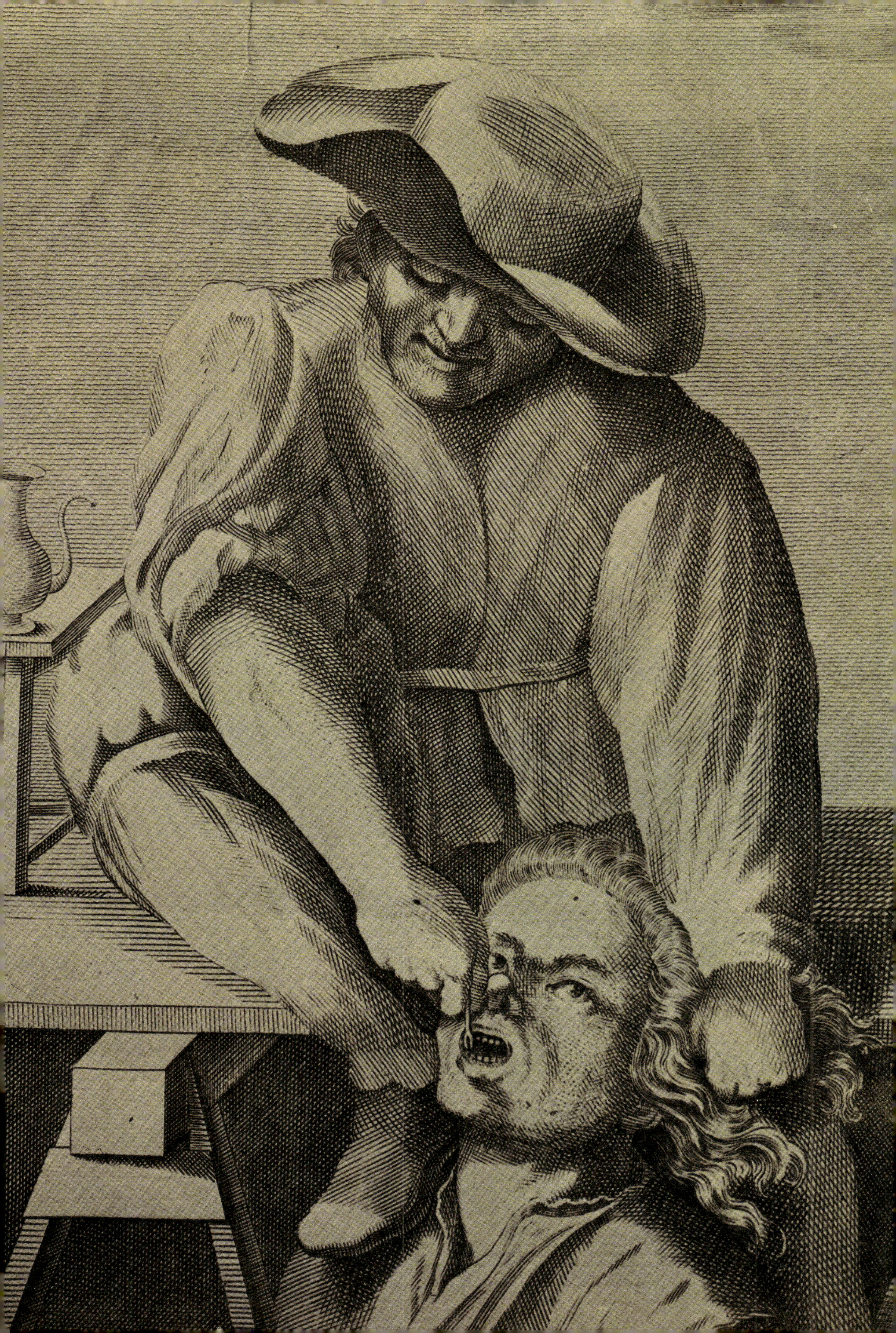

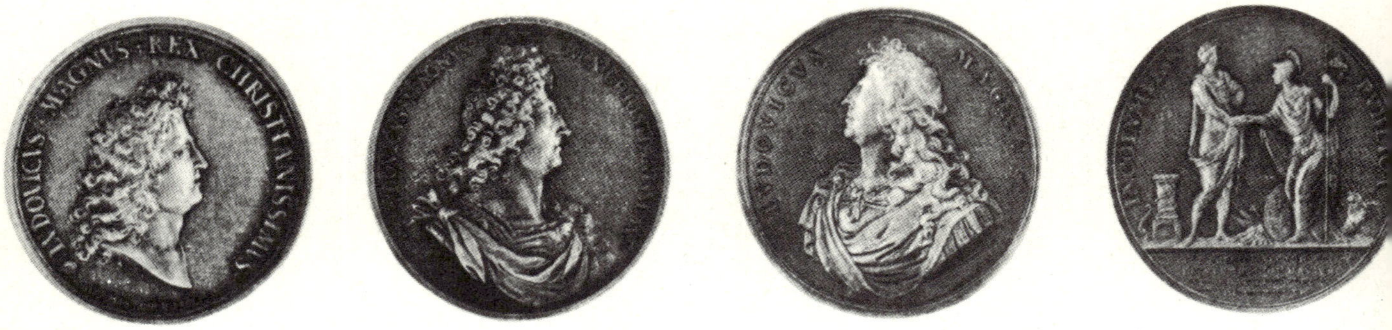

unfortunately caused a patient to die with lacerations of the uterus; he was later successful in introducing the forceps into Holland, but it was many years before the instrument came into general use. In the meanwhile the family, its invention and the secrets and intrigues involved became surrounded by legend.

The greatest obstetrician of the age was François Mauriceau (1637–1709), with whom Pierre Chamberlen clashed in Paris. His famous textbook, which contained the first accurate study of the female pelvis, was the standard work in several languages until well into the eighteenth century.

Although medical practitioners were still in the grip of formal preconceptions and were content with minimal knowledge, the seventeenth century was a period of development in medicine. It was, in contrast, a century of the most grave economic and political crises in Europe and especially in Italy and Germany. After the discovery of America, the great ports of Italy declined because trade was going by the new sea routes. In addition, the peninsula was torn by constant war, and students no longer came from all over Europe to the Italian universities as they had in the Renaissance. The Thirty Years War (1618–1648) ravaged German towns, trade and industry: it began as a struggle between the forces of reaction and reform, but developed into a fight for supremacy between France and the Habsburgs. The discovery of the New World and

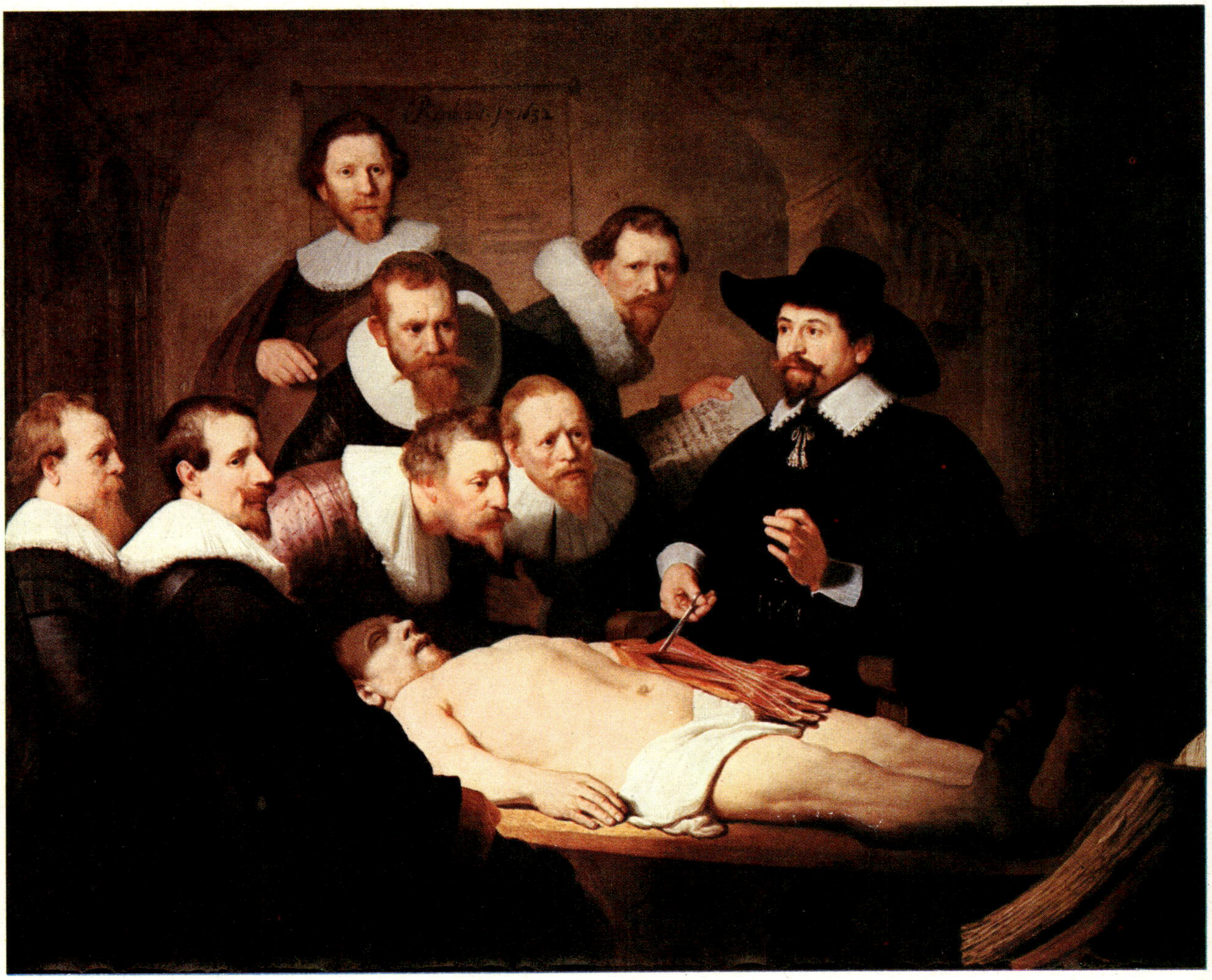

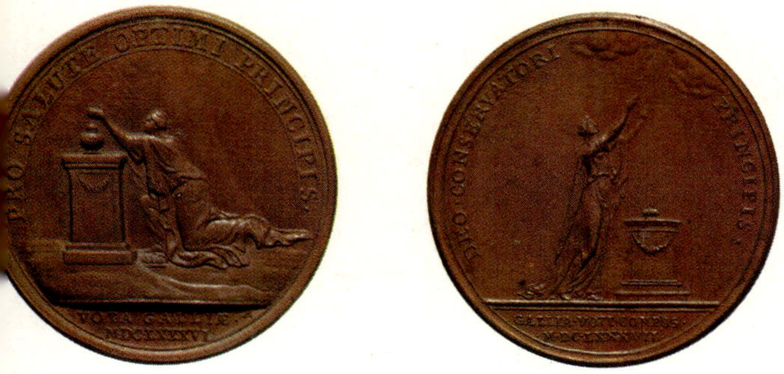

Three commemorative medallions for the fistula operation and cure of Louis XIV. *Cabinet des Médailles, Louvre Museum, Paris.*

The anatomy lesson of Doctor Tulp. *By Rembrandt van Rijn. The Hague Museum.*

Curer of hernias. *Caricature by Larmessin, seventeenth century.*

Frontispiece of a seventeenth-century 'Galenic and chemical pharmacopoeia'.

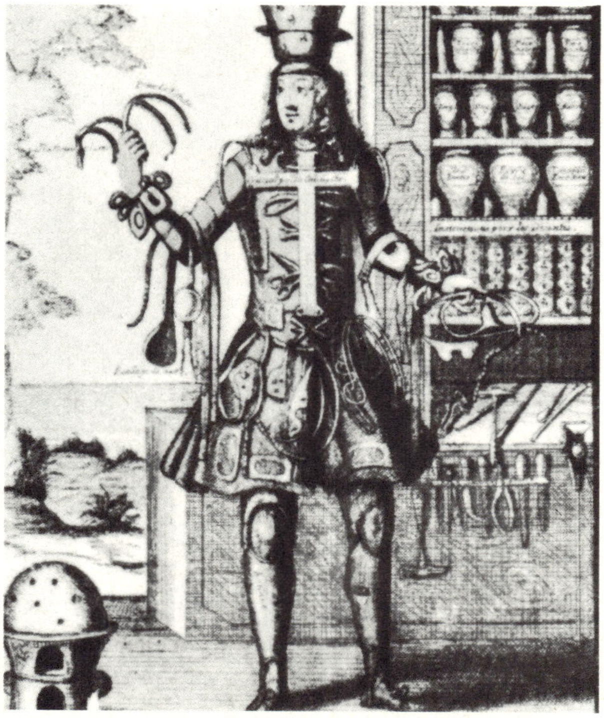

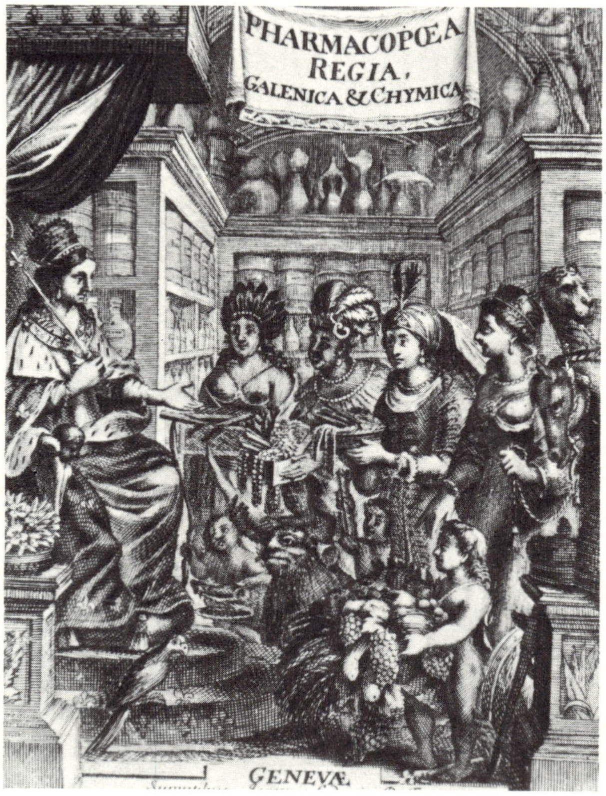

the Thirty Years War led, however, to the rise of England and Holland, which enjoyed economic prosperity and military power, especially sea-power.

While literature and the arts flourished in the Renaissance, the seventeenth century was a golden age for science. The idea of Johann Kepler (1571–1630) that nature 'loves simplicity, loves unity and there is nothing superfluous in it' epitomized this era. The creators of the natural sciences–Kepler, Galileo, Descartes and Newton–stressed the need for direct study of nature in the light of objective criticism and without prejudice and dogma. In the new era of science, diligent and assiduous observation was the first requisite, with experiment as a test of hypothesis and with mathematical methods enabling a great variety of facts to be condensed into fundamental formulae.

Guido de Ruggiero sums up the new movements in this way: 'In contrast with the increasing inward trend of philosophy, there was an expansion in scientific work, gradually but uninterruptedly extending to ever-new spheres; this largely made up for rejection of enquiry into primary causes and the true nature of things by producing a dense network of relationships and connections binding reality together as a whole, thus turning human knowledge into a docile instrument. The secret of this magic lay in the method, the order with which science arranged its thoughts, proceeding from the known to the unknown, from the particular to the general or from the complex to the simple, constructing an all-embracing idea in a logical manner.

'Such order of enquiry and technique, and the scepticism shown over results, soon became a mental habit with research workers, and led to a common nature that was stronger than individual personalities; this made possible the effective communication of work, and joint participation in it, creating from many observers, as it were, a hundred-eyed Argus, in whom the perception of the individual was multiplied rather than averaged.'

The expansion of scientific research was not the only development to characterize the seventeenth century; another resulted from the fact that with Galileo science had become more exact. 'Science is measurement' is a concept which has influenced medical science not less than the other sciences,

Three urine examinations. *Details from : The doctor's visit, by Adriaen van Ostade. Hermitage, Leningrad ; Examining the urine, by Gerard Dou. Library, Vienna ; Proof of chastity, by Godfried Schalten. The Hague Museum.*

Four pulse examinations. *Details from : The lovesick lady, by Jan Steen. Amsterdam Museum ; Doctor visiting a lady patient, by Franz van Mieris. Vienna Museum ; Taking the pulse, by Gerritsz Brekelenkam. Louvre, Paris ; The lovesick lady, by Jan Steen. The Hermitage, Leningrad.*

Lady with dropsy. *Gerard Dou. Louvre, Paris.*

In this age of scientific advance, treatment still rested heavily on blood-letting and purging, diagnosis on examination of the urine and of the pulse ; both these procedures proved popular subjects with the painters of the period, particularly in the Low Countries. Urine-examination was supposed to be able to provide a wide range of information, including the diagnosis of chastity and of love-sickness.

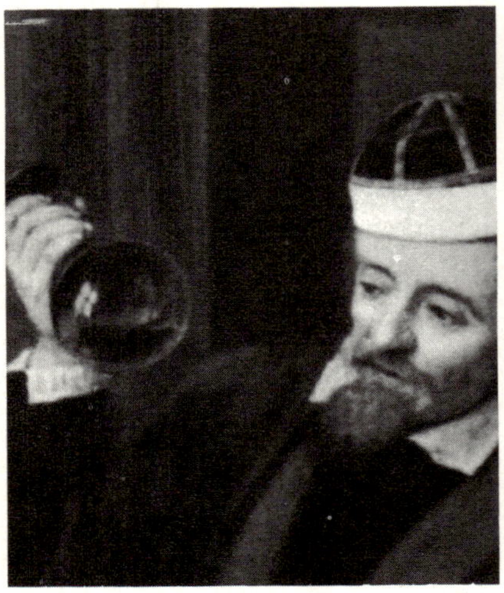

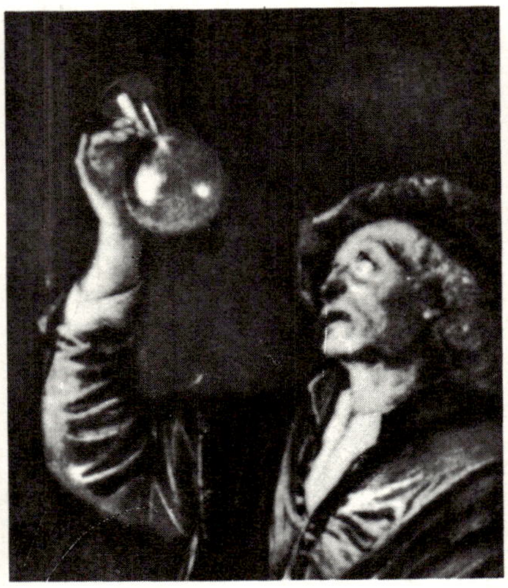

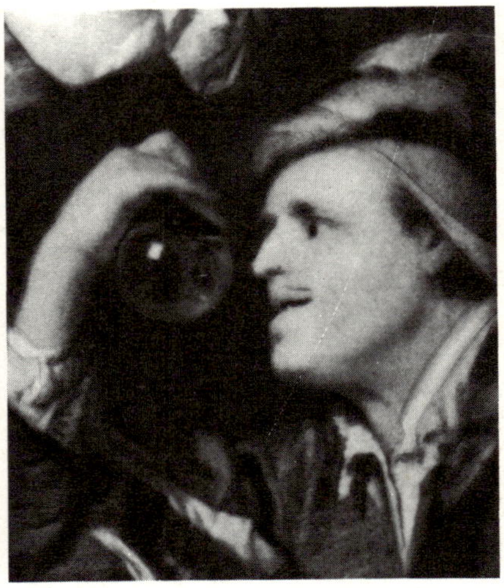

and one which medicine owes to Galileo Galilei.

The need to multiply the perception of the individual led to the rise of scientific associations, the first of which was the Accademia dei Lincei, founded in Rome in the year 1603 by Prince Cesi. In 1635, Cardinal Richelieu created the French Academy. The Accademia del Cimento, (Academy of Experiment) initiated in 1648 under the Grand Duke of Tuscany Ferdinand II, was established by Prince Leopold in 1657 for the purpose of promoting the physical sciences; Redi, Viviani and Borelli belonged to it, but it came to an end after only ten years. Scientific learning transcended national barriers. The Royal Society of London, incorporated in 1662, invited Marcello Malpighi to become a corresponding member. In 1700, Leibnitz influenced Frederick I to found the Berlin Academy of Sciences. The first scientific periodicals were issued in the seventeenth century. Medical contributions appeared in the pages of the *Philosophical Transactions of the Royal Society,* in the *Journal des Sçavans* in France and in the Venetian *Giornale dei Letterati.* The first medical review, entitled *Journal des nouvelles découvertes sur toutes les parties de la médicine,* began in 1679, while it should be noted that the first political newspaper, the *Gazette de France,* was founded in 1631 by a well-known doctor, Theophraste Renaudot, whose name is commemorated in a Paris literary prize.

In the seventeenth century, therefore, medicine turned towards the natural sciences and experimental research. It was an ineluctable development in an epoch dominated by the figure of Galileo, who looked for an exact mathematical law governing every phenomenon, and Descartes, who based his philosophy on the concept that knowledge of one's own was the only absolutely certain fact. A third giant of this era is Francis Bacon, whose work in spreading the new learning must not be forgotten; in particular he stressed the importance of the inductive method in the natural sciences.

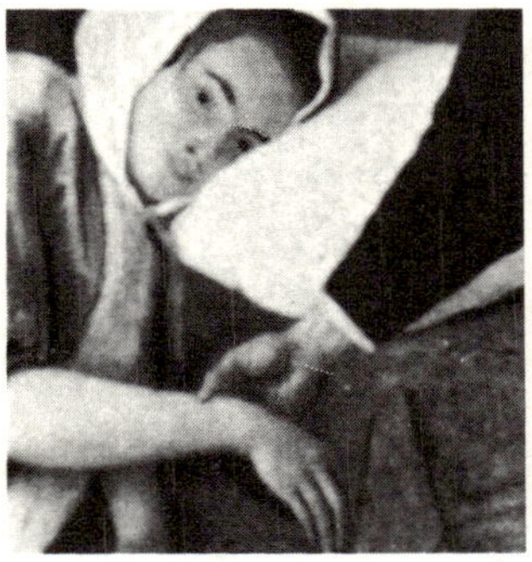

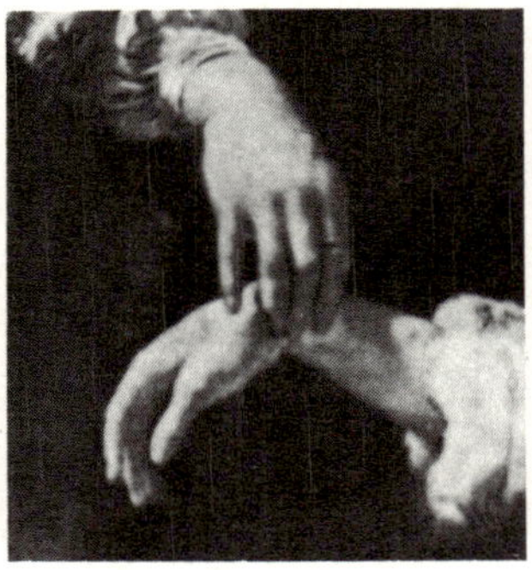

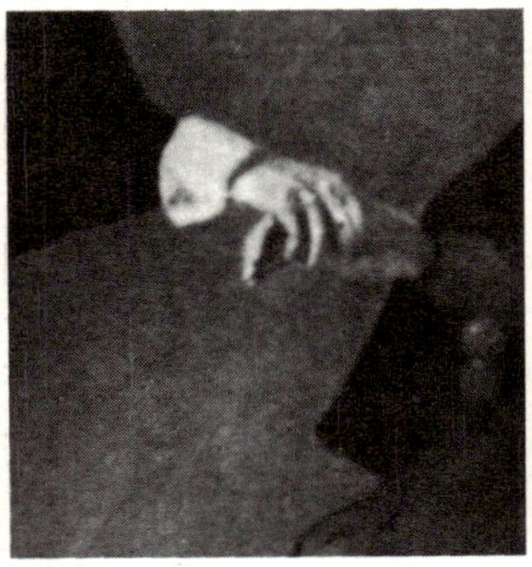

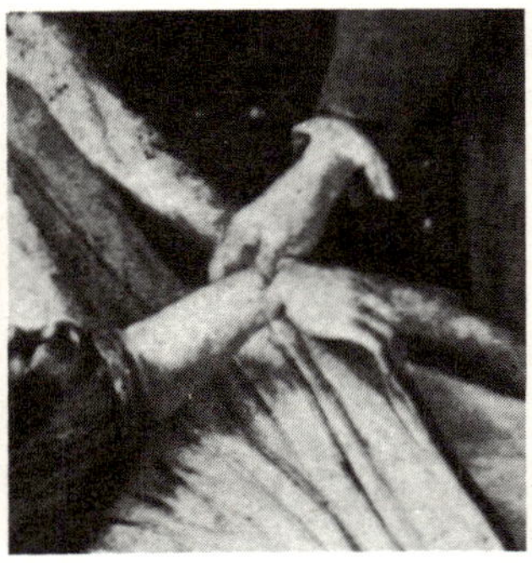

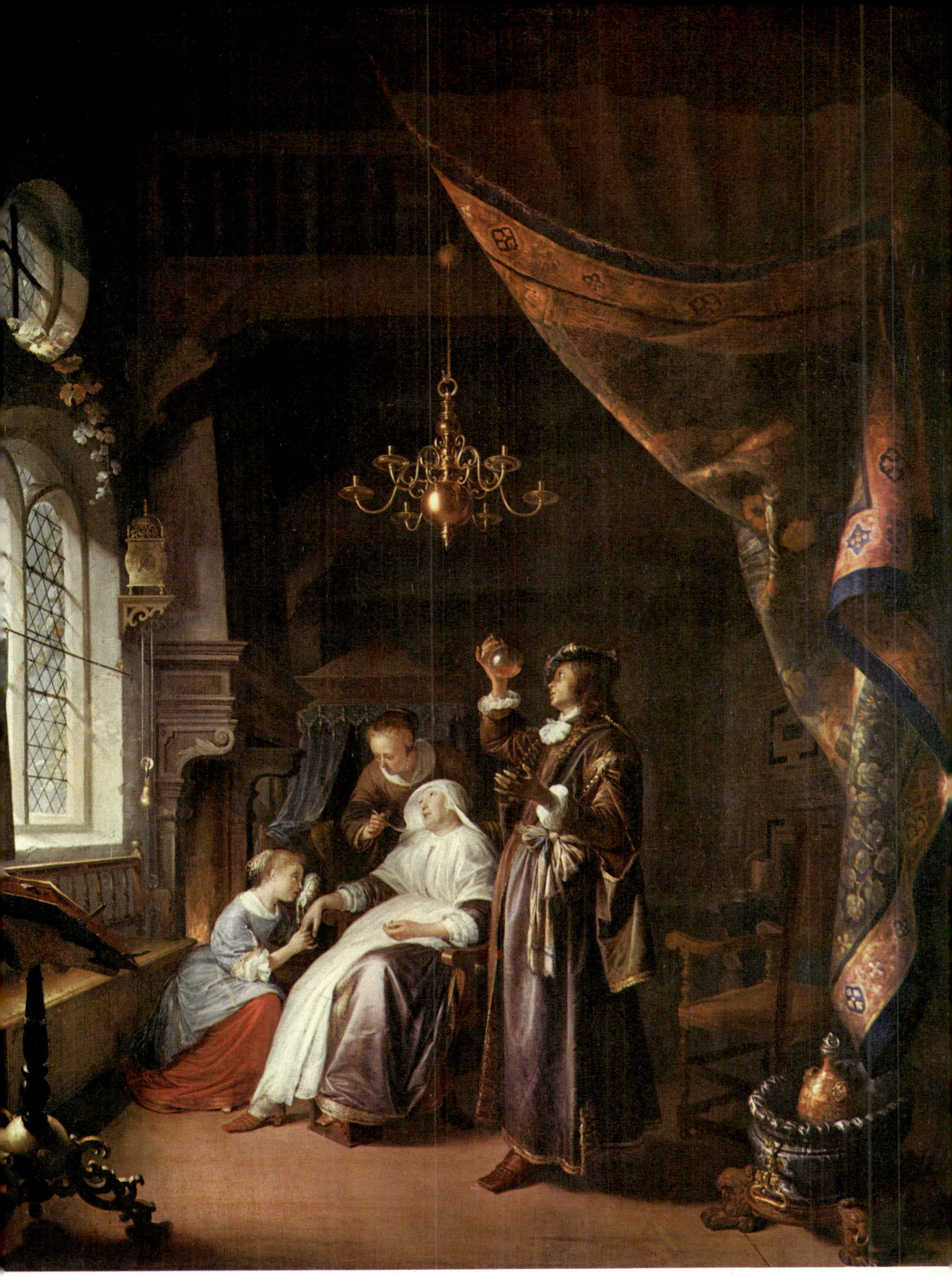

Harvey and the discovery of the circulation

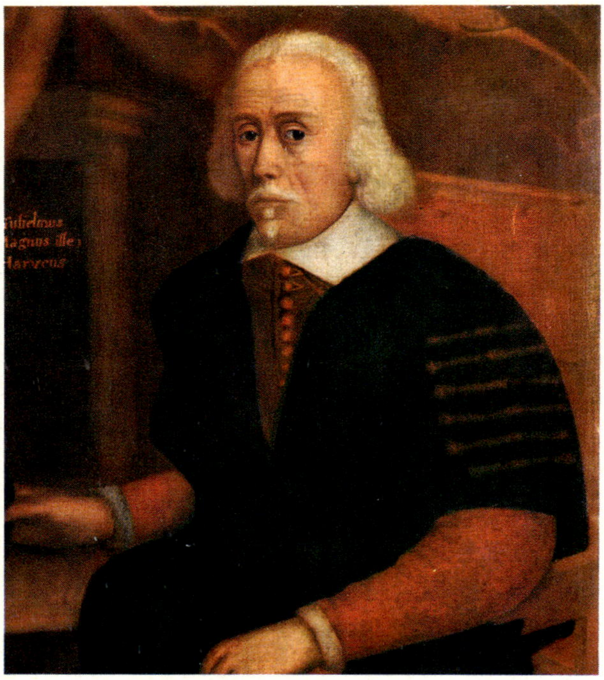

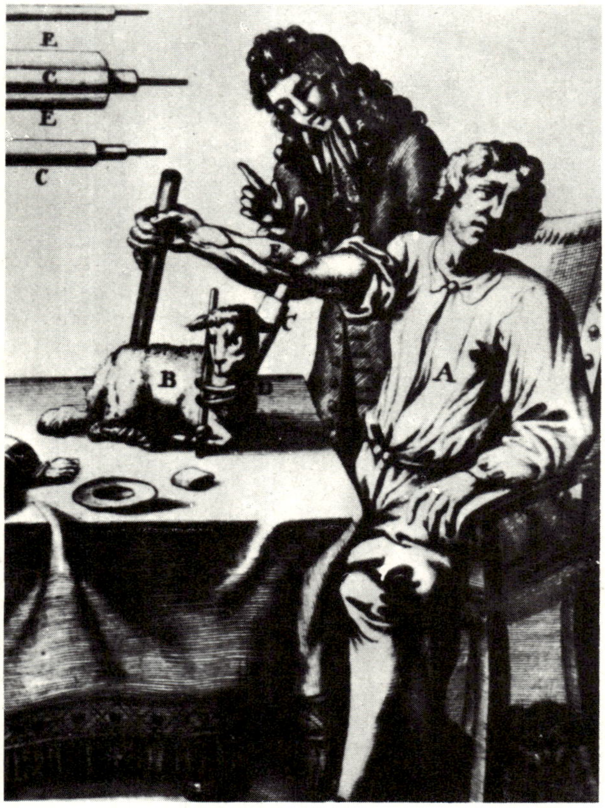

William Harvey was born at Folkestone in 1578; after studying at Caius College, Cambridge, he enrolled at the university of Padua in the year 1598. Galileo was a teacher there and without a doubt, as Busacchi observed, it was in Padua that Harvey's scientific method crystallized. Like other young men he was aware of the influence exercised by Galilean teaching; the atmosphere was one of freedom and he learned from dissection and anatomical observation. In Padua he was a pupil of Fabrizio d'Acquapendente, the first person clearly to describe the valves in veins. When he came back to London in 1602 Harvey married the daughter of Lancelot Browne, physician to Queen Elizabeth and King James I; he joined the staff at St Bartholomew's Hospital and became a reader in anatomy and surgery. Meanwhile he continued his investigation of the vascular system which led to his discovery of the circulation, which he announced in 1616. It was not until twelve years later that his classic work, *Exercitatio anatomica de motu cordis et sanguinis in animalibus,* was published in Frankfurt. He described in this how arterial blood flowed from the left ventricle of the heart to the aorta and was distributed via this vessel to all parts of the body; having become venous, the blood was carried in the veins to the right atrium of the heart, from where it flowed into the right ventricle. This propelled it forwards into the pulmonary artery and from here to the lungs, where the transformation of venous blood into arterial blood took place. After passing through the pulmonary veins, the blood reached the left atrium and from there it returned to the left ventricle.

A number of Harvey's precursors had already refuted the Galenic doctrine according to which the liver was the centre of the circulation. The ancient doctrine maintained that the left ventricle of the heart contained air, or blood mixed with air, which reached it from the right part of the heart through invisible pores in the cardiac septum. Leonardo and Vesalius may have realized the truth. In 1553 Michael Servedo or Servetus (1511–1553), a Spanish theologian and physician, published *Christianismi Restitutio,* a work which earned him death at the stake for heresy against the Trinity. In this work, almost as an aside, Servedo postulated the existence of the pulmonary circulation and denied the porosity of the septum. Realdo Colombo of Cremona (1516?–1559), successor to

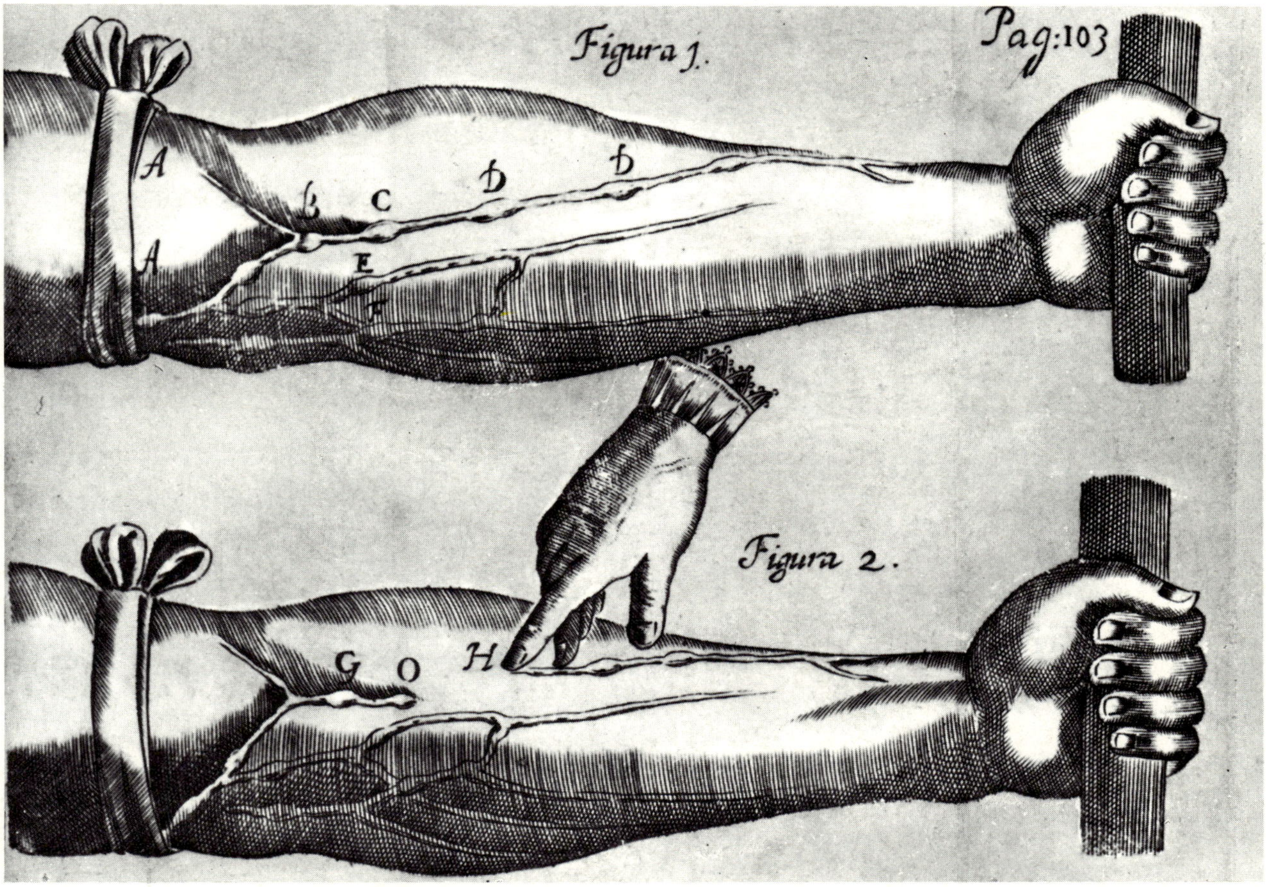
Figura 1.
Pag:103
A
b
C
D
D
A
E
F
Figura 2.
G
O
H

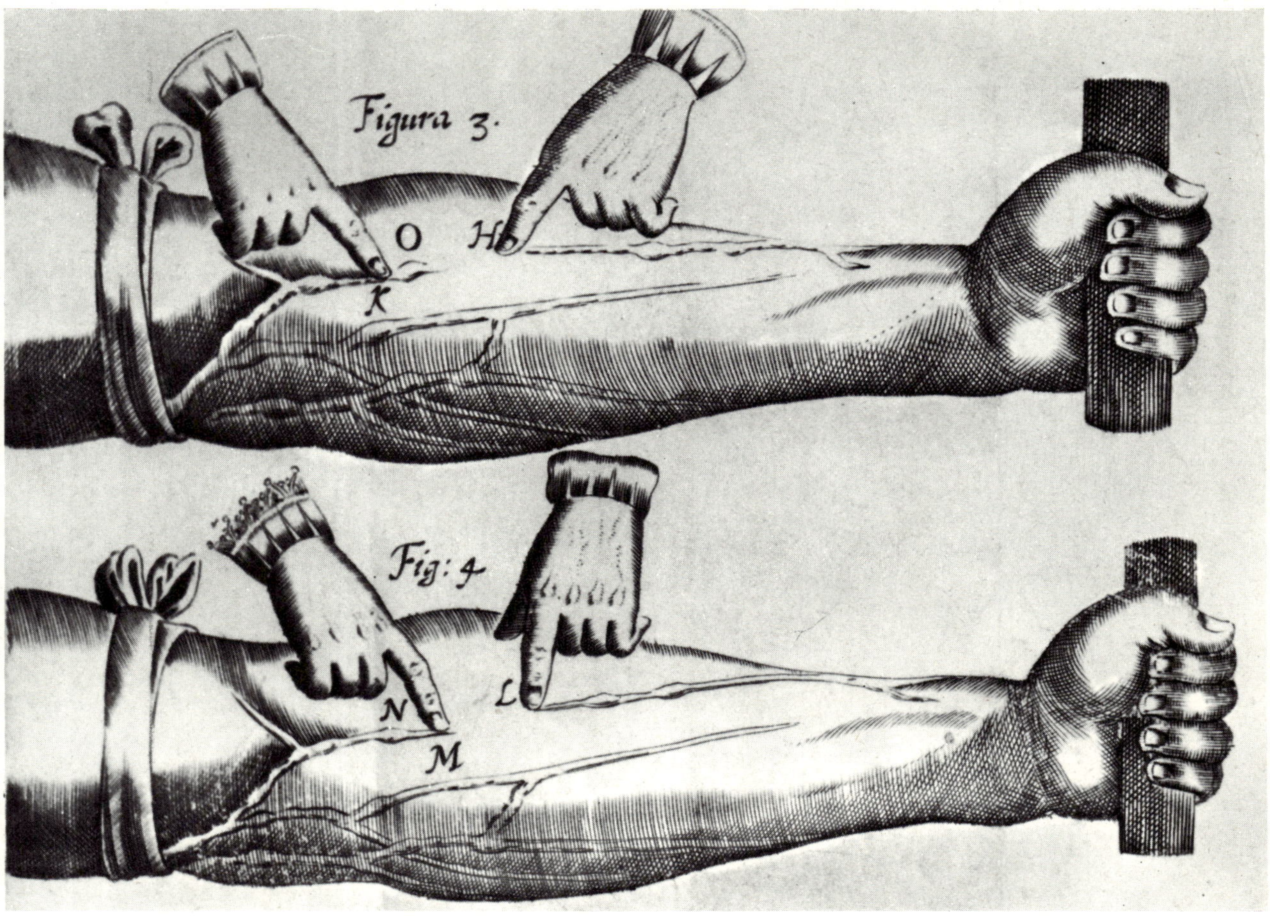
Figura 3.
O
H
K
Fig: 4
N
L
M

Previous pages:
William Harvey. *Contemporary portrait.*

Blood transfusion. *Engraving from Lorbeer-Krantz oder Wundartzney by M G Purmann, 1685.*

Circulation of the blood in the veins of the forearm. *Plate from Exercitatio anatomica de motu cordis et sanguinis in animalibus by William Harvey, Frankfurt, 1628.*

Facing page:
Diagram of circulation of the blood. By Niels Stensen. *Plate from Diaphragmatis structura nova by Caspar Bartholimus, Paris, 1671.*

Frontispiece to William Harvey's work on the circulation of the blood. *Rotterdam, 1661.*

Vesalius in the chair of anatomy at Padua, in *De re anatomica* (published in 1559 but compiled some time before), unequivocally refuted the hypothesis of the permeability of the cardiac wall.

Andrea Cesalpino of Arezzo (1524?–1603), a physician and botanist, professor of medicine at Pisa and discoverer of sex in plants, lucidly explained the pulmonary circulation in his work *Quaestionum peripateticarum* published in 1571 in Venice: 'The orifices of the heart are prepared by nature in such a way that from the vena cava the blood penetrates to the right ventricle of the heart, from which there runs a way out from the heart to the lungs. From the lungs there is in addition another entrance to the left ventricle from which there is in turn an opening giving access to the aorta. Special membranes at the openings of the vessels prevent the blood flowing back so that there is perpetual movement from the vena cava through the heart and through the lungs into the aorta'. These concepts were confirmed in the work *De plantes* published in 1583; the experimental proof was given in *Quaestionum medicarum* published in 1593. His house in Arezzo today bears a plaque which reads 'here lived Andrea Cesalpino, discoverer of the circulation of the blood and first author of a classification of plants'.

What Harvey did was to complete the solution of the problem, putting into a clearly worked-out form ideas which had previously been advanced without the backing of experimental results; with great skill in the design and execution of experiments he was able definitively to confirm his hypothesis. He suggested that the heart was a pump, worked by muscular force; he observed the phenomenon of systole, the contraction of the walls of the heart cavities at the moment when they emptied of blood, and diastole, the dilation of the cavities when filled, and with knowledge of the valves in the heart and veins, and the observation that veins swelled distal to a ligature, he was able to work out the direction of blood flow and so outline the mechanics of the cardio-vascular system.

Harvey died in 1657, leaving behind him a massive epoch-making work. In the structure he created, the only thing lacking was proof of the existence of the capillaries; this was to be provided by Marcello Malpighi in 1661. Other research relevant to the discovery of the circulation was that of Carlo Ruini of Bologna, in whose work *Dell' anatomia del cavallo* (On the anatomy of the horse), published in 1598, was the statement that the heart filled during diastole and emptied during systole, and that of Gaspare Aselli (1581–1626), professor at Pavia, who discovered the chyliferous vessels, which he called venae albae et lacteae; these were known to the ancient Greeks, who did not realize their function or importance. The work of Aselli was completed by a Frenchman, Jean Pecquet (1622–1674), with the discovery of the thoracic duct in the dog, and by the Swede Olaf Rudbeck (1630–1702) who discovered the intestinal lymphatics and their connection with this duct.

Harvey's other great work was published in 1651, six years before his death. This book, *De generatione animalium,* is of much importance in the history of embryology for it contained the theory of 'epigenesis', whereby the organism does not exist as a minute, preformed entity within the ovum but develops from it by a gradual building up of its parts. This theory was confirmed in the nineteenth century by von Baer, who had the advantage of the microscope; just as Harvey's concept of the circulation was limited to theory by one point, the invisible capillaries, so, without the microscope, his painstaking investigation of the embryo reached an impasse. Perhaps for this reason he fell into grave error over the nature of fertilization, which he believed to be something mystical, metaphysical and due to an incorporeal agent, likened by him to the magnetism transferred from one piece of metal to a second. This concept, as Garrison noted, made self-contradictory the famous dictum 'omne vivum ex ovo' by denying the continuity of the germ plasm, but was of value in Harvey's hands in that it went against the ancient idea that life arose from decay and putrefaction.

The most brilliant of Harvey's pupils was Francis Glisson (1597–1677), who worked on the anatomy and physiology of the liver. His name is commemorated in Glisson's capsule, the fibrous sheath of the liver. He also carried out the first major study of rickets, and published his *De rachitide* in 1650.

An important immediate result of the application of Harvey's experimental method to other problems was the elucidation, by four Englishmen, of the physiology of respiration. According to

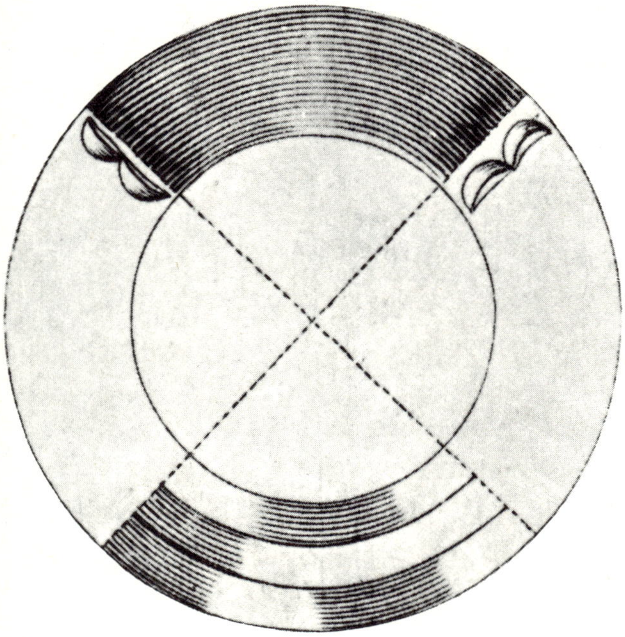

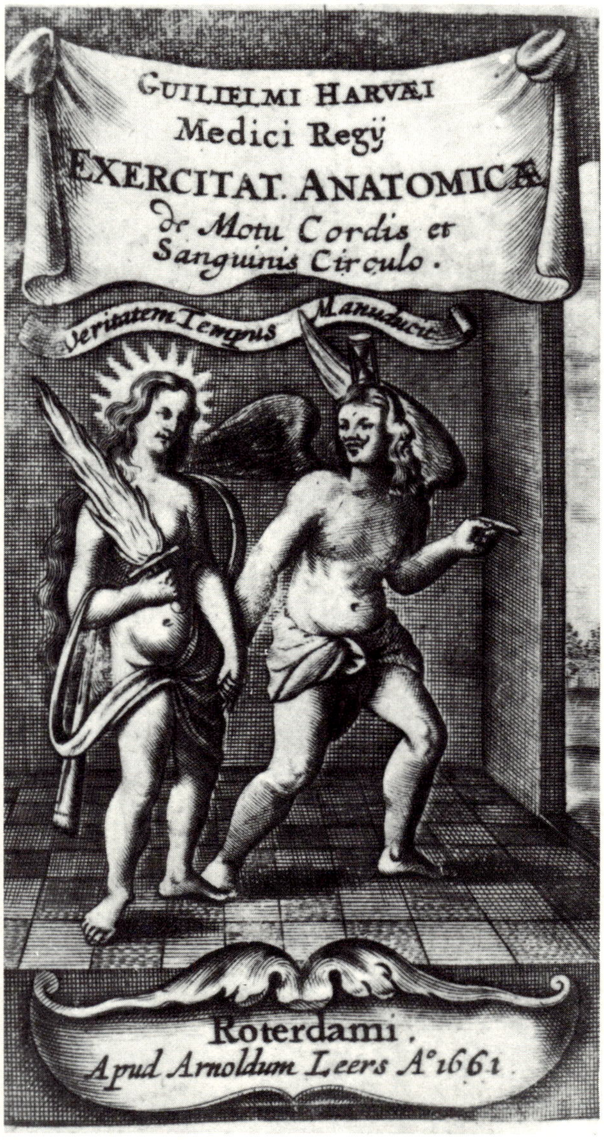

Galen's concept of the circulation had assumed that there was a communication between the two ventricles of the heart through invisible pores. Further discoveries showed that the blood could flow only one way in the veins. Cesalpino explained the pulmonary circulation and almost completed the picture, but it was William Harvey who finally confirmed the hypothesis with a series of ingenious experiments.

Galen, the purpose of respiration was to cool the heart, and the movements of the chest served to introduce air for generating vital spirits and to eliminate the smoky vapours of the heart. This belief was held up to Harvey's time, before when, as Allbutt wrote, 'respiration was regarded not as as a means of combustion but of refrigeration. How man became such a fiery dragon was the puzzle.' A preliminary step in the working out of respiratory physiology was taken when Harvey showed that blood is changed from venous to arterial in the lungs.

The first advance came when Robert Boyle (1627–1691) carried out experiments in 1660 and demonstrated that air was necessary for life as well as combustion, and that in a vacuum neither a flame nor an animal could survive. Seven years later, Robert Hooke (1635–1703), the pioneer microscopist and the first to apply the term 'cells' to the minute units he saw in razor slices of cork, showed that by attaching a bellows to the trachea of a dog in which the chest had been opened, the animal could be kept alive by artificial respiration and without any movement of either chest or lungs. Vesalius had done exactly the same thing over a century earlier, but now it was possible to say that the essential feature of respiration was not the movements of breathing but certain changes of the blood which took place in the lungs.

The next contribution was made by the Cornishman Richard Lower (1631–1691), who was the first person, in 1665, successfully to transfuse blood directly from one animal to another. In 1669 he injected dark venous blood into the aerated lungs of an experimental animal and observed its change of colour to bright red. This colour change must have resulted from some substance absorbed by it from the air in the lungs. Finally John Mayow (1643–1679), who was also a native of Cornwall, showed in a series of experiments that the venous blood was made red by the addition of 'nitro-aerial spirit', a constituent of nitre (potassium nitrate) as well as air. He thus came close to the modern concept of oxygenation of blood in the lungs, and in addition he advanced respiratory physiology by working out the function of the intercostal muscles, showing that maternal blood supplied the foetus with air as well as food, and asserting that heat production was from the muscles of the animal.

Iatrophysics and iatrochemistry

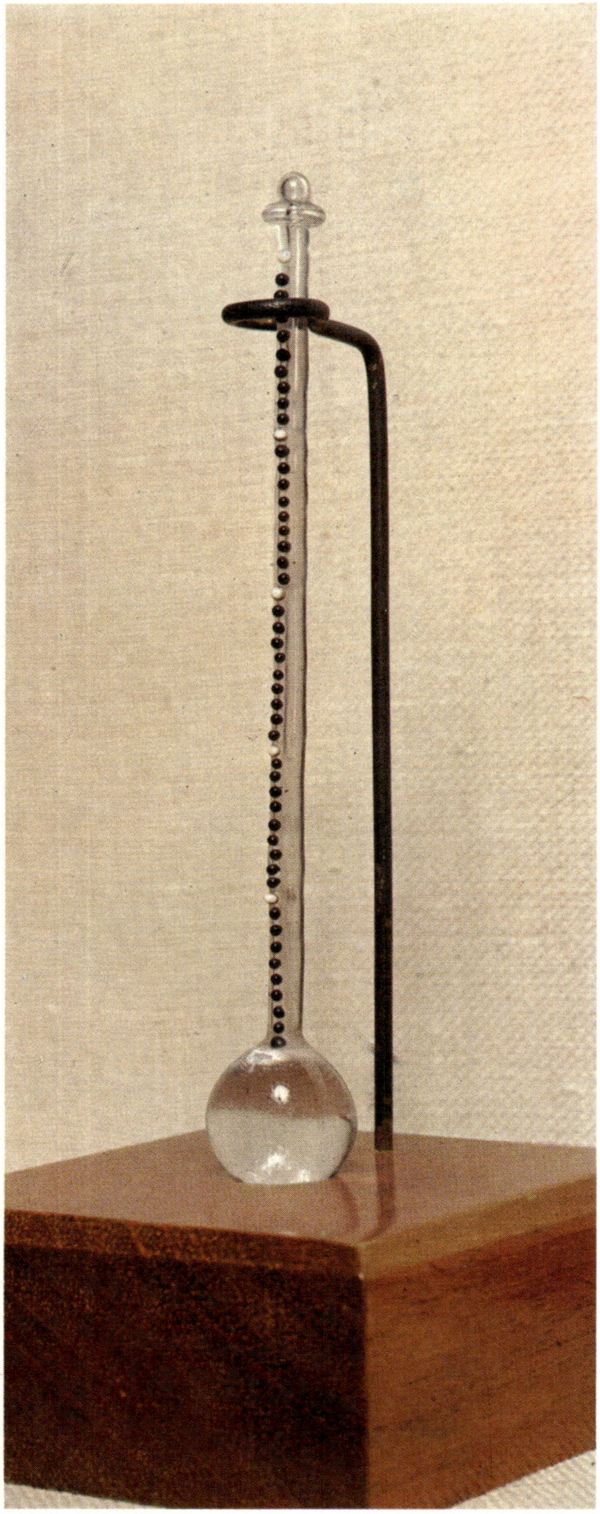

By the mid-seventeenth century, the effort to free medical thought from the doctrines of the ancients was almost complete. The situation was fluid, with many new concepts, more or less tenable. The genius of Galileo led to practical results, with the development of instruments invaluable in the service of medicine. Although unacceptable to pragmatic scientists, abstract arguments such as the mechanist theory of René Descartes (1596–1650) were also valuable.

Descartes carried out studies in anatomy, and immediately recognized the truth of Harvey's discovery. The author of a work, perhaps the first, on physiology, *Tractatus de homine* (1662), he envisaged the human body as a machine activated by the heat collected by the blood. The blood, sent in the direction of the brain by means of the aorta, carried there the purest element, the vital spirit. The vital spirit dilated the brain and enabled it to receive impressions of external objects, that is sensations, and also those of the soul, which Descartes clearly distinguished from matter.

Iatrophysics and iatrochemistry, the study of physics and chemistry in relation to medicine, were born at this time. One of the founders of the iatrophysical or mechanist school was Santorio Santorio (1561–1636), a Dalmatian, who became professor at the university of Padua; he was the inventor of a clinical thermometer and an ingenious platform, bearing both his bed and his work table, which enabled him to measure alteration in body weight at all times. He thus discovered 'insensible perspiration', loss of water vapour from the skin. Santorio published the results of his experiments in a work called *De statica medicina* (1614) which anticipated modern studies in metabolism in its quantitative approach and use of precise measurement.

Another proponent of iatrophysical physiology was Gian Alfonso Borelli (1608–1679), a Neapolitan pupil of Galileo and master of Malpighi, who taught mathematics for twelve years at the university of Pisa. He attempted to explain in mechanical terms the most important facts of animal life and expounded his principles in a great work, *De motu animalium* (1679). Borelli studied the mechanical principles of muscular action and tried to measure the quantity of energy expended in movement. He affirmed that the volume of the muscles increased during contraction through the afflux of a hypo-

Thermometer constructed in 1657 at the Accademia del Cimento in Florence. *Science Museum, London.*

Spiral thermometer from the Accademia del Cimento (1657–67). *Execution attributed to Antonio Alemanni, called The Glassblower. History of Science Museum, Florence.*

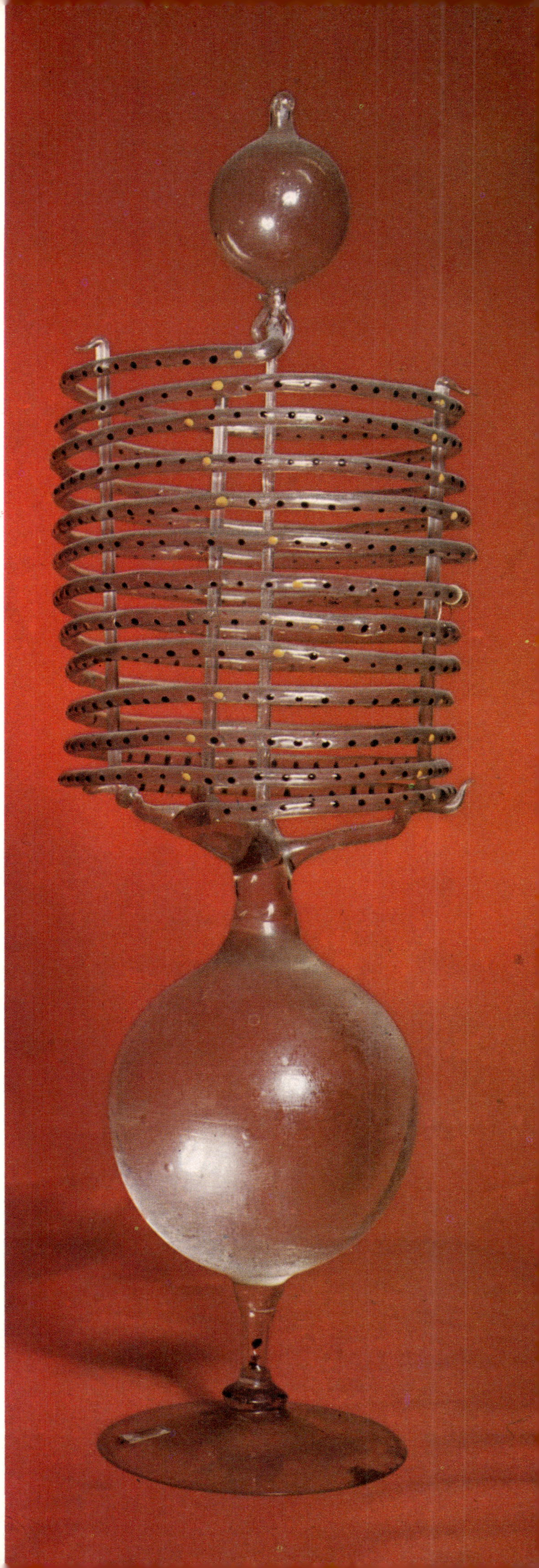

thetical substance which he called succeus nerveus (nerve juice).

When Borelli explained the respiratory mechanism he made valid observations on the function of the intercostal muscles and the diaphragm in breathing. But his theories about the separation of blood from urine in the kidneys and from the bile in the liver, and his theory of fever coming from fermentation of nerve juice belong to 'empty realms of fancy' (Castiglioni).

Giorgio Baglivi (1668-1706), a pupil of Malpighi, represented the extreme development of the iatrophysical doctrine in Italy: he divided the machine of the human body into several smaller machines, comparing the teeth to scissors, the stomach to a flask, the viscera and glands to sieves, and the heart and blood vessels to a waterwork. Baglivi experimented on the physiology of muscles and was the first (in 1700) to distinguish between smooth and striped muscle. But in his work as a physician Baglivi seems to have discarded his theories and is in fact regarded as one of the great pioneers in clinical medicine: his book *De praxi medica* (1696) reveals the powers of observation of a fine clinician, while his lectures at the Collegio della Sapienza in Rome, where Clement XI appointed him to the chair of medical theory, were attended by students from far and wide. Baglivi said: 'The young should know that they will never find a more interesting or instructive book than the patient himself.'

Together with the iatrophysical school there grew up the iatrochemical one, under the leadership of the strange mystic researcher, the Belgian Jean Baptist van Helmont (1577–1644). His biographer Lobkowitz described van Helmont as 'pious, learned and famous; he was the sworn enemy of Galen and Aristotle. The sick never lingered long in his care: within three days, they were dead or they were well again'. His life was a succession of passionate episodes, acts of faith, spiritual revolt and contrition. He related how as a child he had apocalyptic visions in the cloister of the Capuchins at Louvain; he was tempted to take up the practice of magic but then decided to study the Stoic philosophers. Van Helmont next fell under the spell of the doctrines of Thomas à Kempis, which he later abandoned for medicine; he then became

The mid-seventeenth century saw the development of interest in the physical and chemical aspects of medicine–iatrophysics and iatrochemistry. There was a preoccupation with the measurement of all sorts of vital functions, which led to the development of various instruments, notably thermometers, although it was some time before there was agreement on the scales to be used. The body came to be regarded as a machine governed by natural laws and thus capable of finally being understood.

The inspiration for these attitudes came from the brilliant work of the great scientists of the period–like Galileo Galilei, who invented the telescope and whose astronomical discoveries and theories gave rise to a new concept of the universe.

The greatest philosopher of the period was the

influenced with Galen and read every one of his works.

One day a lady dropped her glove and van Helmont courteously picked it up. But the lady had scabies and the young gallant caught it. On referring to Galen, he discovered that scabies came from combustion of the bile and a saline condition of the phlegm, and that a massive purge was the indicated treatment. Van Helmont followed this advice with the result that his resistance was seriously lowered, his scabies remaining unaffected. This made him detest Galen but he did not forsake medicine: indeed, he made an effort to reform it. He was in fact cured of scabies by a prescription from Paracelsus, of whose naturalist philosophy he became an ardent follower.

Van Helmont believed that every living process was guided by a spirit (archaeus) and that all physiological phenomena were determined by ferments and so were of purely chemical origin. He called the divine force which regulates all physical and mental phenomena in man 'archaeus influus', while the vital body force in man, derived from nature, was 'archaeus insitus'. Disease resulted from alteration of the archaeus, for every change

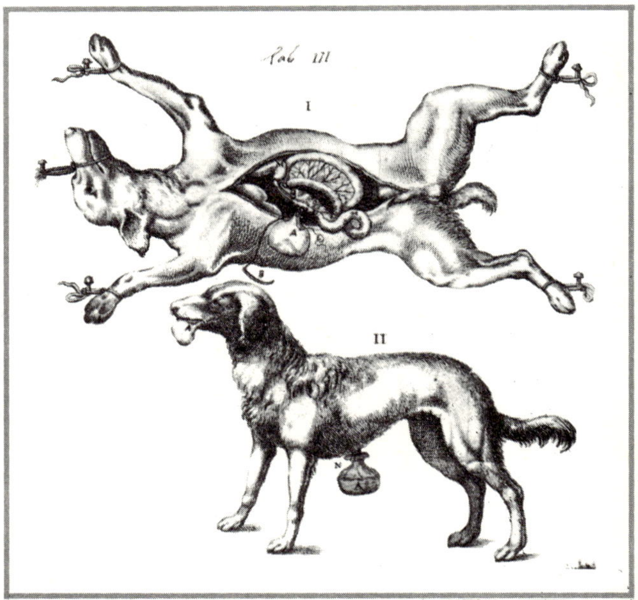

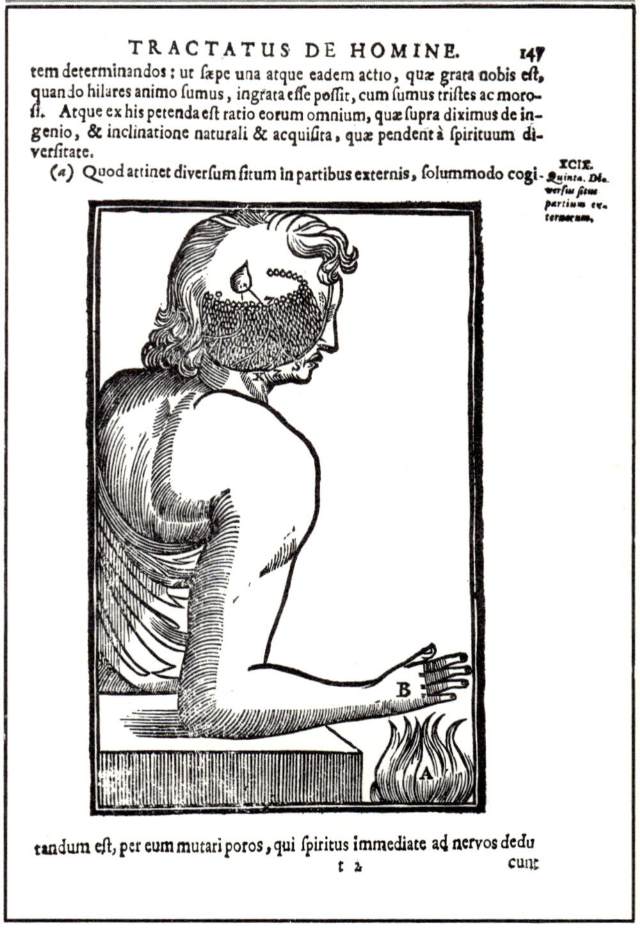

TRACTATUS DE HOMINE. 147

tem determinandos: ut sæpe una atque eadem actio, quæ grata nobis est, quando hilares animo sumus, ingrata esse possit, cum sumus tristes ac morosi. Atque ex his petenda est ratio eorum omnium, quæ supra diximus de ingenio, & inclinatione naturali & acquisita, quæ pendent à spirituum diversitate.

(a) Quod attinet diversum situm in partibus externis, solummodo cogi- XCIX. Quinta. Diversus situs partium externarum.

tandum est, per eum mutari poros, qui spiritus immediate ad nervos dedu

t 2 cunt

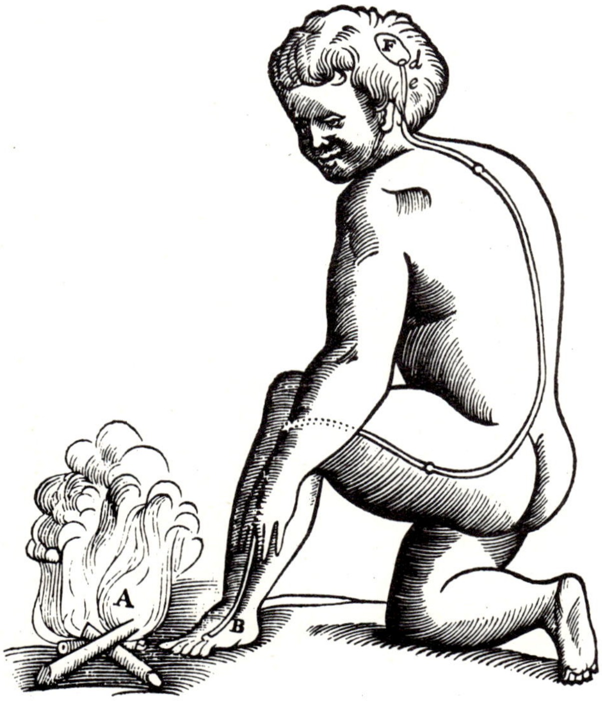

Frenchman René Descartes, who also produced what is often regarded as the first physiology textbook, his famous De homine. *Descartes was perhaps the main supporter of the view of man as a machine, directed by a rational soul located in the pineal gland, which is attached to the brain. But he also gave a correct explanation of the mechanism of reflex action.*

Sensation of heat or pain (centre in the brain). *From De homine by René Descartes.*

Experimental pancreatic and salivary fistulas in the dog. *From Tractatus anatomico-medicus de succi pancreatici natura et usu, by Regnier de Graaf, from his Opera omnia, Leiden, 1678.*

Localization of sensation in the brain. *From De homine by René Descartes.*

Anatomical hall in Leiden. *Engraving by Harewyn, published in 1769.*

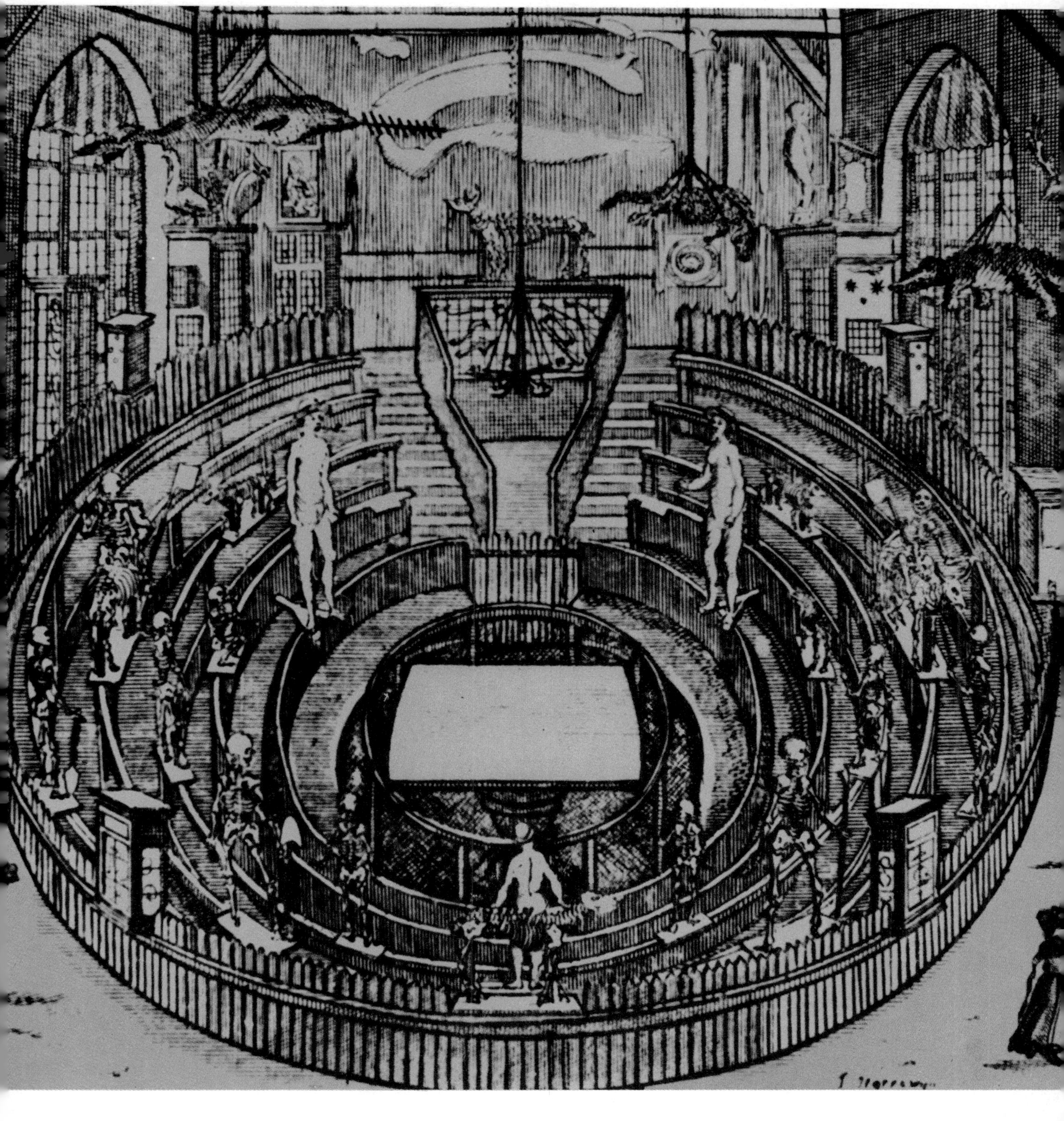

TAV. XVIII

Fig. 40

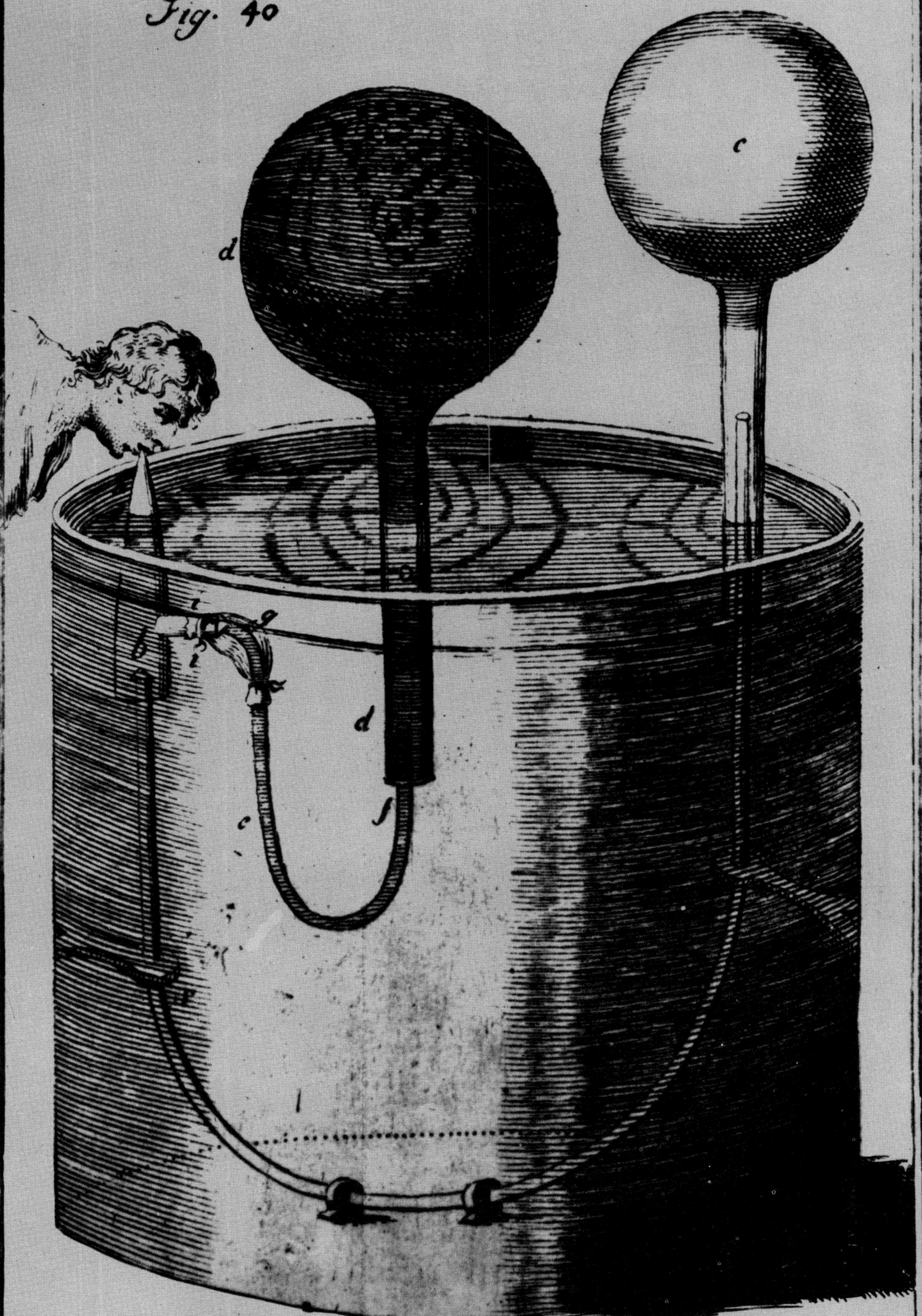

Method to measure air contained in lungs and its elasticity. *Plate from the Statical Essays by Stephen Hales, 1731–3.*

Hermann Boerhaave.

Albrecht von Haller.

Drawings of thermometers. *Plate from the work of Boerhaave, 1737.*

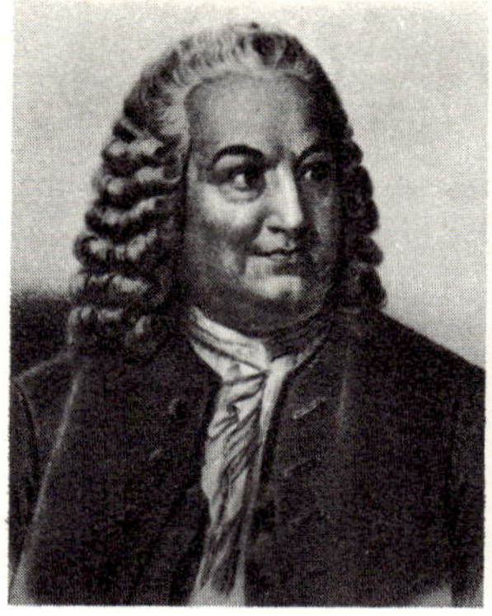

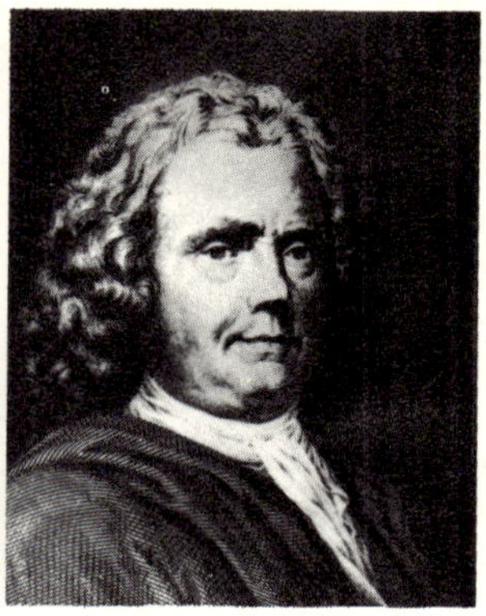

of the regulatory principle brought with it change of matter. In 1624 van Helmont was accused of heresy and brought before the Inquisition; he was imprisoned in 1634 but released two years later.

Today van Helmont's iatrochemical theories are of no more than historical interest. On the other hand, he was a good chemist. He founded pneumatic chemistry and invented the name of gas (derived from 'chaos', as used by Paracelsus in the sense of air). He discovered carbon dioxide, which he called 'gas silvestre', and he made noteworthy contributions to pharmacology. His main work, *Ortus medicinae,* was published in 1648. His son Francesco Mercurio had the book printed in Amsterdam, a Protestant town where there was nothing to fear from the Inquisition.

The iatrochemical school was in fact founded by Francois de la Boe (1614–1672), better known as Franciscus Sylvius; he was born at Hanau in Germany of French parents but was accounted a Dutchman since he lived most of his life at Leiden. He asserted that all physiological phenomena could be explained in chemical terms. From all over Europe pupils came to Leiden to attend his classes. One of his virtues as a teacher lay in his revival of the old custom of Hippocrates, that is of instruction at the patient's bedside. In a way, the school that he founded could be said to have survived him today; many researchers believe that life can be created in the laboratory. The great German chemist Justus von Liebig (1803–1873) inscribed on the door of his study in Geissen 'God created the world with weights and measures', so certain was he that it was possible to explain every phenomenon in material terms.

Iatrochemistry flourished in France, Germany and particularly England, where its chief exponent was Thomas Willis (1621–1675), a member of the Oxford group, which included Boyle, Hooke, Lower and Mayow as well as Christopher Wren, who experimented in introducing food and drugs by intravenous injection.

Willis was born in Wiltshire, the son of a farmer, and graduated from Christ Church, Oxford, in 1639. He was professor of natural philosophy at the university in 1660 and six years later he moved to London, where he acquired the largest fashionable practice of his day. This success was well deserved, for Willis was undoubtedly a fine clinical observer; he was the first to notice the characteristic sweetish taste of diabetic urine (1670), to describe the disease now called myasthenia gravis (1671), and to describe and name puerperal fever. He also made the original observation that some deaf people could hear in the presence of noise (paracusis Willisii), and produced works on nervous diseases, including general paralysis, (1667) and on hysteria (1670). Today Willis is known best for his work on the anatomy of the nervous system, and his *Cerebri anatome* (1664), with illustrations by Wren, was the best book that had yet been written on the subject. It classified the cranial nerves, in an account which was accepted until the end of the next century, describing for the first time the eleventh or spinal accessory nerve (the nerve of Willis) and the group of communicating arteries at the base of the brain known as the circle of Willis.

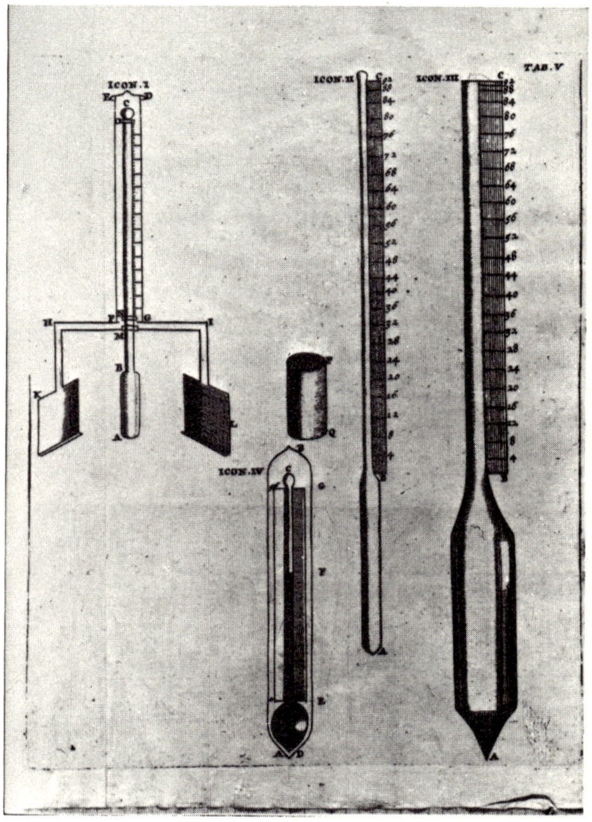

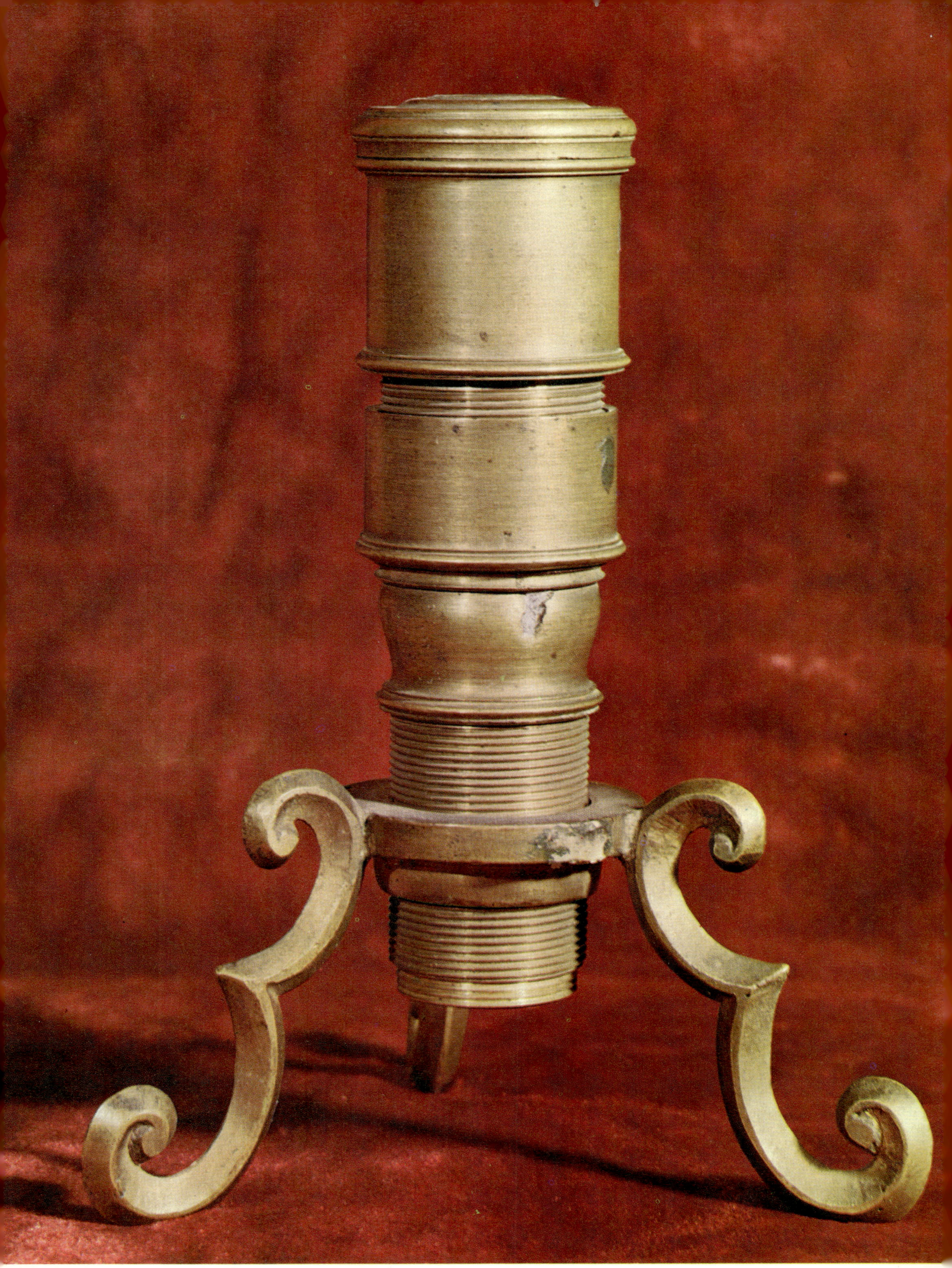

The first microscopists

The quest for scientific knowledge necessitated new instruments. The unaided eye, however keen, could no longer see enough. It was necessary to multiply its power in order to unveil the secrets of nature from the most vast to the smallest. Priority of invention of the microscope was a partisan subject among historians of science for a long time. Now it is admitted that most probably the instrument was invented in 1590 by Johannes and Zacharias Jansen of Middelburg in Holland. In 1610, Galileo was successful in adapting the telescope to visualize small objects, and the instrument was afterwards considerably modified by van Leeuwenhoek, of whom more will be said, who was erroneously described as its inventor. The use of this instrument enabled the natural sciences and medicine to make rapid progress.

The man who worked out basic microscopical technique and discovered many new facts about man, animals and plants was Marcello Malpighi (1628–1694) of Crevalcore. After taking his degree in medicine at Bologna, he taught at the university of Pisa, at the invitation of Ferdinand II, Grand Duke of Tuscany. He became friendly with Giovanni Alfonso Borelli whom he taught anatomy in exchange for mathematics and physics. Three years later he returned to Bologna.

In 1661 Malpighi added the final piece of evidence to Harvey's work on the circulation by direct observation of blood in the capillaries:

'I saw the blood, flowing in minute streams through the arteries, in the manner of a flood, and I might have believed that the blood itself escaped into an empty space and was collected up again by a gaping vessel, but an objection to the view was afforded by the movement of the blood being tortuous and scattered in different directions and by its being united again in a definite path. My doubt was changed to certainty by the dried lung of a frog which to a marked degree had preserved the redness of the blood in very tiny tracts, which were afterwards found to be vessels, where by the help of a glass I saw not scattered points but vessels joined together in a ring-like fashion. And such is the wandering of these vessels as they proceed from the vein on this side and the artery on the other that

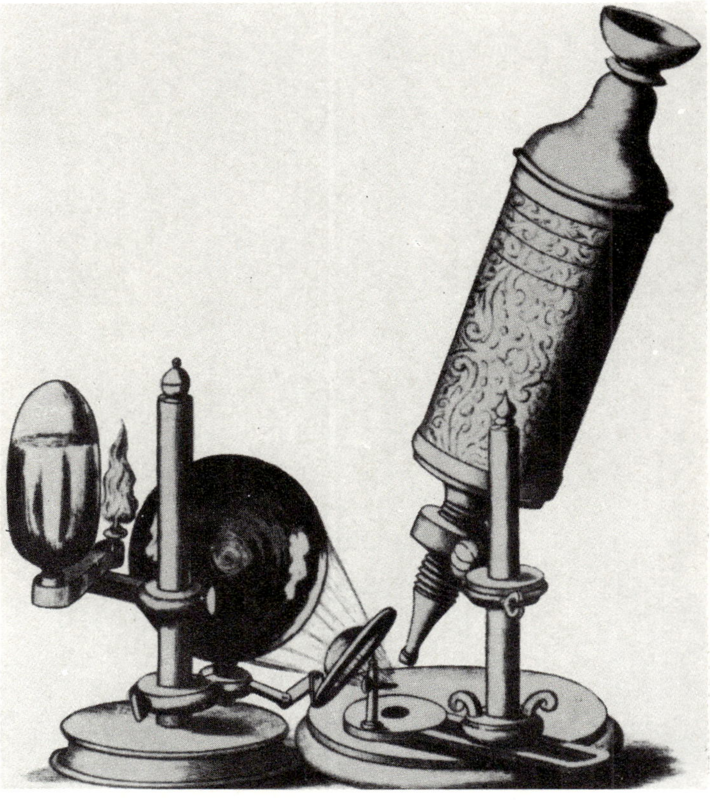

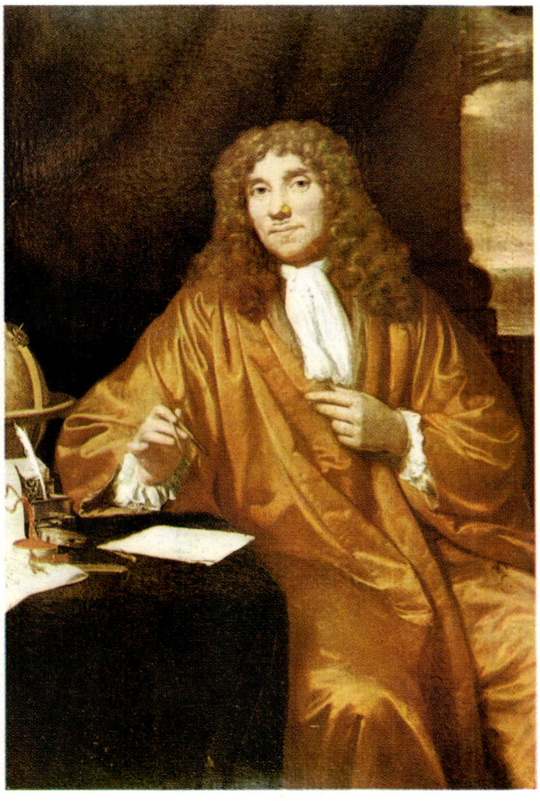

Previous pages:
Eighteenth-century microscope. *History of Science Museum, Florence.*

Robert Hooke's microscope. *Plate from the work Micrographia by Hooke, London, 1665.*

Antoni van Leeuwenhoek. *Portrait from the 1695 edition of his works.*

Facing page:
Marcello Malpighi. *Putti Collection, Rizzoli Institute, Bologna.*

they do not keep a straight path but appear to form a network joining the two vessels. Thus it was clear that the blood flowed along sinuous vessels and did not empty into spaces, but was always contained within vessels, the paths of which produced its dispersion.'

But Malpighi's discoveries did not stop there. He was the first man to see red blood corpuscles, and he also discovered the papillae of the tongue, the intestinal glands, and the pulmonary alveoli. In addition, he made a detailed study of the microscopic structure of the skin, spleen and kidneys, and some of his findings, such as the Malpighian layer of the skin and the Malpighian bodies in the spleen, commemorate his name.

Marcello Malpighi, founder of the microscopic anatomy of animal and vegetable tissues, did not have an easy life. His conservative colleagues in the faculty of medicine at the university of Bologna waged a bitter war with him. Two of them attached him in disguise at his home in Corticella, while the anatomy professors, Giovanni Sbaraglia and Paolo Mini, insulted Malpighi in public and warned students not to practise dissection, on the ground that it was superfluous since Galen had already revealed all the secrets of the human frame. It seems incredible that halfway through the seventeenth century university staff still rigidly upheld the old doctrines, not even yielding when experimental proof stared them in the face.

Obscurantism could not prevail in the long run. The teaching of Malpighi bore rich fruit and was immediately acknowledged outside Italy. His work *Dell'anatomia delle piante* (On the anatomy of plants) was published by the Royal Society in London.

The foremost of Malpighi's pupils was Antonio Maria Valsalva (1666–1723), who in turn became the teacher of the great Morgagni. Valsalva is best known for his studies of the anatomy and physiology of the ear, during which he made hundreds of dissections, distinguishing between the external, middle and internal parts of the organ and describing the functions of the eardrum, ossicles and semicircular canals.

While Malpighi was making his discoveries, Father Athanasius Kircher, a German exile in Rome as a result of the Thirty Years War, was verifying and confirming by means of the microscope the truth grasped by Girolamo Fracastoro: organisms affected by contagious disease contained minute, invisible living creatures which passed into healthy organism and thus reproduced the disease. Kircher believed that the germs were born of the corrupt humours and that in turn they corrupted the humours of the new victims they overcame.

A pioneer of the microscope whose contribution to science was of inestimable value was an amateur. Antoni van Leeuwenhoek was a draper, born at Delft in 1612, who never left his native city and died there in 1723; he is considered the father of protozoology and bacteriology. He was self-taught, had never set foot in a university and knew no Latin or Greek or indeed any language apart from Dutch. He began to use the lens in his business for counting threads of fabric. He built microscopes for pleasure, grinding the simple biconvex lens himself and mounting it between two metal plates. He made over four hundred, continually improving the apparatus and achieving up to two hundred times magnification.

His biographer, Clifford Dobell, in *Anthony van Leeuwenhoek and his Little Animals,* recounts how he spent hours at the microscope without plan or preconceptions, examining bits of material, liquids, tissue, little insects and amphibians. In 1676 he initiated microbiology by discovering infusoria—microscopic ciliate organisms. Many people were indignant at this discovery, seeing it as further evidence of the perverted taste of scientists in attacking the dignity of man. Van Leeuwenhoek wrote that once he was astounded to see graceful little animals, more numerous than all the people of the Low Countries, when he examined a bit of food found between his own teeth.

The astronomers had removed the earth from its place at the centre of the universe and recognized it as no more than a modest planet. It needed only a Dutch merchant to say that there were minute creatures everywhere to reduce to little the value of human life. 'I have often heard it said', wrote van Leeuwenhoek, 'that my reports are drawn from sheer fantasy. It seems that in France someone has actually said that the minute creatures described by me and visible to the eye are inanimate. According to this source, the creatures can be seen moving even when the water containing them has been boiled. Yet I have shown the opposite to many

The instrument which proved to be the most important for the advance of medical knowledge was the microscope, invented in Holland towards the end of the sixteenth century. The invention came into its own in the next century, with the work of two men, Antoni van Leeuwenhoek and Marcello Malpighi. The first was not a doctor, but his technical accomplishment (he ground his own lenses and constructed his own instruments), intelligence and boundless curiosity led him to many original observations; by discovering the minute organisms called infusoria he initiated the science of microbiology. Malpighi is regarded as the founder of the microscopic anatomy of living tissues, and his brilliant observations of the capillaries completed the discovery of the circulation of the blood.

eminent scholars and I dare add that persons foolhardy enough to make such statements do not yet have the experience necessary to pass judgement.'

Van Leeuwenhoek discovered a new world: protozoa, bacteria of various kinds, and spermatozoa, which for a further hundred and fifty years were regarded as infusoria, their true nature being unknown. He also confirmed the capillary circulation discovered by Malpighi, observing it in the tail of a tadpole. 'When I examined the tail of this creature', van Leeuwenhoek wrote, 'I beheld the most exhilarating sight imaginable. While the tadpole was still in the water, allowing me to examine him at my ease with the microscope, I noticed more than fifty points of circulation of the blood. Thus I was able to state that the blood was conveyed through minute vessels from the centre to the sides of the tail, and also that each of these had curves and loops and carried the blood towards the centre of the tail for re-admission to the heart. It made me clearly appreciate this: the blood vessels observed by me are divided into veins and arteries, but in practice it comes to the same thing: they are called arteries when they convey the blood to the furthest parts and veins when they bring it back to the heart.'

Van Leeuwenhoek did not write books: his discoveries received wide publicity through the agency of the anatomist Regnier de Graaf (1641–1673), famous himself for the discovery of the ovarian follicles bearing his name, and for his work on the pancreas and genital organs. De Graaf informed the Royal Society of London about the work of his friend the microscopist, and from 1673 onwards van Leeuwenhoek communicated his observations to that body from time to time in the form of letters, which were published at Leiden in four volumes in 1722. Thus he became celebrated in his own lifetime and was visited by many famous people, including Tsar Peter the Great of Russia.

During his visit to the Low Countries, the Tsar also went to see the anatomist Frederik Ruysch (1638–1731), who had made a famous collection of anatomical preparations, including several complete corpses or 'mummies'. Peter bought part of the collection for use in teaching anatomy at St Petersburg. Ruysch had developed his techniques for preserving specimens from what he learned working with Jan Swammerdam (1637–1680), who was also a microscopist and the first to describe the red cells of the blood. Swammerdam had devised a method of injecting the blood vessels with liquid wax to investigate the circulatory system; Ruysch introduced the idea of using a microscope in the injection of the finer vessels.

By this time, dissection had become established as a means of studying and teaching anatomy, especially in Holland, France and Italy; in England and Germany, where most material for dissection was obtained by grave-robbers (with the full knowledge of the anatomists), the practice still aroused some public apprehension and opposition. This period was also the heyday of Dutch painting, and doctors and dissections became a favourite subject of many of the great masters. Perhaps the most famous of these works is the *Anatomy lesson* of Rembrandt, which portrays Dr Nicholas Tulp, professor of anatomy at Amsterdam, with his pupils.

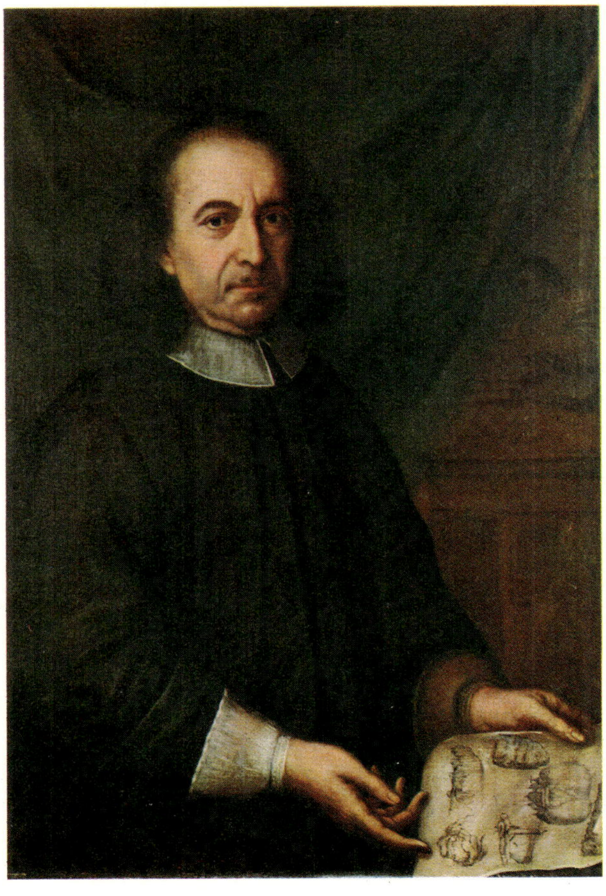

Sydenham, the English Hippocrates

Medicine was now advancing; the discipline of the exact sciences created the environment for future victories over disease. On the other hand laboratory study, research and experiments tended to make many doctors (apart from those practitioners who may well have fitted the image drawn by Molière and Lesage) forget about the people who had the diseases. Thomas Sydenham could not have come at a more opportune time, for he incessantly reminded doctors that their primary duty was to get to know and care for their patients.

The brilliant career of Thomas Sydenham, who was born in Dorset in 1624, was helped by his having been a parliament-man in the Civil War. He obtained his degree in medicine at Cambridge in 1645 'by order from above', after he had been at the university only a year or so. At All Souls he soon became a fellow, replacing one who had been 'purged'. Thus through a politically-motivated injustice he had sufficient authority to launch his necessary campaign in favour of clinical medicine.

Sydenham was profoundly sceptical about the natural sciences and theoretical medicine, because he considered the human mind too limited to be able to deal with fundamental truths. This nihilistic attitude was characteristic of Sydenham, who like all revolutionaries saw all issues in black and white. One day when he was already famous, he was visited by a young man with an introduction. This was Sir

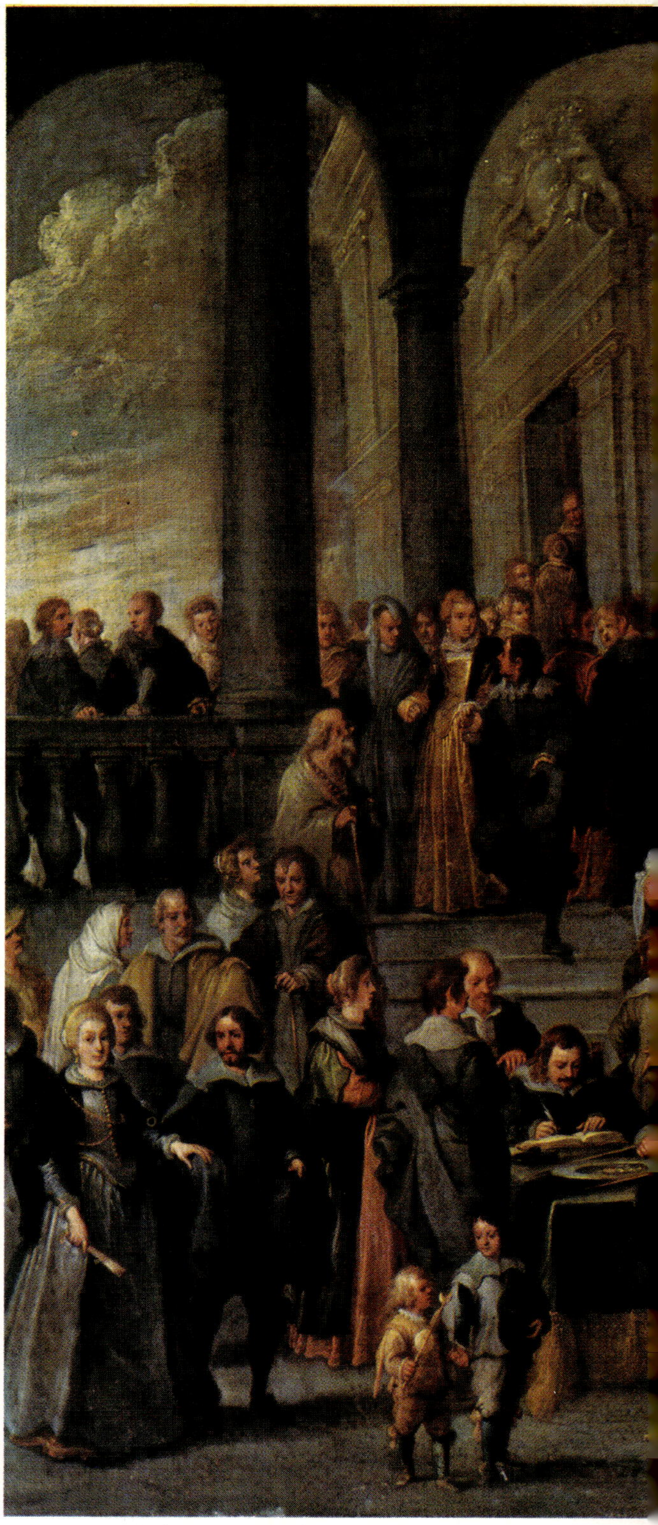

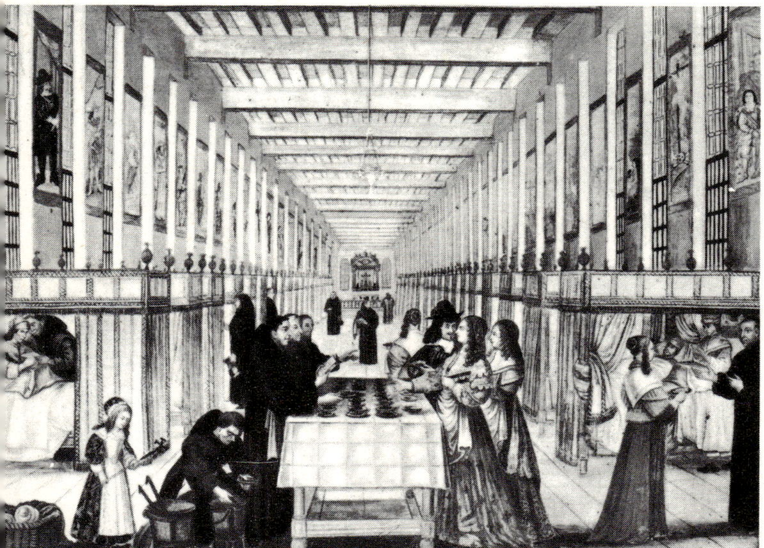

Knowledge of the workings of the human body, in health and in disease, advanced considerably during the seventeenth century. But the theoretical and experimental work which produced this knowledge was accompanied by a tendency of medical men to overlook the people who were actually suffering from the diseases they studied. One man above all redressed the balance of emphasis in medicine—Thomas Sydenham, who is often called the English Hippocrates because of his insistence on the bedside values of the great Greek teacher. In time the importance of clinical teaching was recognized and teaching along Sydenham's lines was widely instituted.

Infirmary of the Hôpital de la Charité, Paris. *Engraving by Abraham Bosse. Carnavalet Museum, Paris.*

Visiting the sick. *By Cornelius de Wael. Palazzo Bianco, Genoa.*

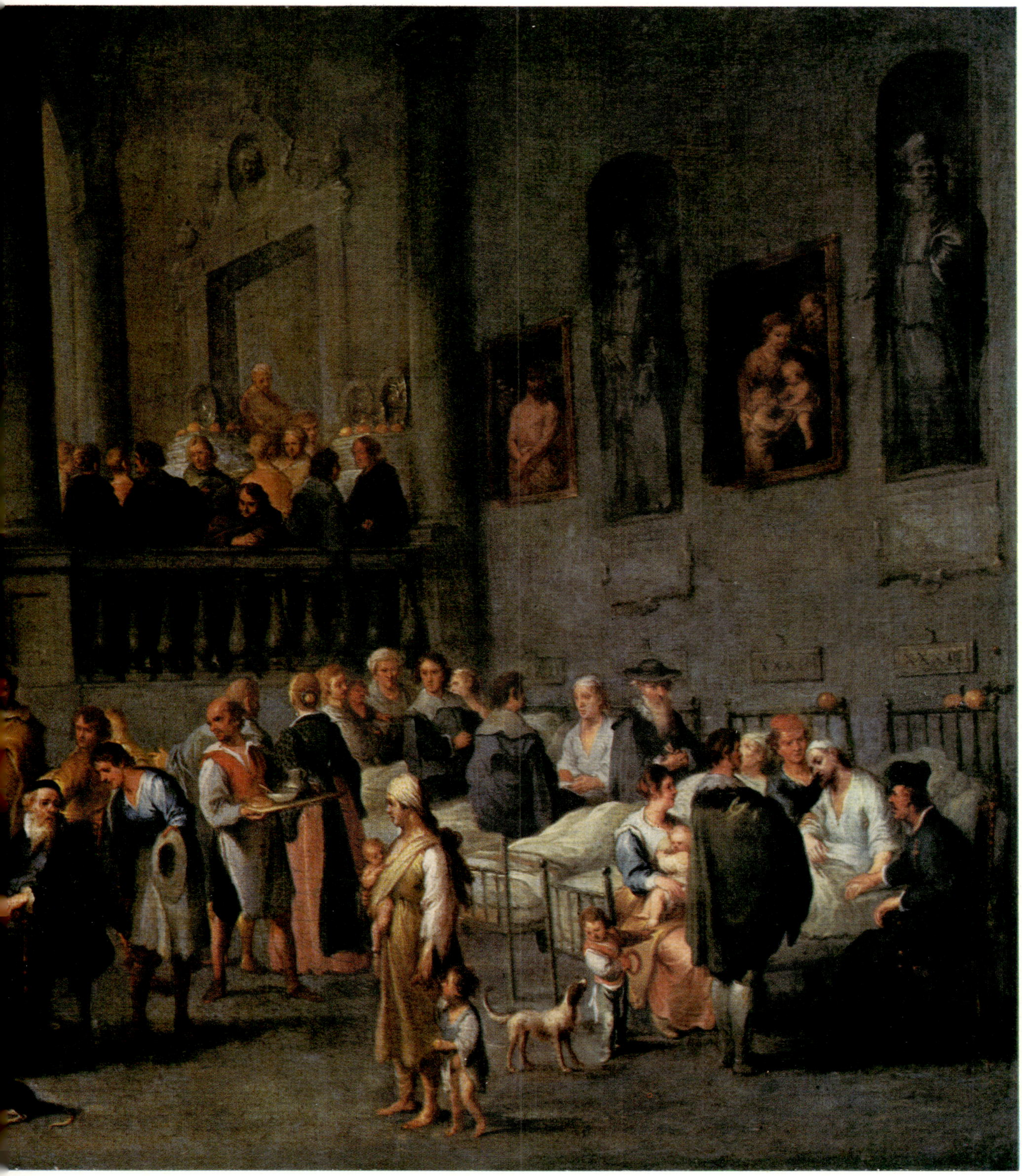

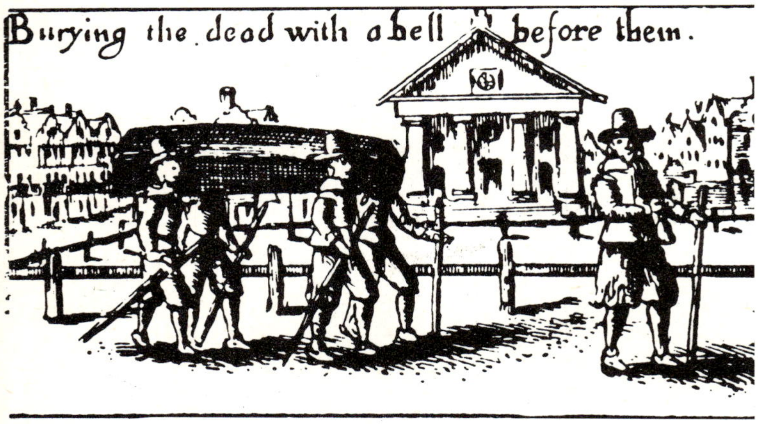

The Great Plague of London, 1665. *Print. Pepysian Library, Magdalene College, Cambridge.*

Fever hospital at Milan. *Seventeenth-century map.*

Plague hospital. *Engraving, 1679.*

Deformed human skeleton. *Seventeenth-century engraving. Bertarelli Collection, Milan.*

Hans Sloane, who in his letter of introduction was described as a good scholar, first-rate botanist and fair anatomist. Sydenham discounted these attainments, remarking that the women in Covent Garden knew more botany and his butcher more anatomy, and exhorted him to forget these matters and go to the bedside, where he could learn something about disease.

Sydenham, 'the English Hippocrates', was a keen observer, describing rheumatic fever and Sydenham's chorea and distinguishing between scarlatina and measles, and giving a classic account of acute gout. He left superb clinical descriptions of such epidemics as smallpox and dysentery. He was very successful as a physician, thanks to the keen attention which he paid to symptoms and the course of illness, without concerning himself with standard professional etiquette. According to Sydenham, disease was something extraneous to the organism, which reacted by attempting to eliminate the disease-bearing substances from the blood. Sydenham held that all acute diseases derived from inflammation of the blood and he shared the faith of Hippocrates in the healing powers of nature. His most outstanding therapeutic successes can be explained by the intelligent use of quinine not long after its introduction into Europe, and a preparation of opium which he devised. This was known as Sydenham's drops, and he regarded it as an excellent treatment for heart disease.

The fact that Sydenham paid little attention to anatomy, physiology and all the scientific advances of his time is irrelevant to his task, and achievement, of re-establishing the dignity of the medical profession.

There was now urgent need for clinical classes in many places, and teaching was instituted (among others) by De la Boe at Leiden and Giorgio Baglivi in Rome. Another celebrated Italian clinician was Giovanni Maria Lancisi (1654–1720), considered as a pioneer of public health, especially for his suggestions about reclaiming marshland. He in turn proposed a radical reform of the study of medicine. Lancisi believed that medical students needed a broadly-based knowledge, should follow long courses of study, and should dedicate themselves to anatomy and pathology and learn the use of the thermometer and microscope. At that period thermometers had come into use; they had been devised by members of the Accademia del Cimento and by Santorio, but no agreement had been reached about the scale. The modern clinical thermometer in fact dates only from the latter half of the nineteenth century, having been introduced into practice by Karl August Wunderlich (1815–1877).

Another sort of medical measurement began

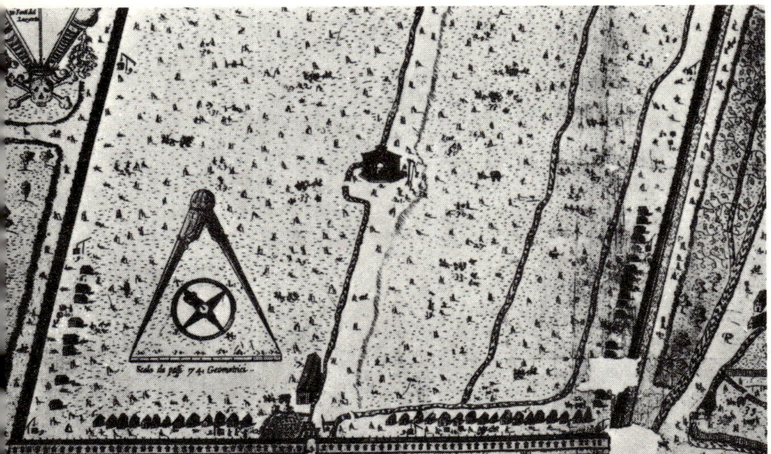

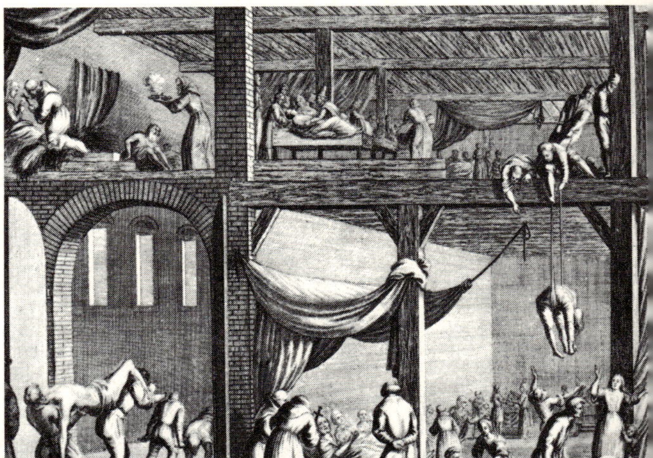

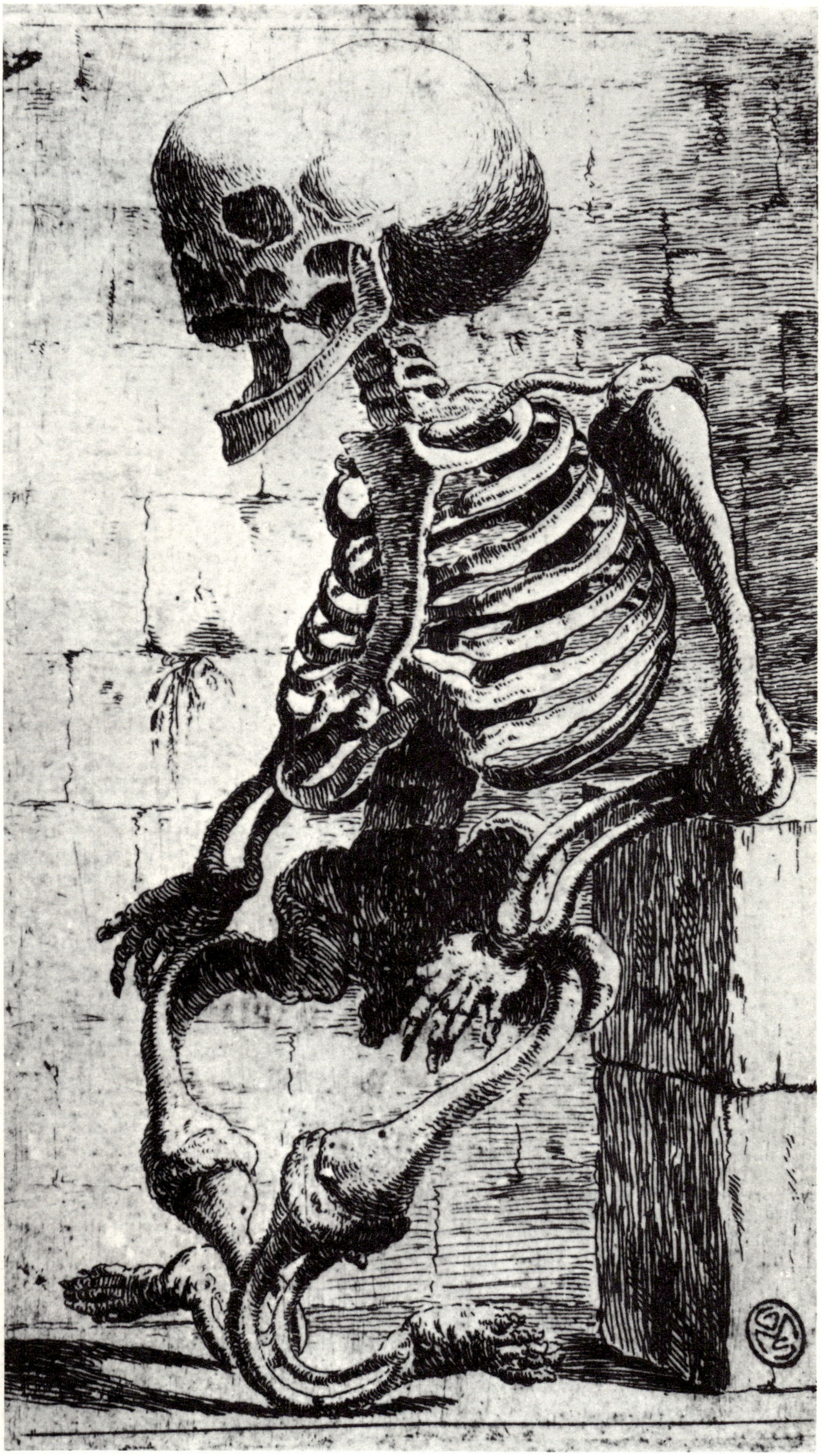

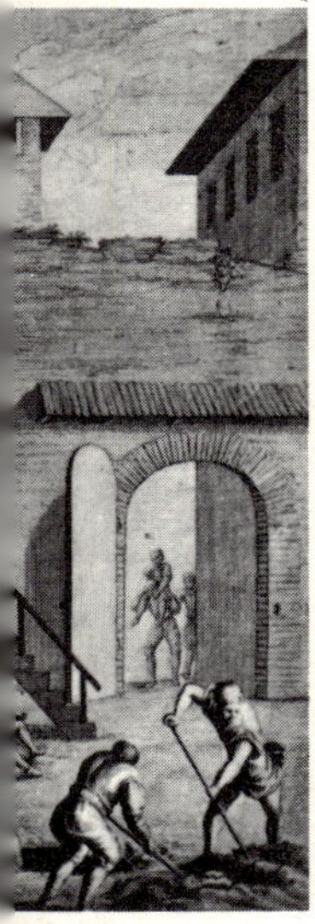

In spite of progress in medicine and improvements in social conditions, seventeenth-century Europe suffered many epidemics as bad or worse than those of the Middle Ages. Scurvy was rife throughout northern Europe and Germany, malaria was epidemic in Italy, while in 1657 an outbreak of fever reduced all England to the state of one large hospital, according to Thomas Willis. Typhus, dysentery and smallpox ravaged the continent, and the latter disease was also common along the Atlantic coast of the American colonies.

Perhaps the worst epidemics were of the dreaded bubonic plague—the Black Death of the Middle Ages—which returned with great virulence and claimed millions of victims, often reducing the populations of whole towns and cities by over a half.

about this period. The first book on vital statistics, John Graunt's *Natural and Political Observations upon the Bills of Mortality* was published in London in 1662. The census may be a very ancient practice, but Graunt was the first person to establish, from bills of mortality, that more boys are born than girls, and that the population can be estimated from an accurate death rate. In his book he described how in Elizabethan England the parish clerk would assign to a number of women the task of finding out who was dead or about to die. Of course, as at the time there was no compulsory notification of births and deaths, any information collected in this way would be of no scientific value. Graunt's work was followed in 1695 by the Breslau table of births and funerals compiled by the astronomer Sir Edmund Halley (1656–1742), which, by estimating mortality rates and the proportion of able-bodied men in a population, was the first scientific work in this field.

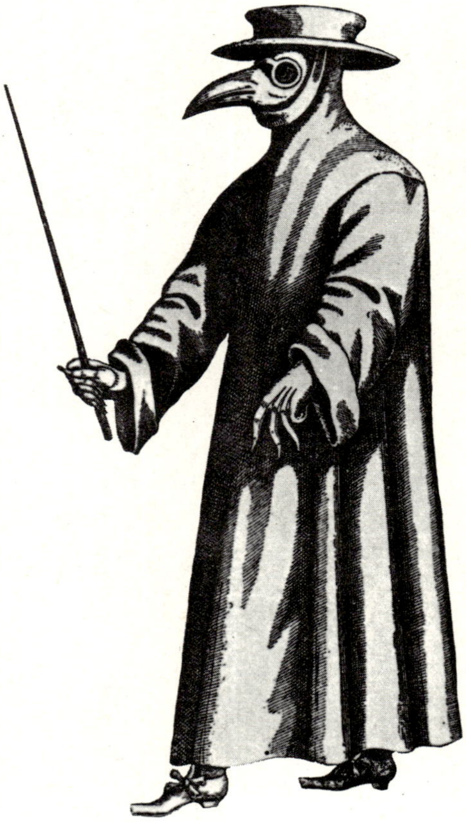

Ineffectual plague doctors were appointed, who wore strange protective clothing, often all of leather – cloak, gauntlets and a mask with glass-covered eye-holes, and a long beak filled with antiseptic substances, and carried a rod to take the pulse. But some physicians, notably Lancisi, made suggestions for the prevention of epidemics, and the end of the century saw significant steps in sanitary legislation.

The plague doctor. *Seventeenth-century print.*

Curing a woman with gangrene of the foot. *From the series of Miracles of St Charles by Cerano in Milan Cathedral.*

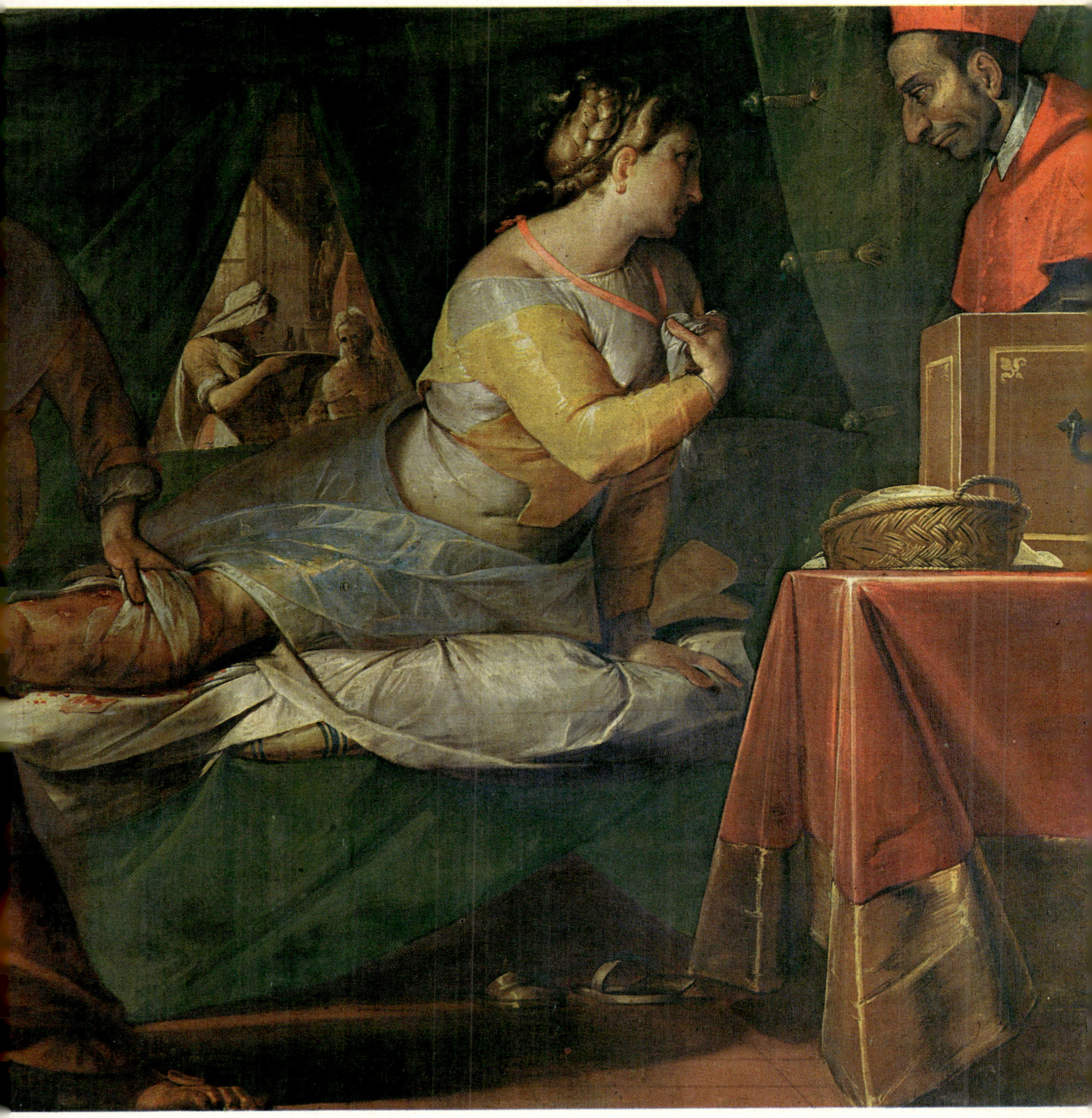

The eighteenth century, socially and politically an age of revolution, saw the emergence of the physician in something of the modern style, his practice based firmly on scientific knowledge. The best doctors of the period, like the Dutchman Boerhaave, were among the finest clinicians of all time; others, like the Frenchman Pinel, made great progress in the field of mental health, so that in this century, for the first time, the insane were to be treated as other sick people rather than locked away like dangerous criminals. Nevertheless, this was also the heyday of charlatans, whose wordly success does not seem to have suffered much from the satires and caricatures of which they were among the most popular targets in this sharply critical age.

The wounded man. *By Gaspare Traversi. Accademia Gallery, Venice.*

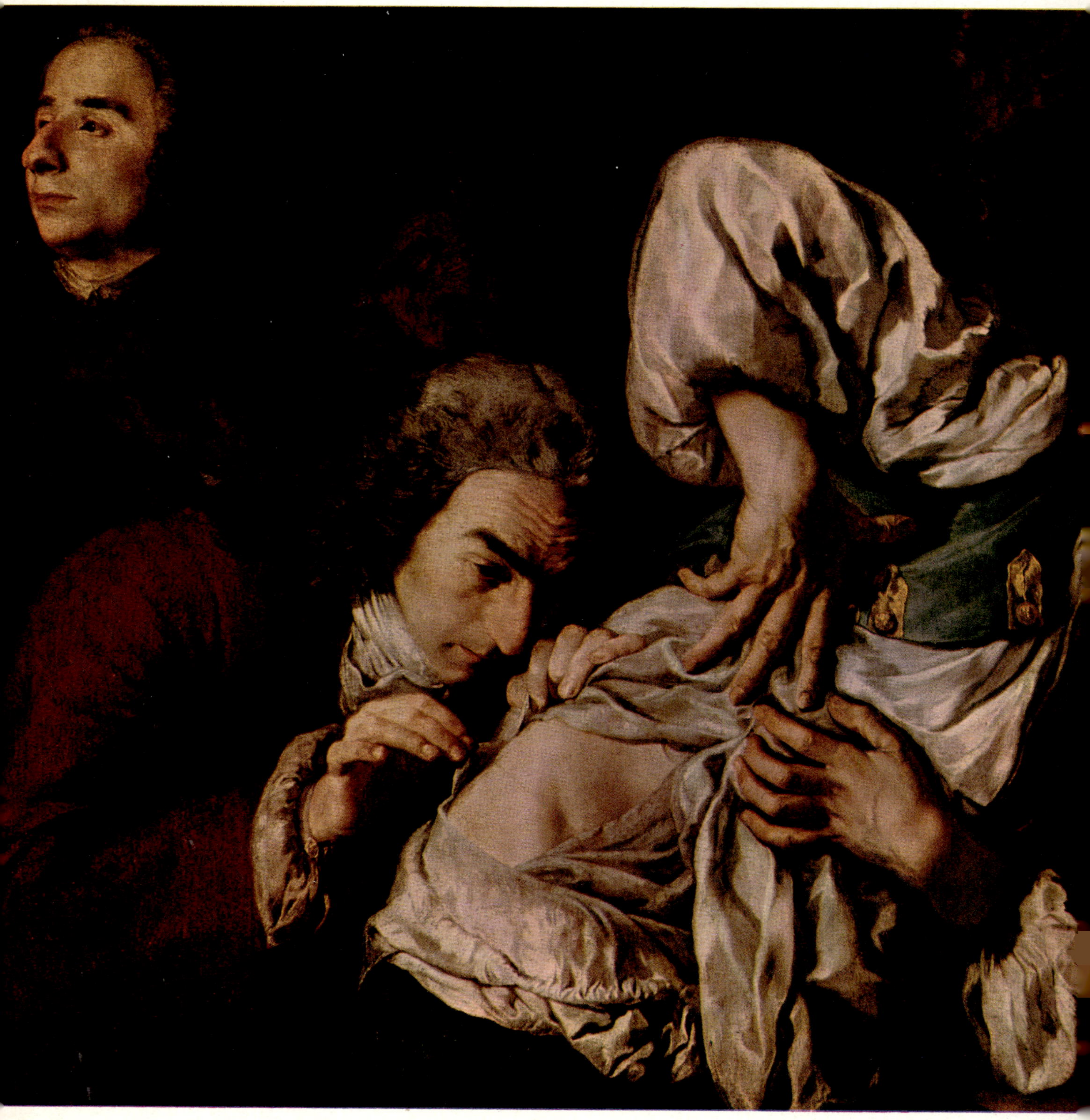

EIGHTEENTH CENTURY
The age of enlightenment

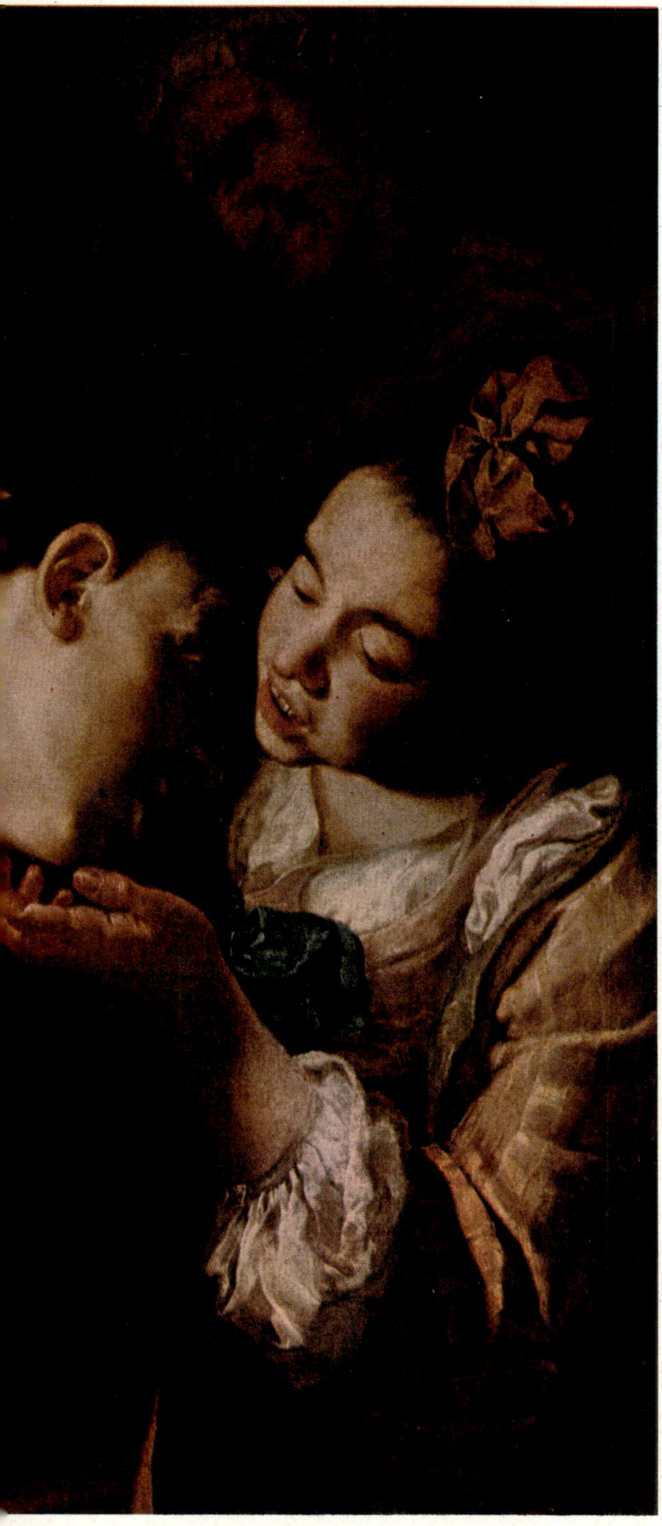

The eighteenth century opened with the War of Spanish Succession and closed with the French Revolution. In between it saw the emergence of the United States, which had seceded from England and drawn up a constitution in 1787. It was a century of political upheaval and revolutionary idealism, which extended to all fields of thought and diminished the influence of academic dogmatism. While Montesquieu and Rousseau were outlining a new social structure, Gottfried Wilhelm Leibnitz, as scientist and mathematician as well as philosopher, was founding the school of German thought which was to be a dominant influence on European civilization.

Eighteenth-century Europeans, besides looking increasingly inwards, came more and more to accept only what was observable directly and reproducible by experiment. This was a result of the increasing regard for the experimental method, the basis of scientific research since Galileo. The conflict between the new ideas and traditional trends of thought was great at the beginning of the century. On one hand there was renewed opposition to the experimental method, and on the other new ideas were gaining ground through direct verification of natural phenomena and formulation of natural laws. The conflict between the opposed ideologies ended with the triumph of the latter, and set the pattern of scientific thought for the nineteenth century. The enlightenment that accompanied scientific progress had many direct effects on medicine and humanity at this time. Increasing awareness of the sufferings of the poor sick led to the foundation of many municipal hospitals and dispensaries. A number of the great teaching hospitals of London date from this period: Westminster (1719), Guy's (1725), St George's (1734), the London (1740) and the Middlesex (1745).

The conflict of two opposed trends of thought led some doctors to oppose the new scientific attempt to influence medical doctrines by upholding animist philosophical concepts; this happened mainly in Germany, and could be linked in a sense with the Romantic movement. Other doctors, especially in Italy, vigorously opposed scientific mysticism and transcendentalism, and looked to new fields for elucidation pf physiological and pathological phenomena. It was through the work of Morgagni in particular that the basis was laid for the anatomical concept of pathology,

Scientists in the eighteenth century had a tendency to construct systems which would explain the phenomena they observed, at the same time devoting themselves to endless experiment and research in an effort to discover the true nature of things. A system which has survived in principle to this day was that devised by the Swede Carl von Linné for the classification of plants and animals, including man, whom he called Homo sapiens.

A strong influence on medicine was that of the philosophers, Montesquieu, Rousseau and Leibnitz, the last of these being the founder of the German school which was to become a dominant force in European thought. Two of the great medical systematists of the period were the Germans Stahl and Hoffman, champions respectively of animism, which opposed materialism, and of a mechanistic system.

which itself was made possible by Malpighi's revelation of normal microscopical anatomy.

The trend towards systematic study was growing in many fields. In the natural sciences, the Swedish doctor and botanist Carl von Linné or Linnaeus (1707–1778) devised a system of classification for plants and animals, and placed man in the order of primates with the name of *Homo sapiens*, in accordance with the binomial nomenclature he devised for all living creatures. Other systematic work

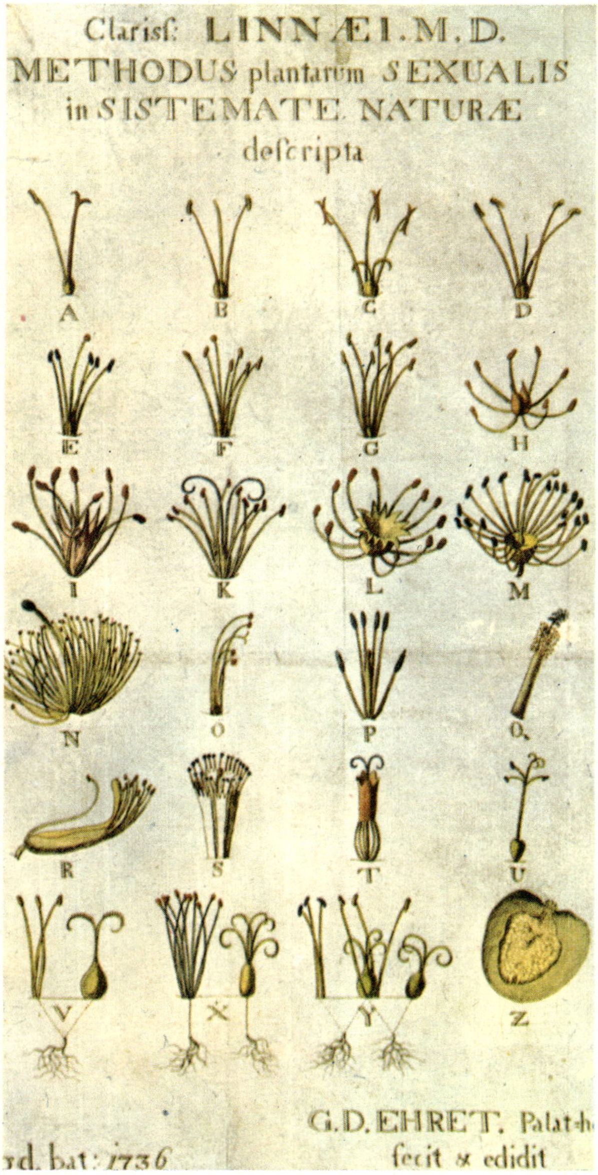

was carried out by Caspar Friedrich Wolff (1733–1794), who evolved a theory of generation; and by George Louis Leclerc, Count Buffon (1707–1788), a writer who popularized more than one science, and was famous for his *Natural history* and for saying that 'the style is the man'.

The old school of thought, however, gained new strength with the revival of animism in the hands of the German doctor and philosopher Georg Ernst Stahl (1660–1734), who declared that illness was a salutary effort on the part of the soul to expel morbid matter from the body. A pupil of G. W. Wedel, a follower of the iatrochemical school, Stahl opposed Descartes' dualism, which divided the life of the body from that of the soul. According to the German doctor, the supreme vital principle was represented by the universal soul, which was the cause of every form of life and came direct from God. When the soul left the body on death the body putrefied. Illness was the tendency of the soul (which became identified with nature) to re-establish order in bodily functions. Stahl's animism was expounded in his *Theoria medica vera,* published in 1708.

Vitalism was distinct from animism. It occupied an intermediate position between the materialist doctrine and the spiritualist, and embodied the concept of a special principle distinct both from the body and the rational soul. The most notable exponents of vitalist thought in medicine were the Frenchmen Theophile de Bordeu (1722–1776), who taught that health was the co-ordination of the separate life of each organ of the body, Joseph Barthez (1734–1806), who introduced the term 'vital principle' and maintained that disease was each and every abnormality of normal function, and Philippe Pinel (1756–1826), the great reformer of psychiatry, pupil of Barthez, who anticipated Bichat in showing that certain tissues were subject to certain disease.

While Stahl was teaching medicine, botany and pharmacology at the university of Halle he had a difference of opinion with his friend and colleague Friedrich Hoffman (1660–1742), another of Wedel's pupils, over the direction medicine ought to take. A fervent believer and rigid personality, Stahl was opposed to the materialism of his time, and pursued the aim of stressing the unity of the living organism with arguments that unfortunately were unacceptable to science. Hoffman, on the other hand,

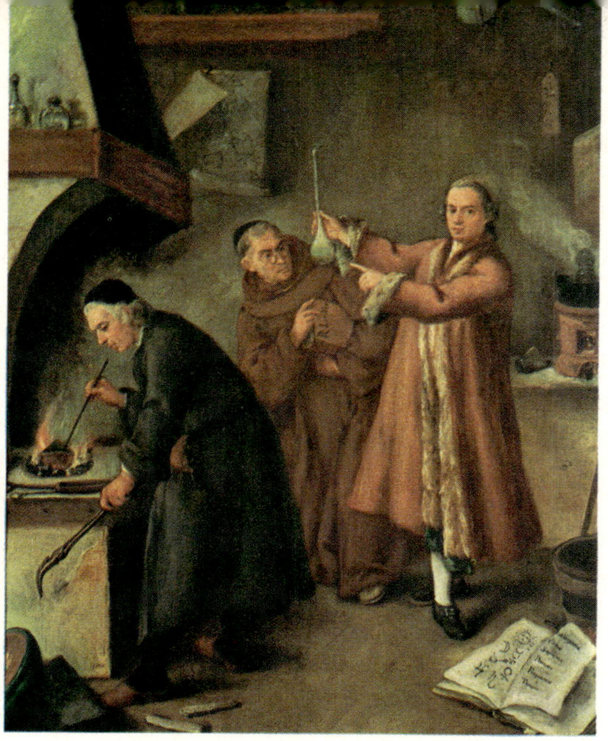

Plant reproductive organs. *Plate from Methodus plantarum sexualis in sistematae naturae descripta, by Linnaeus, 1736.*

The alchemist. *By Pietro Longhi. Correr Museum, Venice.*

A surgeon and surgical instruments. *Eighteenth-century print. Bertarelli Collection, Milan.*

created a rational system on a mechanical basis and expressed his concept in a nine-volume work, *Medicina rationalis systematica,* published between 1718 and 1740. A follower of the philosophy of Leibnitz, he affirmed that our minds could not grasp ultimate causes and that our knowledge was limited to what could be gained through the senses.

All the energy of matter was conceived in terms of movement. According to Hoffman, life was movement, and especially the movement of heart

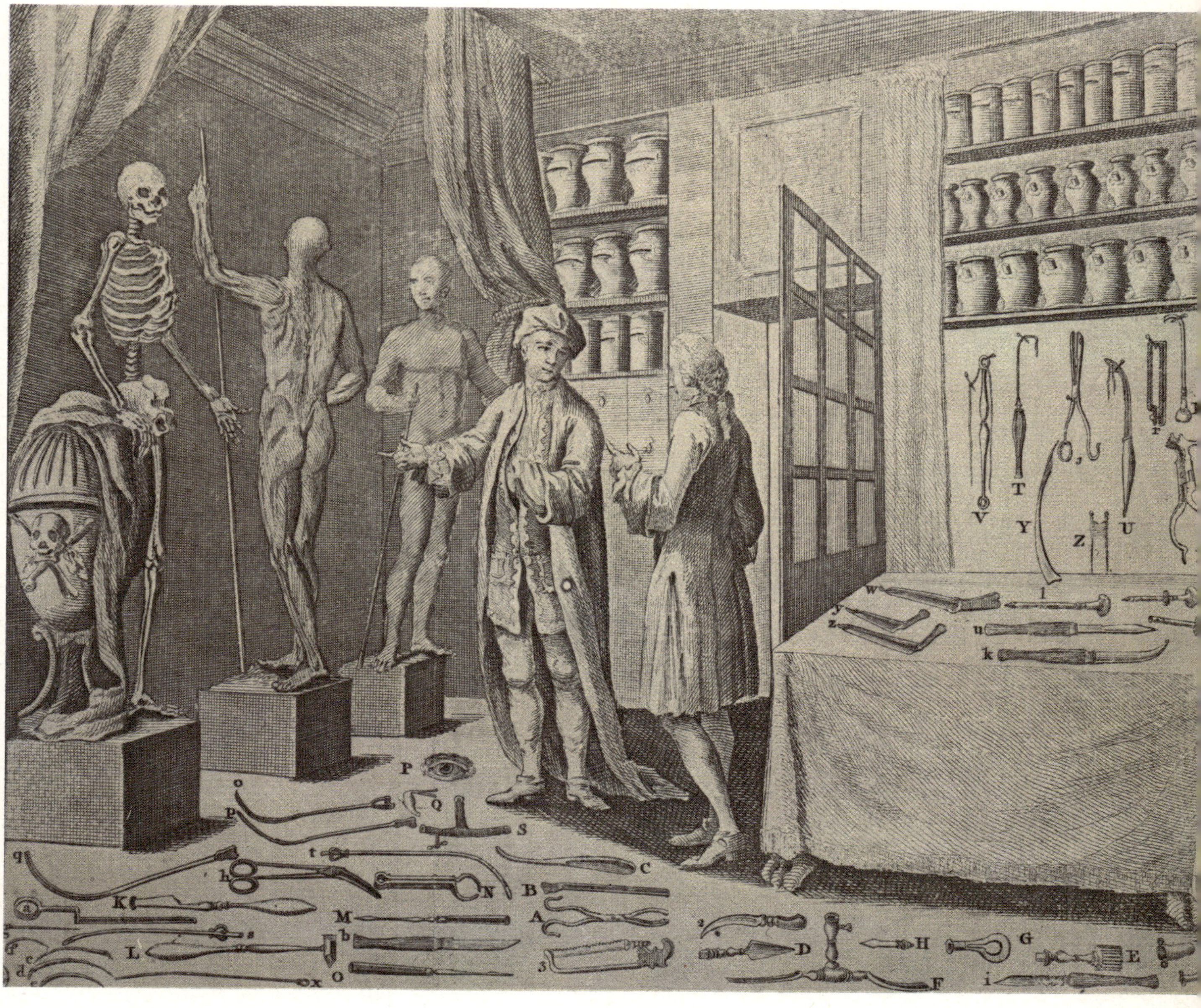

By the eighteenth century, the teaching of anatomy was fully established in the medical schools of Europe, the subject being still mostly in the hands of the surgeons. During the previous century, Holland had become the centre of anatomical studies, but now the schools of Paris and Edinburgh came to the fore. Edinburgh, under the teaching of three successive generations of surgeons, all called Alexander Monro, father, son and grandson, remained a dominant influence for over a century; the standard of teaching declined under the last Monro, who is said to have used his grandfather's lecture notes word for word, including remarks such as: 'When I was a student at Leiden in 1719.'

Doctors in consultation. *By Louis Boilly, 1760.*

Professor Roell's anatomy class. *By Cornelius Troost. Rijksmuseum, Amsterdam.*

and blood, while death was the definitive cessation of all movement. The human body was formed of fibres with the ability to contract or dilate under the influence of a nervous fluid secreted by the brain and distributed throughout the body through the nerves. The chief cause of disease was plethora (fullness), which acted indirectly through the stomach and intestines, at which therapy should therefore be directed. Hoffman's remedies derived partly from Hippocrates, but were partly of his own devising, for example Hoffman's Drops and Anodyne which are still to be found in some pharmacopoeias. Treatment of chronic diseases by 'tonics' such as quinine and iron originated with him and is employed to this day by some doctors.

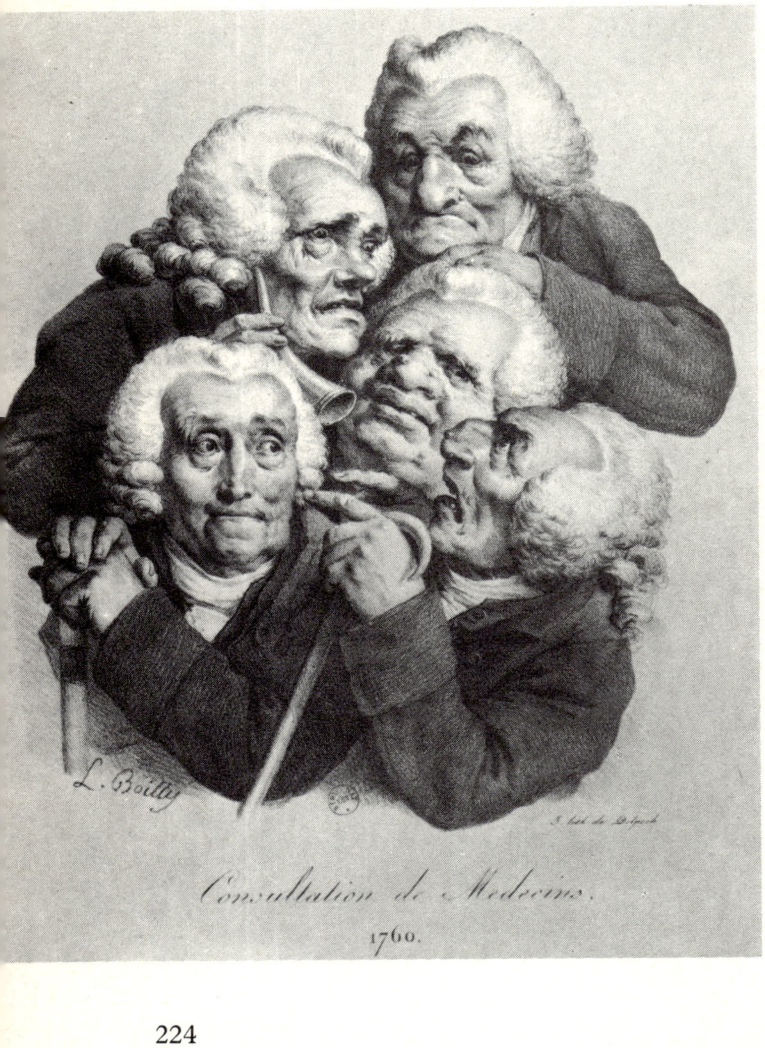

Friedrich Hoffman is noteworthy as a modern scholar, in the sense that he was in contact with colleagues all over Europe for the purpose of exchanging useful scientific information; he rightly believed that science was international. He was especially friendly with the Englishman Robert Boyle and the Italian Ramazzini.

Bernado Ramazzini (1633–1714) was born at Carpi, near Modena, and was professor at the university of Modena, then at Padua. He was an outstanding general clinician, but it is as the founder of occupational medicine that he has gone down in history. In his work *De morbis artificum,* Ramazzini systematically assembled his careful observations on working conditions and the causes of diseases in hundreds of trades and callings; among other things he noted the lethal effects of such metals as mercury and antimony. Ramazzini was not too proud to investigate the humblest or dirtiest work. 'On visiting a poor home, a doctor should be satisfied to sit on a three-legged stool in the absence of a gilt chair, and he should take time for his examination; and to the questions recommended by Hippocrates he should add one more–"What is your occupation?"'

Hoffman should also be remembered for the importance he attributed to the nervous system in pathogenesis. William Cullen, the Edinburgh 'neuropathologist' also held that the nervous system regulated all the vital functions. Cullen's pupil John Brown (1735–1788) in turn produced a theory that life was ultimately not a spontaneous state but one imposed by continual stimuli: these might be internal, such as sensory perception, muscular contraction, thought and emotions; or they might be external, such as air, diet and atmospheric temperature. Good health was determined by an exact dosage of stimuli combined with normal excitability of the organs. In contrast, ill-health was caused by over- or under-excitation, as a result of some imbalance between stimulus and excitability. The morbid state could thus be sthenic, if the excitation were excessive, or asthenic if deficient. Therapy was straightforward–sedatives for sthenic illness and stimulants for asthenic. The remedies John Brown preferred were laudanum and whisky. Though he died of alcohol at the age of 53, his system–Brunonism–outlived him, for its extreme simplicity made it easily comprehensible and so had many followers.

Boerhaave and his disciples

The outstanding clinician of this period was a Dutchman who through his practice acquired an immense personal fortune, leaving over ten million florins when he died, and who in his lifetime was admired, even adored, not only by his pupils but by the public in general. This man was Hermann Boerhaave (1668–1738), called by one of his pupils, the great Haller, 'The Common Teacher of all Europe'. Boerhaave's clinics were attended by students from all over the continent, and his *Institutiones medicae* (1708), a 'physiology textbook', and *Aphorisms* (1709) went through a huge number of editions and translations, including one in Arabic.

Hermann Boerhaave was born at Voorhout near Leiden in 1668. His father was a clergyman and wished his son to make the church his career, and so Boerhaave studied theology and philosophy. He then changed to medicine, qualified, and in 1701 became professor of medicine and botany at the university of Leiden, which was the first to change the traditional methods of teaching. Boerhaave was greatly respected for his intelligence and a character which enabled him to ignore defects in others and live without envy, selfishness of mistrust.

As a doctor he was eclectic, accepting some concepts formulated by the iatrophysicists and the

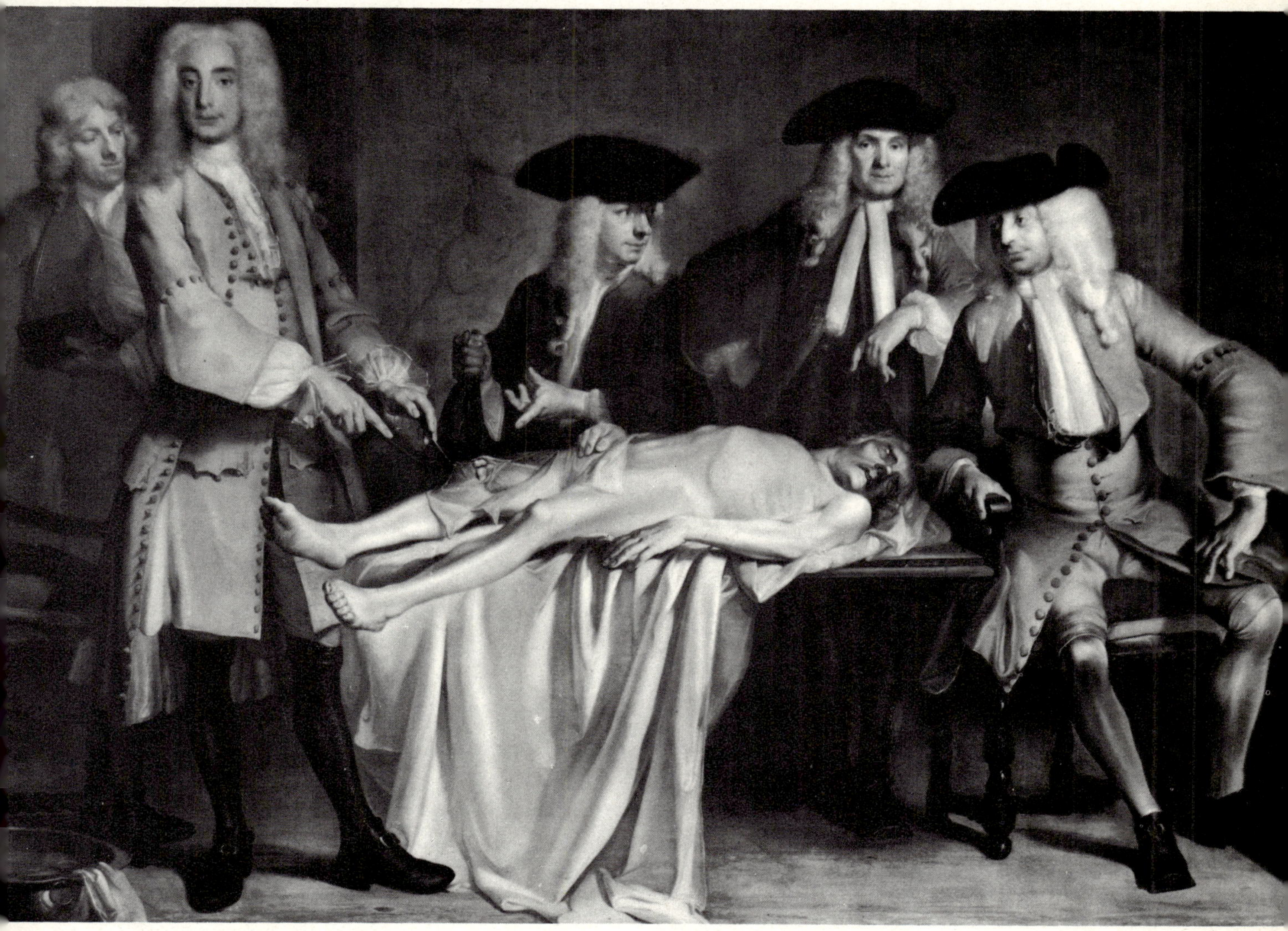

The greatest physician of the century was the Dutchman Hermann Boerhaave, who like Sydenham upheld the Hippocratic doctrine of therapy depending on the curative powers of nature, and thus restated the importance of the doctor at the bedside.

One of Boerhaave's greatest pupils was Albrecht von Haller, who had been a child prodigy and who started his medical studies at the age of fifteen. Haller studied very widely and wrote an enormous number of books, on physiology, anatomy, surgery, botany, and theology, as well as several poems and works of fiction. His scientific works were mainly in the encyclopaedic style popular in the eighteenth century, which saw the publication of the Encyclopaedia Britannica *and similar attempts at a comprehensive account of current knowledge by the Frenchmen Voltaire and Diderot.*

iatrochemists. His basic idea was pre-eminently Hippocratic and governed his teaching: the aim of medicine was to cure the sick and the doctor at the bedside must set aside all academic preconceptions and assess the situation calmly for himself. When a patient died, Boerhaave went with his pupils to investigate the cause of death at autopsy. To speak of his theories would be to detract from his greatness; it was for his teaching that he was most renowned and this was imparted at the courses held in the small hospital at Leiden. Every day with his students he went over the notes of each patient and visited him, taking his temperature and examining excreta.

His disciples Albrecht von Haller and Gerhard van Swieten in turn became famous. Haller was born at Berne in 1708 and was a child prodigy, compiling a Greek and Hebrew dictionary at the age of nine. He began to study medicine at Tübingen when he was fifteen and he continued studying at Leiden; he was still under twenty when he qualified, with a thesis confuting the statement of Professor Coschwitz of Halle that the lingual vein was a salivary duct. He also studied in London, Paris and Basle, where his teacher was the celebrated Jean Bernoulli (1667–1748) of the Swiss mathematical family, a man of extraordinarily prolific talent who made important discoveries in mathematics, worked in chemistry, physics and astronomy, and wrote *De motu musculorum* (Basle, 1694). Haller began to practise medicine in his native Berne in 1729. Seven years later he was appointed professor

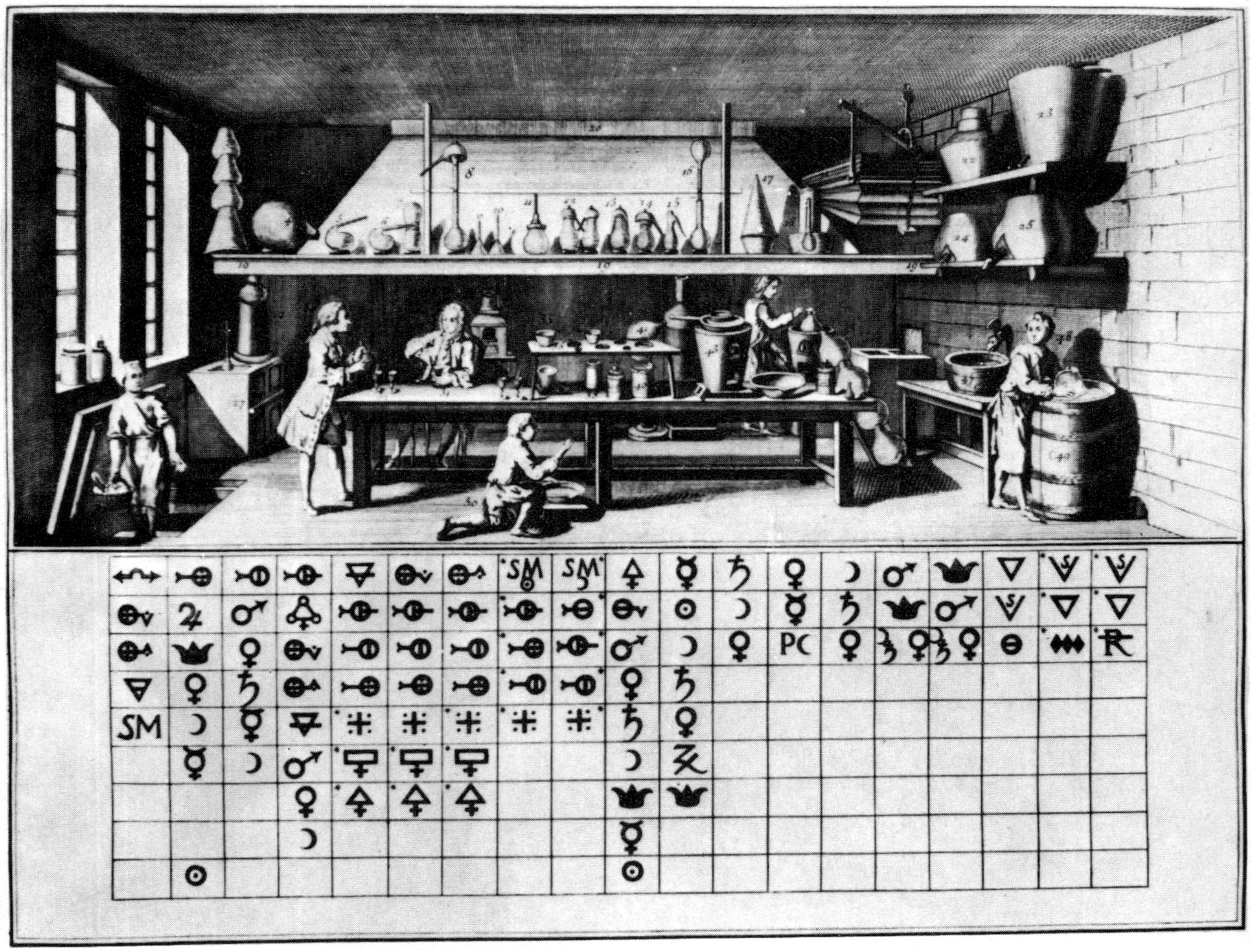

Chemist's laboratory and chemical symbols. *Plate from Diderot's Encyclopaedia, Recueil des planches sur les sciences et les arts, 1772. Bertarelli Collection, Milan.*

Doctor preparing prescription. *Detail from The dentist, by Pietro Longhi. Accademia Gallery, Venice.*

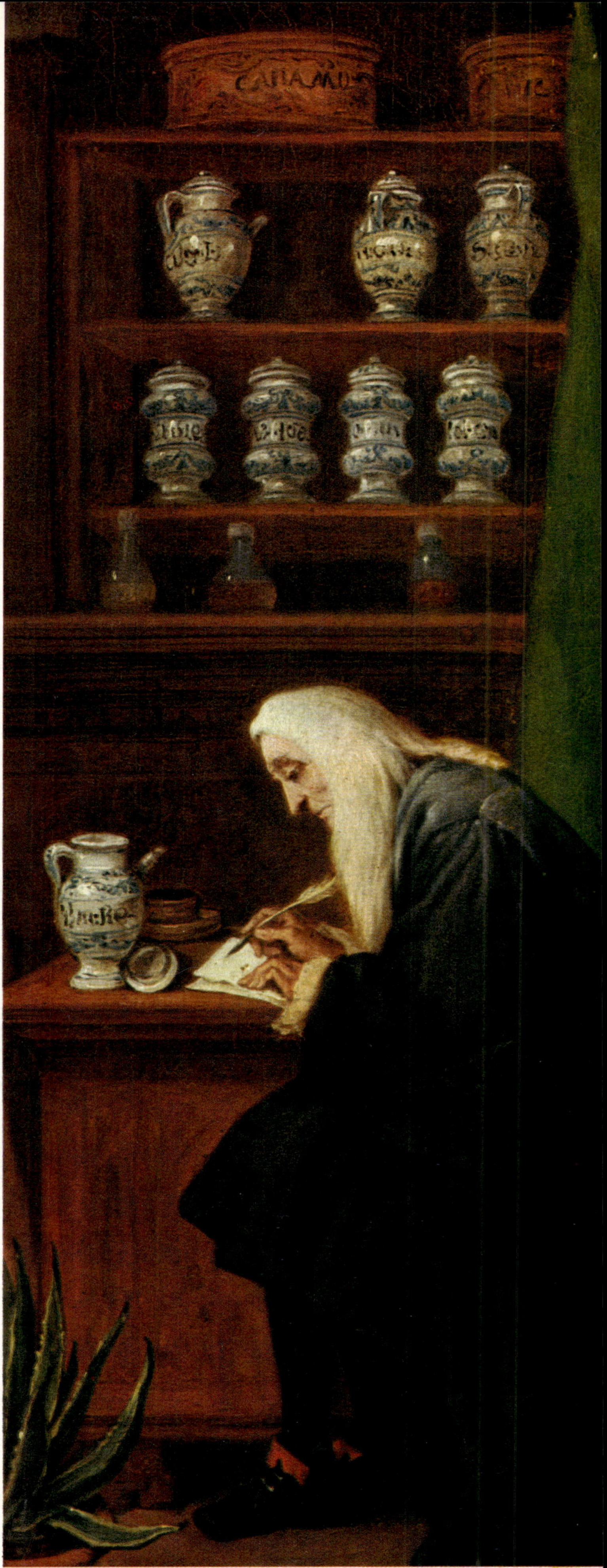

of botany, medicine and anatomy at the university of Göttingen. He remained there for seventeen years and then returned to Basle.

Haller's output was enormous. He taught all branches of medicine, did an undefinable but certainly prodigious amount of work in anatomy and physiology, and created and directed botanical gardens. He also found time to write twelve books on physiology, four on anatomy, seven on botany, two on theology and four historical romances and limitless reviews in a scientific periodical at Göttingen, together with ten volumes of bibliography on botany, the medicinal properties of herbs, anatomy, surgery and medical practice; he also wrote poetry (something he had in common with a great neurophysiologist of modern times, Charles Sherrington). When one reads his great work *Elementa physiologiae corporis humani* (1757–1766) one realizes that at last the modern era had begun, for the eight encyclopaedic volumes review the subject, discuss old concepts and present current views in the same way as a present-day work. Haller's most valuable contribution related to the physiology of the blood vessels and the nervous system.

Galen asserted that all sensibility was bound to the nervous system, while Glisson declared that irritability or excitability was a property of all fibres in the body. Haller gave purely experimental definitions to irritability (which was present when contraction was observable) and sensibility (where stimulation was consciously noted–in man–or caused unrest–in animals) and showed by a long series of experiments that these two properties were distinct and independent, the former being a characteristic of muscle fibres and the latter of parts supplied by nerves. Xavier Bichat (1771–1802) went on to state that these two phenomena were the basic characteristics of life. Haller is thus one of the founders of neurophysiology, but his studies embraced the anatomy, functions, and physical and chemical properties of all parts of the body as well as critical evaluation of all current experimental work.

Another of Boerhaave's pupils was the Dutchman Gerard van Swieten (1700–1772), who founded the old Viennese school. At that period the Austrian empire stretched westwards to Flanders and included a great part of northern Italy to the south. In 1744, the sister of the Empress Maria

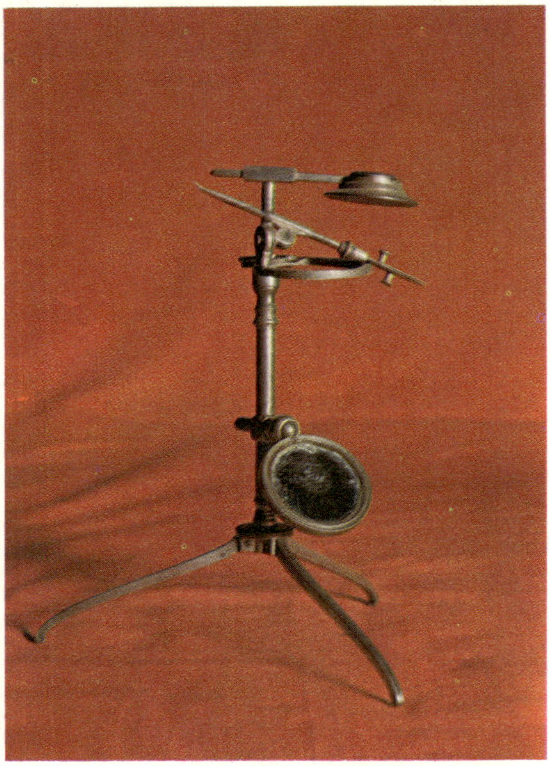

Another of Boerhaave's pupils was his countryman Gerard van Swieten, who perpetuated his master's teachings when he was given the job of reorganizing the medical faculty at the ancient university of Vienna. Van Swieten was a great clinician like Boerhaave and many of his reforms were in the hospital wards, but he also built a chemistry laboratory and instituted an anatomy department separate from that of surgery.

Theresa fell ill in Brussels and van Swieten was called in. The Empress was deeply impressed and invited him to become her personal doctor. The Dutchman was logically the successor to Boerhaave but he realized that as a Catholic his chances of obtaining the post in Protestant Leiden were small. He therefore accepted the offer and went to Vienna, where, soon afterwards, he was given the job of reorganizing the faculty of medicine. The university of Vienna had been founded in 1365 but had no medical tradition, so that this was not a case of salvaging an old foundation by measures of reform, but of creating a new structure.

Van Swieten separated the teaching of anatomy from that of surgery; he created a chemistry laboratory and an anatomy department; he foun-

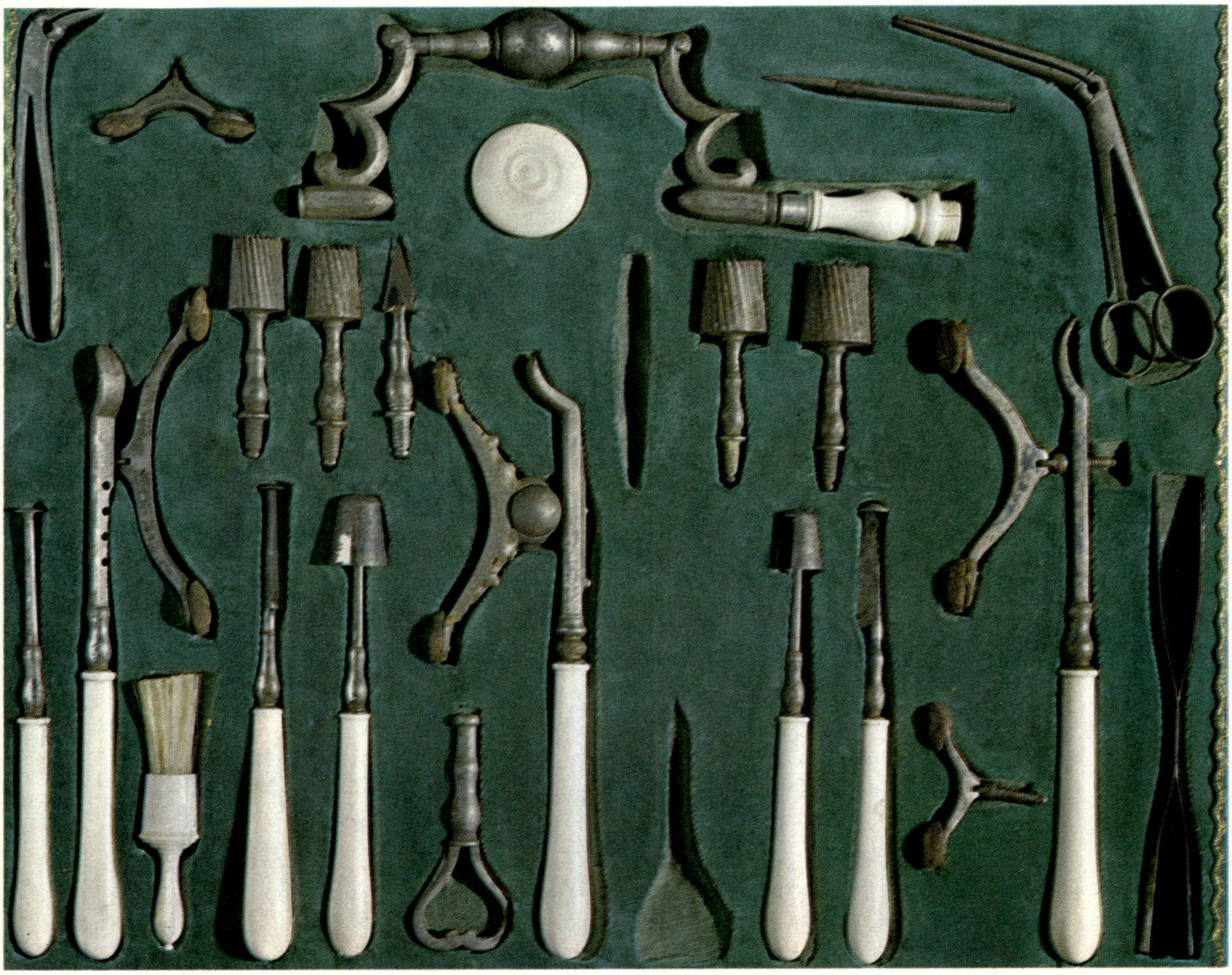

Van Swieten, in fact, founded the first university clinic. The importance of proper clinical methods was now recognized; Boerhaave had taught his pupils to use the thermometer and to examine faeces. It was a doctor of the old Vienna school, Leopold Auenbrugger, who gave physical diagnosis the status of a science by his development of the method of percussion, interpreting the note produced by tapping the chest.

Silver microscope of the nineteenth century. *History of Science Museum, Florence.*

Surgical instruments for trephining the skull, *c* 1700, sent by Emperor Joseph II to his brother Pietro Leopoldo, Grand Duke of Tuscany, for the S Maria Nuova Hospital. *History of Science Museum, Florence.*

Leopold Auenbrugger with his wife. *Portrait by an unknown artist, c 1770. Putti Collection, Rizzoli Institute, Bologna.*

ded a botanical garden. Faithful to the system of his master Boerhaave, he had two wards at the hospital, one for male and one for female patients, reserved for the teaching of clinical medicine. The professors were no longer to be appointed by the faculty but by the state, which paid their salaries and also granted diplomas to those who studied medicine. Van Swieten was a celebrated clinician as well as an intelligent administrator with a long-term outlook. When he was still Boerhaave's assistant at Leiden, he noted down in his own hand the master's day-by-day comments on the cases, and he used this material in the compilation of five typically Hippocratic volumes entitled *Commentaria in Hermani Boerhaave aphorismos.*

The most distinguished doctor of the old Vienna school was Leopold Auenbrugger (1722–1809), who founded the science of physical diagnosis by developing percussion as a diagnostic method. The son of an innkeeper, he got the idea from the practice of tapping wine casks to find out how much they contained. He described the new technique of percussion in a little book, *Inventum novum,* published in 1761: by tapping lightly on the chest with the fingertips a note would be produced, the depth of which would indicate how much air was present in the thoracic cavity and whether or not the lungs were diseased. At first the discovery went almost unnoticed, but after Napoleon's doctor, Jean Nicolas Corvisart, translated Auenbrugger's work into French the new technique spread throughout the world.

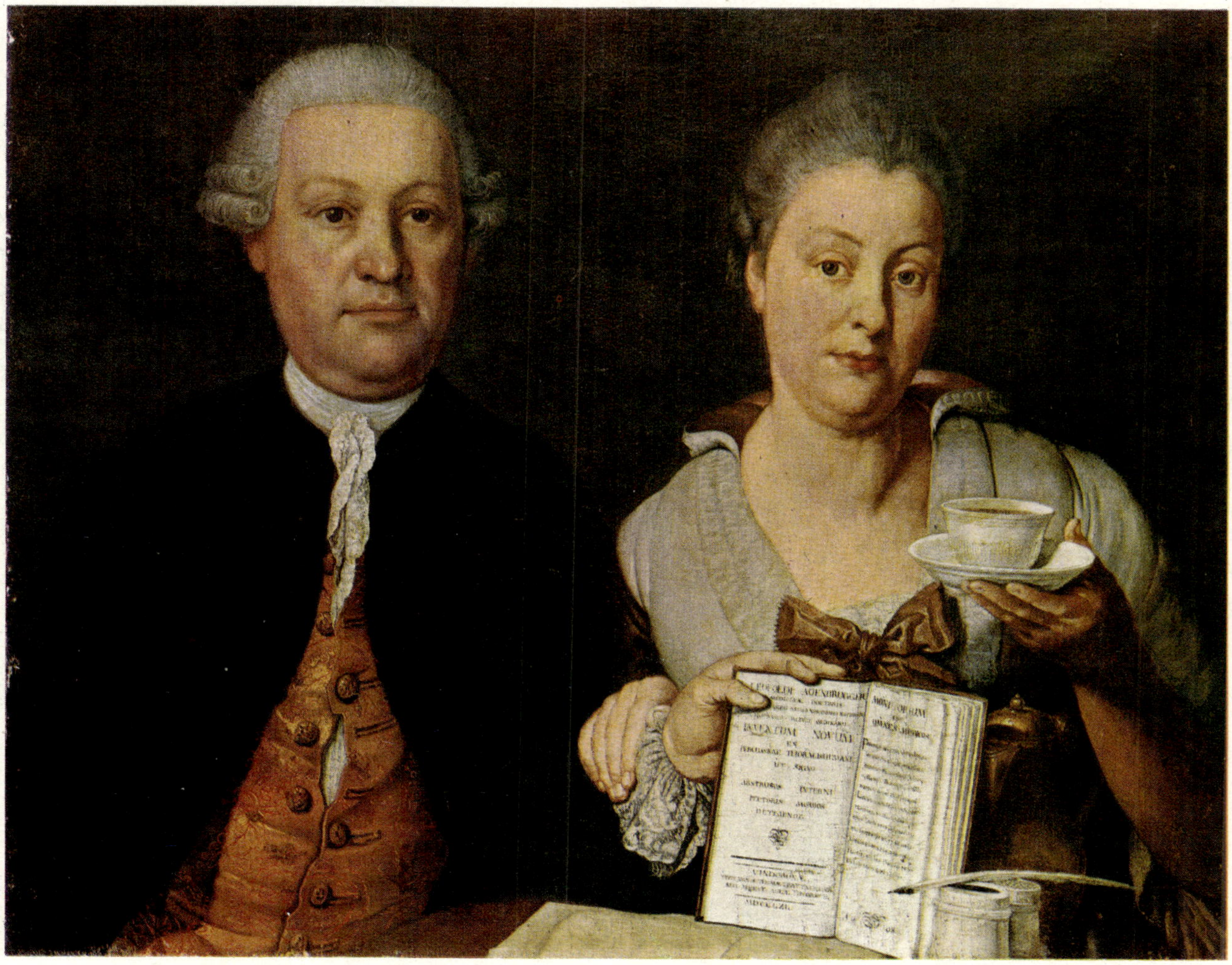

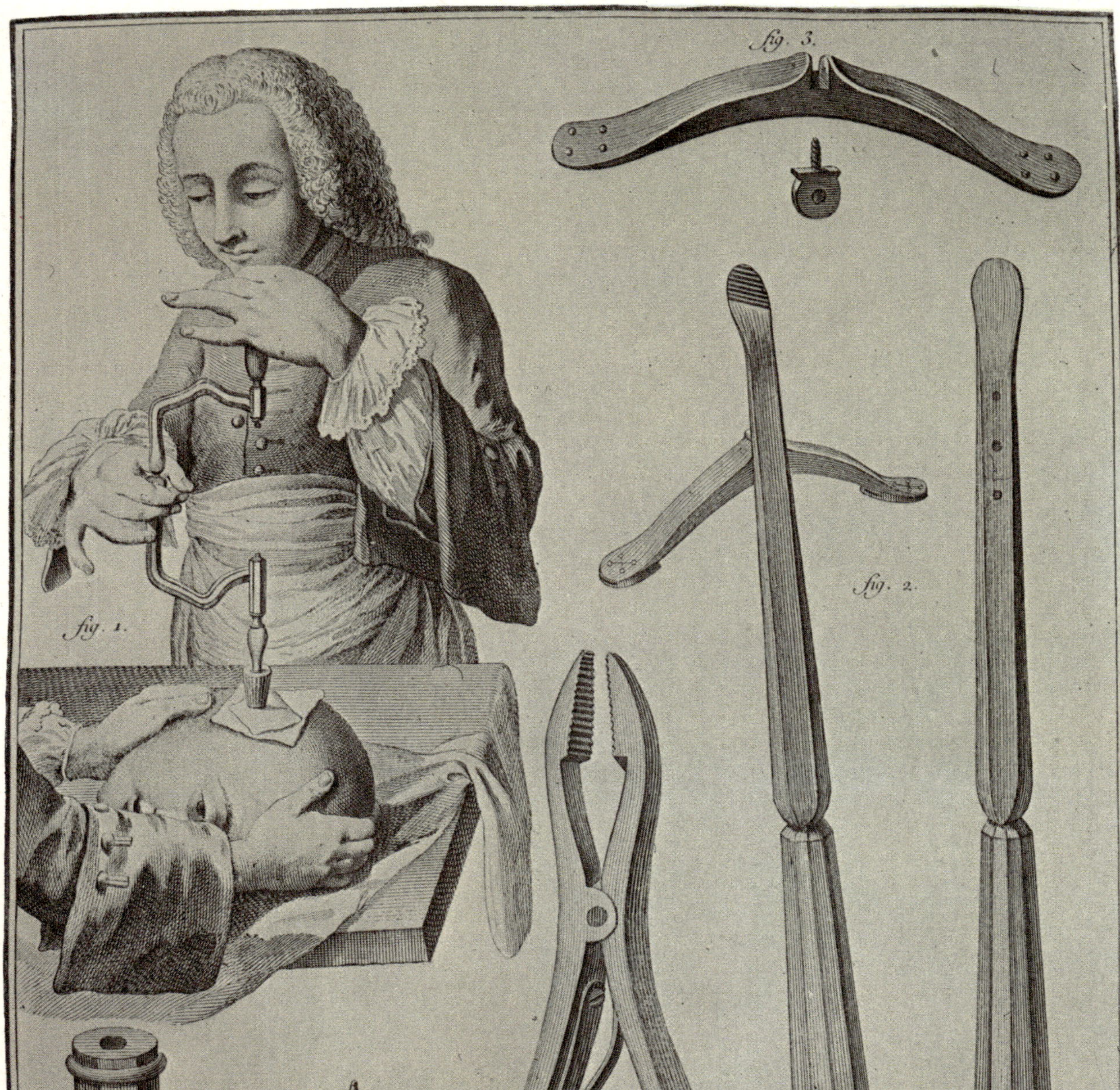
fig. 3.
fig. 2.
fig. 1.
fig. 11.
fig. 3.
fig. 4.
fig. 9.
fig. 10.
fig. 5.
fig. 6.
fig. 7.
fig. 8.

Morgagni, founder of modern pathology

In 1761, a work entitled *De sedibus et causis morborum* (On the sites and causes of diseases) was published in Italy. Its author was Giovanni Battista Morgagni (1682–1771), professor at the university of Padua, and it laid the foundations of pathological anatomy. Morgagni was also a fine archaeologist and author of a biography of his teacher, Antonio Maria Valsalva, remembered for his work on the anatomy and physiology of the ear; he made a great many discoveries, so that his name is often encountered in anatomical textbooks attached to various parts of the body. He studied the anatomical difference between the unhealthy and the healthy body and showed that every anatomical alteration in an organ was accompanied by an alteration in function.

Castiglioni puts Morgagni among the few who were great not only in medicine but also in the history of science. His discoveries are too many to enumerate. He made classic descriptions, to name only a few conditions, of angina pectoris, myocardial degeneration, and subacute bacterial endocarditis, and distinguished postmortem blood clots in the chambers of the heart from vegetations formed in life. Morgagni made original observations on tuberculosis of the lungs and described vividly a tubercle in the process of liquefaction. His work on tumours of the pylorus is noteworthy. He showed that urethral discharge (as in gonorrhoea) occurs independently of penile ulcers (as in syphilis).

Morgagni stated that strokes did not come primarily from a lesion of the brain but rather from changes in the cerebral blood vessels. He was the first to connect syphilis with disease of the cerebral arteries and he noted that hemiplegia affected the

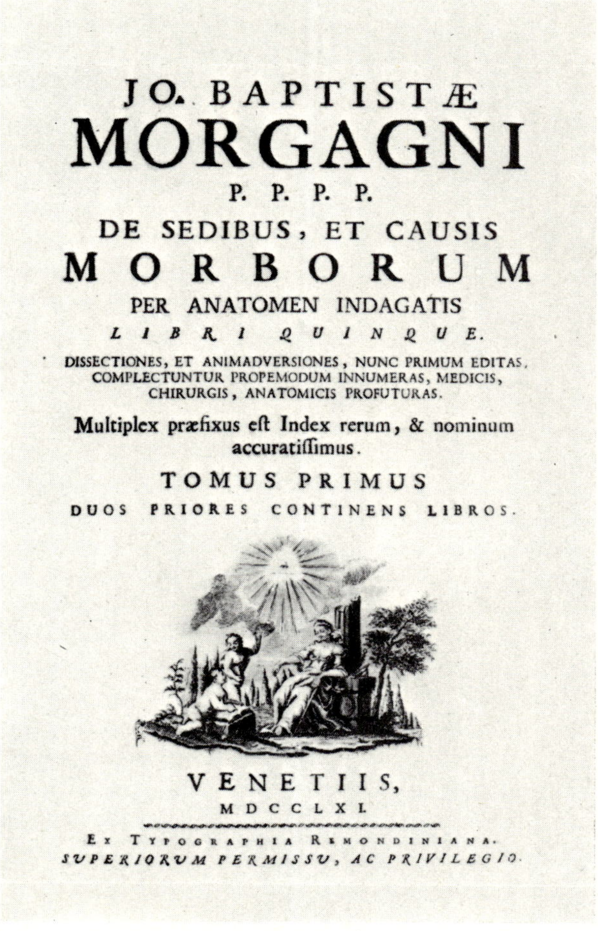
JO. BAPTISTÆ
MORGAGNI
P. P. P. P.
DE SEDIBUS, ET CAUSIS
MORBORUM
PER ANATOMEN INDAGATIS
LIBRI QUINQUE.
DISSECTIONES, ET ANIMADVERSIONES, NUNC PRIMUM EDITAS, COMPLECTUNTUR PROPEMODUM INNUMERAS, MEDICIS, CHIRURGIS, ANATOMICIS PROFUTURAS.
Multiplex præfixus eſt Index rerum, & nominum accuratiſſimus.
TOMUS PRIMUS
DUOS PRIORES CONTINENS LIBROS.
VENETIIS,
MDCCLXI.
Ex Typographia Remondiniana.
SVPERIORVM PERMISSV, AC PRIVILEGIO.

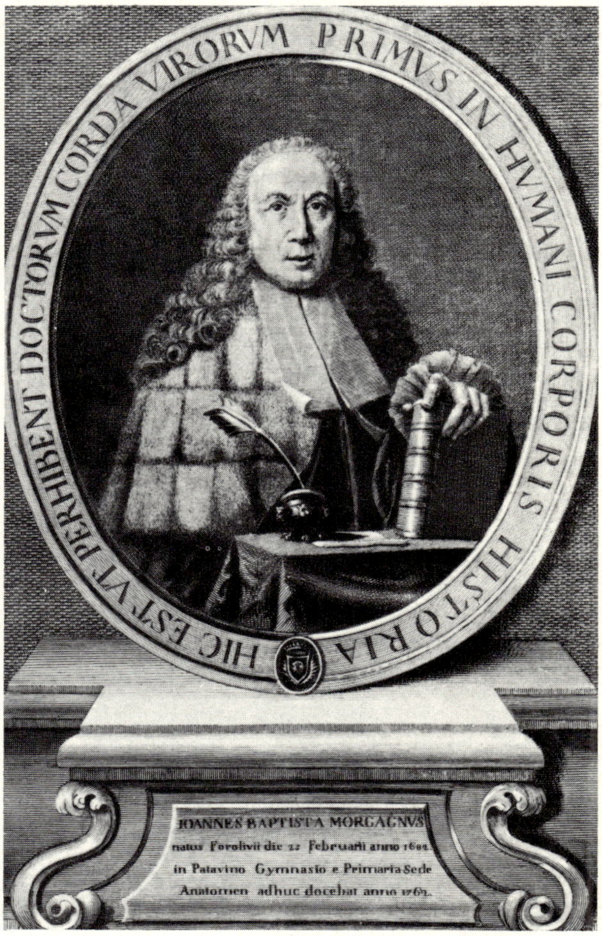

Previous pages:
Trephining the skull and the instruments used. *From Diderot's Encyclopaedia, Recueil des planches sur les sciences et les arts, 1772. Bertarelli Collection, Milan.*

Frontispiece of Giovanni Battista Morgagni's Opera omnia (1765) with his portrait.

These pages:
Operation for cataract. *From Diderot's Encyclopaedia, 1772. Bertarelli Collection, Milan.*

Medallions of Pietro Leopoldo of Lorraine, Grand Duke of Tuscany (1765–1790). *From the porch of the Regolamento del Regio Arcispedale di Santa Maria Nuova di Firenze, 1783.*

Operating chair. *From Diderot's Encyclopaedia, 1772. Bertarelli Collection, Milan.*

side of the body opposite that of the cerebral hemisphere which had been damaged, and that hemiplegia did not result from lesions of the cerebellum. It should be noted that crossed hemiplegia had been noted in Smith's papyrus, in Hippocrates' *On cranial fractures* and in Aretaeus of Cappadocia; the pyramidal decussation had been anatomically described by Mestichelli of Rome in 1710. On reading his work one finds that there is no aspect of pathological anatomy in which Morgagni did not excel. Almost two centuries have passed and his work remains alive and complete, so that one can today give exact diagnosis to the cases that he describes.

Morgagni had many distinguished students. Leopoldo Caldani (1725-1813) succeeded to his chair at Padua and introduced into Italy the doctrine of excitability formulated by Haller. Antonio Scarpa (1752–1832), in the company of Spallanzani and Volta, gave lustre to the university of Pavia. Lazzaro Spallanzani was born in 1729 at Scandiano, near Reggio Emilia, and taught natural history for a period of twenty years at Pavia, where he died in 1799. He carried out remarkable biological work and made fundamentally important contributions to the study of the digestion, circulation, regeneration and reproduction. The concept of spontaneous generation, that is of the birth of animals from decomposing matter, was still actively discussed. Francesco Redi of Arezzo (1626–1698) had denied in vain spontaneous generation of certain insects; the upholders of the concept remained numerous. Spallanzani confirmed the thesis of Redi in the case of frogs by showing that spermatozoa from the male were needed for fertilization of the female ova. His experiments were logical and simple.

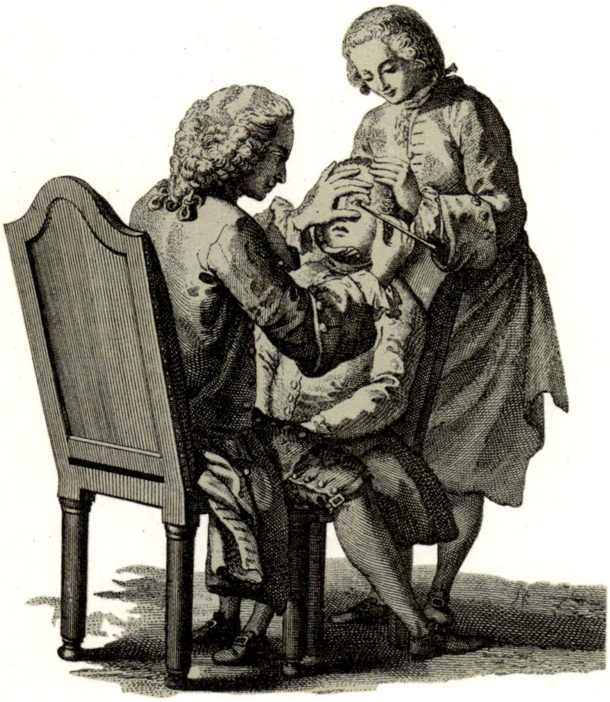

Harvey had written that all living beings shared in common an origin either from the seed or the egg, leaving the question of whether the seed or egg derived from beings of the same species unanswered. Spallanzani demonstrated that the frog, placed on the back of the female, showered the eggs with sperm as they were produced. He then showed that the fertilizing power of the male fluid was suppressed if its direct contact with the eggs was prevented by covering the male parts with waxed cloth, but that the male fluid so obtained, when placed in contact with the eggs, fertilized them.

Spallanzani employed a method devised by René de Réaumur (1683–1757), inventor of a scale for thermometers and of the alcohol thermometer. On lines already used by members of the Accademia del Cimento, Réaumur prepared metal tubes closed at either end by a fine metal mesh and, having filled them with food, he made kites ingest them; these birds regurgitate what they have not digested. Spallanzani experimented similarly with birds and confirmed Réaumur's findings that digestion was not a process of trituration and putrefaction of food, as was then believed, and went further to show that gastric juice dissolved food. Spallanzani, making use of Lavoisier's discoveries, increased knowledge of the physiology of respiration, and showed that asphyxiated animals died, not from cardiac arrest, but from damage to the brain produced by lack of oxygen.

Antoine-Laurent Lavoisier, born in Paris in 1743, was not only the father of modern chemistry but also an eminent physiologist. He died on 8 May 1794, a victim of the French Revolution. His friend Lagrange commented, 'It takes only a second to sever a head. Perhaps a century will pass before there is another like his.' Lavoisier

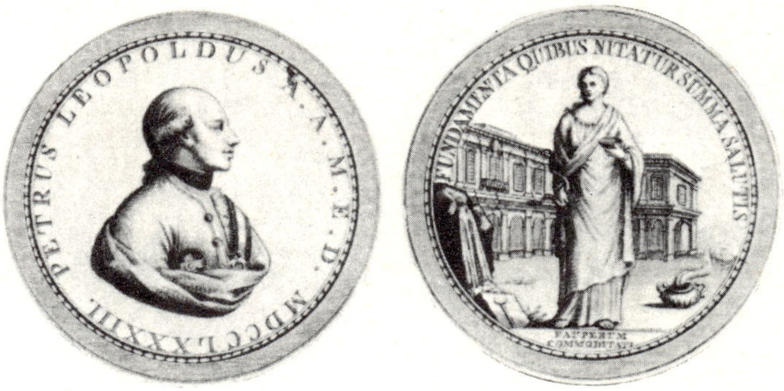

Morgagni is regarded as the founder of scientific pathological anatomy – the study of the appearance of the body in disease. Whereas before pathology had been no more than a collection of isolated individual observations, Morgagni rebuilt it on a system of logical reasoning. The other great developments of this period were the completion of the theory of respiration by Lavoisier, and the study of biological electricity.

showed that respiration was a process of combustion, with the utilization of the oxygen in the air and the production of carbon dioxide. Lavoisier applied his discovery to public health, and demonstrated the need for a certain quantity of air per head in confined inhabited spaces.

Lavoisier's work was the culmination of extensive studies on the physiology of respiration carried out during the eighteenth century in several countries, notably in England. The different gases of the atmosphere had been discovered: carbon dioxide by Joseph Black (1728–1799) in 1757, hydrogen by Henry Cavendish (1731–1810) in 1766, nitrogen by Daniel Rutherford (1749–1819) in 1772. Joseph Priestley (1733–1804) had isolated oxygen in 1772, but was confused by Stahl's theory, whereby substances were supposed on burning (oxidation) to lose something called phlogiston – even though an increase in weight was observed; Priestley called oxygen 'dephlogisticated air'. It was Lavoisier who finally discovered the true nature of the process by which oxygen is taken up by the blood in the lungs.

Spallanzani also made a study of the electric ray, a fish with electric organs formed by little neural units, divided by walls of insulating connective tissue, which functioned in a way similar to the elements of an accumulator. The electric ray and certain other fishes are provided with these electric organs, which as Redi put it 'make the hand that touches them numb and limp', in order to stun and kill their prey.

Special study began at this time on the electrical phenomena of muscles and nerves. When muscles contract, energy, heat and electrical activity are generated. When the nervous impulse passes along a nerve it is manifested by an electrical phenomenon, the action potential. The electrical changes in these tissues can be detected in various ways, both directly and in other parts of the body. The investigation of animal electricity began with the experiments of Luigi Galvani of Bologna (1737–1798) and Alessandro Volta of Como (1745–1827). Using a skinned frog, Galvani observed that by touching the nerves or the muscles with a piece of metal connected to an electrostatic machine, the muscles could be made to contract. The interpretation of this phenomenon was the cause of a long but polite difference of opinion between Galvani and Volta, who repeated the experiments and became convinced that electricity was not inherent in the organism but was due to the contact of the different metals of the conducting circuit.

Volta developed his concept and invented the battery; electric current was thus produced for the first time. Electrophysiology advanced some years later when, in 1841, the Italian physiologist Carlo Matteucci (1811–1868) showed that all muscular activity was accompanied by an electrical phenomenon. He placed the sciatic nerve of a frog in contact with muscle fibres of another thigh. By stimulating the nerve of the second thigh, Matteucci produced a secondary contraction in the muscles of the first. These experiments laid the foundations of neurophysiology and electroencephalography, while they were applied in practice in electrotherapy, with benefit in some neuromuscular disorders.

Through the development of modern techniques of investigation, such as the cathode oscillograph and valve amplification, it is now known that all cells possess an electric charge, the inside of a cell being a few thousandths of a volt negative in relation to the outside.

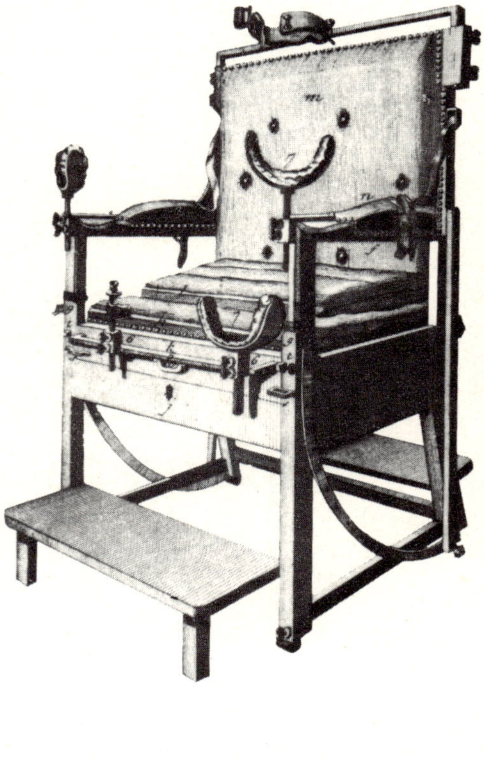

Mesmerism and homeopathy

Franz Anton Mesmer (1734–1815) qualified in medicine at Vienna with a thesis entitled *De planetarum influxu,* which showed how the planets exercised an influence on the tissues of the human body both in health and disease. This influence was thought to be due to a mysterious fluid which he later named 'animal magnetism'. Subsequently, Mesmer elaborated a doctrine according to which every living creature possessed a magnetic fluid, from which emanated special energy that animates both the living and the inorganic world and produces connections between living beings. He introduced magnetic therapy, which derived from the laying of hands on the sick patient, a method which he claimed to have produced remarkable cures.

Mesmer was born in a village on Lake Constance. After qualifying in Vienna, he settled there and married the young and wealthy widow of a court official. He became a friend of Mozart and a fashionable figure. The elector of Bavaria asked his opinion about the cure obtained at Monaco by the priest Johann Gassner (1727–1779), who 'compelled the demon to leave the body of the sick person' by the laying on of hands. Mesmer did not throw doubt on the honesty of the priest but said that there was nothing miraculous in his cures, asserting that they were due to animal magnetism. Early in 1763 he became a controversial figure when the sight of a girl was partly restored by his methods; the girl, Maria Paradies, had been blind since the age of three and a half. Doctors in Vienna started intriguing against him and it became necessary for him to emigrate to Paris.

In the French capital he soon became one of the most popular physicians on account of his power of healing the sick and ending pain by inducing a state of trance. Mesmer earned vast sums and enjoyed the patronage of Queen Marie Antoinette. Louis XVI offered him an income of twenty-thousand francs to remain in Paris and a further ten-thousand francs if he opened a Magnetic Institute there. But a dispute with established French physicians obliged Mesmer to forgo the king's attractive offer and he retired to Spa. However his pupils were very numerous and they formed an association in his support, collected 340,000 francs and agitated for his return.

Mesmer's fame was such that his clients included famous writers, aristocrats, generals and politicians, and they had to book their appointments weeks in advance. He received them in magnificent consulting rooms where they found others around a bath of dilute sulphuric acid from which curved iron bars protruded. The lights would dim, perfume would fill the air and distant music would create a suitable atmosphere. The patients grasped the bars, joined hands and formed a circle. Then Mesmer would appear in a scarlet silk gown and touch each patient in turn in different spots, producing a hypnotic state in which he would suggest that they were cured. On returning home, his visitors would be convinced that they were better.

A commission was set up with four members of the Academy of Medicine and five from the Academy of Sciences, including Benjamin Franklin and Lavoisier. They conducted an enquiry into Mesmer's system of treatment and gave an unfavourable verdict. 'Nothing proves the existence of magnetic animal fluid; imagination without magnetism may produce convulsions; magnetism without imagination produces nothing.' Despite official disapproval, Mesmer could not be accused of chicanery for he acted in all good faith. On the other hand, his enthusiastic admirers–including the famous general Lafayette–must themselves have believed sincerely in animal magnetism. Today Mesmer may be assessed dispassionately, that is without the enthusiasm of immediate followers and the sneers of doctors of the period, undoubtedly jealous of his success and income, to cloud the judgment.

One of Mesmer's pupils, Puysegur, observed that the greatest benefit occurred in the case of patients who were unconscious during the sessions of any other stimulus, and concentrated all their attention on the magnetizer, accepting without question everything that he suggested to them. When they came round, these patients remembered nothing of what had taken place. This is characteristic of the state produced by hypnosis, the most important aspect of Mesmer therapy. Later on, hypnosis was to hold the attention of many eminent doctors, including the great French neurologist Jean Martin Charcot (1825-1893), whose classes at the Salpêtrière were attended by Freud and Breuer.

Certainly, in the wake of Mesmer came many quacks and adventurers who earned themselves a great deal of money by playing on the gullibility of others. One of the best known of these was a

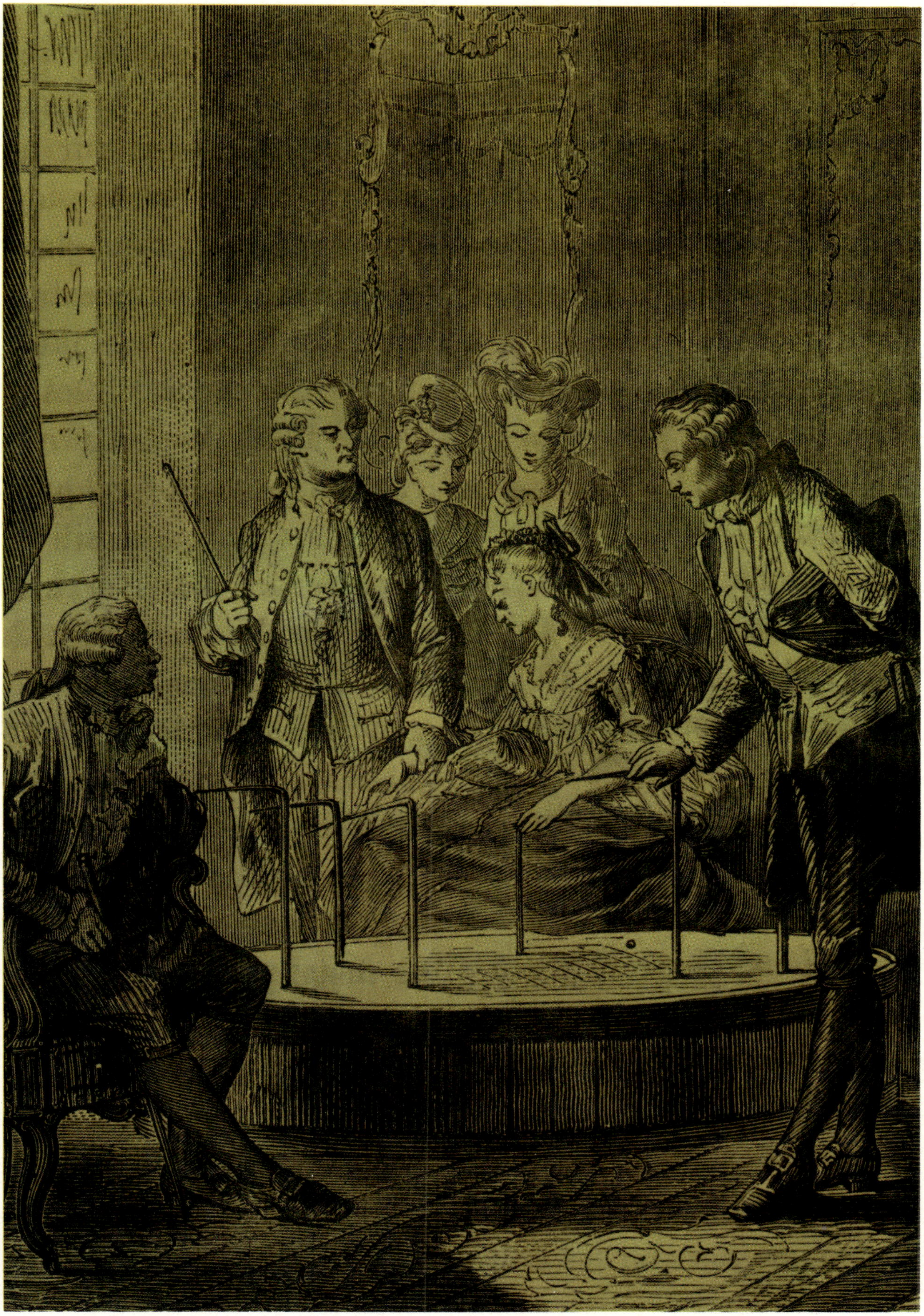

Previous pages:
Mesmer's tub. *Contemporary print.*

These pages:
Dr James Graham's mud baths, 'a new way of preserving health and beauty.' *From Rambler's Magazine, June, 1786.*

The use of suggestion in therapy appeared in the eighteenth century in new forms, showing the influence of the scientific discoveries of the age. In mesmerism, the ancient practice of the laying on of hands became confused with the study of magnetism: the central feature in Mesmer's consulting rooms was the magnetic tub, filled with dilute sulphuric acid and fitted with curved bars which the patients

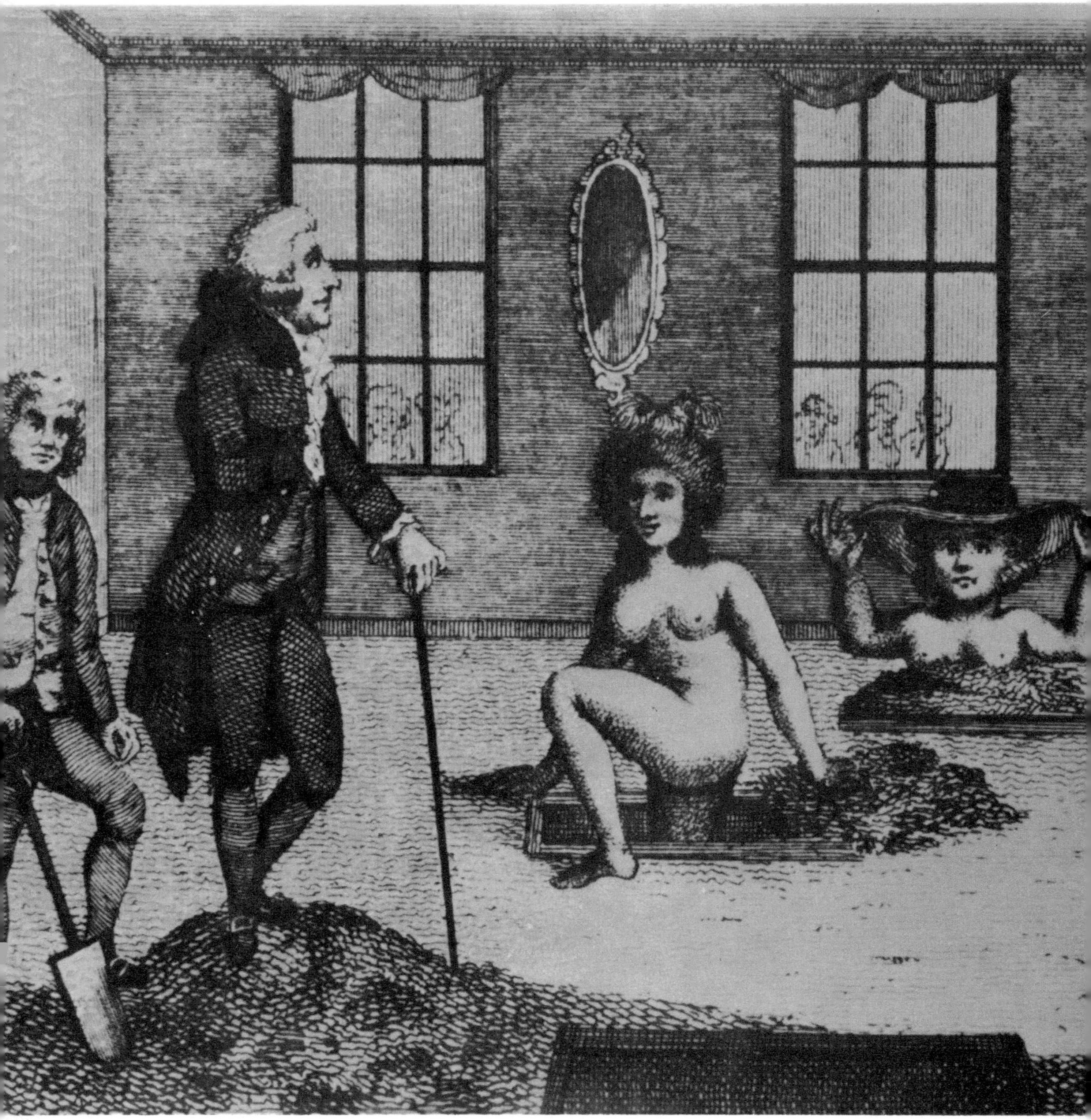

grasped in order to receive the magnetic currents. Mesmer himself touched each patient and his cures, which seem to have had great success, undoubtedly depended on his great powers of suggestion.

Electricity and magnetism were exploited by the most notorious of the innumerable quacks operating in England at this time, Dr James Graham (1745–1794) of Edinburgh. Graham had studied some medicine and had picked up something of Benjamin Franklin's experiments with electricity in America. In succession, he instituted 'celestial beds' for restoring virility and fertility, a 'temple of health' in London in 1780, then, when this fraud was exposed, mud-baths, which he himself entered for several hours a day—only to die at a comparatively early age.

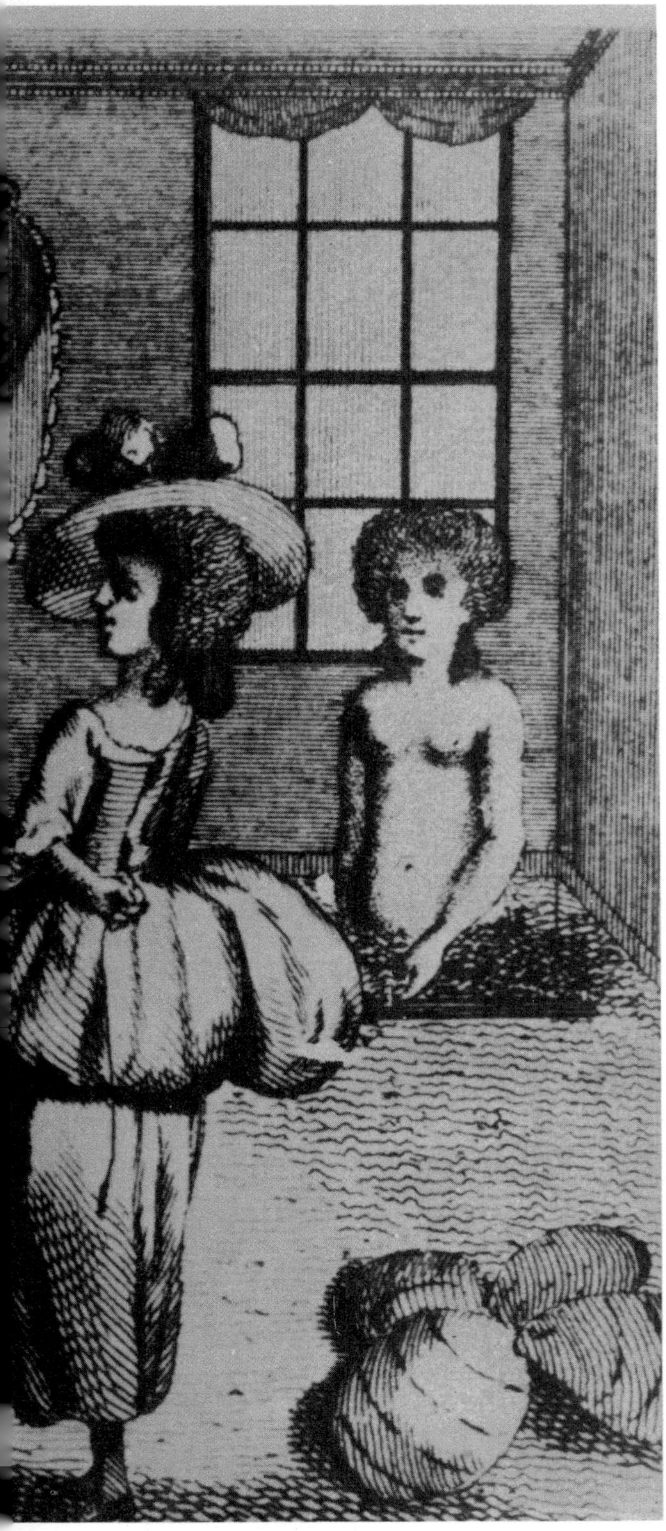

native of Palermo, Giuseppe Balsamo (1743–1795) or Count Alessandro di Cagliostro. A doctor and occultist to whom miraculous cures were ascribed, he was a fashionable physician at Louis XVI's court in Mesmer's time. He was involved in a scandal with the Cardinal de Rohan and Countess de la Motte, a lady of fortune in the service of Marie Antoinette, and he then fled to Rome. Later he was arrested as a heretic, freemason and swindler, and imprisoned in the castle of San Leo near Rimini, where he died. Mesmer's career ended with the French Revolution; the famous inventor of animal magnetism fled to London, and then to Vienna and finally to Frauenfeld, on the shores of his native lake. He died a forgotten man, in 1815, at the age of 81.

In this period another system emerged which, according to Castiglioni, was of greater importance than is usually allowed by historians: this was homeopathy. Homeopathic therapy consisted essentially in the use, at minimal dosage levels, of substances which in a greater dose provoked symptoms similar to those of the disease they were supposed to cure. The founder of this system of treatment was the German Samuel Friedrich Hahnemann (1755–1843), who upheld the principle 'similia similibus curantur' (like is cured by like), after having experimented on himself with various medicines. Thus hot compresses were used for burns and opium for sleepiness. Hahnemann introduced the 'theory of potencies', by which the greater the dilution the more powerful was the effect of the drug. For liquids he recommended use of the thirtieth potency, in which two of a tincture were added to ninety-eight of alcohol, one drop of the diluted solution mixed with ninety-nine of alcohol, and so on for thirty times. As a famous British pharmacologist remarked, this would give you one molecule of the drug in a sphere the size of the orbit of Venus!

The doctrine of Hahnemann met with more opposition than support at the outset, and is now virtually abandoned, although some homeopathic doctors and pharmacies still exist. However, from the historical point of view, as Premuda observed, homeopathy was not an entirely negative influence, for it restrained the use of blunderbuss treatment and powerful polypharmacy; this benefited the praiseworthy principle, that should never be forgotten, of 'primum non nocere' (first do no hurt).

Jenner and the discovery of vaccination

Edward Jenner (1749–1823), who was born at Berkeley in Gloucestershire, is certainly among the most admirable and likeable figures in the history of medicine. It was sometimes said that he was lazy and of only fair intelligence. This opinion probably came from the sophisticated doctors of London who underestimated the honest countryman that he remained all his life.

From his boyhood Jenner was determined to become a doctor. At the age of thirteen he became a surgeon's assistant near Bristol, where he remained for a period of six years. One day a young countrywoman came to the surgery and the conversation turned to the subject of smallpox; she said 'I cannot take that disease, for I have had cowpox'. This phrase impressed itself on Jenner, who observed its truth in his practice among farmers and their families. When he was twenty-one he went to London, where he became the pupil and friend of the celebrated Scots surgeon John Hunter (1728–1793), founder of pathological anatomy in England, inventor of a method of

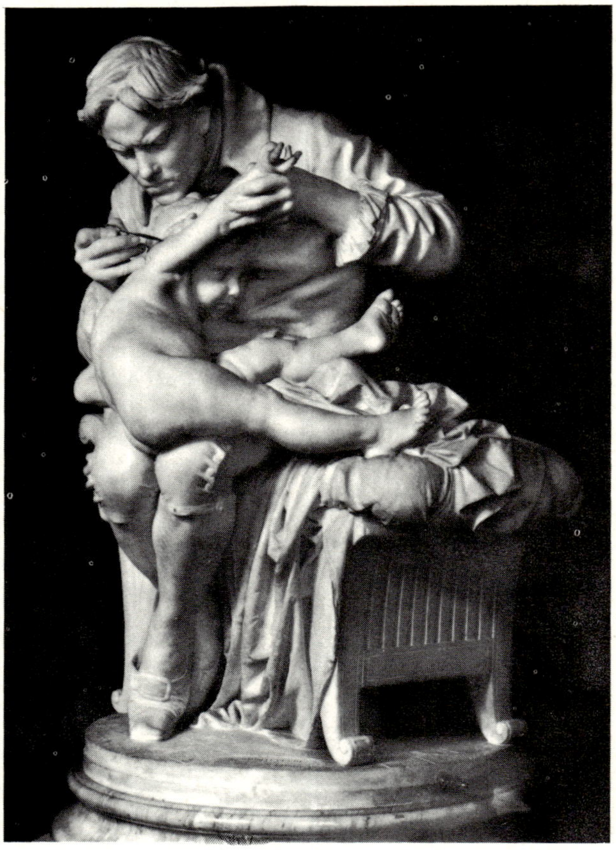

ligating aneurysms and creator of an anatomical museum.

A former naval surgeon, John Hunter was not an academic but a fervid and intelligent experimenter, who became the victim of one of his own experiments. In an attempt to find out if gonorrhoea and syphilis were two different diseases or merely two forms of the same disease, he inoculated himself with pus from a patient. As luck would have it, he had chosen a patient infected with both conditions. This circumstance led him to state, erroneously, that gonorrhea and syphilis were one and the same; and it also produced a syphilitic aortic aneurysm, which killed him.

Hunter's elder brother William (1718–1783) was the most noted British anatomist of the eighteenth-century and author of a great and monumental work, *The Anatomy of the Gravid Uterus,* published by the famous Birmingham printer John Baskerville; the work contained 34 copper plates that were masterpieces of anatomical illustration.

Jenner spent two years at John Hunter's but then, tired of London life, he went back to Berkeley to live according to his vocation, as a country doctor. In Gloucestershire, it had long been common knowledge that milkmaids who caught cowpox were immune from smallpox. This must have been known the length and breadth of England, for smallpox had been commonplace for at least two hundred years. Although its origins in this country are obscure, there are scattered mediaeval references to 'pockes', which may have been smallpox or various other skin conditions. It came gradually into prominence, but did not reach epidemic importance until the reign of James I. For some reason, later champions of vaccination argued that it was devastating and widespread in the earliest times, while opponents maintained that the disease was new to England in the sixteenth century. Anyhow, it became increasingly common and, as Creighton wrote in his *History of Epidemics in Britain* (1894), 'It first left the richer classes, then it left the villages, then it left the provincial towns, to centre itself in the capital; at the same time it was leaving the age of infancy and childhood.'

It has been calculated that smallpox claimed a total of sixty million lives in eighteenth-century Europe, averaging six hundred thousand lives a year in the one continent, which was far less densely populated than it is today.

E D I T T O

A RIPARO DELLE CONSEGUENZE DEL MALE DELL' ETISIA.

Riflettendo l'Imperial Consiglio di Reggenza a i molti disordini, e pregiudizi, che vengono a risultare alla pubblica quiete, e sicurezza dalla frequenza delle Tisi Polmonari, che si scuoprono giornalmente, e da non prendersi contro il suddetto male veruna di quelle precauzioni, che sono necessarie per impedirne il progresso, e la dilatazione; anzi che facendo vedere l'esperienza, che le robe istesse servite all'uso de i Tisici, o sia per l'avidità di cavarne qualche ritratto, o sia per allontanarle più presto, che sia possibile dalla propria Casa, senza alcuna cautela, e senza il minimo riguardo all' altrui pregiudizio, poste in contrattazione cagionano di poi danni, e conseguenze luttuose alla salute di coloro, ne i quali perciò coll' uso delle dette robe si dilata la malignità del suddetto male.

E credendo il Consiglio in un oggetto così importante di essere in necessità di provvedere a i suddetti inconvenienti, e alla troppo libera, e dannevole contrattazione delle robe servite all'uso de i Tisici, e di dover cautelare efficacemente la pubblica salvezza da quegli ulteriori perniciosi avvenimenti, che potrebbero in avvenire derivare dalla continuazione di un contegno così irregolare, ha incaricato perciò il Magistrato di Sanità di Firenze di dare i provvedimenti più utili al riparo di tali inconvenienti.

Perlochè in adempimento de' Supremi Voleri, il Magistrato di Sanità di questa Città di Firenze Ordina, Stabilisce, e Comanda, che in avvenire dal giorno della pubblicazione della presente Legge, ciascheduno Medico, e Cerusico del Gran-Ducato di Toscana sia tenuto, ed obbligato indispensabilmente a denunziare al Tribunale della Sanità di questa Città di Firenze ogni Ammalato, che sia vero Tisico confermato, niuna Persona di qualsivoglia sesso, grado, stato, e condizione eccettuata, con specificare nell'atto di detta denunzia il Nome, Cognome, e Luogo dell' abitazione del detto Ammalato, ad oggetto di potersi con tali notizie ordinare quelle diligenze, che saranno necessarie, e che restano prescritte a pubblico benefizio, sotto pena in caso di trasgressione, e di mancanza nel fare le dette denunzie, di scudi cento per ogni volta, da applicarsi per un terzo all' Accusatore segreto, o palese, e ogni restante alla Cassa del Magistrato medesimo in sgravio delle spese, con più l'arbitrio di detto Magistrato di Sanità.

E per maggior comodo, e facilità de i Medici, e Cerusici, che esercitano fuori della Città di Firenze, e così in tutto il rimanente dello Stato, Ordina, e Vuole il Magistrato, che siano tenuti li medesimi sotto l'istesse pene di sopra prescritte a fare le suddette denunzie a i Governatori delle respettive Provincie, nelle quali abiteranno, Commissari, e Iusdicenti, che hanno Giurisdizione Criminale, i quali saranno obbligati di dare avviso al Magistrato predetto di Sanità di Firenze delle denunzie, che saranno loro fatte da i Medici, e Cerusici delle respettive loro Provincie, e di fare in seguito a i suoi luoghi, e tempi eseguire con tutta l'esattezza le precauzioni, e diligenze degl' espurghi, che sono notati in appresso.

Avutesi dal Magistrato le sopraddette ordinate denunzie da i Medici, o Cerusici, procederà il medesimo a far fare da' suoi Ministri a ciò deputati l'Inventario di qualunque cosa esistente nella Camera dell' Infermo attaccato dal precitato male, e che fosse, o potesse servire per uso del medesimo, e in specie de' Panni lini, e lani, materasse, sacconi, coltroni, coperte, e altro, che si ritrovi nel letto, vasi, sedie, e di ogn' altro utensile, niuno eccettuato, per procedere in caso seguisse la morte del predetto Infermo a farne fare i necessari espurghi a cautela della pubblica salute, e di coloro nelle mani de' quali potranno passare le dette robe, Quale Inventario, ed espurghi dovranno farsi con tutta la moderazione a proprie spese de i Ricchi, e Benestanti, e per i Poveri a spese della Cassa del Magistrato loro; dovendosi l'istesso regolamento, fare osservare inviolabilmente fuori della Città di Firenze da' Governatori, Commissari, e Iusdicenti dello Stato, con previa partecipazione, e ordine del Magistrato medesimo di Sanità.

Si vuole in oltre, che subito seguita la morte di qualunque Tisico come sopra, siano tenuti, ed obbligati sotto l'istessa pena di scudi cento, ed arbitrio, gli Congiunti del Defunto, e la Persona, o Persone, che averanno assistito al medesimo, alla cura di alcuno de' quali nel formarsi il suddetto Inventario verranno consegnate le Robe inventariate, di denunziarne la morte in Firenze al Tribunale di Sanità, e fuori a i respettivi Governatori, Commissari, o Iusdicenti, affinchè possano essere dati immediatamente gl' ordini opportuni per l'effettuazione degl' espurghi stati prescritti.

Ed afine d'impedire, che il suddetto male dell' Etisia maggiormente si dilati, e serpeggi da un luogo all' altro, onde ne restino infettate altre case, che quelle dove abitano i Tisici, Proibisce espressamente il Magistrato di Sanità a i Proprietari delle Case, nelle quali abitano i Tisici di potere in veruna forma licenziare dalle medesime i Pigionali, che fossero stati dati in nota per attaccati d' Etisia, per assicurarli eziandio dal rischio, in cui sarebbero di non trovare altro luogo, ove potersi ricoverare.

Resta parimente proibito agli Eredi di quelle Persone, che saranno morte del suddetto male di Etisia, di poter vendere a i Rigattieri, Rivenditori, o altri alcuna cosa di quelle, che hanno servito ad uso de' predetti Ammalati durante il termine di un mese dopo la loro morte, dentro il quale dovranno farsi le purgazioni espresse ne i seguenti Capitoli, sotto la detta pena di scudi cento per ogni volta a i trasgressori da applicarsi come sopra, ed a i Rigattieri, Rivenditori, o altre simili Persone della Carcere ad arbitrio del Magistrato di Sanità.

E perchè siano palesi le cautele da praticarsi nel decorso del male della Tise, e le diligenze degl' espurghi, che saranno fatti eseguire dopo la morte, afine d'impedire ogni progresso, e dilatazione del suddetto male, si Ordina, e prescrive quant'appresso.

Siccome l'esperienza fa chiaramente vedere, che l'aria stagnante accresce molto qualunque putrefazione, così dovrà esser cura di quelli, che assistono al Tisico, di lasciare di tempo in tempo l' ingresso libero all' aria nella Camera del medesimo; Siccome di procurare, che l' ammalato non sputi altrove, che in Vasi di vetro, o di terra invetriata, e questi spesso si mutino, e si lavino, avendo anche il pensiero di allontanare ogni giorno dalla Camera dell' Infermo le altre separazioni, afine di togliere qualunque causa di maggiore putrefazione.

Dovranno dopo la morte essere lavate almeno due volte col ranno bollente le Biancherie, che hanno servito a i Tisici. E l' istesso dovrà esser fatto a tutti i Panni di lana lavabili, ed a i gusci delle materasse, e de i guanciali, con lavare anche la lana, e battendola, ed esponendola all' aria, il che dovrà farsi anche alla Piuma.

Si spiegheranno all' aria in luogo ventilato le vesti, ed ogni genere di Tappezzeria non lavabile, e si scuoteranno, e spazzoleranno, astergendole superficialmente con panni lini puliti.

I Mobili di legno, e di metallo, vasi, e strumenti, che averanno servito all' Infermo, saranno lavati, e stropicciati almeno due volte, tenendogli pure esposti all' aria per qualche tempo.

Il Pavimento della Camera sarà lavato almeno per due volte, e le muraglie rubiancata tutta, tenendo per qualche tempo le finestre, e le porte aperte, acciò possa l' aria dissipare affatto ciò che restasse d' infezione nella Camera medesima.

Riservandosi il Magistrato di supplire con ulteriori cautele, e provvedimenti a misura delle circostanze, sempre che il bisogno lo richiedesse.

La presente Legge, e tutti gl' Ordini, e determinazioni in essa contenute, le quali sono dirette alla conservazione della pubblica salute dovranno essere in avvenire puntualmente eseguite, ed osservate in tutte le Città, e Luoghi del Gran. Ducato di Toscana, non ostante &c.

E contro i Trasgressori si procederà sommariamente, ed omessa ogni formalità di ragione & ex officio.

E tutto &c. mand. &c.

Urbano Pierattini Cancelliere.

Bandito da me Niccolò Ulivi pubblico Banditore ne' Luoghi soliti di questa Città di Firenze questo dì 11. Novembre 1754.

In Firenze. L' Anno 1754. Nella Stamperia Imperiale.

Previous pages :
Edward Jenner vaccinating a child. *Marble group by Giulio Monteverde. Genoa.*

Edict announcing preventive measures against tuberculosis, Florence, 1754.

These pages :
Cowpox. *Engraving from the Treatise on vaccination by Luigi Sacco, Milan, 1809.*

English cartoon against Jenner. *Late eighteenth-century engraving.*

Vaccine eruption on arm. *From Sacco's Treatise, Milan, 1809.*

Three early nineteenth-century French prints on vaccination.

Variolation or variolization was known in England from 1717, when Lady Mary Wortley Montagu, the wife of the English ambassador in Constantinople, who had seen it practised among the Turks, described it in detail in a letter to a friend. Variolation was carried out by inoculating material from persons suffering from mild varieties of smallpox, in order to reproduce the benign form of the disease and thus prevent more serious forms from developing. Although this procedure provided a defence it was also very risky, sometimes producing a serious infection even when the primary disease was ostensibly benign.

Given that smallpox was a variable disease, inoculation of infected material offered the possibility of preventive treatment. Jenner studied the problem systematically; it took him twenty years to complete his work with a decisive experiment. This was carried out on 14 May 1796, when he extracted the contents of a pustule on the hand of a milkmaid affected by cowpox and inoculated it into the arm of a healthy eight-year-old boy. This had no ill effects, and the experiment was a success, for six weeks later Jenner inoculated the child with material from human smallpox pustules and the boy did not catch smallpox. Jenner repeated the experiment on others; when he was quite certain that he had made a valid discovery, he referred the matter to the Royal Society, of which he had been made a fellow for his zoological work. His report was returned to him with a covering note explaining that Jenner would do best not to endanger the reputation he had earned for his previous studies by continuing with his present work. But the country doctor was confident of his observations and did not take the well-meant

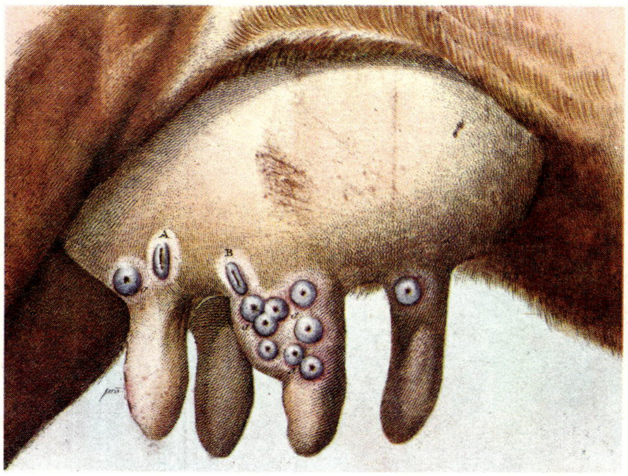

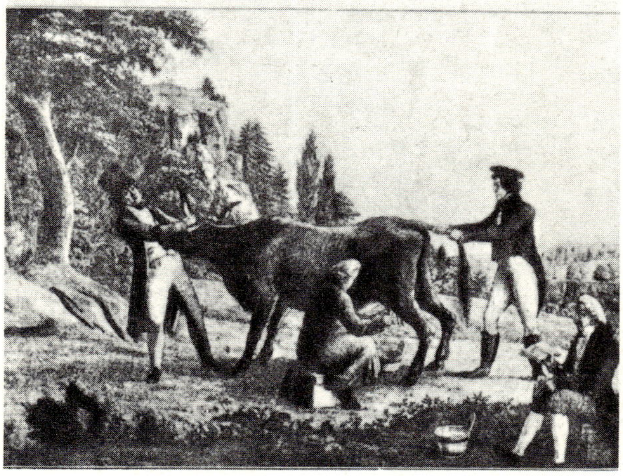

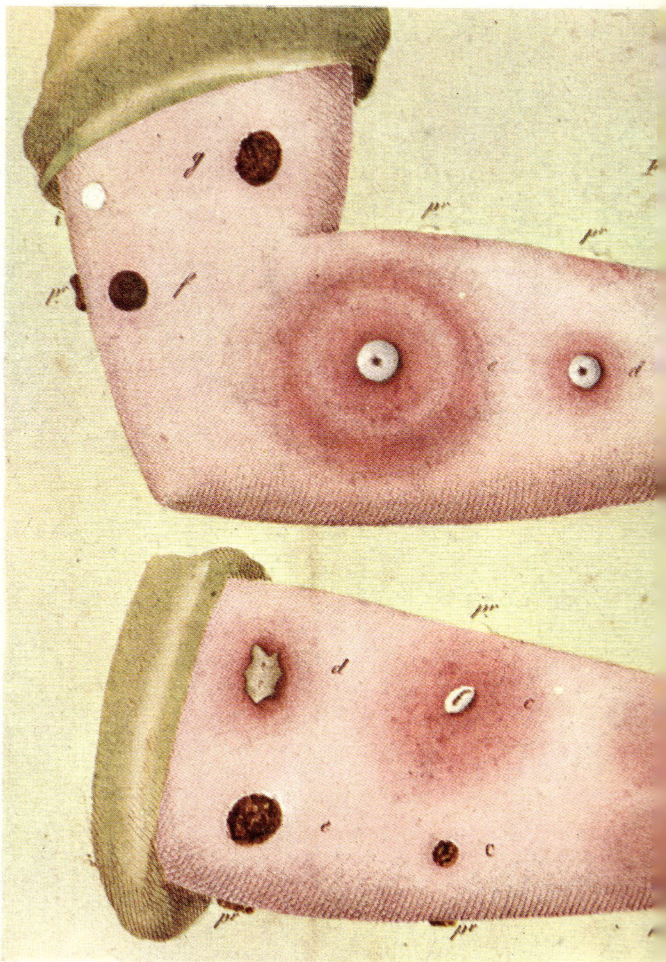

A new era of preventive medicine began in 1796, when Edward Jenner pioneered the use of cowpox vaccine to produce immunity to smallpox. The practice was at once widely adopted, soon diminishing a disease which had previously been one of mankind's greatest plagues. In spite of its obvious effectiveness (and safety), vaccination was for long a target for ill-informed and superstitious popular criticism.

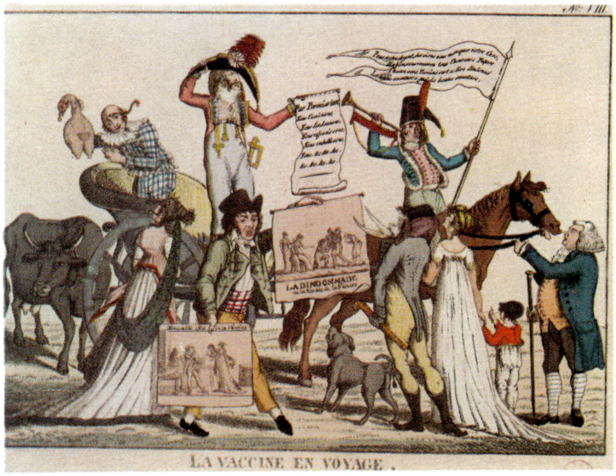

advice. His study was published in 1798 under the title, *An Inquiry into the Causes and Effect of the Variolae Vaccinae.*

The treatise aroused violent emotions, but all that mattered was that smallpox vaccination became known and practised everywhere within a short space of time. Jenner gained just recognition, and in 1802 Parliament voted him a grant of £10,000 and in 1808 he was appointed by the government as director of the newly-formed institute for vaccination. His discovery resulted from masterful experience and observation, although Jenner himself was constantly saddened by his inability to explain why his system worked. It was another hundred years before the basic features of immunity were revealed, but Jenner's genius and perseverance nevertheless produced in his time an empirical triumph of preventive medicine.

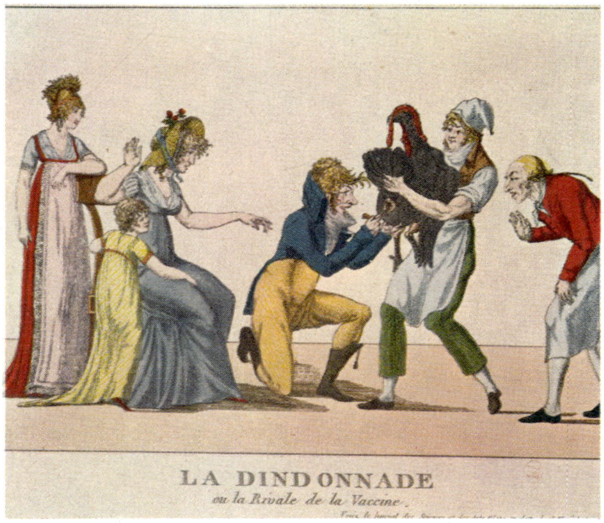

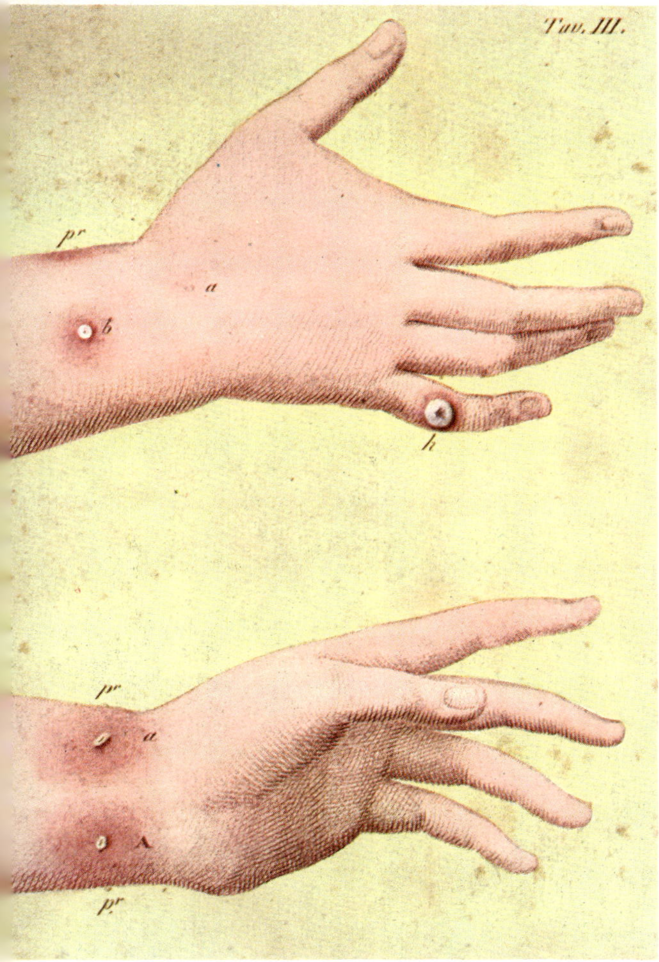

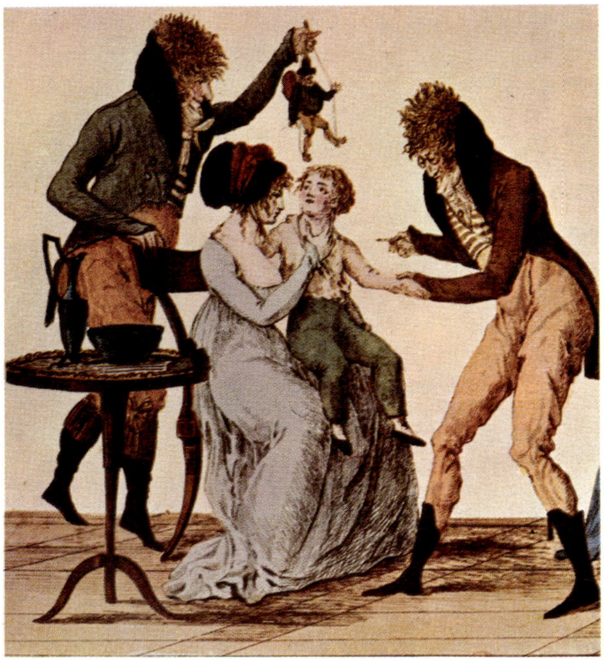

THE MODERN PERIOD
The era of great conquests

With the end of the eighteenth century and the triumph of the French Revolution, the revolt against dogmatism was total and scientific thought and enquiry pervaded all branches of knowledge. The universities began to be free of ecclesiastical and political control, and study there became possible for members of social classes formerly excluded. University College, London, was founded in this liberal spirit in 1828. Under the impetus of Auguste Comte (1798–1857), positivism emerged and confronted romantic idealism with a methodical approach; it was based on scientific fact and a philosophy of scientific synthesis. The great English naturalist Charles Darwin (1809–1882) gave the theory of evolution a scientific foundation by correlating masses of biological data within the framework of a single idea. Julian Huxley has referred to him as the Newton of biology; in his work *On the origin of species* (1859), Darwin expounded the law of natural selection, which opened new horizons in medicine. Of vital importance, too, were the discovery in 1845 of the law of the conservation of energy by Robert Jules Mayer and by James Prescott Joule, and of a fundamental law of genetics by Gregor Mendel (1822–1884).

Mechanization and industrial development in the early nineteenth century benefited medicine directly through the invention of new diagnostic and therapeutic instruments. One of the earliest of these was Laënnec's stethoscope, the origins of which are described later; another of great import-

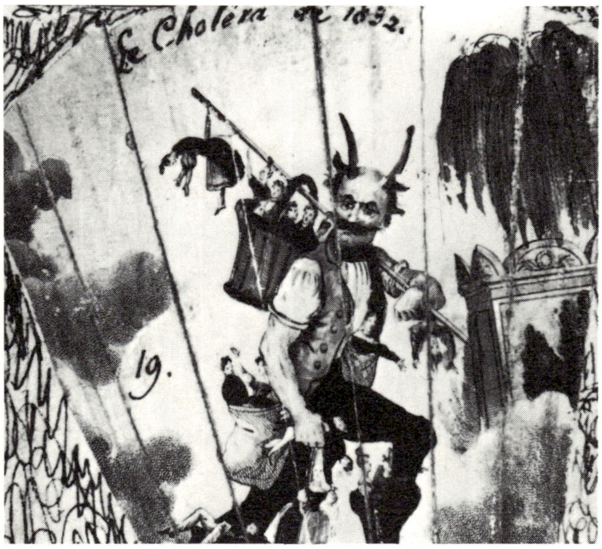

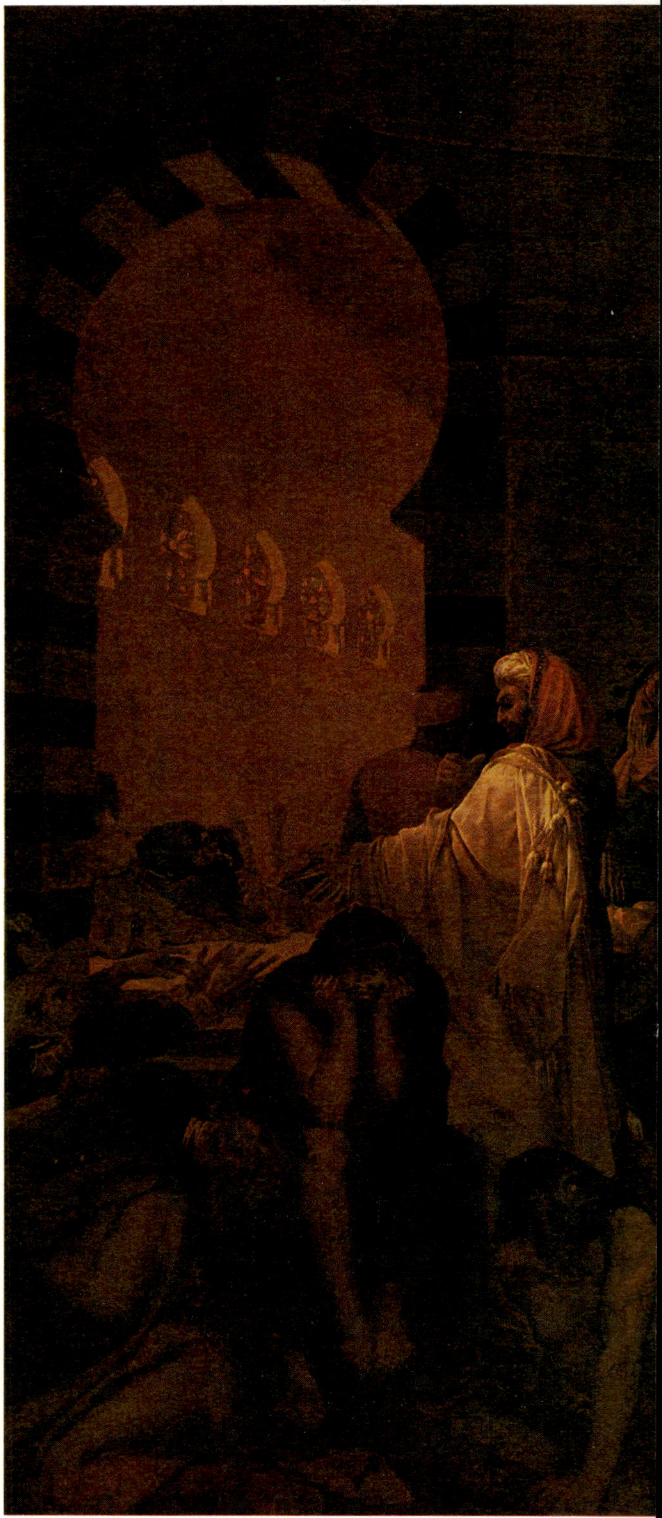

The nineteenth century was a period of rapidly accelerating change and development. Scientists made countless discoveries and formulated many basic laws, while the Industrial Revolution saw the application of the new knowledge on something like the modern scale. At the same time, overcrowding in the new industrial towns brought health problems that recalled the Middle Ages. But now more effective measures could be taken: in 1854 a London cholera epidemic was checked when Snow traced the infection to drinking water; and in 1874 Max von Pettenkofer (1818–1901) suggested quarantine for travellers from the Orient, where cholera and plague were endemic.

Popular cartoon of 1832 showing cholera as a demon.

Napoleon among the plague-stricken at Jaffa. *By Baron Gros, 1799. Louvre, Paris.*

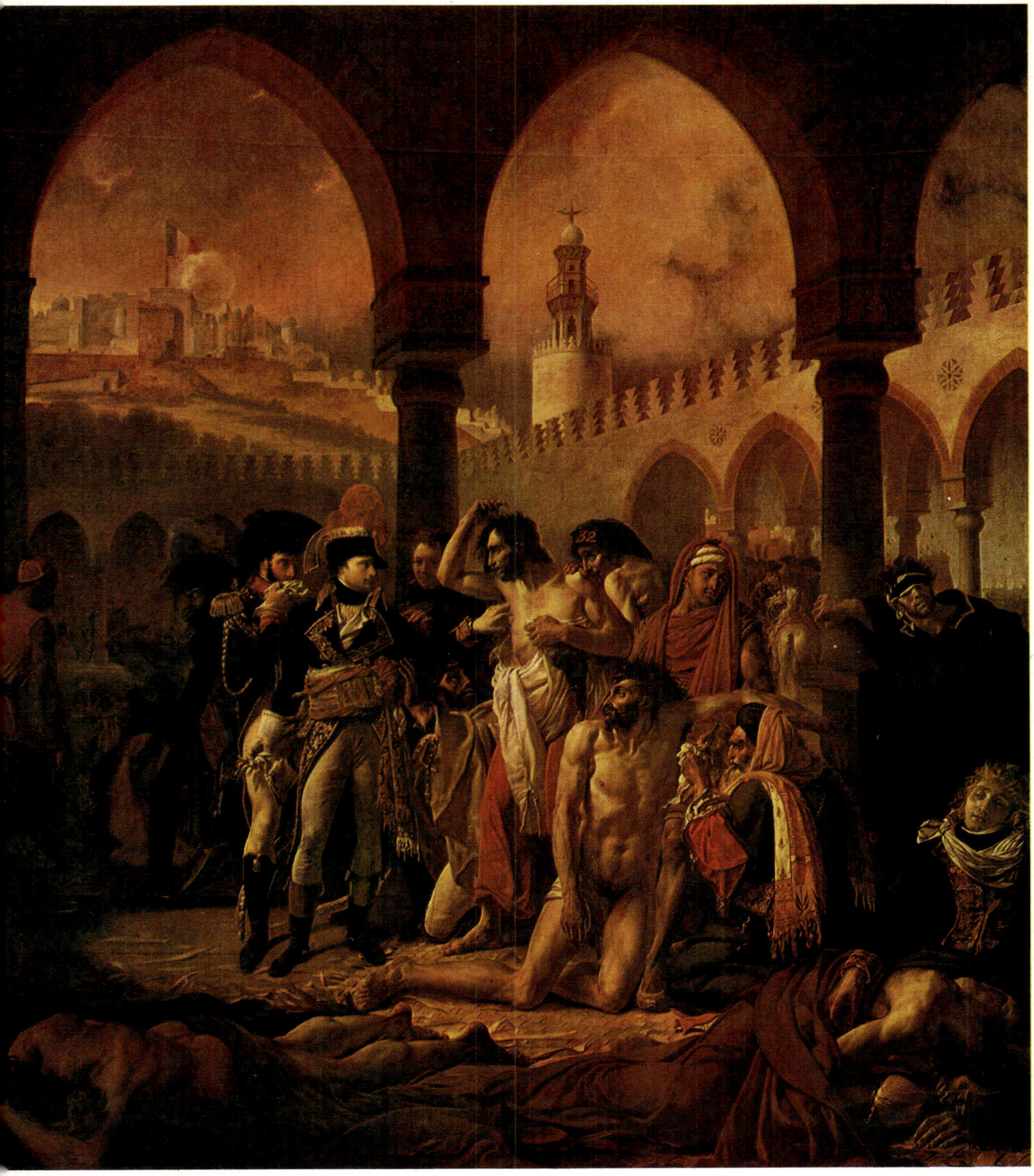

The nineteenth century saw the emergence of the United States of America as a centre for original scientific study. Although still culturally dependent on Europe, where many of its doctors and scientists were trained, in time it began to produce figures of international repute. Perhaps the greatest of these was Benjamin Franklin (1706–1790), statesman, writer and scientist, famous for his studies of electrostatics and lightning (he invented the first lightning conductor), who contributed to medicine his invention of bifocal spectacles, suggestions for the treatment of paralysis by electricity, and papers on lead-poisoning, gout, sleep, deafness, the infective nature of colds, infant mortality and medical education. Franklin was the principal founder and first president of the Pennsylvania Hospital in Philadelphia (1751). The

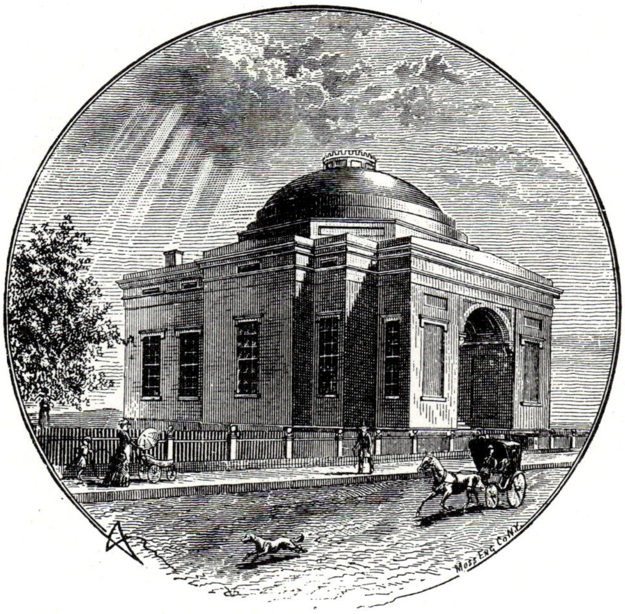

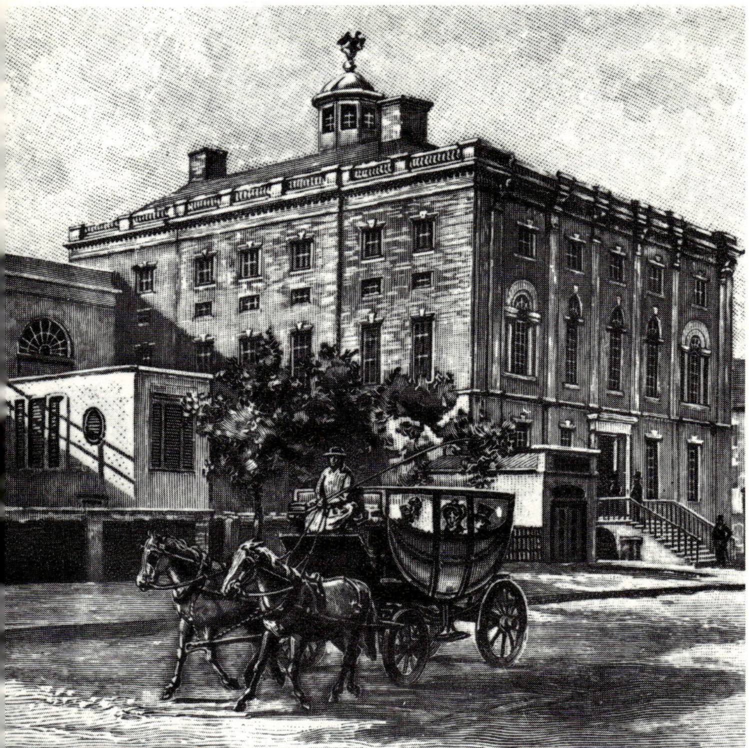

ance was Helmholtz's ophthalmoscope. The introduction of the hypodermic syringe in 1853 by the Frenchman Charles Pravaz and Alexander Wood of Edinburgh was a medical landmark, for doctors now had an entirely new means for the administration of drugs.

The first years of the nineteenth century saw the development of modern chemistry and particularly biochemistry. Much of the important work in this field was accomplished in Germany, which retained its lead for many years. An epoch-making event, which is echoed today by the production of viruses in test-tubes, was the laboratory production of urea from an inorganic substance, ammonium carbonate, by the German Friedrich Wöhler (1800–1882) in 1828. Following the work of the English chemist John Dalton, Justus von Liebig (1803–1873) investigated many organic chemical compounds, both in and derived from food and in waste-products, and discovered among other things chloral and chloroform.

Before 1828 it was believed that organic compounds, the chemicals of life, could be formed only by living tissue and were totally distinct from mineral or inorganic substances. After Wöhler's synthesis the two great classes became inseparable, and today organic chemistry is no more than the chemistry of carbon compounds. At the time, it must have seemed as if a veil had been lifted from the mystery of life.

The Industrial Revolution created a new society, with rural populations shifting to the towns. Cities developed so fast that public health suffered; slums grew up, with unhealthy and overcrowded dwellings. Lavoisier found that in a closed environment the air soon deteriorated through the utilization of oxygen and expiration of carbon dioxide, and he remarked on the need for living space to be made the subject of legislation. But this was a liberal era—'laissez faire, laissez passer'—and no controls were imposed, even over water and food. Perhaps anticipating this turn of events, the Austrian Johann Frank (1749–1821), for ten years a professor at Pavia, wrote in his work *Medicinisches Polizei* that it was the duty of the state to supervise public health at all times, not only during epidemics.

The new United States of America was ready to contribute to all fields of knowledge, but especially to medicine. Its first medical school had been founded in 1765 at Philadelphia by John Morgan *first medical school in the United States was founded at the University of Pennsylvania in 1765.*

The greatest historical figure in American medicine, called the American Sydenham, was Benjamin Rush, a graduate of Princeton and Edinburgh, physician to the Pennsylvania Hospital and professor at the College of Philadelphia. His name was given to Rush Medical College, Chicago, chartered in 1837.

Rush Medical College, Chicago, in 1843, its opening year. (It merged in 1898 with the University of Chicago to become the faculty of medicine.) *Nineteenth-century woodcut. Department of History of Medicine, University of Kansas.*

The first school of medicine in the United States: Pennsylvania University in Philadelphia. *Nineteenth-century woodcut reproduced in History of Medicine in the United States, by Packard, New York, 1931.*

(1735–1789) on the best European models. Morgan worked in London with the Hunter brothers, qualified at Edinburgh, lived in Paris and travelled through Italy where he made the acquaintance of Morgagni.

The most popular doctor of the War of Independence was Benjamin Rush (1745–1813) 'the American Sydenham', a product of the Philadelphia school. He was well known in Europe for his work on yellow fever, the vector of which he believed to be the mosquito, and as a pioneer in physiotherapy. He wrote an important psychiatric work, but at the time of Pinel's reforms he advocated the use of a barbarous 'tranquilizing chair'. He seems to have been the first to suggest that such conditions as rheumatism and epilepsy could be relieved by the extraction of bad teeth.

Ephraim McDowell (1771–1830) is remembered as one of the first to remove diseased ovaries. His first patient, Mrs Crawford of Danville, Kentucky, was operated on under the primitive conditions of a remote village, without antiseptics or anaesthesia. She sang hymns while he removed her tumour, with a crowd waiting anxiously outside. McDowell enjoyed phenomenal success at the time and became famed across the Atlantic when eight of his thirteen patients were cured.

The most internationally famous American doctor was William Beaumont (1785–1853). He developed in a unique way from a frontier surgeon to a physiologist specializing in the mechanism of digestion. In 1812 Beaumont was licensed to practise by the medical society of Vermont, having served a two years' apprenticeship. He became camp surgeon at Fort Mackinac, and the incident marking the turning-point in his career took place there in 1822. At Mackinac Island, situated at the confluence of Lake Huron and Lake Michigan, Red Indians and French-Canadian trappers sold their pelts and bought supplies.

One day in June a drunken group was talking outside the American Fur Company, which bought the skins, when a gun went off accidentally. Alexis Saint Martin, a nineteen-year-old trapper, was hit in the stomach. The man responsible for the accident sought out the priest to administer the last sacrament as the young man lay dying. Beaumont arrived, dressed the severe wound and gave his opinion that Saint Martin had only a few hours to live. But the patient survived the wound and a difficult operation was carried out successfully.

The surgeon looked after him medically for a long period. In two years Alexis had recovered, but with a permanent gastric fistula. Beaumont was able to see directly into the cavity of the young man's stomach, and he began one day to study the digestive process at work. Although without academic training, his research was impeccably methodical and successfully provided accurate information, which led to the formulation of theories that are still valid. Pavlov and Claude Bernard both acknowledged later their indebtedness to Beaumont. In fact the American surgeon studied the whole field of gastric physiology, observing carefully the contractions of the stomach and various changes in its lining in different phases of digestion. He investigated the manifestations of hunger and thirst. He described the appearance and properties of gastric juice and determined the presence of hydrochloric acid and other active substances in the stomach. He found that in fact the stomach was a contractile sac, separated from the duodenum by the pylorus, which periodically opened like a valve to allow food digested by the gastric juices to pass onwards. Peristaltic contractions had two functions, to mix the food with gastric secretions and to enable the stomach to empty the products of digestion.

In the nineteenth century, medicine developed rapidly in Europe and America on account of the work of a far greater number of researchers than in previous centuries, when science was still esoteric and of no practical importance to the population as a whole. Until the nineteenth century, advance in medicine was episodic, with triumphs and sidetracking observations and concepts intermixed with long periods of stagnation. Now developments came so quickly that knowledge of all aspects of medical science became impossible for individuals to attain, and specialization, a new phenomenon, appeared at this time. Medical knowledge, now embracing huge and diverse fields, split into several distinct branches. Claude Bernard wrote, apropos of modern science, that 'the names of its main artificers disappear in the general pattern and science becomes more detached and impersonal the farther one goes'. We will thus find that we are dealing more and more with schools, trends and specialities and less with individuals, though advances in any field have frequently come from the initial work of a genius.

The school of Paris

It might be said that Napoleon was an important and permanent influence on medicine; undoubtedly he encouraged the work of a number of great clinicians and scientists in the first years of the nineteenth century and so laid the foundations of a great school. The first giant of this Parisian school was Marie François Xavier Bichat (1771–1802), who carried out work of fundamental importance before his premature death. In his *Anatomie generale,* Bichat showed that all the different organs were made up of a smaller number of tissues, which he described both in the healthy and diseased state. In the masterly *Recherches physiologiques sur la vie et la mort,* Bichat distinguished two types of functions, those of vegetative and those of animal life. Through the latter, higher organisms were able to perceive the external world, respond to stimuli, move and display desires and emotions. Through the vegetative functions, that is the circulation of the blood, respiration, digestion, metabolism and temperature regulation, they took in and utilized materials from outside (food, water, air) and then excreted the waste products.

Bichat had a strong influence on the most celebrated clinician of the First Empire, Jean Nicolas Corvisart (1755–1821), Napoleon's personal physician, who as noted earlier translated Auenbrugger's book on percussion and so led to the general adoption of the technique. He was a cardiologist, defining symptoms due to heart diseases and distinguishing them from pulmonary symptoms. It is said that one day he was looking at a portrait and remarked, 'If the painter was right, the man in this picture died of heart disease'. Someone

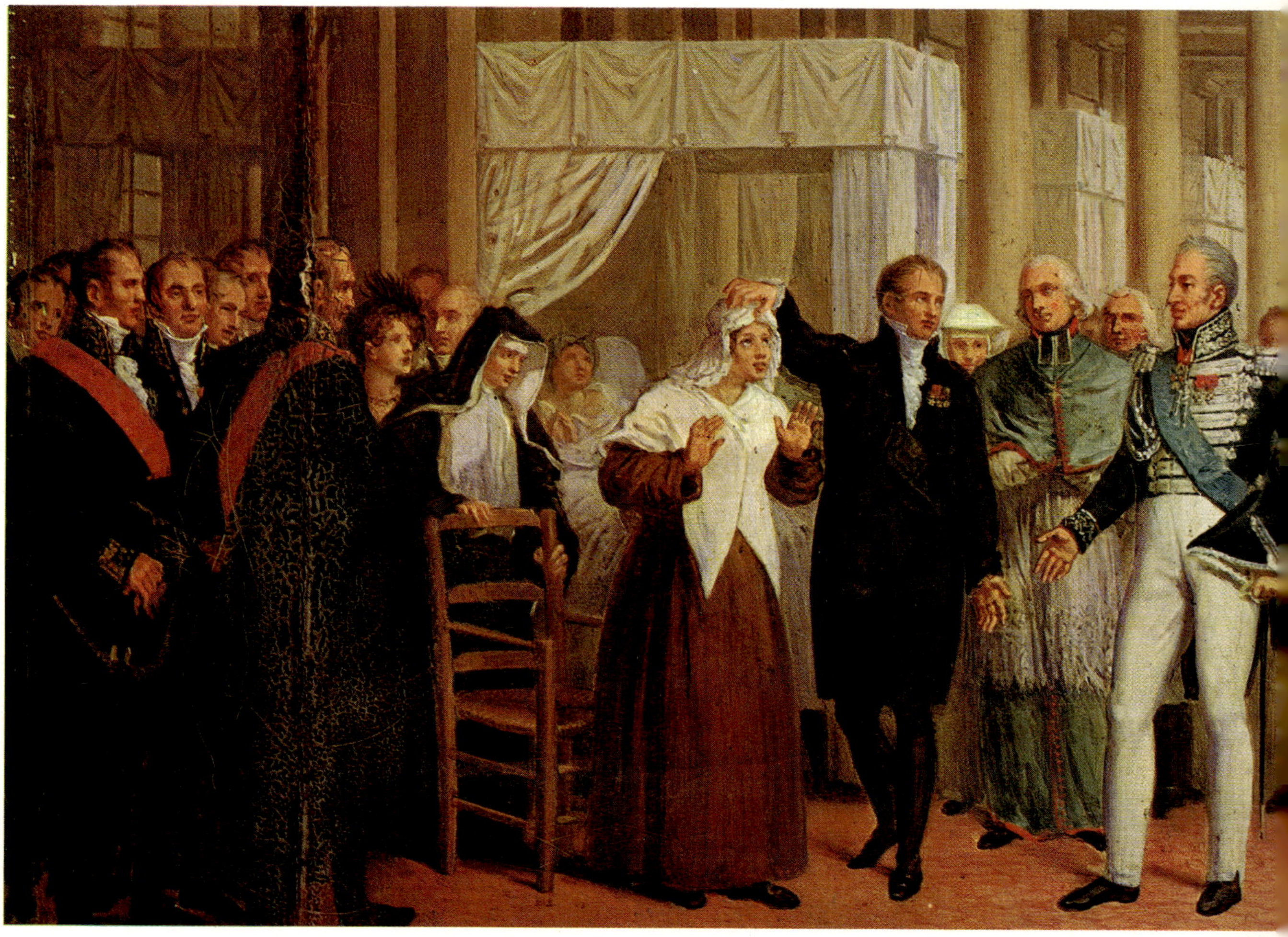

In the period when France under Napoleon dominated Europe politically and militarily, French doctors, too, led in many fields. The great Paris school, founded on the teachings of Bichat, a pioneer of pathology, was the foremost centre of medical learning. Bichat's pupil Corvisart was an outstanding clinician and personal physician to the emperor, while the surgeons Larrey and Dupuytren were among the greatest of their day. Corvisart's own pupil Laënnec, a superb diagnostician, invented the stethoscope.

Dupuytren demonstrating a cured patient at the Hôtel-Dieu, Paris.

The room of a man with tuberculosis. *Nineteenth-century engraving. Bertarelli Collection, Milan.*

Laënnec visiting a patient at Necker Hospital. *Department of History of Medicine, University of Kansas.*

found out about the portrait and Corvisart's diagnosis was shown to be perfectly correct.

Another favourite of Napoleon, who stood by him at his abdication and awaited his return in 1815, was Jean Dominique Larrey (1766–1842), the chief doctor of the Grande Armée, biographer of Paré and author of interesting works about his own life as an army surgeon. Larrey was the first to institute field units to give first aid and immediate surgery to the wounded. He took part in all Napoleon's great battles and was wounded three times. In November 1812 when Napoleon's troops were combating the Russian army under Kutusov, he performed two hundred and two amputations within the space of twenty-four hours and without getting any sleep. The emperor, who said of him 'C'est l'homme le plus vertueux que j'ai connu',

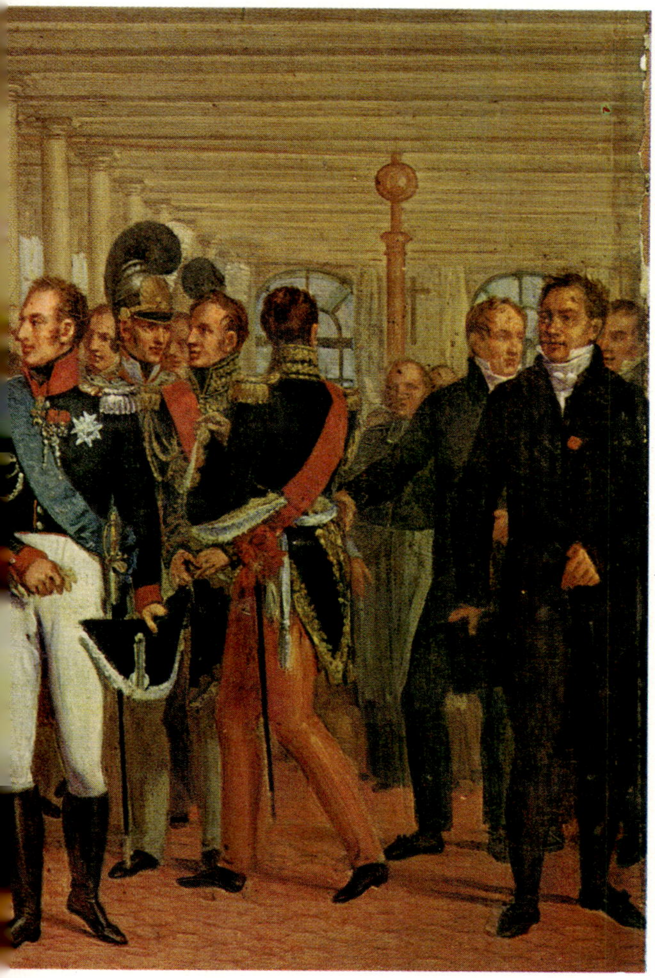

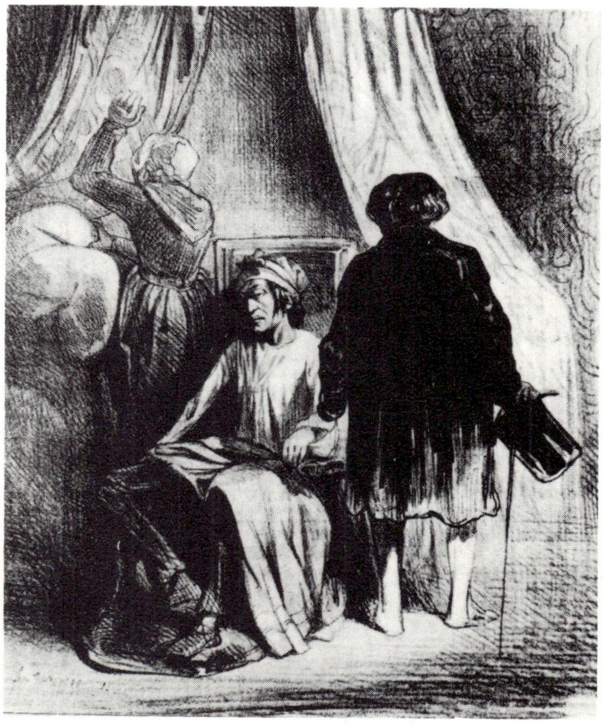

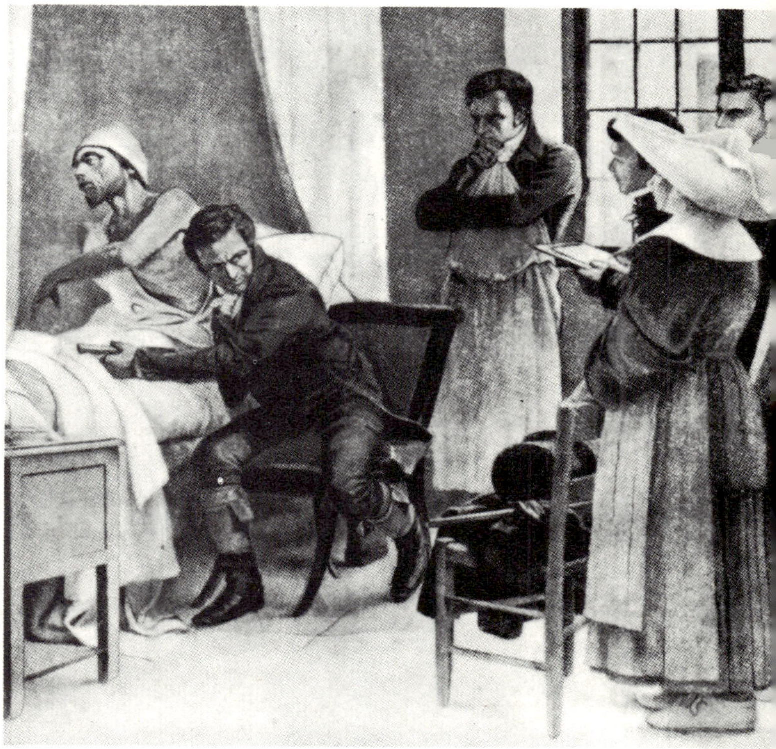

Bichat showed that the organs of the body were made up of numerous types of tissues, each serving a different function. The idea of specialization was carried along an erroneous path by the German Franz Joseph Gall (1758–1828), founder of the system variously called craniology, phrenology or organology. Gall maintained that certain areas of the brain were concerned with certain intellectual functions, the strength of which could be judged by the size of protuberances on the skull over the areas. A similar theory was advanced by a Swiss clergyman and physician, Johann Lavater (1741–1801).

Lavater's anatomical and physiological research. *Lithograph after a drawing by Lavater. Bertarelli Collection, Milan.*

Craniological system, with portrait of Franz Joseph Gall. *Bertarelli Collection, Milan.*

left Larrey a legacy of one hundred thousand francs after having made him a baron.

Napoleon also conferred baronies on Corvisart and on two surgeons–Pierre François Percy (1754–1825), the chief surgeon of the army and author of the important *Manuel du chirurgien d'armee* (the army surgeon's handbook), and Guillaume Dupuytren (1777–1835), who was the chief surgeon at the Hôtel-Dieu.

Dupuytren was an extraordinary man who worked his way up from humble origins to become the leading surgeon of France and a millionaire. At the age of eighteen he became an anatomy prosector, at thirty an assistant surgeon and four years later professor of operative surgery at the Hôtel-Dieu. His clinics were extremely popular with students and he had a practice of about 10,000 patients outside his hospital work. But in his ambitious struggle Dupuytren was a hard and overbearing man who persecuted and intrigued against rivals, had no friends, and was more respected and even feared than loved: Percy called him the first of surgeons and the least of men.

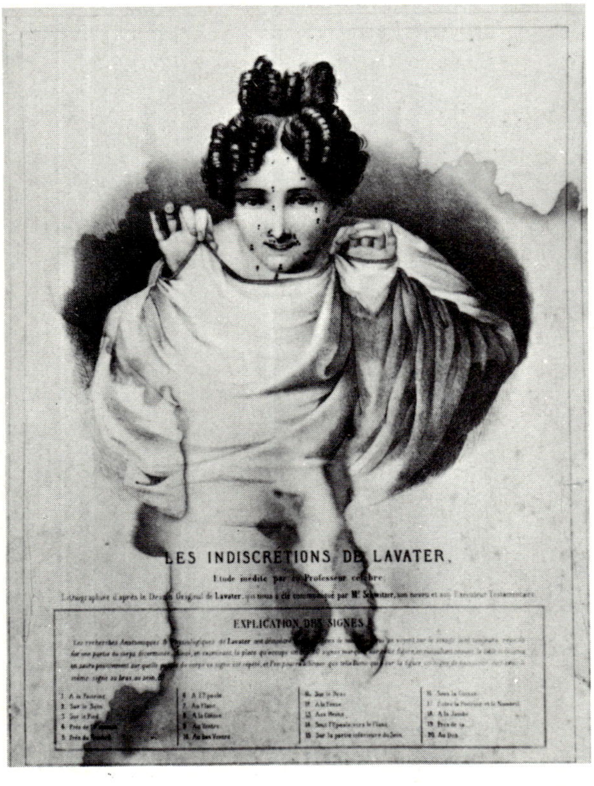

Dupuytren left classic descriptions of the characteristic flexion of fingers caused by contraction of ligamentous tissue in the palm (Dupuytren's contraction) and of fracture of the lower end of the fibula (Dupuytren's fracture).

Corvisart's greatest pupil was René Theophile Hyacinthe Laënnec (1781–1826), the inventor of the stethoscope and the first man to create a complete diagnostic system for pulmonary and cardiac complaints. For many years he was obsessed with a desire to hear clearly the noises of opening and closure of the heart valves in systole and diastole, in order to achieve accurate diagnosis. It is said that one day, while Laënnec was crossing the courtyard of the Louvre, he saw a boy listening with his ear at the end of a wooden beam to signals tapped by another child with a nail on the other end. At the first opportunity, Laënnec, during the examination of a patient put a roll of paper to his chest: he heard the heart sounds with great clarity, and even better when he replaced the roll of paper with a cylinder of turned wood, to which he gave the name stethoscope. Laënnec's name is remembered too in association with cirrhosis of the liver, a condition which had been recognized since the time of Hippocrates. He also left many superb writings and was said by the English physician Thomas Addison to have contributed more toward the advancement of the medical art than any other single individual.

Laënnec was a native of Quimper in Brittany. Another Breton, whose influence on medicine was negative rather than positive in the long run was François Broussais (1772–1838), who enjoyed great popularity for a while. He served as a sergeant in the Republican army and as a mariner before obtaining his medical degree in 1803, and for the next three years he travelled with Napoleon's army as a military surgeon. His theory was derived from Brunonism in maintaining that life was dependent on irritation and especially on heat, which enhanced the chemical processes taking place in the body. He held that disease was the result of some localized irritative process occurring in a particular organ, especially the stomach and the intestines, and he denied that specific poisons or extraneous substances were responsible for individual illnesses. Thus 'gastroenteritis' of one sort of another was the cause of a wide variety of ailments (compare Cullen's implication of 'neurosis'): believing that nature had no healing power, and that active

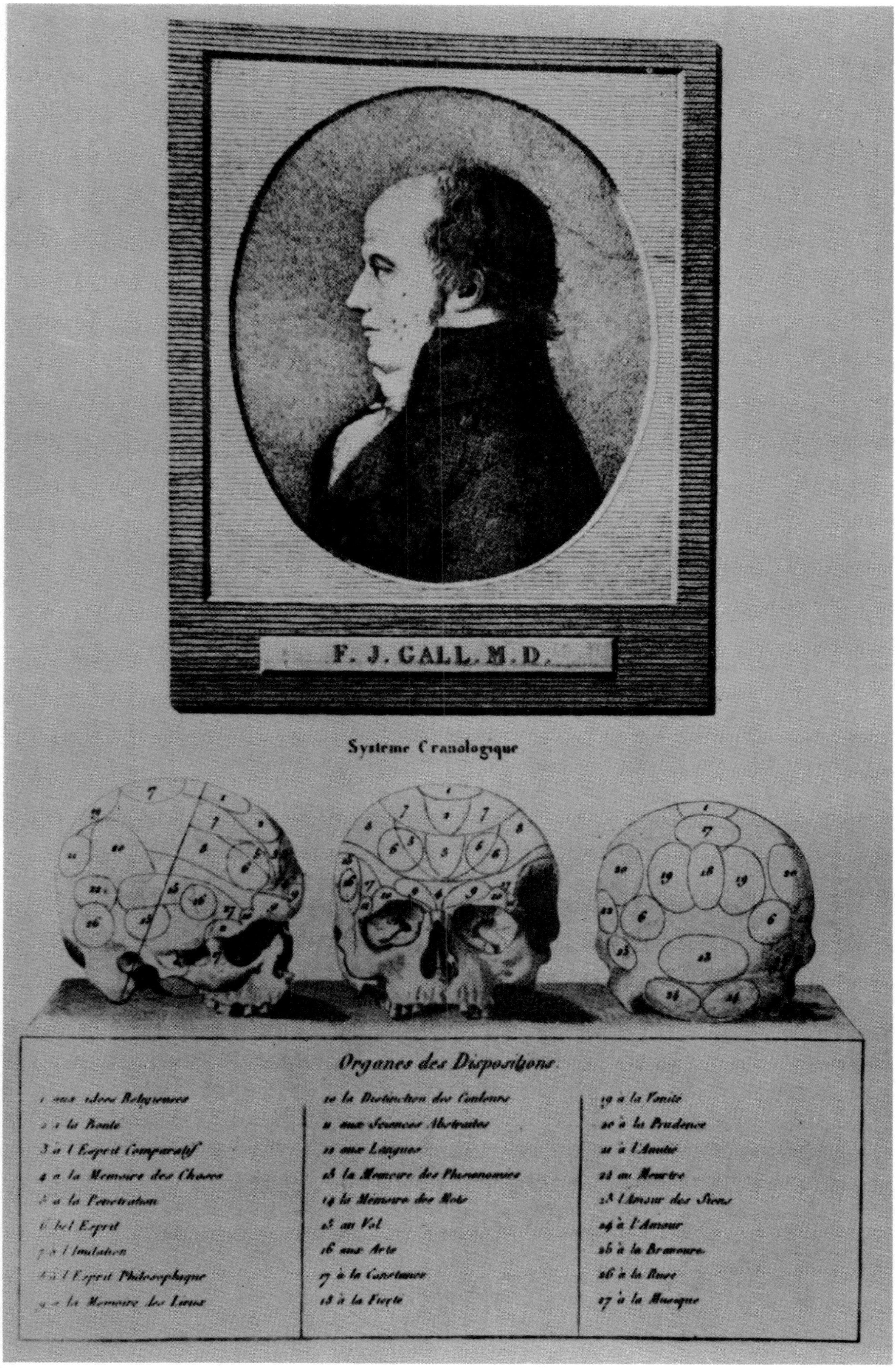

F. J. GALL. M.D.
Systeme Cranologique
Organes des Dispositions.
3 à l'Esprit Comparatif
4 à la Memoire des Choses
6 bel Esprit
10 la Distinction des Couleurs
11 aux Sciences Abstraites
12 aux Langues
13 la Memoire des Phisionomies
14 la Mémoire des Mots
15 au Vol
16 aux Arts
17 à la Constance
18 à la Fierté
19 à la Vanité
20 à la Prudence
21 à l'Amitié
22 au Meurtre
23 l'Amour des Siens
24 à l'Amour
25 à la Bravoure
26 à la Ruse
27 à la Musique

Medical science flourished in the early nineteenth century, especially in the field of physiology. France was the main centre of study in this subject, and its greatest pioneer was François Magendie, who emphasized the importance of an experimental basis for research; he is said to have refused to believe any statement that had not been confirmed by experiment. In demonstrating the action on animals of strychnine and morphine, Magendie was also a founder of modern pharmacology. He performed innumerable experiments on animals (he was the arch-enemy of the anti-vivisectionists), but made no attempt to draw any general conclusions from what he observed; Magendie described himself as a 'rag-picker' who gathered any information he found in his path.

The synthesis of experimental facts into funda-

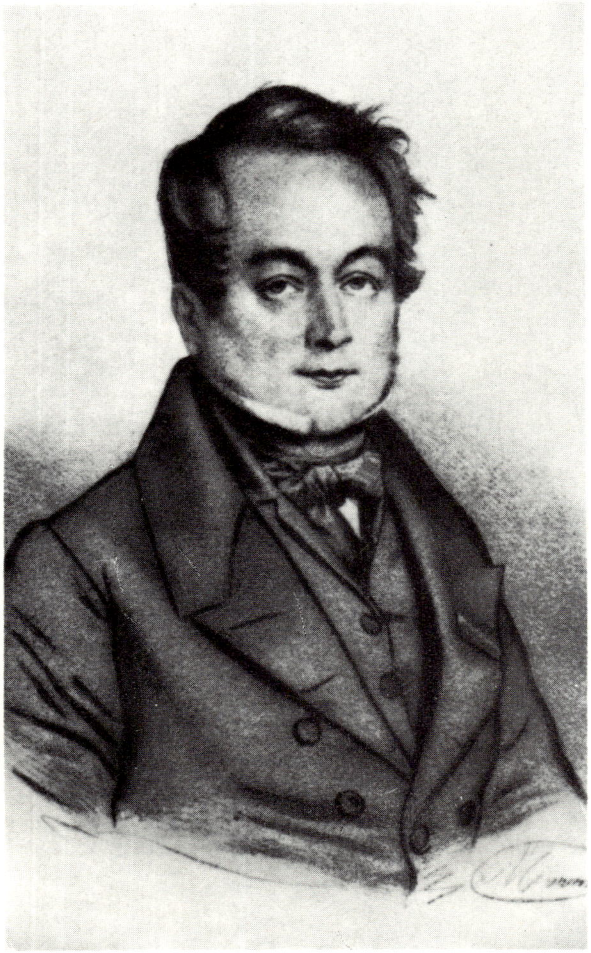

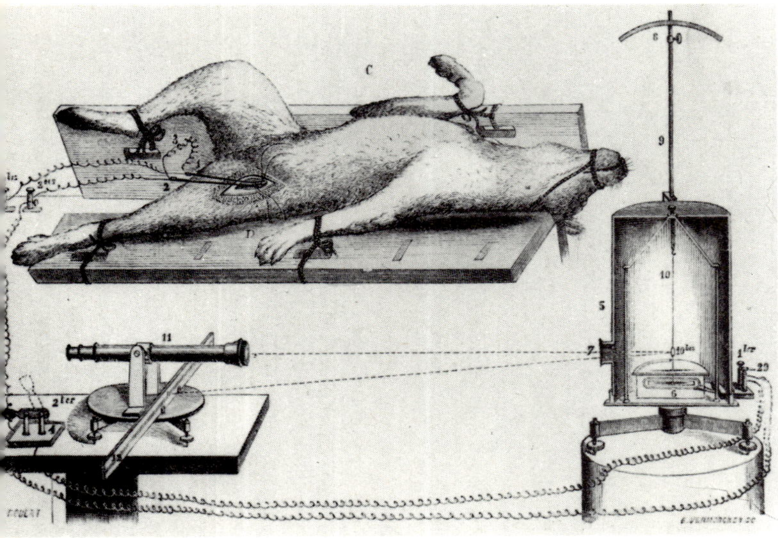

measures were indicated, he tried to counter disease with a regime that debilitated the patient and involved semi-starvation and the furious application of leeches–up to fifty at a time–to all parts of the body. Enthusiasm for his method resulted in a shortage of leeches: in 1833 41,500,000 were imported into France and only nine or ten million exported, while in 1824–1825, two or three million met the requirements of the nation's doctors. As he grew older and more dogmatic, Broussais let more and more blood, and the younger generation of physicians, influenced by the moderate and intelligent ideas of Laënnec and others, gradually abandoned his doctrines.

Broussais' ideas were finally overthrown by Pierre Louis (1787–1872), who is remembered today as the person who introduced statistical methods into medicine, and in the 'angle of Louis', the prominence in the upper part of the breastbone. As a young man Louis spent six years in Russia and he became disillusioned by the powerlessness of the medicine he knew and practised to cope with severe epidemic infections. He returned to Paris to study and spent the rest of his life in hospitals, carrying out research and teaching. In the course of his work he became firmly convinced that fallacious theories or arguments could be refuted by a careful statistical analysis of the medical evidence, and that statistics could be used to give a convincing result on occasions where experiments could not be carried out. He was thus the father of medical statistics, that branch of science which has become familiar to everyone through Doll and Hill's work on smoking and lung cancer. In fact the use of statistics in medical research was first suggested by the astronomer Laplace, while in Jules Gavarret's *Prinçipes generaux de statistique* (1840), special consideration was given to therapeutic problems, but Louis was the first to apply mathematical methods to a range of medical uses, receiving little support or encouragement in his lifetime. His work, although including some superficial and inaccurate conclusions, has proved of lasting value: an early application was when Fournier and Erb showed by means of statistics that tabes dorsalis and general paralysis of the insane were consequences of infection with syphilis, and later Louis' methods were used to determine the effectiveness or otherwise of new treatments for particular diseases. His chief works were his *Recherches anatomico-physiologiques sur la mental doctrines was the achievement of Magendie's favourite pupil, and his successor at the Collège de France, Claude Bernard. Among the most important of the discoveries made by this outstanding figure, who began his career as a pharmacist's assistant, was the role of the autonomic (involuntary) nervous system in controlling the flow of blood to different parts of the body under varying conditions.*

François Magendie. *Lithograph by Maurin. From an impression in the Wellcome Historical Medical Museum, London.*

Experiment to measure the temperature of the blood in the crural vessels. *Plate from Leçons de physiologie operatoire, by Claude Bernard, Paris, 1879.*

Claude Bernard. *Portrait by Jean-Baptiste Antoine Guillemet.*

phthisie (1825), which were based on nearly 2,000 cases and showed the frequent occurrence of tuberculosis in the apex of the lung, his *Recherches* on typhoid fever (1829) which gave the disease its present name, and his attack on Broussais (1835) which included a statistical proof that blood-letting was of negligible value in pneumonia.

The physiologist Joseph François Magendie (1783–1855) made a number of important discoveries, which however he never attempted to synthesize. He affirmed the necessity of obtaining knowledge from animal experiments. 'The aim of science', he said, 'is to substitute facts for appearances and demonstrations for impressions'. Today Magendie is remembered for his discovery of the sensory function of the posterior roots of spinal nerves (together with Charles Bell, the Edinburgh surgeon who was one of the founders of the Middlesex Hospital Medical School in London, and who confirmed the motor function of the anterior spinal roots). But he was also the founder of modern pharmacology, because by animal experiment he showed the mode and site of action of such substances as strychnine and morphine, this knowledge giving a scientific basis for the clinical use of these drugs. In fact modern therapy had begun some years earlier with the publication (1786) of the Birmingham practitioner William Withering on the effectiveness of digitalis in certain heart conditions. Soon afterwards, the pharmacopoeia of the Royal College of Physicians of London had at last discarded the archaic remedies that included animal organs and excreta, while in the first decades of the nineteenth century quinine and atropine as well as morphine and strychnine were isolated.

Magendie's favourite pupil was Claude Bernard. At the ceremony in 1913 commemorating the centenary of his birth, A. Dastre, the official speaker, remarked that 'Bernard chased away the phantasms that were still haunting physiology. Physiology had been the humble handmaid of medicine; he made her an independent science with methods and purpose of her own'. Bernard's achievements embraced every branch of physiology, and with the imagination of genius he was able to synthesize the findings from his superb experiments into fundamental doctrines.

Claude Bernard was born in 1813 in the village of Saint Julien, near Villefranche, Rhône. At the age of eighteen he went to Lyons and found work as a pharmacist's assistant. Pharmacy was not to his liking, and he took up literature and playwriting, his works in his medium including an entertainment called *La Rose du Rhône,* and a five-act drama entitled *Arthur de Bretagne*. The pharmacist dismissed him, and Bernard went to Paris. In his pocket was a letter of introduction to Saint-Marc Girardin, a celebrated critic, to whom Bernard took the manuscript of his *Rose* and the first act of the drama. The critic, a professor at the Sorbonne, said, 'My dear boy, you have been working in a pharmacy and your head is full of ideas. It is science you want, not the theatre'.

Bernard then enrolled in the faculty of medicine, and, on completion of his studies, he became Magendie's assistant, demonstrating experiments and lecturing at the Collège de France. His lectures were published in a number of volumes between 1854 and 1878, the year of his death. One of his first discoveries was based on his observation that

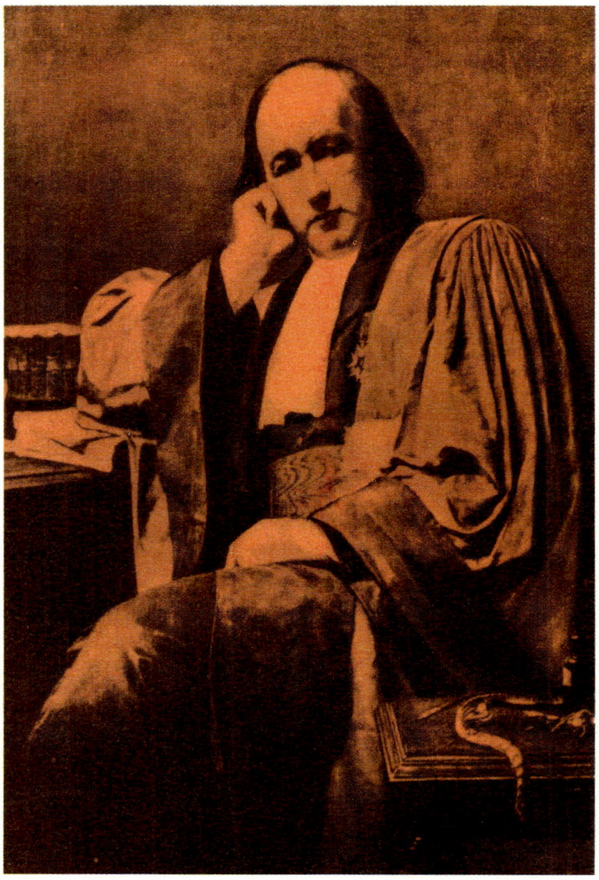

Claude Bernard's crowning achievement was his concept that the body has an 'internal environment' which is kept constant by several interacting, self-regulating mechanisms. The nervous system constituted one of these mechanisms, another was provided by the hormones. Study of these 'chemical messengers' was pioneered by Bernard's work on glycogen metabolism (which is regulated by the secretions of the pancreas) and continued by his successor at the Collège de France, Charles Brown-Séquard. Valuable work was also done in England by Thomas Addison, of Guy's Hospital, on malfunction of the adrenal gland.

As in many fields of medical study, these investigations did not bear fruit, in terms of effective therapeutic measures, until the twentieth century. Adrena-

sugar was found in the blood coming from the liver of a dog whether the animal was fed meat or sugar. The liver thus had a glycogenic (sugar-forming) function, and Bernard initiated modern metabolic studies by showing the synthesis and breakdown of a substance (glycogen) in the body.

Equally important was his work on vasomotor nerves, which constrict and dilate blood vessels and so control the flow of blood under varying conditions to different parts of the body. By cutting the sympathetic nerves he showed that they cause constriction, while the parasympathetic nerves were necessary for glandular secretion as they increased blood flow. By producing a pancreatic fistula he discovered that pancreatic juice was important for digestion (previously thought to occur only in the stomach), breaking down fats, starch and protein. But perhaps his greatest achievement was his last published work, *Leçons sur les phenomenes de la vie* (1878), in which he stated his doctrine of the constancy of the 'internal environment'. This concept was neglected for many years, but with the accretion of knowledge of interdependent hormones and the equilibria of many bodily processes ('homeostasis') it is now accepted as one of the fundamental principles of physiology.

Bernard's attitude to experiment and observation is contained in his aphorism about taking off one's imagination on entering the laboratory as one would take off an overcoat (putting it on, of course, when leaving). He stated his intellectual outlook in his *Introduction a l'étude de la médecine experimentale* (1865): 'One must break the bonds of philosophical and scientific systems as one would break the chains of scientific slavery. Systems tend to enslave the human spirit'.

Claude Bernard won high recognition in his lifetime from the government of his country and the scientists of the world. In 1855 he succeeded to Magendie's post at the Collège de France. He was admitted to the academy of medicine in 1861 and to the Académie Française in 1868. He was made a senator one year later and died in 1878.

Bernard's successor at the Collège de France was Charles Edouard Brown-Séquard (1817-1894), born on the island of Mauritius of an American sea captain father and a French mother. He studied medicine in Paris and travelled a great deal in America and England, teaching at Harvard and practising at the National Hospital, Queen Square, London, returning after Bernard's death to Paris. Claude Bernard wrote, 'It may be held that the total internal secretions constitute the blood which should thus, in my opinion, be held to be a true product of internal secretion'; thus anticipating the discovery of hormones, the blood-borne secretions of the endocrine glands. Brown-Séquard took note of Addison's observations on the effects of disease of the adrenals and by experiment proved that these glands were essential to life, and was thus a pioneer of endocrinology.

Since his time, two hormones have been found to be produced by the adrenal medulla: adrenaline (isolated in 1901 by Takamine and synthesized in

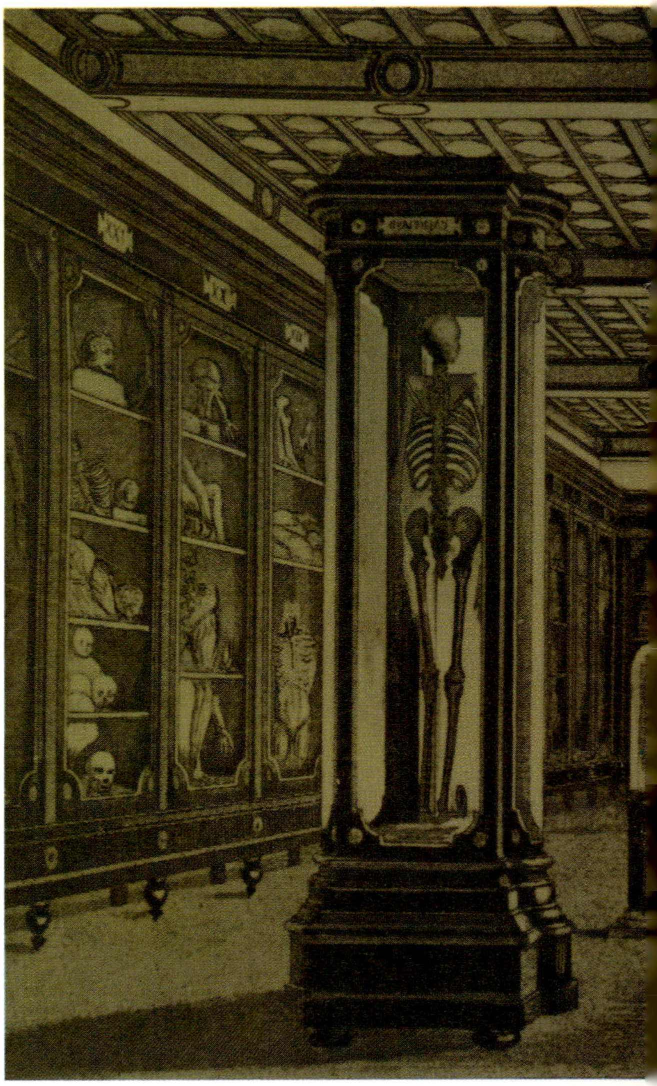

line was isolated from the adrenal medulla by Takamine in 1901 and synthesized by Stolz in 1904. Loeb demonstrated the important functions of the adrenal cortex, from which Kendall isolated various cortical steroid hormones in 1936, when Reichstein also discovered cortisone. Insulin, which regulates sugar metabolism and is used in the treatment of diabetes, was isolated from the pancreas by Banting in 1921.

1904 by Stolz) and noradrenaline. The former produces constriction of the skin and digestive blood vessels and relaxation of visceral muscles, while the latter is the true mediator of sympathetic nerve impulses.

After Jacques Loeb (1859–1924) showed the important function of the cortical (outer) zone of the adrenal glands, Kendall and his colleagues succeeded (1936) in isolating various cortical steroid hormones. In the same year Reichstein also discovered a number of corticosteroids, among them cortisone, which has found many applications in the treatment of inflammatory and some malignant conditions as well as in Addison's disease.

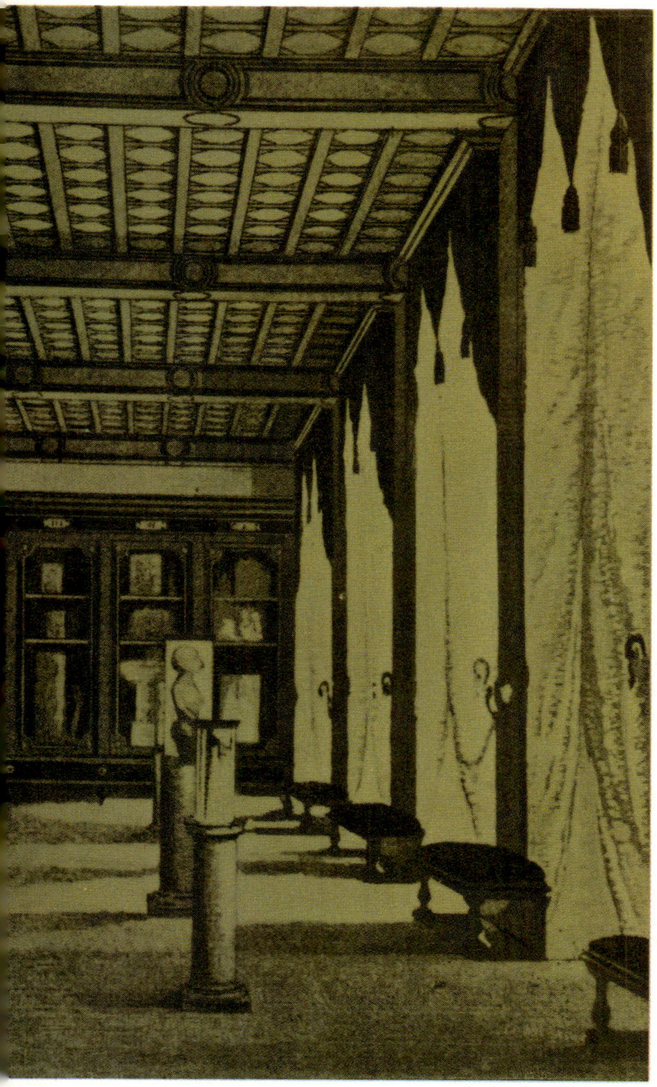

Anatomy museum. *Nineteenth-century engraving. Bertarelli Collection, Milan.*

The term hormone was used for the first time in 1902 by Bayliss and Starling, who discovered secretin, a substance produced by the duodenal mucous membrane and passed directly into the blood, thus determining the secretion of pancreatic juice without the intervention of the nervous system. Insulin, the active principle of the islets of Langerhans in the pancreas, which regulates sugar metabolism, was isolated in 1921. Merit of discovery belongs to the Canadian Frederick G. Banting (1891–1941), who in 1923 won a Nobel prize. Insulin came into therapeutic use at once as a treatment for diabetes, where deranged sugar and fat metabolism results from its deficiency.

Modern endocrinology is thus seen to be derived from the concept of Claude Bernard, according to which the glands responsible for the constancy of the internal environment produce secretions which go directly into the bloodstream rather than into ducts and so to the outside.

Repeated mention of Thomas Addison (1795–1860) should prompt us to consider briefly what might be called the Guy's school, which flourished in London in the middle of the nineteenth century. The three great men of Guy's, if John Keats is excluded, were Addison, Richard Bright (1798–1858) and Thomas Hodgkin (1798–1866), and each is remembered with an eponymous disease.

Addison produced early accounts of appendicitis and toxicology. His essay, published in 1855, *On the constitutional and local effects of disease of the suprarenal capsules,* contained descriptions both of Addison's disease and pernicious anaemia, but the significance of his observations remained largely unrecognized during his lifetime.

Richard Bright, whose name is attached to glomerulonephritis, was an Edinburgh graduate like Addison, travelled in Iceland and Hungary, as artist, naturalist and geographer, collected engravings and left lucid descriptions of many diseases. He established at Guy's in 1842 what may have been the first clinical research unit, with two wards for kidney patients and an attached laboratory and consulting room. The third great name, Hodgkin, was a pathologist rather than a clinician. His skill is attested by re-examination of his specimens of Hodgkin's disease–enlargement of lymph nodes and lymphatic tissue–which survive to this day. The microscope, which he did not use, confirms his diagnosis.

Anaesthesia

Surgery, as we have seen, was in decline during the Middle Ages and until the late Renaissance to the point of becoming simply a skilled manual craft in the hands of barbers, and at this time it was regarded as unworthy of the attention of the medical profession proper. With progress in anatomy, the knowledge of which is the basis of surgery, a revival took place. Great anatomists such as Fallopio, Vesalius, Berengario da Carpi and Fabrizio d'Acquapendente also had great surgical skill. It was Paré who gave surgery its professional dignity. Morgagni's eighteenth-century pathological studies represented a further surgical advance; later, as has been described, pathology flourished especially in France, where there were many excellent surgeons during Napoleonic times.

Nevertheless, surgery at the beginning of the nineteenth century had limited horizons. The solution of four difficult problems–pain, sepsis, haemorrhage and post-surgical shock–had not been found. Of these, pain was the gravest handicap to the surgeon's task.

A few attempts were made at using 'mesmerism' to produce oblivion to pain. The Scottish surgeon James Braid (1795–1861) showed by experiments that genuine sleep could be induced by fixed staring at a bright object. Hypnosis was first used in surgical operations by John Elliotson (1791–1868), who published his results in 1843. Two years later, James Esdaile (1808–1859) performed 261 painless operations (with only 5.5 per cent mortality) on Hindu prisoners in Bengal; but afterwards found that his fellow Scots were less susceptible to the trance state.

The pharmacological relief of pain produced today by anaesthetics has a very long history. Sleep-inducing drugs of various kinds have been used since the earliest days–these include Homer's nepenthe, the hemp used by the inhabitants of the East, Dioscorides' potion and the mandrake used by the thirteenth-century surgeon Hugh of Lucca. No single drug was consistently effective, and in Europe up to the middle of the last century the only relief for the agony of the operation might have been a heavy dose of alcohol.

Anaesthesia has the two functions of eliminating pain and inducing a state of muscular relaxation in the patient, thus making easier the task of the surgeon. Before its discovery surgeons attempted to overcome their difficulties by operating as fast as possible: the great Larrey, surgeon to Napoleon's army, once performed more than two hundred amputations in the space of twenty-four hours.

The problem of pain relief was solved not by the surgeons but by chemists. In 1772 Joseph Priestley discovered nitrous oxide; the analgesic and exhilarating effects of this gas were described in 1800 by Sir Humphrey Davy, who suggested tentatively that it might be used with advantage in surgical operations.

The first person to prove that the pain of surgical operations could be abolished by the inhalation of gas was Henry Hill Hickman (1800–1830) who published at Ironbridge, Shropshire, in 1824 *A letter on suspended animation, containing experiments showing that it may be safely employed during operations on animals, with the view of ascertaining its probable utility in surgical operations on the human subject*. Hickman made animals unconscious by depriving them of air and then giving them carbon dioxide, after which he was able to amputate limbs painlessly and with good results. His discovery was received without enthusiasm and was not taken up. In fact it was not until 1842 that modern surgical anaesthesia began, with the use of ether (the anaesthetic properties of which had been discovered by Faraday in 1818) by Crawford W. Long (1815–1878) of Jefferson, Georgia. The information is to be found in the doctor's records: James Venable, 1842, administration of ether and removal of tumour–2 dollars'. Long, a modest country practitioner, did not make known his results until 1849, by when he had used ether successfully a number of times and its effectiveness had been proved by the work of Morton and others. In 1844 Horace Wells (1815–1848), a dentist of Hartford, used nitrous oxide with good effect in removing teeth. He demonstrated the discovery at Harvard Medical School but the demonstration failed, and, a broken man, Wells eventually committed suicide by cutting a vein and inhaling ether.

William Thomas Green Morton (1819–1868), of Charlton, first used ether at the Massachusetts General Hospital in 1846. He began his career in dentistry as Wells' assistant, and then enrolled at the Harvard Medical School where the chemist Charles Jackson supplied him with ether and suggested he should try it to allay pain. On 30 September, 1846, after experiments carried out on dogs, Morton anaesthetized a patient before extracting a

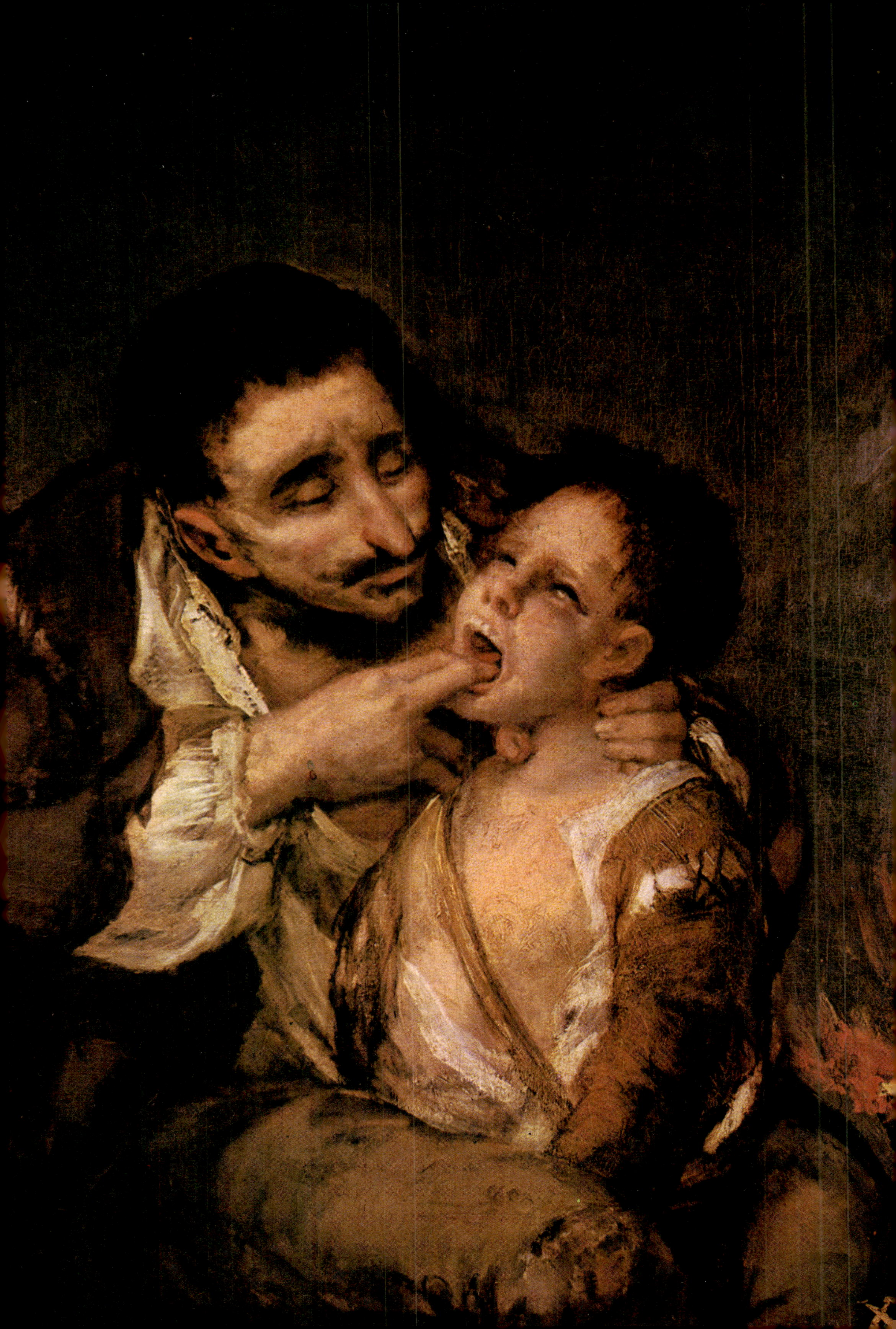

Previous page :
Il garrotillo (diphtheria). *By Francisco Goya. Mme Dolores Maya de Maranon Collection, Madrid.*

These pages :
Lüer's apparatus for spraying disinfectant liquids.

Richardson's apparatus for local etherization.

Charles Jackson experimenting on himself with ether. *Engraving, 1843.*

With advances in anatomy in the early nineteenth century, surgery had reached a considerable level of proficiency. But it had come up against the barrier of pain. Over the centuries, various drugs had been used to provide relief, but modern surgical anaesthesia began in 1842, when an American doctor, Crawford W. Long, removed a tumour from a patient under ether.

tooth and the news was published in the *Boston Daily Journal*. Then John Collins Warren, chief surgeon at the Massachusetts General Hospital, allowed Morton to try ether at the hospital. On 16 October, 1846, Morton etherized a patient who then fell into a profound sleep, during which Warren excised a tumour of the neck. The patient woke up shortly after the wound had been sutured and admitted that he had not felt any pain during the operation. The use of ether as an anaesthetic was publicized within a month by H. J. Bigelow and within another month ether was being used in London.

Unaware of Long's work, Morton at first

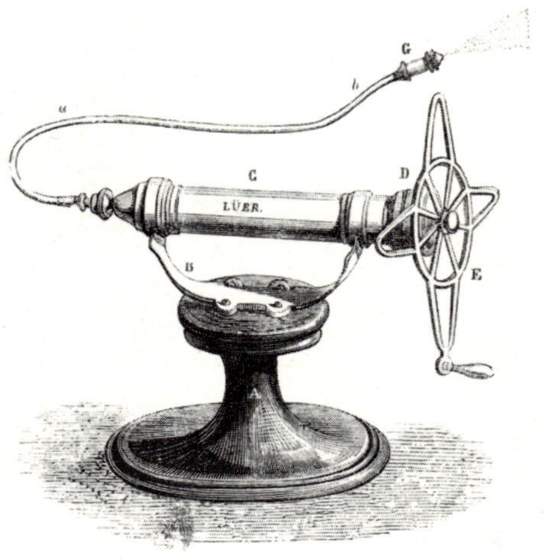

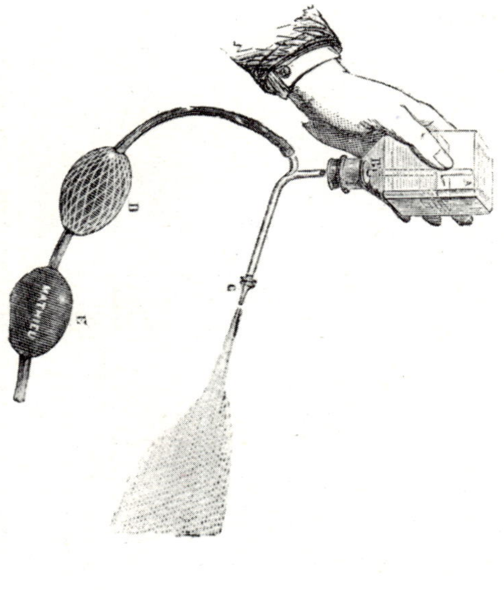

attempted to patent his discovery under the name of 'Letheon'. As the nature of this substance became widely known within a short space of time Morton soon dropped the idea. Later he gave up his lucrative practice to work full-time on the study and publicization of surgical anaesthesia, spending more than £20,000 and reducing himself to poverty in the process. His sacrifice was recognized in the United States and a public subscription was organized to assure him of comfort in his last years.

A number of names were given to the new discovery before the famous American clinician Oliver Wendell Holmes found an acceptable one: anaesthesia. The term was derived from Greek and meant insensitivity, and was in fact an ancient one, used by Plato and Dioscorides. Dioscorides' potion alleviated pain and was made thus: 'boil roots of mandrake in wine until the liquid is reduced to one third; then administer the decoction in a cup to a patient before operation or cauterization, so that the person is in a state of insensitivity'. The word used in the original was indeed anaesthesia.

Mandrake, which often has a forked root (hence its name), contains an alkaloid, mandragorina, which like hemp and poppy was widely used in antiquity to assuage pain. Recourse to all these drugs was prohibited during the Middle Ages, perhaps because they were dangerous. These alkaloids are all strong poisons, but as remedies they were only partly effective.

As we have seen, ether made its entry into Europe as a general anaesthetic at the end of 1846. The Scottish obstetrician Sir James Y. Simpson (1811–1870) was not satisfied with the action of ether, which he used with great success, because of its persistent and strong smell and the bronchial irritation it caused. After many experiments, Simpson adopted a new anaesthetic, chloroform, which had been independently described by Eugène Soubeiran and Justus von Liebig in 1831, and by the American Samuel Guthrie in 1832. In November 1847, he informed the association of surgeons of Edinburgh about his discovery, thus incurring the wrath of the Scottish clergy. The Calvinists maintained that Genesis stated, 'with pangs shall you give birth to children'. Simpson replied by reminding his opponents that God made Adam fall into a deep sleep before taking the rib from him; in other words God anaesthetized him. When some doctors of Philadelphia wrote to him protesting that the

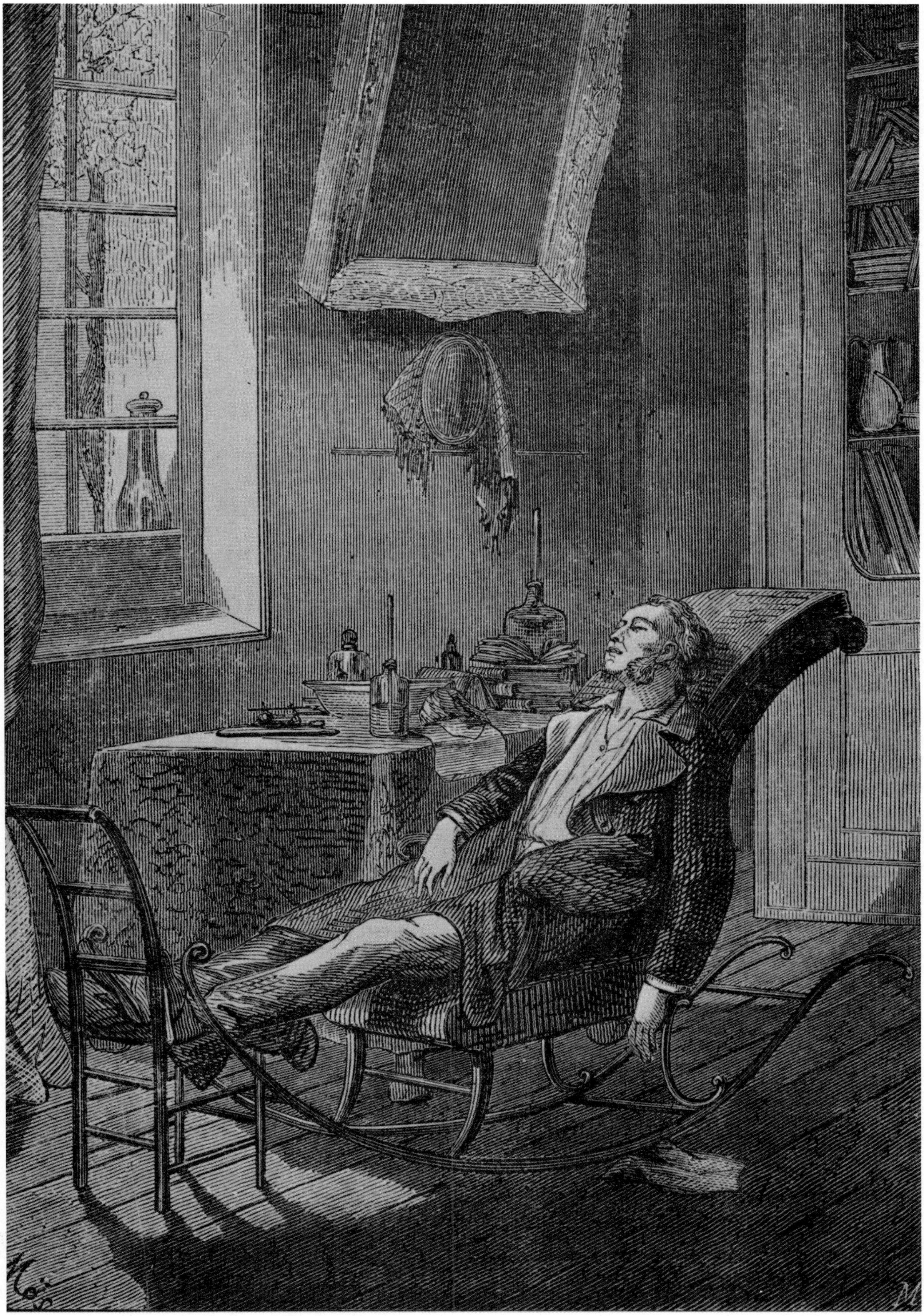

Before the discovery of effective anaesthetics, surgeons had to try to operate as quickly as possible because of the pain (the great Larrey once performed over two hundred amputations in twenty-four hours), but now time became a less important factor and the scope of surgery widened accordingly. After the little known pioneering work of Long, others continued to experiment. In 1846, William Morton, at Harvard Medical School, where he was supplied with ether by the chemist Charles Jackson, successfully removed a tooth from a patient. Later he etherized a patient for the surgeon John Warren, who removed a tumour from his neck.

The anaesthetic properties of ether had been discovered in 1818 by Michael Faraday, but other substances were also known and used from the

pain of childbirth, as a spontaneous, natural and therefore necessary manifestation, should not be eliminated, Simpson advised them not to take the train next time they went to New York, if they wished to be spontaneous and natural, but make the journey on foot.

Simpson's victory was complete when Queen Victoria required administration of an anaesthetic for the delivery of Prince Leopold, her seventh child. With royal assent, anaesthesia became at once fashionable and acceptable. The Queen was delivered by John Snow (1813–1858), whose work on chloroform and other anaesthetics put the subject on a scientific basis.

After Simpson had overcome the objections raised by reactionaries and uninformed public opinion, anaesthesia was adopted in every hospital. Technical developments and the introduction of new anaesthetics helped to overcome some of the initial difficulties. Ether irritated the respiratory tract. Chloroform could damage the liver and cardiac muscle and cause circulatory failure. A mixture of oxygen and nitrous oxide was less toxic, but this did not produce deep narcosis or sufficient

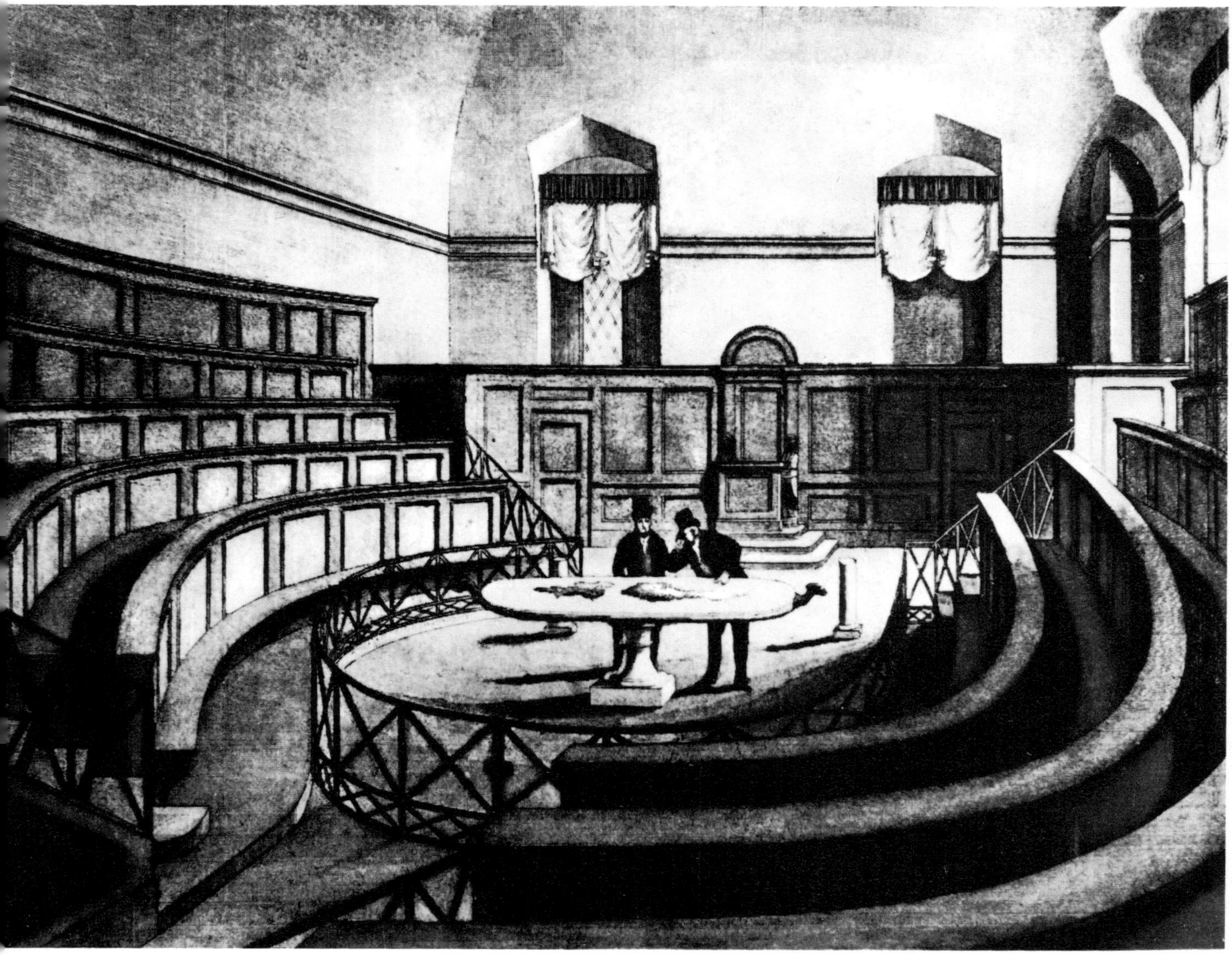

earliest days of anaesthesia. In 1800, Humphry Davy (1788–1829) had experimented on himself with nitrous oxide (laughing gas) and had suggested that it might 'be used with advantage in surgical operations in which no great effusion of blood takes place'. In 1844, an American dentist, Horace Wells, used the gas successfully in removing teeth, though he later took his life when one patient died.

Anatomy theatre. *Nineteenth-century engraving. Bertarelli Collection, Milan.*

Humphry Davy's experiment with nitrous oxide, Clifton, 1799.

Horace Wells with patient who has had a tooth extracted under anaesthesia, before students at Boston Medical School, 1829.

muscle relaxation. The action of ethyl chloride (introduced by Heyfelder in 1848) was too short-lived. Surgeons needed an anaesthetic that was not only non-toxic but also non-inflammable, for new electric surgical instruments were introduced in operating theatres, and these made sparks which could lead to an explosion in atmospheres impregnated with the vapour of the anaesthetic. Of the new anaesthetics, cyclopropane, introduced in 1929, had the disadvantage of being readily inflammable; trichlorethylene was first used in 1934, and was found to have the twofold advantage of reducing awareness of pain without eliminating consciousness, and was thus suitable for use in childbirth.

Among the improvements brought about in the administration of anaesthetics, reference may be made to endotracheal tubes (first used by Kühn about 1900) and to the closed-circuit system (1934). Intravenous anaesthesia was achieved by Oré of Bordeaux in 1874, using chloral, but came into general use after 1902 when Emil Fischer performed the synthesis of Veronal. After Veronal, many other barbiturates were introduced, and of these thiopentone is generally used today for the induction of anaesthesia. These substances have a very effective sedative action but do not produce insensibility to pain, so they have been used in association with other anaesthetics.

After 1945 two other drugs came into use in anaesthesia: curare and succinylcholine, both of which produce muscular relaxation. South American Indians poison their arrows with curare: the prey, wounded but not killed, is unable to escape because its muscles are paralysed by the poison. Curare in fact prevents the nervous impulse from reaching the muscles, blocking, at the neuromuscular junction, the nerve transmitter substance (acetylcholine). The curare used in anaesthesia is tubocurarine, one of the active principles extracted from the bark of *Strychnos toxifera*. Succinylcholine on the other hand neutralizes the action of acetylcholine, which it resembles, by reproducing its effect at the neuromuscular junction and remaining there instead of being rapidly broken down like acetylcholine.

Another type of anaesthesia, in many instances much more advantageous for the patient, had long been sought by surgeons: local anaesthesia. This was achieved in 1884 by the Austrian Karl Koller (1857–1944). The discovery is sometimes accredited to Sigmund Freud, who later wrote:

'In the autumn of 1886 I began to practise medicine in Vienna and married a girl who had waited more than four years for me in a distant town (Hamburg). Now I realise it was my fiancee's fault that I did not become famous at that time. In 1884 I was profoundly interested in the little-known alkaloid of coca, which Merck obtained for me to study its physiological properties. During this work, the occasion presented itself of going to see my fiancée, whom I had not seen for two years. I hurriedly finished my work on cocaine, confining

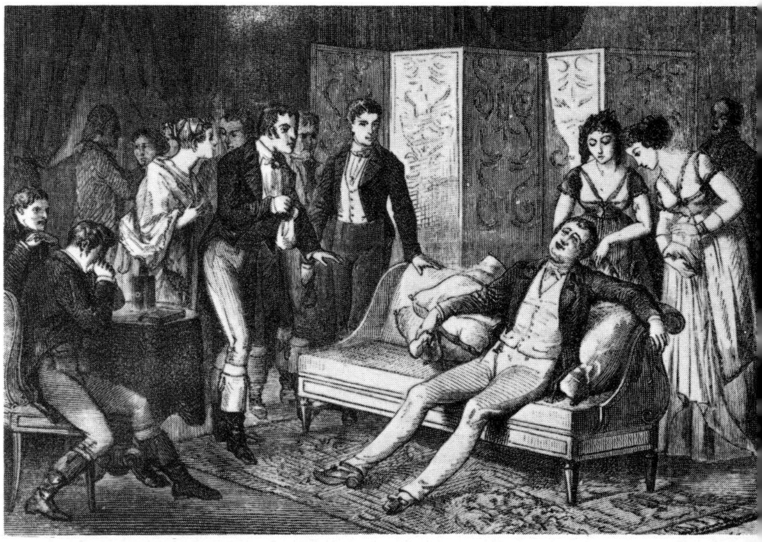

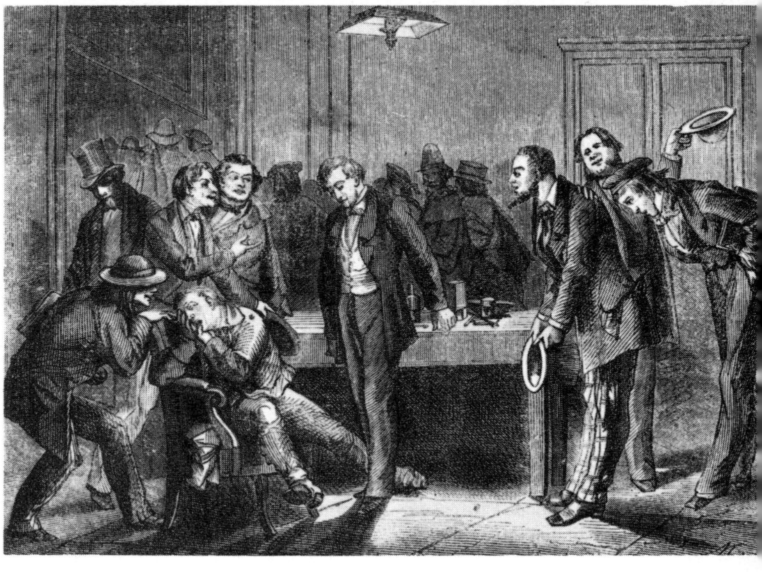

Ether, although effective, caused bronchial irritation, while nitrous oxide did not have profound enough effects. A new anaesthetic, chloroform, which had been described in 1831, was first used by the Scottish obstetrician Sir John Simpson in 1847. He used it, as he had earlier used ether, to relieve the pains of women in childbirth : a few whiffs of the vapour were sufficient to produce the required effects. A few years later, Queen Victoria was delivered under chloroform by John Snow. But chloroform in turn was found to have dangerous properties, and the search for new anaesthetics continued. Discoveries included cyclopropane, the barbiturates, and local anaesthetics, notably cocaine. New techniques for administration were also developed, such as spinal injection to produce anaesthesia of the lower part of the body.

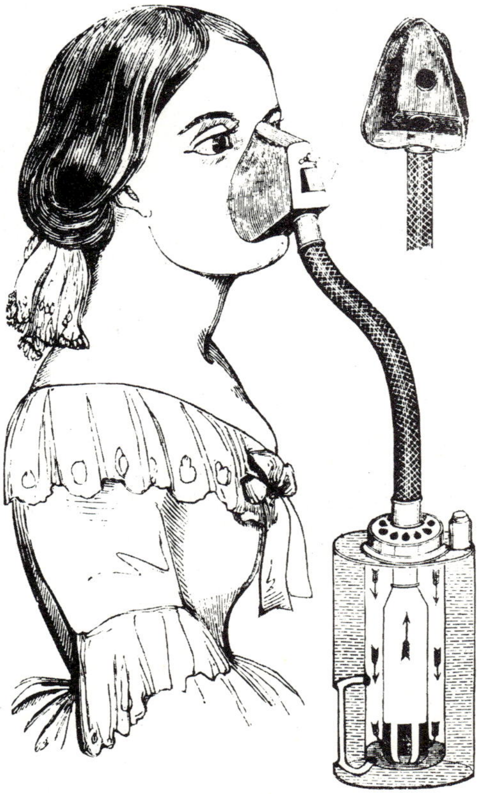

myself in my report to remarking that it would soon be put to new uses. At the same time I suggested to my friend Königstein the ophthalmologist that he should experiment with cocaine on some eye cases. When I came back from holiday, I found that it was not to him but to another friend, Karl Koller, that I had spoken about cocaine; Koller had completed the research on the eyes of animals and demonstrated the results to the ophthalmological congress at Heidelberg. Quite rightly, the discovery of local anaesthesia by cocaine, of such importance in minor surgery, was thereafter attributed to Koller. But I bear my wife no grudge for what I lost.'

Today cocaine is used only in eye and throat operations but the drug is only really effective when applied to surfaces, and, for other procedures, more effective and less toxic substances, such as procaine and lignocaine, are preferred. Local analgesia has the advantage of sparing the patient the pre- and post-anaesthetic unpleasantness. Again, it enables operations to be carried out that would not be possible under general anaesthesia. Local anaesthesia is often combined with the administration of a hypnotic such as a barbiturate.

In 1898 August Karl Gustav Bier (1861–1949) of Greifswald injected cocaine into the vertebral

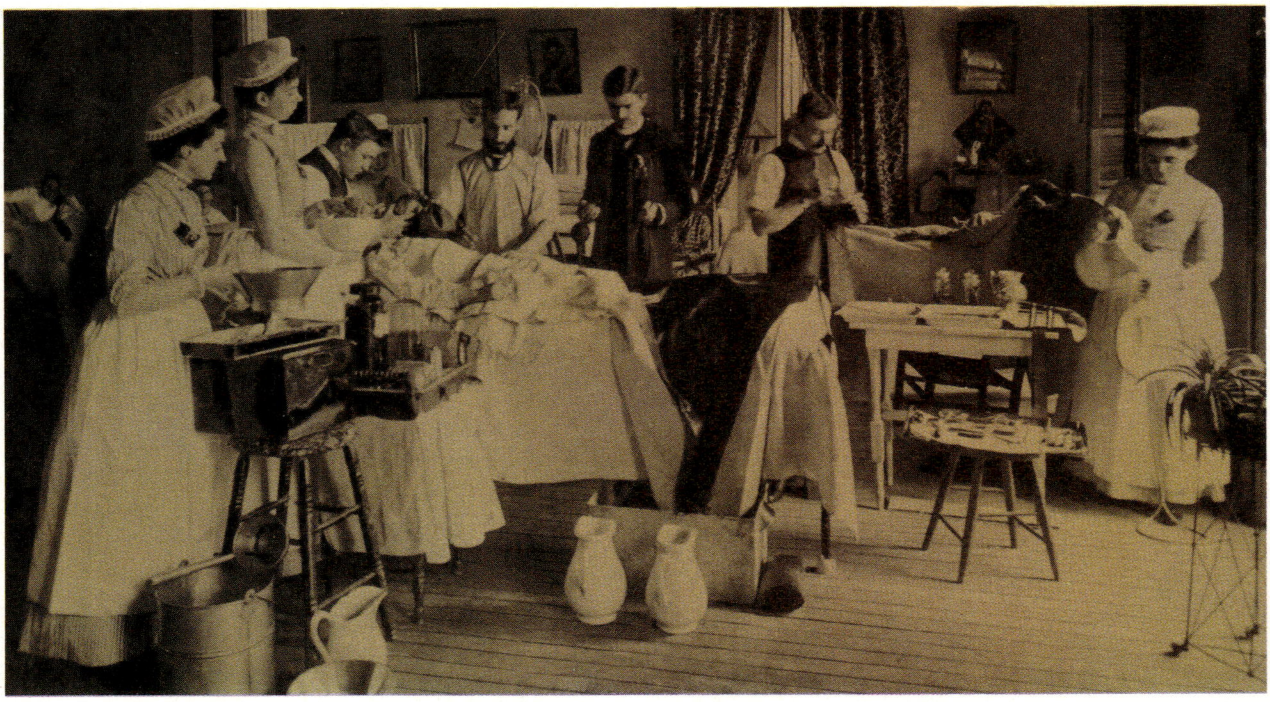

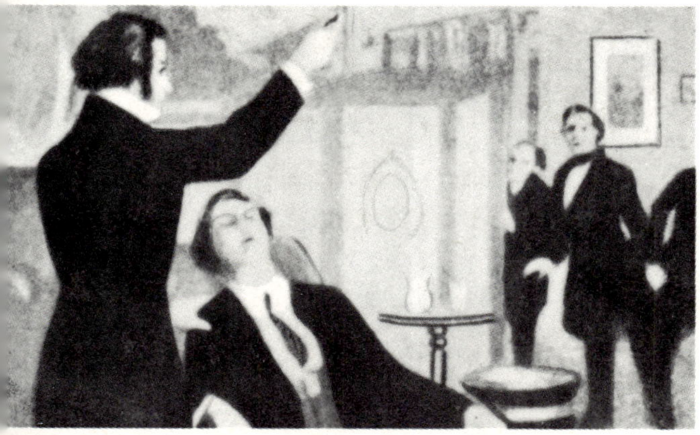

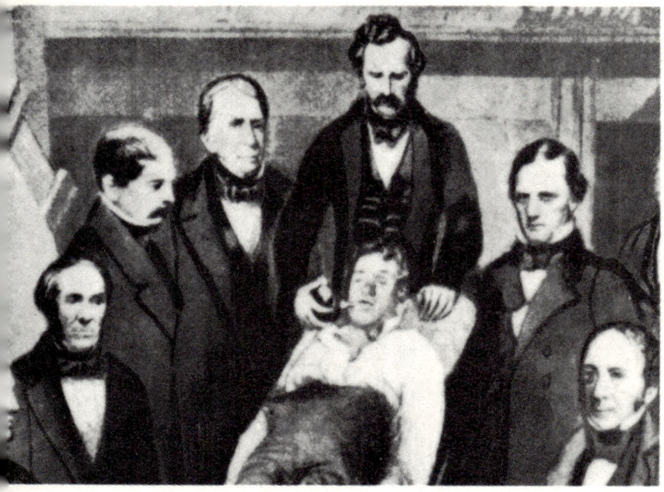

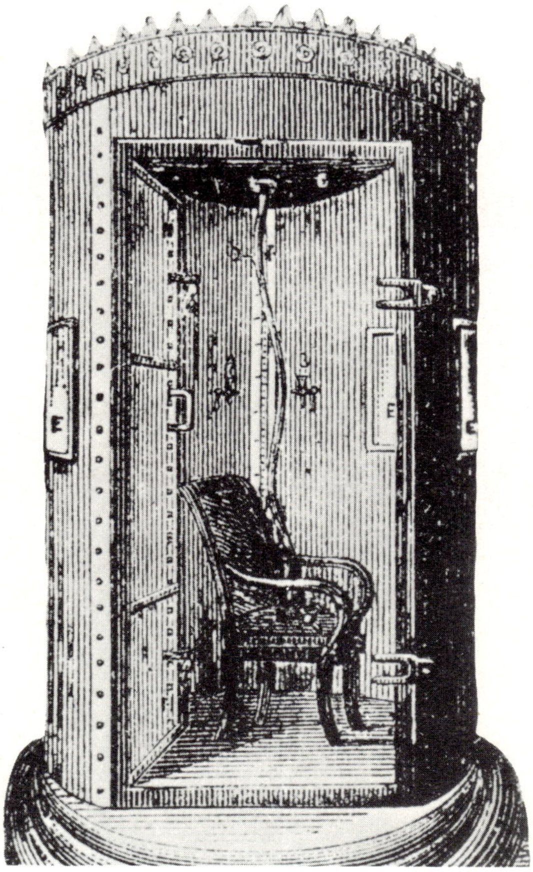

Inhaler for chloroform, invented in England *c* 1858.

An operation with anaesthetic but without disinfection, at Bellevue Hospital, New York, *c* 1870.

First extraction of tooth with anaesthetic.

First public demonstration of surgical anaesthesia, performed at Boston, 16 October, 1846, by Professor John Collins Warren. *From the painting by Keller.*

Compressed-air booth for dental operations, 1881.

canal and obtained analgesia of the lower extremities; then he used the method in surgical operations, and since then spinal anesthesia has become widely used. Another method of administering anaesthetics was first achieved in 1847 by the Russian surgeon Nikolai Ivanovich Pirogov (1810–1881), who introduced ether into the rectum; this substance proved too irritant – of various substances tried since, Avertin (introduced by Butzengeiger in 1927) has come into general use.

Another modern procedure which reduces the risks of major surgical operation is hypothermia, whereby the temperature is lowered from 37°C to 30° or 32°C (98.4°F to 86° or 88.6°F). Larrey and other surgeons of Napoleon's great army found during the Russian campaign that freezing permitted painless amputation. But it was of course not this which led to the development of the technique, but rather the fact that by reducing the temperature the oxygen consumption of the tissues is lowered and vital parts, such as the brain, can be deprived of blood for longer than would otherwise be possible without major damage. This facilitates heart and brain surgery in particular, and there is the additional benefit, derived from lowered metabolism and blood pressure, of reduced operative bleeding.

Hypothermia is achieved by cooling the patient with ice, wet sheets and fans. But these are not enough, for the temperature-regulating mechanisms of the body, centred on the part of the brain called the hypothalamus, result in shivering in an attempt to maintain constancy. Therefore these mechanisms must be inhibited, and this is done with the use of such drugs as chlorpromazine and promethazine, which also have a tranquilizing effect.

Anaesthesia has been a speciality of medicine for over a century. The task of the anaesthetist is a complex one, for he must not only administer and regulate the anaesthetic but also control respiration at every moment of the operation, especially when the patient has been given drugs that, like curare, cause relaxation of all the muscles (including those of respiration). In addition, the anaesthetist must at all times be prepared to intervene with suitable drugs to correct any excessive fall or rise in blood pressure, and indeed with these drugs to alter the blood pressure if bleeding becomes excessive or the patient shocked.

Military medicine and modern nursing

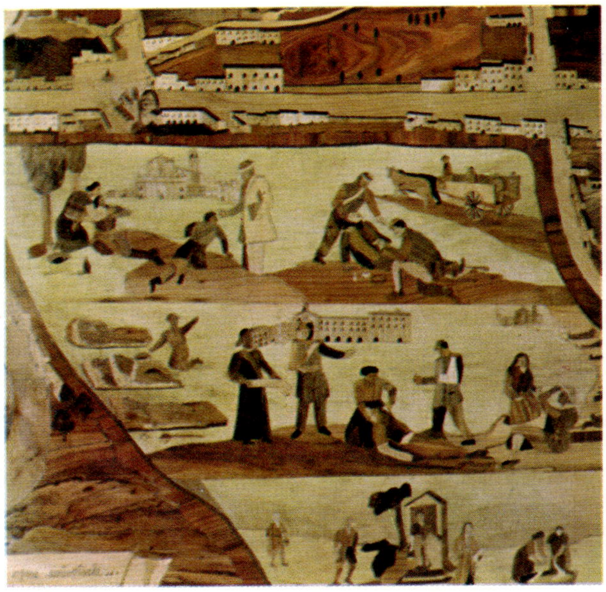

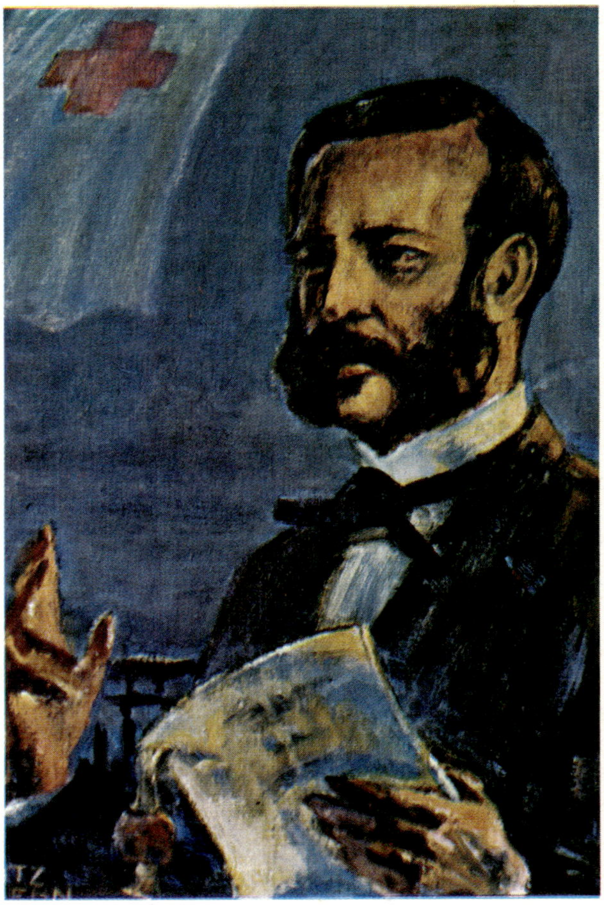

In centuries of warfare armies have been defeated as often by epidemic diseases as by battle wounds, for the destructive effect of war on hygiene and order has always favoured the spread of infections. Military medicine, aiming to treat the sick as well as the wounded soldier, developed slowly. Only at the end of the eighteenth century did the medicine of warfare become incorporated into the army, with the formation of such things as permanent medical corps and the establishment of army hospitals and field stations. It is impossible to estimate what proportion of the six million French and allied men lost in the Napoleonic Wars died in battle or from their wounds and what proportion died otherwise, but this loss was a physical disaster of the first magnitude for France and brought home the need for really efficient medical care in wartime. The Crimean War emphasized this for the Allies, for wretched hospital standards–later raised by Florence Nightingale's work–resulted in enormous and unnecessary losses. The same occurred in the American Civil War, in which over twice as many soldiers died from disease as from battle wounds.

The event which was to alter this picture for subsequent wars occurred in 1864. Henri Dunant (1828–1910), a Swiss philanthropist, was present at the battle of Solferino and was so outraged and moved by the sufferings of the wounded and dying participants that he wrote his *Souvenir de Solferino,* which was published in 1862. This was read widely and aroused such popular support that an International Conference of Red Cross Societies, each a national organization formed to aid the wounded of its country, was held in Geneva in 1863. Following this, on 22 August of the next year, the Geneva Convention was signed: according to the Convention, all sick and wounded, as well as the army medical and nursing staffs, were to be regarded as neutrals on the battlefield. Fourteen different nations were signatory; the Red Cross movement was widely supported from its inception, and today every country has its Red Cross Society to give relief in times of flood, famine and earthquake as well as war.

Not only the Red Cross, but advances in preventive medicine have improved the lot of the soldier. Vaccination and immunization have played a particularly important part, as is illustrated by the incidence of smallpox in the Franco-Prussian War. Garrison notes that the frequently vaccinated

The institution of proper nursing services was something which had to wait until the nineteenth century, when it was prompted above all by huge losses to disease on the battlefield. Throughout history there had been individuals of great charity, like St Vincent de Paul (1581–1660), who founded a nursing order and asylums for helpless infants in France. But the Red Cross was founded in 1864, on the initiative of Henri Dunant, a Swiss philanthropist who was horrified by what he had seen at the battle of Solferino.

The Battle of Solferino, with Henri Dunant aiding the wounded. *Castiglione dello Stiviere, Mantua.*

Portrait of Henri Dunant, founder of the Red Cross. *Castiglione dello Stiviere, Mantua.*

The story of St Vincent de Paul. *Popular print.*

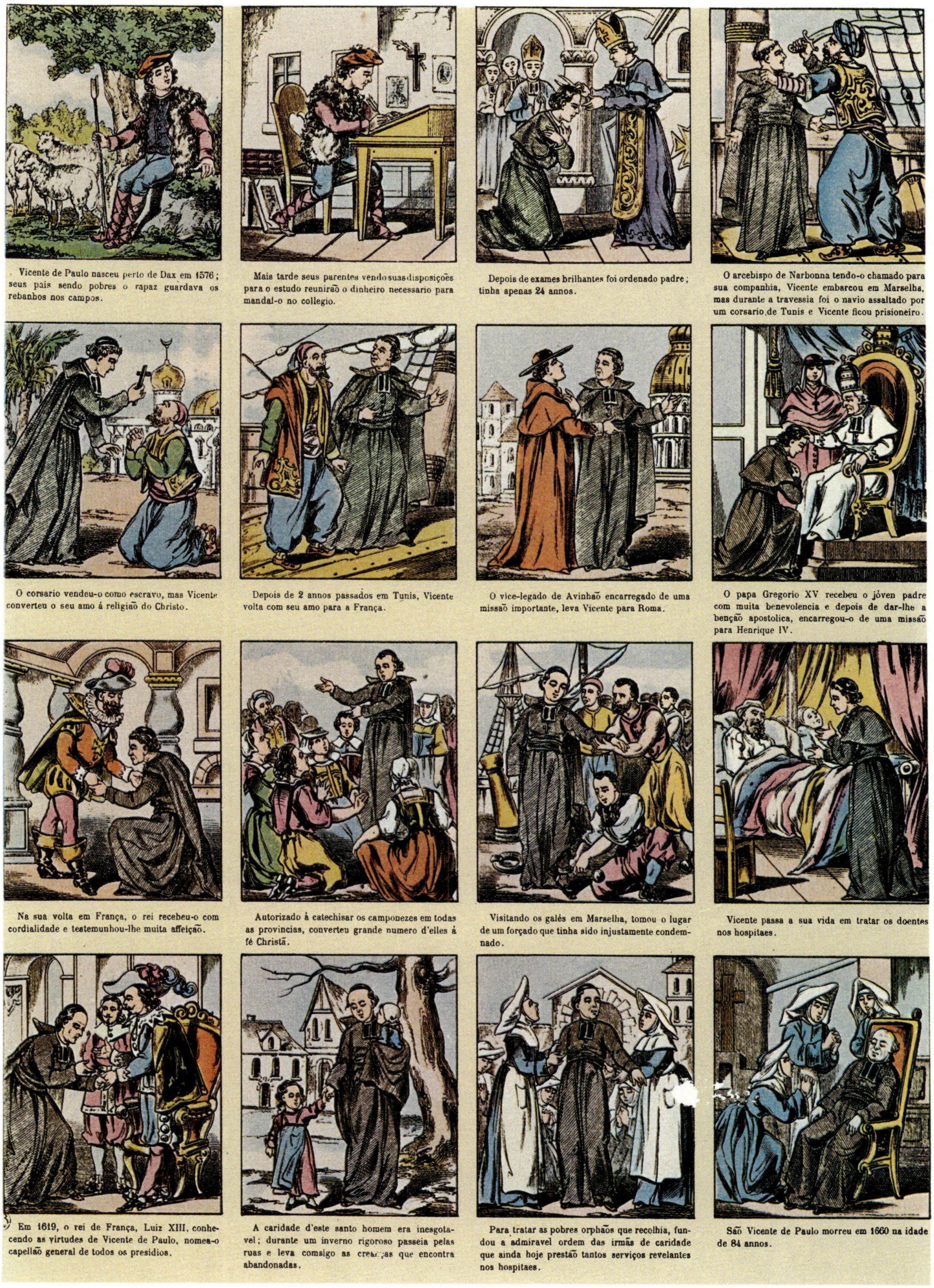

The need for trained nurses was first recognized in England, and it was probably a visit to this country which inspired a German pastor, Theodor Fliedner (1800–1864), to found the first nursing school in 1833. One of the school's helpers was Florence Nightingale, the Englishwoman who revolutionized the nursing service. She went to the Crimea with the British forces in 1854, and within ten days of her arrival was feeding nearly 1,000 men from her kitchen; in three months, she was providing clothes and other necessities for 10,000.

Nursing school at Centre de l'Assistance Publique, Paris, 1900.

Florence Nightingale in a field hospital during the Crimean War (1854–6). *Gernsheim Collection.*

The Italian camp after the Battle of Magenta. *Detail from the work by G Fattori. Modern Art Gallery, Florence.*

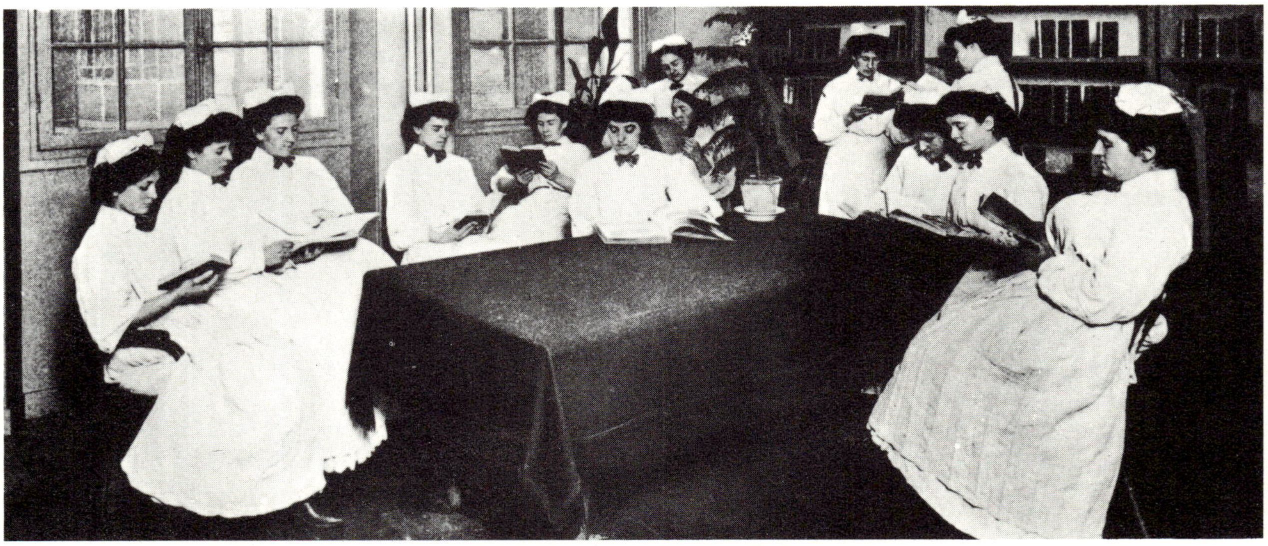

German troops had only 483 cases, while the largely unvaccinated French had 4,178 with 2,000 fatalities. In addition, proper asepsis and good nursing gave the Germans advantage over their opponents.

Perhaps the most famous figure in the history of nursing was an Englishwoman called Florence Nightingale. Born in Florence, Italy, in 1823, Florence Nightingale devoted her whole life to nursing and her reforms were fundamental in making it the admirable institution it is today. In March 1854, at the outbreak of the Crimean War, she was asked by the Secretary of War, Lord Sidney Herbert, to go with some of her nurses to take charge of the barrack hospital at Scutari, where her tireless care for the wounded and sick at all hours won her the affectionate title of the 'lady with the lamp'. Florence Nightingale's work was so successful that on her return to England £50,000 was raised to establish a school for nurses at St Thomas' Hospital, London, which was opened on 15 June, 1860.

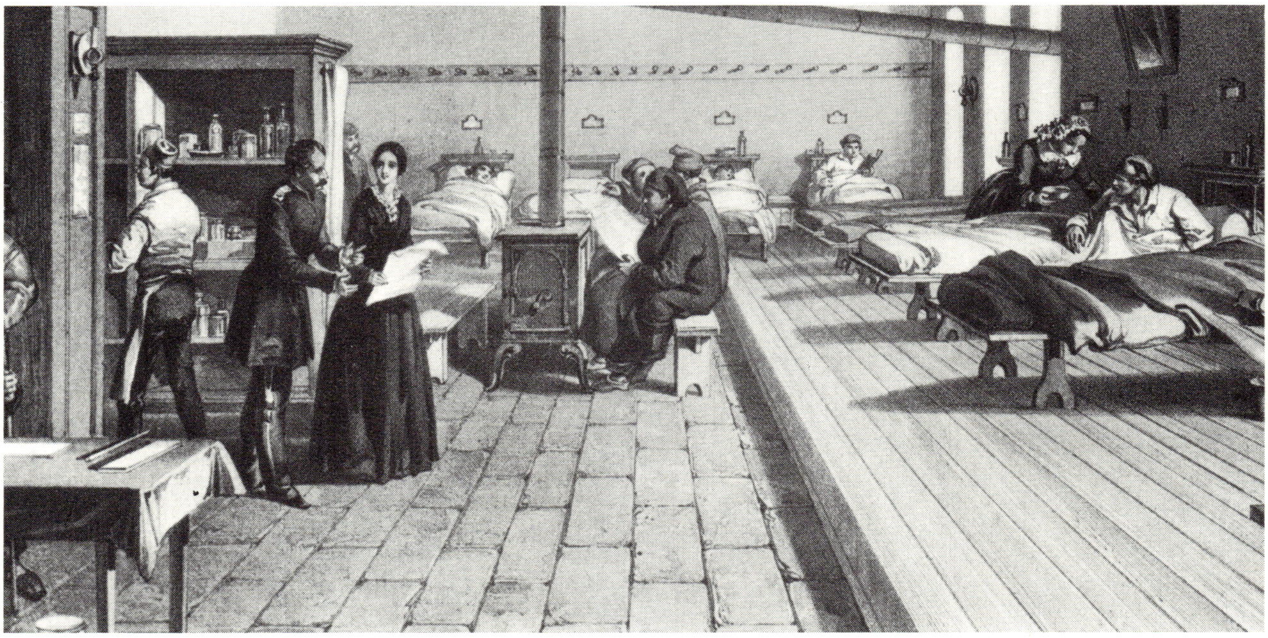

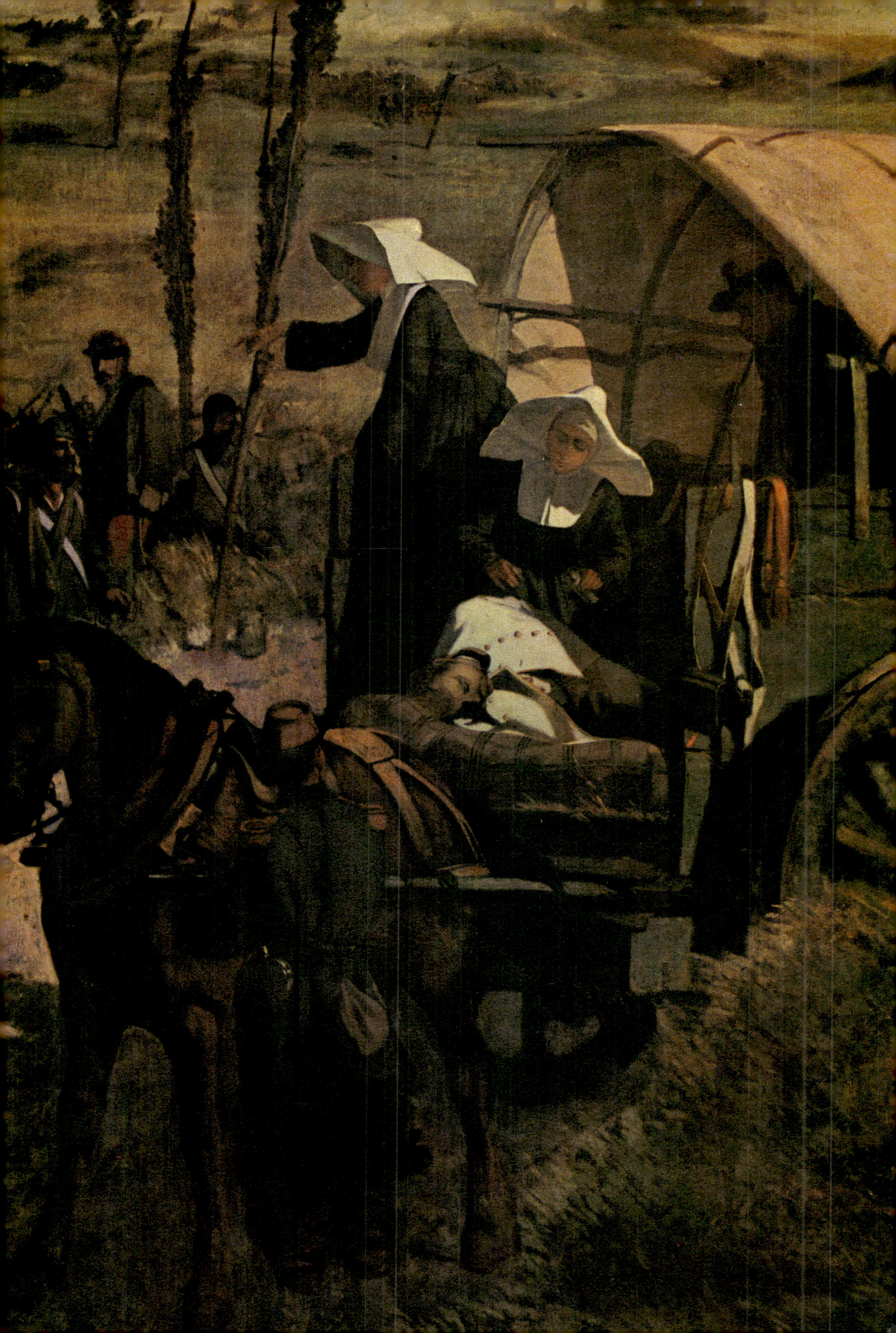

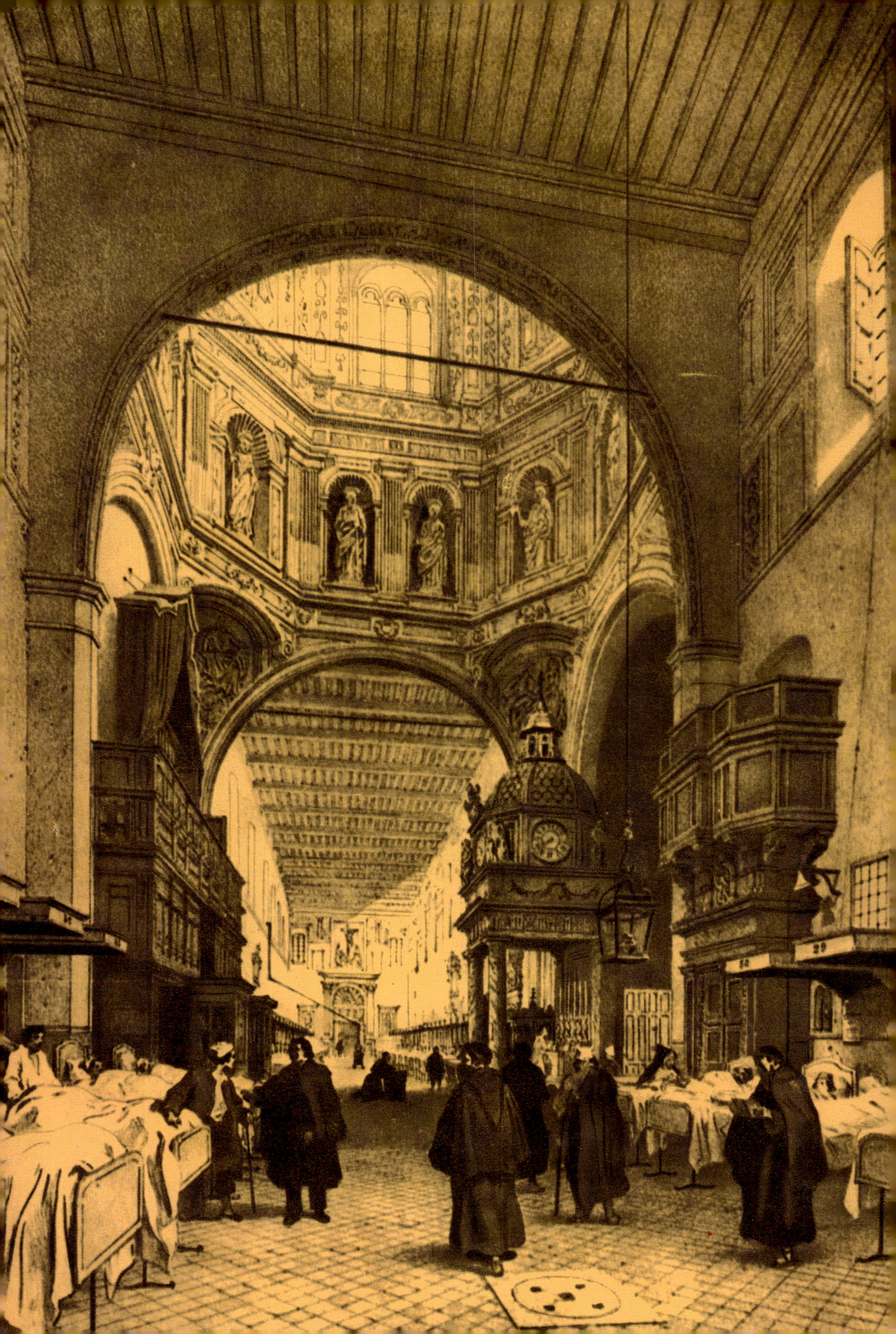

Antisepsis and asepsis

In the first half of the nineteenth century, infection of wounds very frequently complicated surgical operations, and led to disaster in cases which might otherwise have been successfully treated. After operations, healing of wounds by first intent, that is with scar formation unaccompanied by an inflammatory response, was very unusual. So great was the toll of infection that mortality amounted to forty-five per cent in cases of amputation. After the operation, the patient faced not only secondary haemorrhage but also tetanus, erysipelas and septicaemia. Innumerable women died of puerperal sepsis a few days after giving birth. The cause of the high death-rate in the surgical wards of the hospitals was still unknown at the middle of the last century. It was often postulated that it was something in the air, a poisonous vapour.

If the cause of pus formation and inflammation was still obscure, the mechanism of these processes began to be understood at this time. Simpson of St Andrews was the first to suggest (in 1722) that pus came from capillaries; this suggestion was confirmed by observations of Augustus Waller and Thomas Addison (1849) and by the great experimental pathologist Julius Cohnheim (1839–1884). Cohnheim, who in addition to new methods of investigation introduced a number of important histological techniques, saw white blood cells escaping through vessel walls in the damaged mesentery of a frog, together with widening of the vessel and slowing of the circulation within it.

The theory of poisonous vapour was disproved by the Hungarian obstetrician Ignaz Philipp Semmelweiss (1818–1865), one of the most sympathetic figures in the history of medicine and one whom Castiglioni describes as 'one of the greatest medical benefactors to humanity'. He studied at the university of Vienna, where he qualified in medicine in 1844. Two years later Semmelweiss joined the staff on the first maternity ward at the Vienna Krankenhaus as assistant to Klein, a well-known obstetrician. He was at once disturbed by the many deaths among the newly-delivered women: in his first month in his department, 36 died out of a total of 208. Semmelweiss in search of clues to this disastrous mortality observed that in one year, 1846, the number of deaths in the first maternity ward was of the order of 451, whereas in the second ward the number of deaths from puerperal fever was only 90. It seemed unlikely that the hypothetical 'invisible vapour' in the first ward was more of a killer than in the second ward. His attention was drawn to the post-mortem room; it was then the custom for obstetricians to carry out early in the day autopsies on their patients who had recently died, and after this to go on with their ward work. The post-mortem room and the frequent deaths seemed to be connected; for the second ward, where deaths were far less frequent, was staffed by midwives who never came to see autopsies.

Semmelweiss went to Venice in 1847 for a brief holiday and when he returned he discovered that his colleague Kolletschka, the assistant of the great pathologist Rokitansky, had died from septicaemia after wounding himself with a scalpel during an autopsy. He attended the post-mortem and noted that the lesions were similar to those he had observed on so many occasions in women with puerperal fever. It was the scalpel that had transferred the 'invisible poison' from the corpse to the unfortunate Kolletschka.

Convinced that the infection was transmitted in this way, Semmelweiss issued stringent orders: before visiting a patient, everyone was to wash his hands carefully and the wards were to be cleaned with calcium chloride. After this precaution had been taken the mortality rate from puerperal fever in the first ward fell rapidly from twelve per cent, and within two years was almost zero. He then communicated these findings and his discovery that puerperal fever was a septicaemia to the medical society in Vienna; the communication was at once attacked by his colleagues. Semmelweiss found that they were almost all against him; only a few non-obstetrical professors supported him, but these included three great figures, the pathologist Karl Rokitansky (1804–1878), the physician Josef Skoda (1805–1881), who was among the most famous doctors of his day for his diagnostic ability, and a pioneer of the use of percussion and auscultation, and the dermatologist Ferdinand Hebra (1816–1880).

Despite their support, Semmelweiss was dismissed from his post, and returned embittered to Budapest. In the first maternity ward of the Vienna Krankenhaus, doctors and students stopped washing and disinfecting their hands after autopsies and the death-rate among the newly-delivered women soared back to the old level. In Hungary, Semmel-

Page 266 :
Hospital interior. *Nineteenth-century engraving. Bertarelli Collection, Milan.*
This page :
Surgical operation with anaesthetic and antiseptic. *Illustration from Antiseptic Surgery, by W W Cheyne, London, 1892.*
Autoclave installed in Paris for sterilization of surgical equipment, late nineteenth century.
Course for nursing volunteers, instituted in Paris at the end of the nineteenth century.

Surgical pain had been overcome by the discovery of anaesthetics, but the problem of infection continued to complicate the tasks of surgeons and physicians. The new nursing methods, by themselves, did not reduce the countless deaths in hospitals. It was the pioneering work of a Hungarian obstetrician that finally provided the answer: Ignaz Semmelweiss showed that the contagion that killed many women after

weiss continued to practice antisepsis: he ordered doctors, nurses and midwives to disinfect not only their hands but their instruments and the patients' dressings, and he persuaded the hospital administration to provide fresh bed-linen for each patient and periodic disinfection of the wards and bedding. He thus succeeded in removing puerperal sepsis from the maternity ward of the old hospital of St Roch in Budapest.

Ultimately, Semmelweiss published his work *Die Aetiologie, der Begriff und die Prophylaxis des Kindbettfiebers* (1861), which stands as one of the epoch-making books of medical literature. It is written without style and with a mass of barely comprehensible statistics. His biographer, Sir W. J. Sinclair, asserted that if he had written like Oliver Wendell Holmes–who was the first (1842) to prove the contagious nature of puerperal fever–his book would have conquered Europe in twelve months. As it happened, the work was given an unrelievedly hostile reception by the medical profession. Even Virchow, the giant of pathology, refuted its arguments on purely theoretical grounds. When Semmelweiss in 1864 visited Hebra in Vienna, he showed clear signs of mental instability; he was subsequently removed to an asylum, where he died a few months later. An autopsy revealed that he had died from organic brain disease. It was twenty years before his ideas were accepted; later still, in 1894, a monument to him was erected in Budapest.

Joseph Lister, one of the greatest names in the history of surgery, introduced disinfection to the hospital at Glasgow at the time when Semmelweiss' work was rejected. A man of extraordinarily noble nature, Lister (1827–1912) had been a student of the famous surgeon Syme in Edinburgh and was already familiar with the work of Pasteur on micro-organisms when he started to work on antisepsis. Determined to reduce post-operative infections and hospital gangrene, he adopted one of the three measures shown by Pasteur to combat the growth of micro-organisms–disinfection. He thus insisted on meticulous cleanliness of his wards and instruments and the patients' dressings, and used a variety of antiseptics, including Condy's fluid (sodium and potassium permanganates) before selecting carbolic acid (phenol), which he tried out on cases of compound fracture. He had observed that simple fractures healed without complications, whereas those accompanied by laceration of the skin were subject to suppuration and gangrene. The skin was thus an effective barrier against infection, the agents of which were presumably pathogenic bacteria, although this was not yet proven. Thus another barrier, a chemical one, was needed as a replacement when the natural cutaneous one was impaired. Lister's system was simple: with forceps he introduced into the wound a piece of linen soaked in carbolic acid; he placed a second piece, also soaked in dilute phenol, on top of the wound, and secured it with plaster; and he covered the dressing with metal foil to reduce evaporation of the antiseptic. Before starting an operation, Lister had carbolic acid sprayed in the operating theatre and so disinfected not only the instruments but the operative field of the patient's skin as well. He first used this method on 12 August, 1865, and he published his results in a series of articles in the *Lancet* in 1867. It is likely that many readers did not grasp the full implications of these papers, for the first series was entitled *On a new method of treating compound fractures, abscess, etc., with observations on the conditions of suppuration,* although it was concluded that carbolic acid was a suitable preparation for the treatment of fractures by virtue of its bactericidal properties; two further papers were entitled *On the antiseptic principle in the practice of surgery,* and with the preceding articles represented an epoch-making advance in surgery. Lister's results were so strikingly good that the new method caught on at once and spread all over the world.

A great number of surgeons were then famous for their technical ability and the speed with which they operated. In contrast, Lister became famous because most of his patients survived the operations and recovered within a short period of time without complications. Antisepsis and anaesthesia between them changed the whole nature of surgery.

Lister's work was rewarded with the highest honours. In 1869 he succeeded Syme at Edinburgh and in 1877 he was appointed professor of surgery at King's College, London, and he was knighted by Queen Victoria and then raised to the peerage, thus becoming the first doctor to sit in the House of Lords.

The era of antisepsis was followed by the era of asepsis. At a certain point surgeons felt hampered by antiseptics; instead of destroying micro-organisms and at the same time damaging the *childbirth was carried on dirty hands and instruments and could be banished with cleanliness and the antiseptic effect of calcium chloride. Later, Lord Lister used carbolic acid to prevent suppuration in operative wounds. Eventually, the idea evolved of excluding harmful bacteria in surgery, using instruments and towels sterilized by superheated steam in an autoclave : antisepsis gave way to the era of asepsis.*

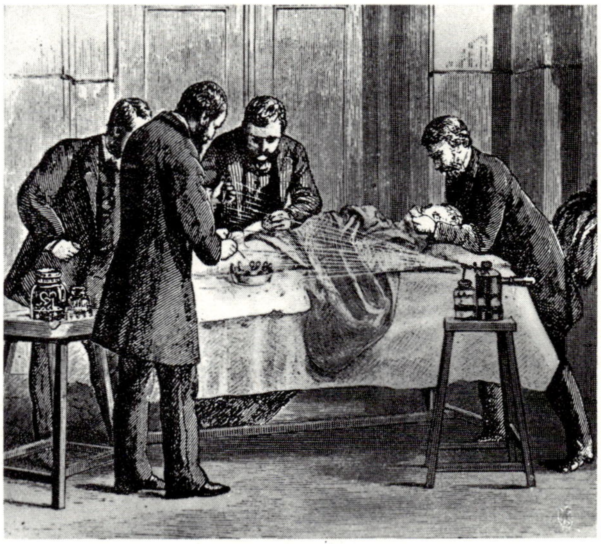

patient's tissues, they aimed to exclude bacteria totally from the operating theatre. Asepsis made use of another of Pasteur's combative measures – heat. In 1886 the German Ernst von Bergmann (1836–1907) introduced steam sterilization of dressings, and four years later the American W. S. Halstead (1852–1922) initiated the use of sterile rubber gloves during operations.

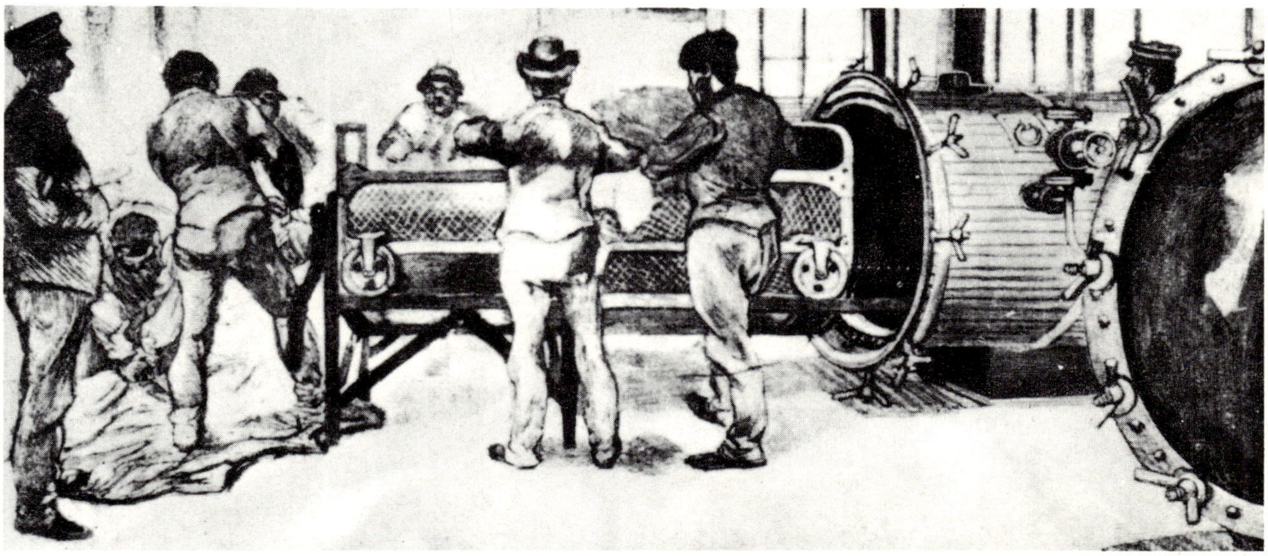

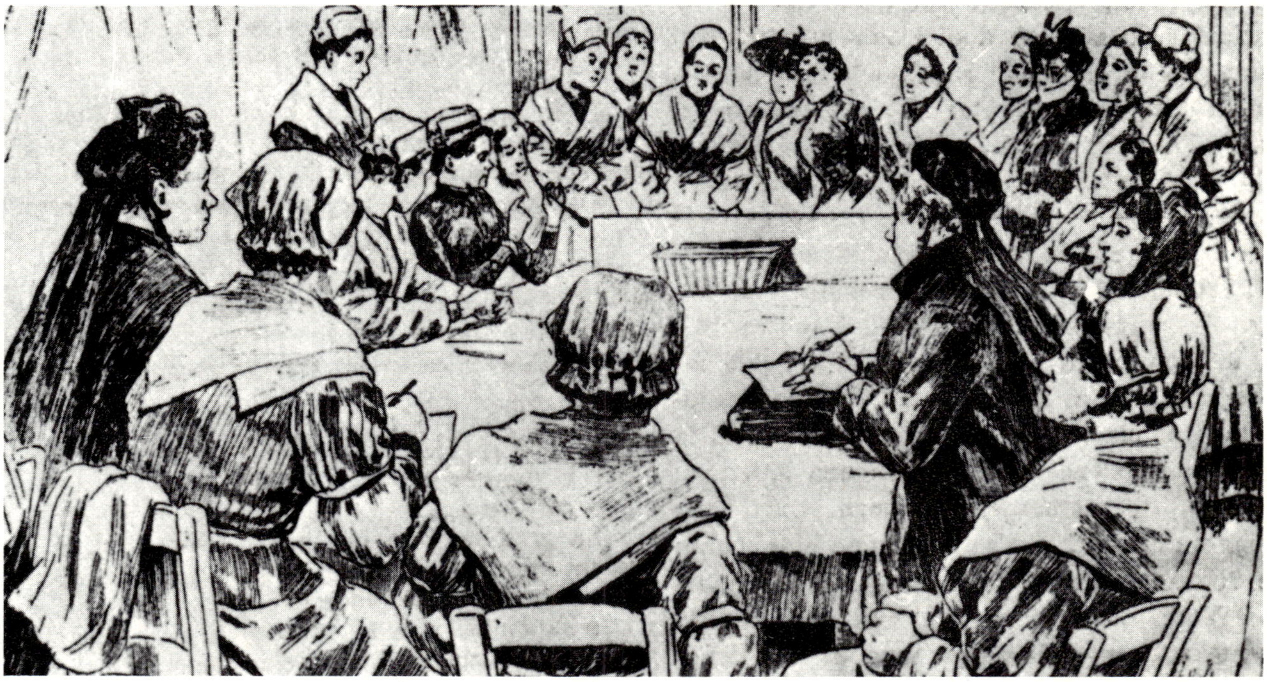

Victory over infection

In the second half of the nineteenth century, revolutionary developments in microbiology had a profound effect both on knowledge of the causation of disease and the approach of doctors to illness. In Germany especially, where bacteriological investigation was conducted with great enthusiasm and thoroughness, hospitals were provided with the facilities for all fields of research. The leading German clinicians began to attach the greatest importance to laboratory investigation, sometimes to the detriment of clinical observation. Since the German school at that time led the world, clinical medicine in a number of other countries began to take second place to laboratory research.

The foundations of scientific medicine in Germany were laid by Johannes Müller (1801–1858), a versatile and able investigator in many fields, including zoology, anatomy, physiology and pathology. Among his achievements were studies of colour vision, sensation and speech, while through his influence on such pupils as Schwann, Henle, Kölliker, Virchow, Du Bois-Reymond, Helmholtz and Brücke, as Garrison remarked, 'we may trace the main currents of modern German medicine'. Jakob Henle (1809–1885) discoverer of the renal tubules that bear his name, was among the first to uphold that micro-organisms caused infectious disease. In his treatise *On miasms and contagions,* he wrote 'the substance of contagion is not only organic but living, and endowed with a life of its own, which has a parasitic relation to the sick body'. Henle's colleague and friend Theodor Schwann (1810–1882) had previously demonstrated that putrefaction was caused by living bodies that could be killed by heat.

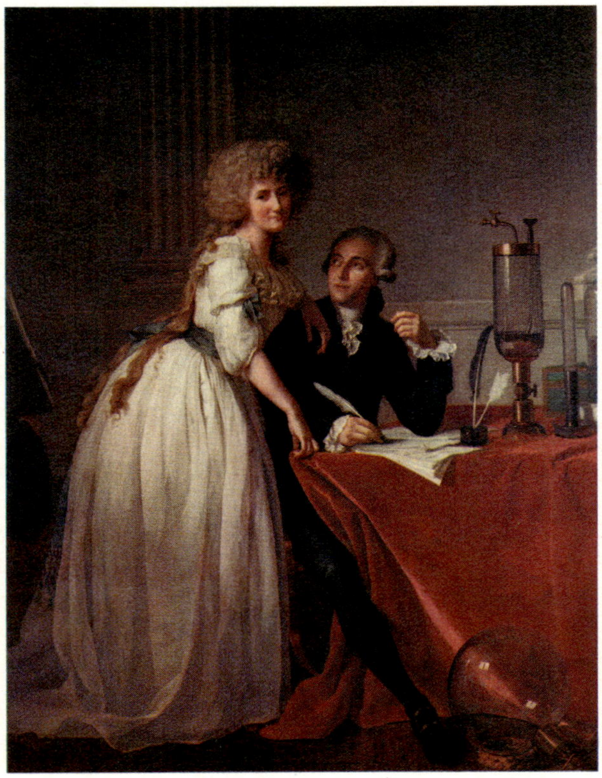

Even before the work of these two Germans, new paths in microbiology had been opened by Agostino Bassi of Lodi (1773–1857), who studied the silkworm disease 'mal del segno' (muscardine) and found it was caused by a living micro-organism, *Botrytis paradoxa.* Under the microscope, Bassi observed white marks, like tiny daubs of plaster, on the bodies of affected worms and established that the disease was produced by 'a living vegetable cryptogamous parasite'.

The discovery was followed by many other experiments which led Bassi to assert in 1846 that 'while many, if not almost all scientists, thought and still think that contagion is a substance of a special kind, in fact it is a living substance, that is to say a species of animal or vegetal parasite'. This was the decisive enunciation of a great truth ten years before Pasteur's discovery of the cause of infectious disease. It was appreciated by Henle and passed on to his pupil Robert Koch.

The microscope, which was of course of essential importance to the advance of knowledge in this field, underwent considerable development in the early part of the nineteenth century. Compound microscopes, that is, instruments with two lenses, were limited by the prismatic properties of the lenses, which produced fringes of colour around the image (chromatic aberration); the seventeenth-century workers concentrated on simple microscopes or magnifying glasses. Around 1825, Giambattista Amici (1786–1863), the Italian naturalist, astronomer and mathematician, improved the achromatic lens (which reduced aberration). Much greater improvements were achieved in 1830 by Joseph Jackson Lister, a London wine-merchant and amateur microscopist, father of the great Lord Lister, and further work was done by Charles Chevalier (1804–1859), who also invented the

Antoine Lavoisier and his wife. *Portrait by Jean-Louis David. Rockefeller Institute for Medical Research.*

Microscope constructed at Milan in 1726. *History of Science Museum, Florence.*

Beck's binocular microscope. *London, late nineteenth century. History of Science Museum, Florence.*

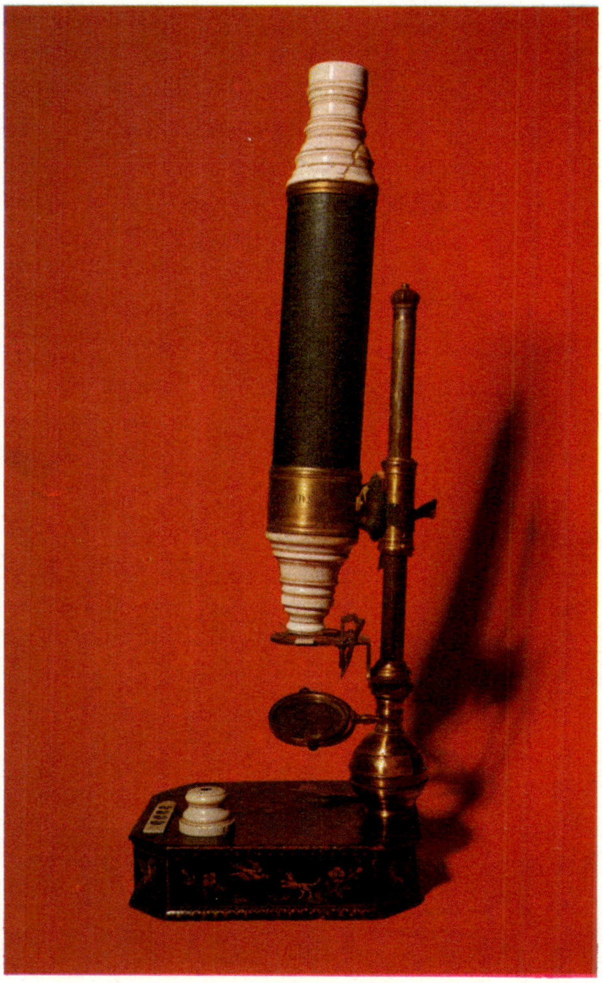

compound objective (lower) lens. Amici later introduced the technique of immersing the objective in water, which allowed greater magnifying power without excessive distortion. The refinement of oil-immersion was added by Ernst Abbé.

Rudolf Ludwig Karl Virchow (1821–1902) dominated medicine for more than half the nineteenth century and is without doubt one of the greatest pathologists ever. If Rokitansky, as has been suggested, may be considered the successor of Morgagni in the study of gross morbid anatomy, it was Virchow who extended and completed this work. Born in 1821 in Pomerania, he studied medicine at the university of Berlin and in 1846 began to teach pathological anatomy, writing that 'pathological anatomy and clinical medicine, the justification and independence of which we fully recognize, have particular value for us as the source of new problems, the answers to which belong to physiopathology'. In 1849, Virchow was sent to Silesia to study an epidemic of exanthematous typhus and he published an indignant account of the miserable

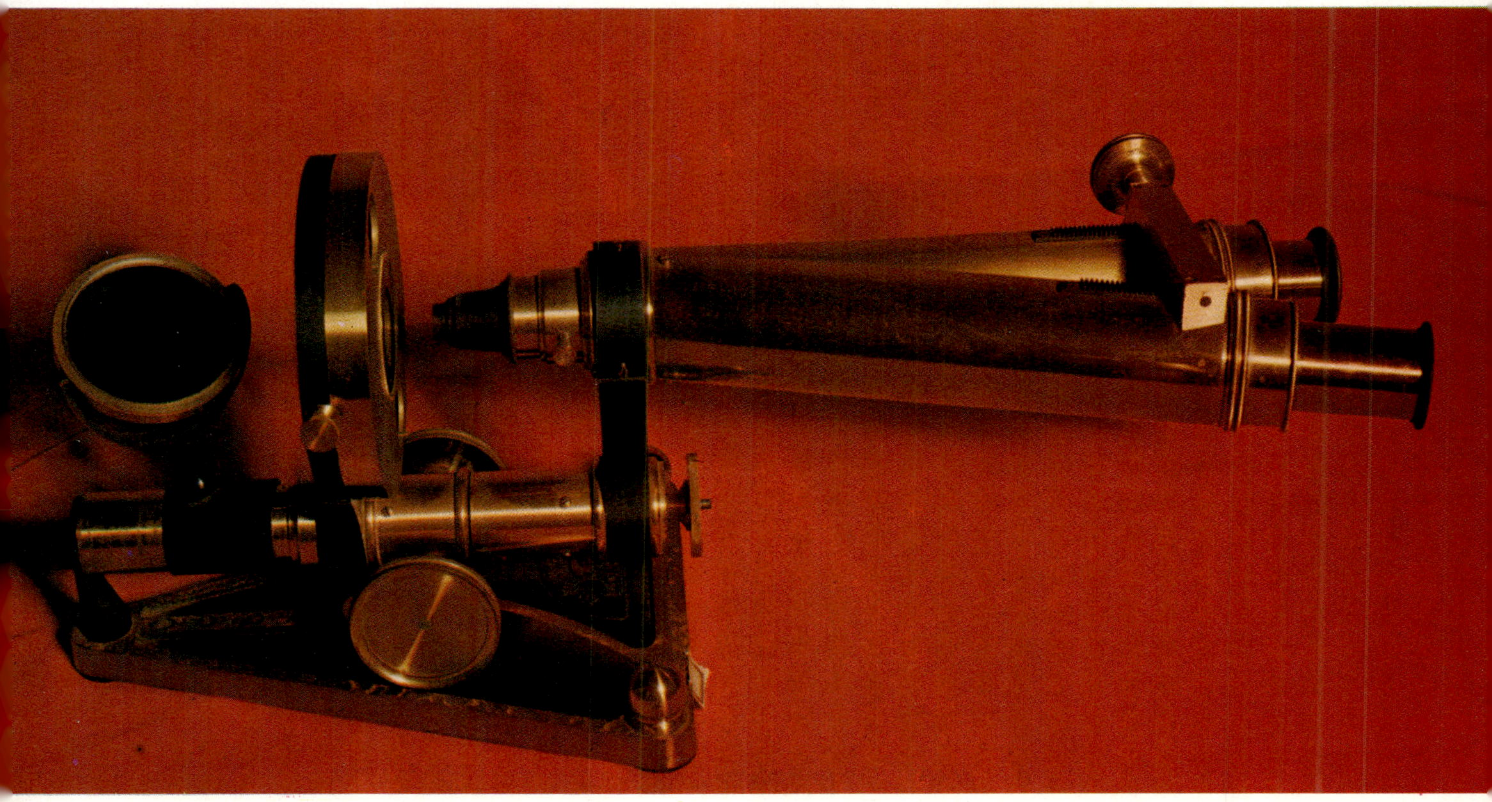

Increasing awareness of the nature of contagion led to a search for the agents which actually caused the diseases. The microscope, which had now been brought to an advanced stage of development, allowed close study of the appearance of the tissues in health and disease. Knowledge of the structure and function of the body at the cellular level progressed rapidly, especially in Germany. Hospitals were given facilities for all fields of research; pathological studies proliferated. The greatest name in nineteenth-century pathology was Rudolph Virchow, who sytematized the subject and stated that diseases were manifested in the cells, not in invisible and intangible humours, as was still generally believed.

Professor Henri Vaquez at la Pitié Hospital. *By Edouard Vuillard, 1921. National Academy of Medicine, Paris.*

conditions in which the workers lived; this account, which characterized his freedom of political utterance, displeased the authorities and he was forced to resign from his post. He spent seven years at Würzburg, during which time he laid the foundations of his great work, and then returned to Berlin where he became professor and director of the Institute of Pathological Anatomy of the Charité Hospital, a post he held until 1902, the year of his death. During his career at Berlin, he carried out and supervised an enormous amount of work in autopsies, the collection of pathological specimens, and pioneer microscopy.

In 1858 he published his great work, *Die cellularpathologie,* in which, taking as a starting point his phrase 'Omnis cellula e cellula' he asserted that the seat of disease should always be sought in the cell, while the macroscopic and microscopic changes in the organism in disease were nothing but the manifestation of the reaction of cells to the cause of disease. This doctrine opened the way for the microscopic study of tissues and at the same time replaced the ancient concept of the humoral nature of disease; it applied to all living structures, and it was based on anatomical knowledge – positive investigation of visible change superseded metaphysical speculation. He later wrote 'The essence of disease, according to my idea, is a modified part of the organism or rather a modified cell or aggregation of cells (whether of tissue or of organs). . . . In fact every diseased part of the body holds a parasitic relation to the rest of the healthy body to which it belongs, and it lives at the expense of the organism'.

At the time when he founded his doctrine Virchow did not know the nature of the extraneous forces which he held responsible for many diseased states. This was explained by Louis Pasteur, who showed that micro-organisms caused disease and themselves came from micro-organisms, thereby demolishing for ever the theory of spontaneous generation.

The son of a tanner who had been a sergeant in Napoleon's Grande Armée, Louis Pasteur was born on 27 December, 1822, at Dôle in the French department of Jura. From the college at Besançon he went to Paris to study chemistry at the Ecole Normale and took his degree in 1848. His early study on the polarization of light in tartaric acid crystals was important in that it led to the development of stereochemistry, and it secured him a teaching post at Dijon; in 1852 he went to Strasburg as professor of chemistry and two years later he moved to Lille. In his inaugural lecture at the university of Lille he made his famous remark, 'In the field of observation, events favour only those who are prepared', which so often applied to his discoveries. In 1857 he became director of scientific studies at the Paris Ecole Normale and his most important work began.

A manufacturer of alcohol was dissatisfied with his product and asked Pasteur for advice. Pasteur began to study fermentation, which until then had been regarded as a process caused by the chemical breakdown of dead yeast. Pasteur showed, on the contrary, that it was produced by living micro-organisms. He ascertained that yeasts in sugar solution took up oxygen from the air and multiplied rapidly, producing little alcohol. Introduced into the same solution but not exposed to air, the organisms utilized the oxygen in the sugar, liberating a large quantity of alcohol. Pasteur continued his research and found that vinegar was the product of the decomposition of wine, brought about by living organisms; and that milk, by an analogous process, was transferred into lactic acid. This process was called fermentation when the product was useful and putrefaction when it was harmful. His discovery of the lactic acid bacilli was soon followed by that of the bacteria responsible for butyric acid fermentation. These could not only live without oxygen but actually flourished in an atmosphere of carbon dioxide, and were thus 'anaerobic' as distinct from 'aerobic' organisms.

In 1864 Pasteur was invited by the wine producers to investigate the reasons for the souring of wine and to suggest a remedy. He discovered that bacteria-free fluids remained free of bacteria if properly protected, and one of the means of protection was heat; he showed that heating the wine for a short while to 60°C (108°F), killed the organism *(Mycetum aceti)* that was responsible for the formation of vinegar without injury to the quality of the wine. This system was also applied to other products and came to be known as pasteurization, in honour of the man who discovered it. In 1865, Pasteur saved the French silk industry from ruin, by throwing light on pébrine, a disease that was destroying silk worms; he found the cause to be a germ present in moths and their ova as well as worms, and showed that removal of infected ova

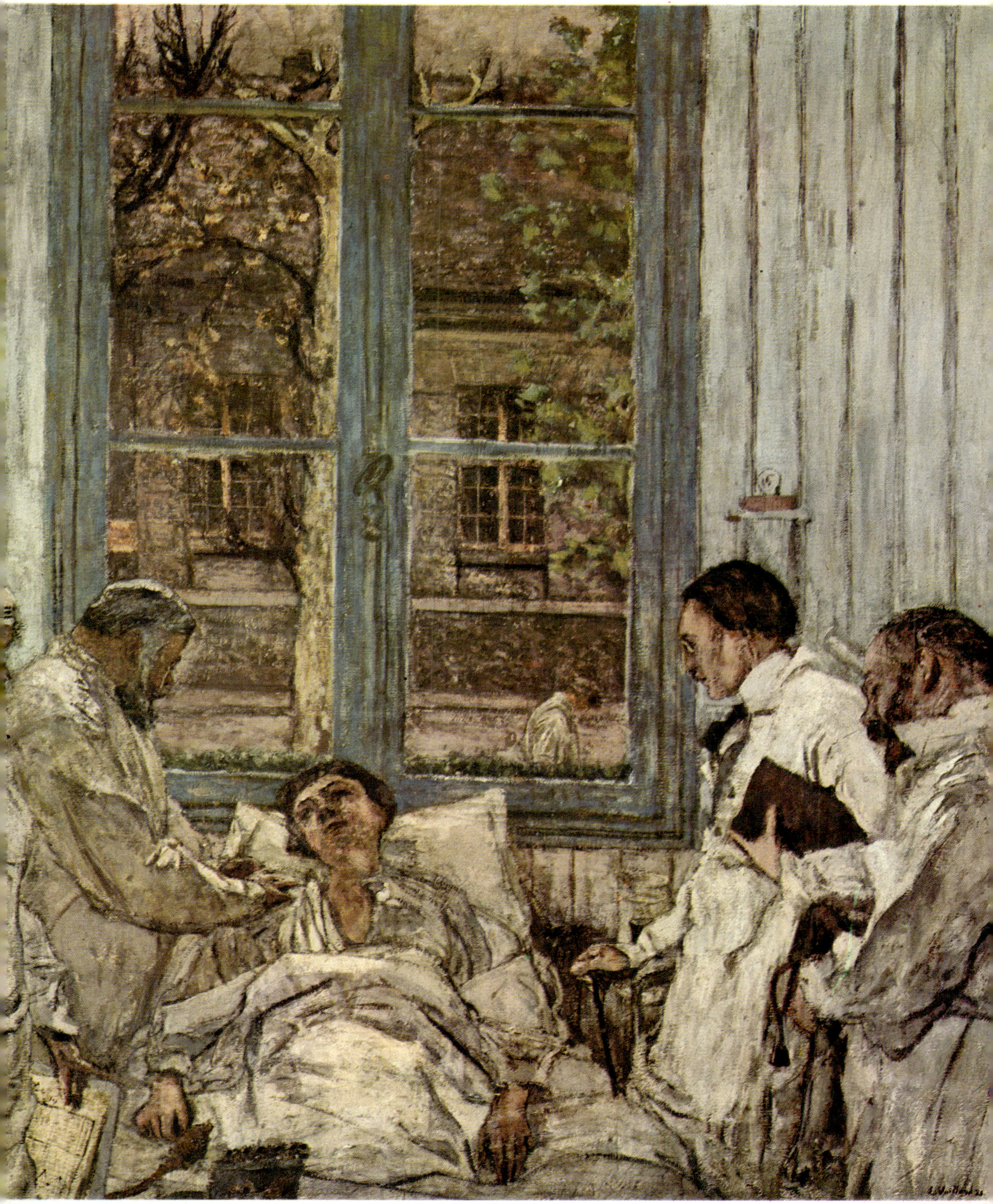

Semmelweiss had demonstrated that in contagious disease there is a tangible agent that could be spread by doctors themselves, Virchow that physical signs of disease could be observed in the body tissues, but so far no one had really identified the agents that caused infection. One man who came near to this was Agostino Bassi, who showed that a certain silkworm disease was due to a minute parasite and maintained that infections in general were due to such organisms.

But the science of bacteriology, which concerns the identification and classification of bacteria–the type of infectious agent first discovered–really began with the work of Louis Pasteur. Born in 1822 of humble parents, Pasteur became a hero and a legend in his lifetime–he was once voted the greatest Frenchman in a popular poll, ahead of Napoleon and Charle-

prevented the spread of disease. He next studied cholera in chickens, a disease that was raging in epidemic form in several areas of France. He succeeded in isolating the pathogenic organism and discovered that old cultures lost their virulence and that when injected into poultry made them immune from virulent germs. This 'attenuation' of the organism made immunization possible against other diseases.

He studied anthrax, an infectious disease of ruminants and horses which was transmitted to man through infected meat or hides. He made the causative bacilli less virulent by heating them to a temperature of 42°C (75.6°F) and then inoculating sheep with them; when the sheep were subsequently injected with virulent bacilli, they did not develop anthrax. In the spring of 1881, Pasteur repeated his experiments in public at Melun with forty-eight sheep. Before a crowd of farmers, veterinary surgeons and journalists he injected virulent anthrax bacilli into twenty-four sheep previously immunized with an injection of a culture of attenuated bacilli and twenty-four sheep not thus immunized. After forty-eight hours, twenty-two of the second group were dead, whereas all the vaccinated animals were perfectly healthy.

Although he had a stroke which left him partly paralysed on the left side, Pasteur continued his memorable work, and as his last achievement discovered a means of treating rabies. Two rabid dogs were brought to his laboratory, and in working out the cause and mode of transmission of the disease, he found that the rabies virus was present not only in the saliva but in the nervous systems of the sick animals, and could be attenuated by drying the spinal cord. He injected healthy animals with a suspension of nervous tissue from infected dogs and demonstrated to a government commission that they were immune from rabies. Pasteur's one regret at this stage was that he could not try the system on human beings.

In the summer of 1885, a woman came to him from Alsace with her nine-year-old son, Joseph Meister, who had been bitten by a rabid dog two days earlier. The disease would have developed in the child from three to six weeks after the dog bite,

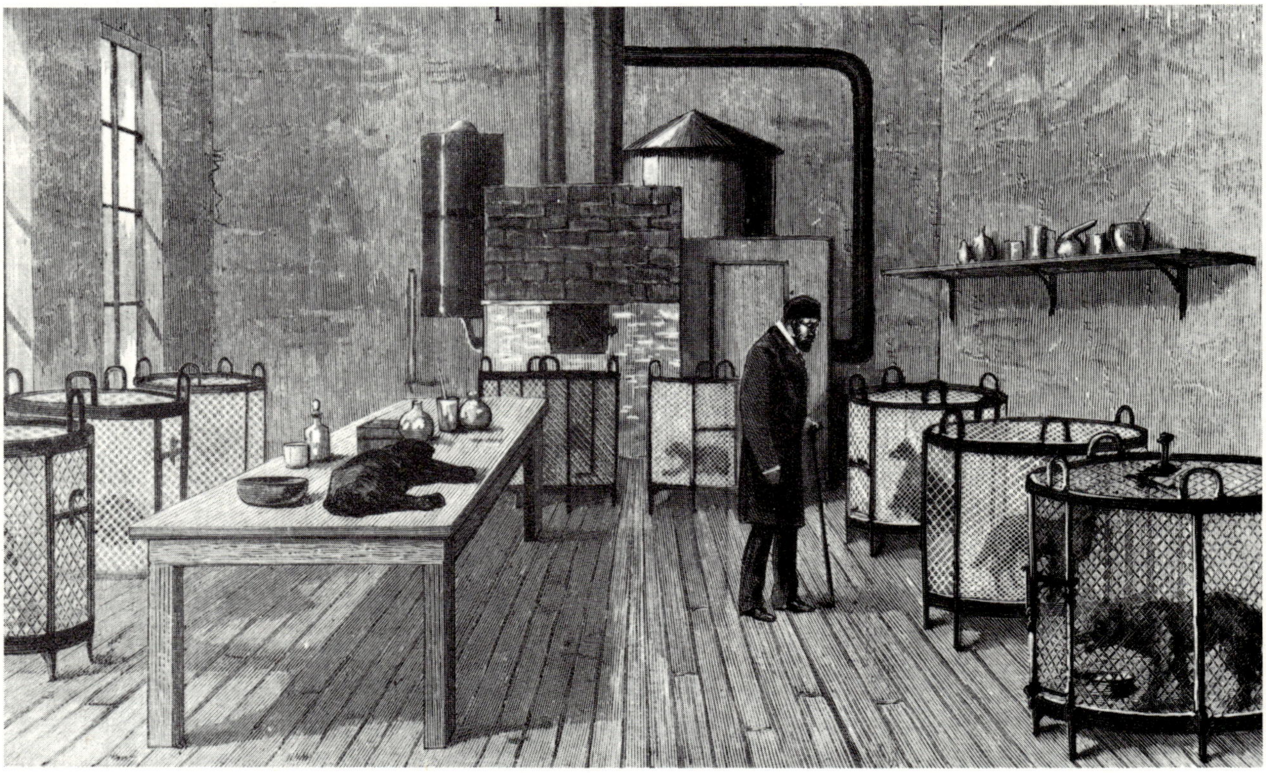

magne. While studying the fermentation of yeast, Pasteur discovered that the process depended on the presence of air-borne organisms, which could be destroyed by heat—'pasteurization'. Later, he applied this technique therapeutically: he injected bacteria partly destroyed by heat to produce immunity, first to anthrax, then to rabies, both times with great success.

Louis Pasteur during one of his experiments. *Centre d'Optique et d'Electronique de l'Assistance Publique, Paris.*

Pasteur in his laboratory. *By Edelfeldt. Pasteur Institute, Paris.*

the symptoms including fever, malaise, nausea and a sore throat, then spasms of the muscles of mouth and throat, at first on drinking but later at the mere sight of fluid (hence the name hydrophobia) followed by severe spasms and convulsions, maniacal behaviour, and finally paralysis, coma and death. On 16 July, ten days after the boy had come to him, Pasteur began inoculation with a suspension of dried spinal cord of rabbits which had been infected with rabies. On 26 October, he was able to inform the Académie des Sciences that Joseph Meister was safe.

Pasteur's last achievement was received with great enthusiasm, and the Institut Pasteur was set up in Paris to enable him to continue his work in discovering new pathogenic agents and preparing new cultures for immunization against disease. There he worked tirelessly to the end of his life, gathering around him a school of famous pupils. Universally honoured, he became a hero and a legend in his lifetime: it is said that in a French newspaper questionnaire he received more votes, as the greatest Frenchman, than Napoleon and

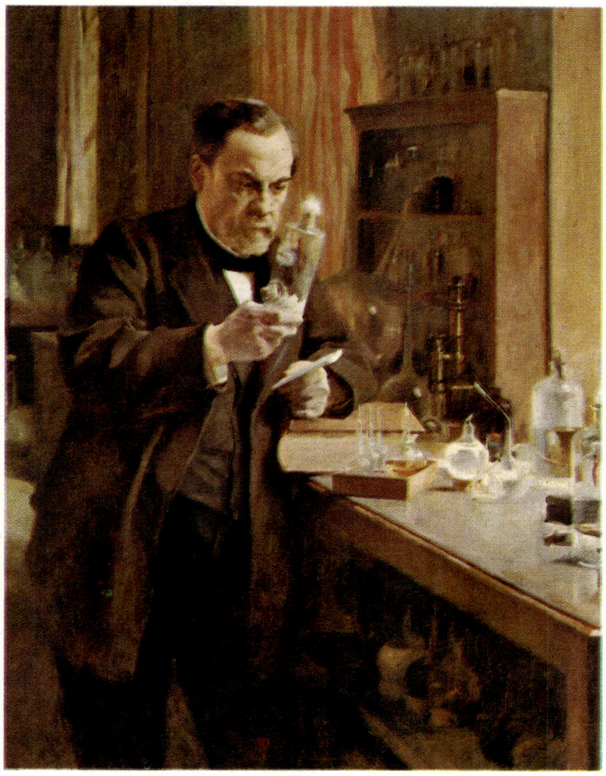

Charlemagne. Recognized throughout the world as a great scientist and benefactor of mankind, Pasteur died at the age of seventy-three in September, 1895.

Pasteur's pupils in turn secured a place for themselves in the annals of microbiology. His friend and successor as director of the Institut Pasteur was Pierre Paul Emile Roux (1853–1933), a pioneer of the study of filterable viruses; together with Yersin he carried out fundamental work on the diphtheria bacillus and on the treatment of this disease with antitoxin, and in collaboration with Metchnikoff demonstrated the experimental transmissibility of syphilis in monkeys. G. A. E. Yersin (1863–1943) discovered at the same time as Kitasato the bacillus of bubonic plague; Albert Calmette (1863–1933), first director of the Institut Pasteur of Saigon and chief medical officer to the French navy, discovered a protective serum against snake bite and the method of antituberculosis vaccination known as B.C.G. (bacillus Calmette-Guérin); and the Russian Metchnikoff became famous for his theory of phagocytosis, and was a Nobel prize-winner in 1908. Elia Metchnikoff (1845–1916), by studying comparative physiology, was the first to shed light on the essential nature of the infective process and immunization. In 1883 he published a classical description of the defence process in the lower invertebrates. He was attracted to Messina in Sicily by the rich marine life and made a special study of the sandhopper (Daphnia) a crustacean sufficiently small and transparent to be observed alive under the microscope. The spores of a simple type of fungus, present in the biologist's aquarium, after ingestion by the sandhopper, perforated the digestive tract and entered the body cavity. At this point cells in the fluid of the coelomic cavity of the crustacean went into action, attacking the intrusive spore by phagocytosis ('cell-eating'). But sometimes the phagocytic cells succumbed and the sandhopper died.

From this observation the Russian biologist argued that every form of animal was equipped with phagocytes adapted to defend the organism against the assault of micro-organisms. On the basis of the doctrine of phagocytosis (a function of the white blood cells in higher creatures), other workers were able at a later stage to investigate the mechanism of immunity in the human body.

Robert Koch (1843–1910) carried on the great bacteriological work begun by Pasteur. He was

Robert Koch carried Pasteur's work further with his own great discovery of the tubercle bacillus, the organism causing tuberculosis. This bacillus has a waxy coat which makes it difficult to stain by methods which suffice for other bacteria, and it is also a difficult one to culture. Koch's work extended the field of bacteriology by introducing new methods of staining, to make more organisms visible under the microscope, and also new ways of culturing bacteria. With these new methods, Koch was able to succeed with Mycobacterium tuberculosis, *where others had failed, and his work won him the highest honours, including the Nobel prize in 1905.*

Convalescence. *By Luigi Nono.*

born at Klausthal, Hanover, and in 1866 he qualified in medicine at Göttingen where one of his teachers was Jakob Henle. Koch showed an extraordinary technical flair for research and, like Pasteur, his investigations were stimulated by immediate practical problems. Thus when anthrax was rife among the stock in Wollstein, Prussia, the district where he worked, he studied this disease intensively and succeeded in discovering the bacillus in the blood and spleen of a dead animal. He cultured the organism and was able for the first time in history to work out its complete life cycle. Koch grew it on artificial media and by studying its spores clarified the question of the start and duration of the disease.

His success led him in 1876 to take his results to Ferdinand Cohn, professor of botany at the university of Breslau, and he was invited to give a demonstration at the Silesian institute of sciences, which published Koch's lecture in a biological review.

Pasteur repeated Koch's work and confirmed his findings of the development of the spores from the bacilli, the transformation of the spores into bacilli and the occurrence of the disease in animals injected with pure cultures.

In 1878 Koch published a monograph on the aetiology of infections in traumatic cases, *Untersuchungen über die Aetiologie der Wundinfektionskrankheiten,* which established the fact that specific bacteria were responsible for the infection of surgical wounds; and in 1880 he was appointed to an important office in Berlin at the Kaiserliches Gesundheitsamt (imperial health department). His assistant was Friedrich Löffler, who was the first to cultivate the bacillus of diphtheria, discovered also by Edwin Klebs.

Koch made many technical advances in the study of bacteria and originated most of the methods used today. He introduced transparent and solidifiable media (like agar and gelatin) to grow cultures of a single bacterial species. He developed staining and microscopical technique, using the oil-immersion lens invented by Abbé in 1878, to obtain photographs of such perfection that minute cilia on bacteria are revealed.

In 1868 the French pathologist Jean Antoine Villemin had demonstrated the main features of the morbid anatomy of tuberculosis and had shown that the disease was transmissible in animals by means of tuberculous material. In 1882 Koch cultivated the tubercle bacillus, and presented his results to the Berlin Physiological Society in a paper which also included 'Koch's postulates': 1, that the organism must always be found in a given disease; 2, that the organism must not be found in other diseases or in health; 3, that the organism must be cultivated artificially and reproduce the given disease after the inoculation of a pure culture into a susceptible animal; 4, that the organism must be recoverable from the animal so inoculated. This famous set of rules must be obeyed if it is to be proved that a specific organism is responsible for a specific disease. Eight years later Koch announced that he had discovered a cure for the disease – tuberculin, derived from the pathogenic organism – but it was soon seen that his discovery was ineffective, although of value in diagnosis.

In 1891 Koch became director of the Institute of Infectious Diseases, and worked out methods of controlling water-borne infections by filtration. One of these diseases was cholera, the agent of which he had discovered in 1884. He later went, as head of a scientific mission, to German East Africa, Rhodesia and Japan, to study indigenous transmissible disease. Nobel prize-winner in 1905, member of the Prussian academy of sciences and honoured throughout the world, Koch became, like Pasteur, the head of a school of brilliant pupils, although unlike the Frenchman he was far from universally admired in his country.

Through the impulse Koch gave to microbiology, many discoveries in Germany followed his work, culminating in the work of Emil von Behring and his colleague the Japanese Baron Shibasaburo Kitasato; two papers, published in 1890, proclaimed the discovery of antitoxins and their immunizing power in relation to tetanus and diphtheria, and laid the foundation for all subsequent studies of passive immunity.

Paul Ehrlich (1854–1915) was an outstanding scientific genius who produced the scientific basis for immunology and founded chemotherapy. The son of a Jewish merchant from Strehlen in Silesia, he was a poor scholar, passing his examinations with difficulty: his professors at the faculty of medicine at Beslau university thought him backward, for during classes his attention would wander to the detriment of acquiring knowledge. He went from one university to another, studying at Strasburg and Freiburg before enrolling at Leipzig,

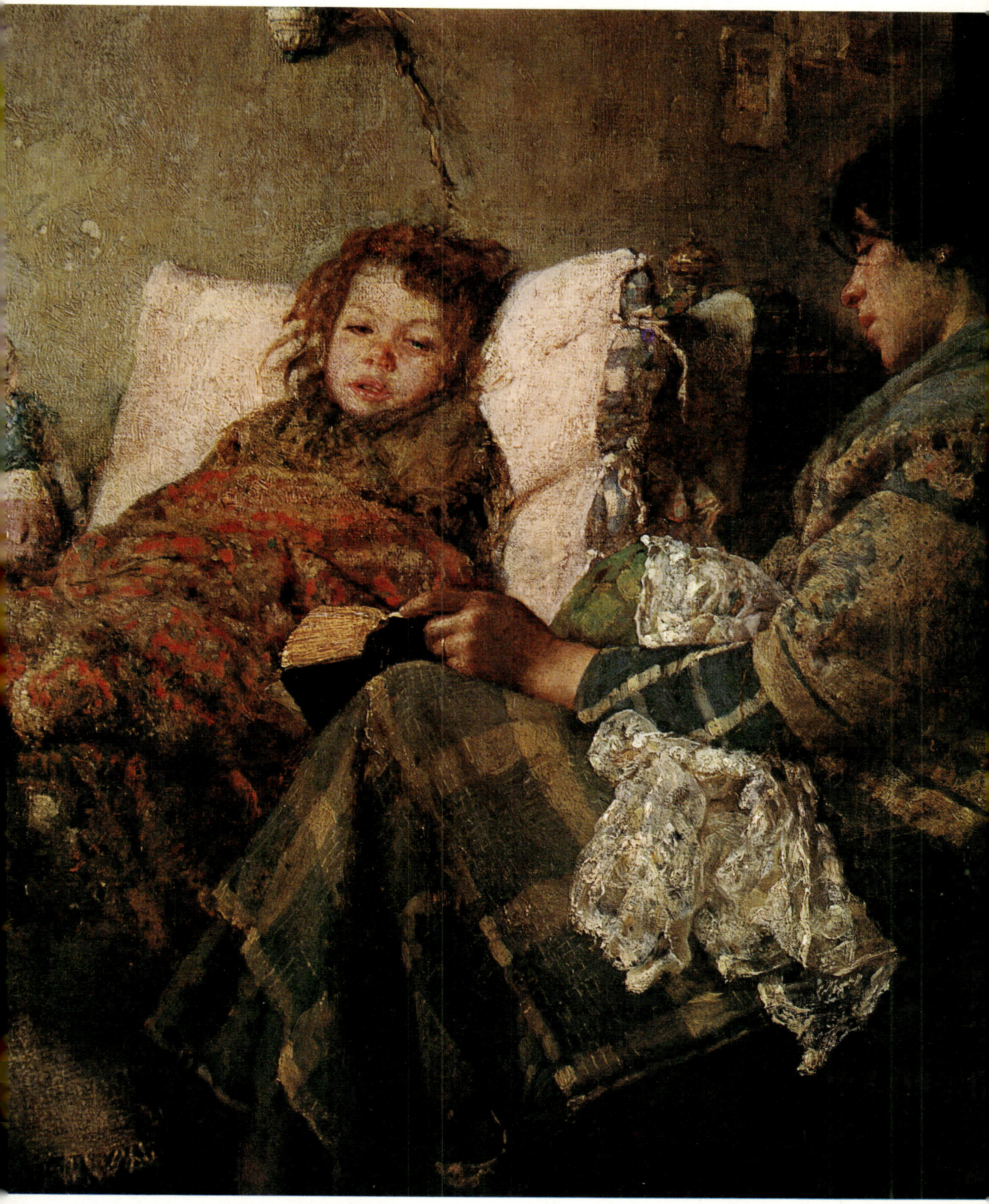

Koch failed to derive an effective treatment for tuberculosis from his cultures. The founder of modern chemotherapy and of immunology was Paul Ehrlich, who prepared substances, such as salvarsan, whose toxic effects on bacteria far outweighed those on the human body, thus providing a powerful new type of therapy. Immunology extended into practice with the preparation of vaccines from animals for use in man.

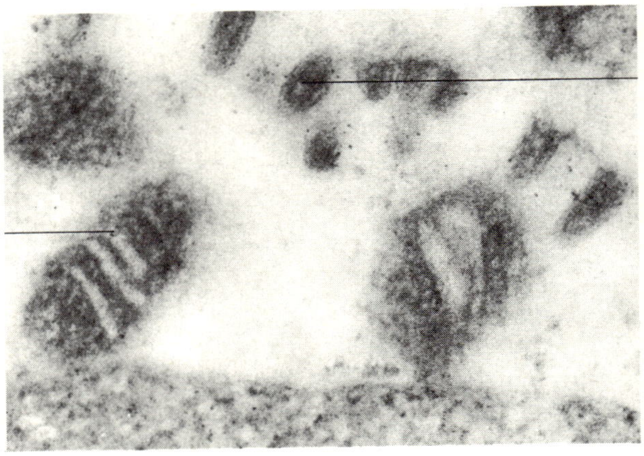

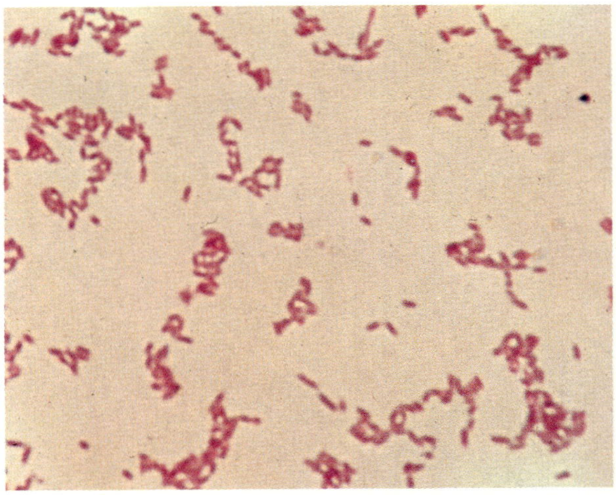

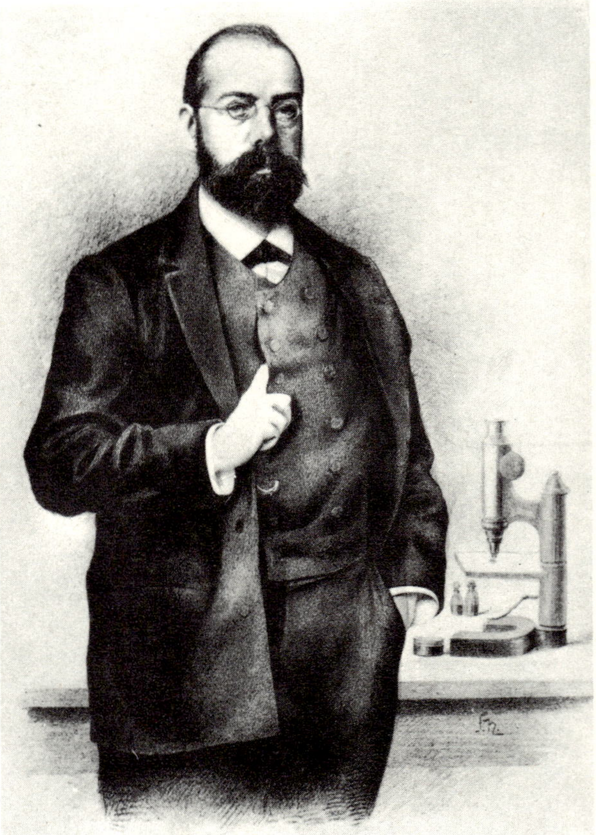

where he qualified in 1878. Even as a student Ehrlich experimented with dyestuffs and tissue staining, and he was the author of a brilliant doctoral thesis on the staining of histological specimens for examination under the microscope. He showed that some of the white blood cells were selectively stained by basic dyes, that the urine of typhoid patients reacted with diazo dyes, and that tubercle bacilli retained the colour of carbol-fuchsin after treatment with acid. His work led him to believe that certain tissues had an elective affinity for certain chemical substances and certain staining materials.

Ehrlich argued that if divers tissues have specific components to which dyes are attached, it ought to be possible to make dyes perform tasks in various parts of the body. Thus to ascertain that an anaesthetic reached nervous tissue, all that would be necessary would be to colour it with methylene blue. He also formulated the hypothesis that dyes, as well as having an affinity for specific tissues, could select pathogenic micro-organisms. By studying trypanosomes, the parasites transmitted by the tsetse fly and causing sleeping sickness, he found the dye trypan red, which has some effect against these organisms.

In 1910, Ehrlich discovered salvarsan. This compound was known as 606 because it was the six hundred and sixth arsenical product to be synthesized in his chemotherapeutic institute, founded three years earlier. Organic arsenicals were produced as potential treatments for syphilis. Shortly before, Fritz Schaudinn (1871–1906) had discovered *Treponema pallidum*, the agent causing the disease, and August von Wassermann (1866–1925) had devised his diagnostic test. Ehrlich equated treponeme and trypanosome, and began tests on a long series of coloured arsenobenzole compounds. Salvarsan was of some therapeutic value, but neither this nor neosalvarsan, '914', was successful in conquering syphilis; that victory was won by penicillin.

Ehrlich's work on immunity laid the foundations for the science of immunology. Early in his career he showed that the specific anti-toxic effect of immunizing serum (i.e. capable of antagonizing disease-producing bacterial substances) could be shown not only in animals but in the test-tube. In collaboration with Julius Morgenroth (1871–1924) he showed in 1899 that immune sera were effective

Photomicrograph of *Pasteurella pestis*.

Robert Koch. *Early twentieth-century engraving.*

The Anopheles mosquito.

Three drawings showing the preparation and inoculation of anti-diphtheria vaccine. *From a popular medical review of the late nineteenth century.*

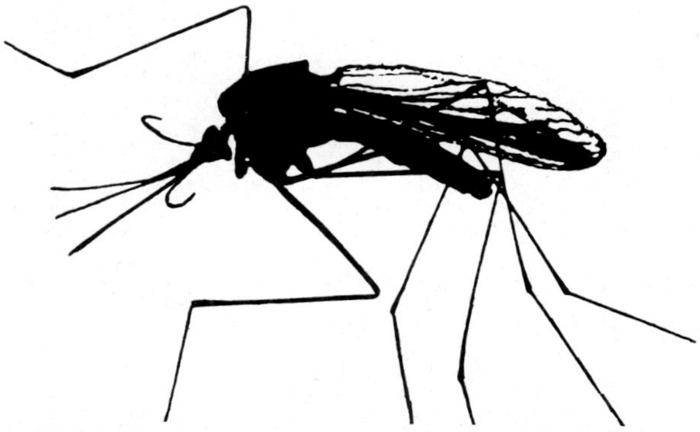

by virtue of a heat-stable 'immune body', which we now know to be the specific antibody to the particular disease, and a thermo-labile substance which they named 'complement'.

The actions of antibodies on harmful organisms were worked out by others. Thus Richard Pfeiffer (1858–1945) showed that in a guinea pig that had been immunized against cholera, the vibrios that caused the disease, when injected into the peritoneal cavity, were dissolved (bacteriolysis). The substances responsible for this process, bacteriolysins, were antibodies to the antigens of the cholera. In the reaction between antigen and antibody, 'complement', a substance also present in normal serum, was used up. This applied not only to bacteriolysis but also to such phenomena as agglutination and haemolysis, seen after transfusion of incompatible blood. Complement fixation, as this was called, was studied by Jean Baptiste Vincent Bordet (1870–1961), who with Octave Gengou (1875–1959) worked out the complement fixation test which formed the basis not only for the Wassermann reaction but also for such diseases as gonorrhoea and glanders.

Departing from his immunological observations and introducing concepts of chemistry to these studies, Ehrlich developed his side-chain theory, whereby the protein molecule was conceived as analogous to the six-carbon benzene ring whose formula was devised by August Kekulé (1829–1896). In this formula, unstable side-linkages are assumed to join together adjacent atoms of the molecule; in the case of proteins, unstable side-links could act as chemo-receptors, combine with bacterial toxins and neutralize them. The immune protein would appear in the blood in response to the presence of an antigen (an infecting agent, or incompatible red blood cell) and persist for as long as the stimulus remained. Although the side-chain theory has been superseded by the suggestions of Haurowitz and Linus Pauling, it remains one of great historical importance.

It followed that there were two possible means of protecting an individual against the effect of pathogenic organisms: active immunization, whereby a living organism of reduced virulence was introduced, and the individual manufactured his own antibodies in response to it, and passive immunization, whereby antibodies were given, in serum from an animal that had been infected.

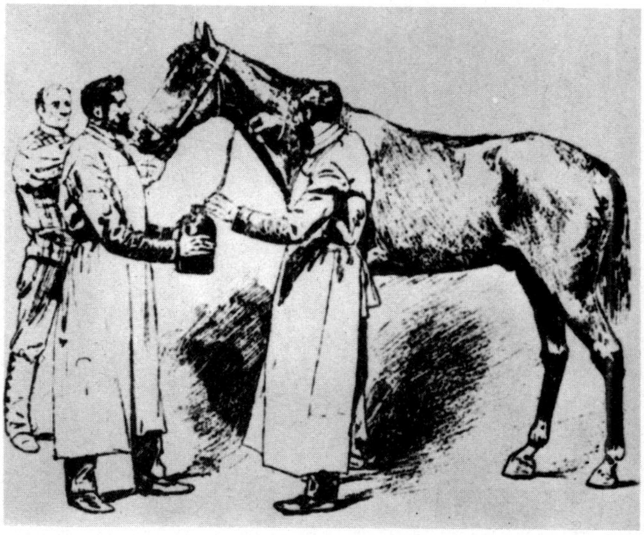

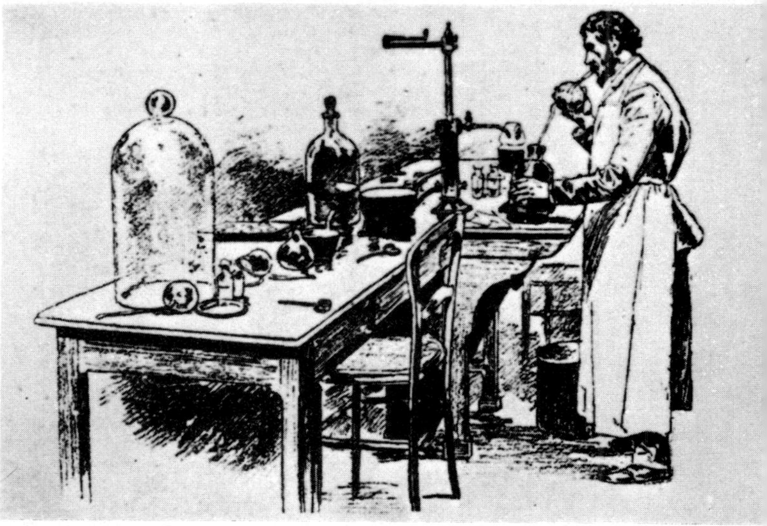

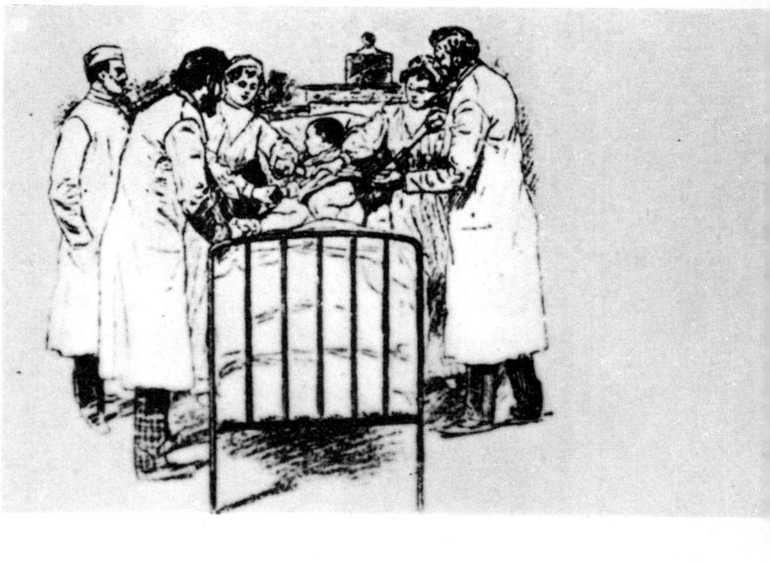

The end of the nineteenth century saw the discovery of a new type of micro-organism—the virus. Viruses are smaller than bacteria and have totally different biological and chemical properties. A few can be visualized poorly with the highest magnification of a light microscope, but it required the invention and development of the electron microscope for their fuller investigation. With the light microscope, a magnification of 1,800 times is all that can usefully be obtained; with the new instrument, in which an electron beam and magnets replace light rays and glass lenses, 180,000 times is a commonplace.

Study of viruses was prompted above all by a series of terrible epidemics in this century, which were traced back to these organisms. The worst was the great influenza pandemic of 1918 to 1919,

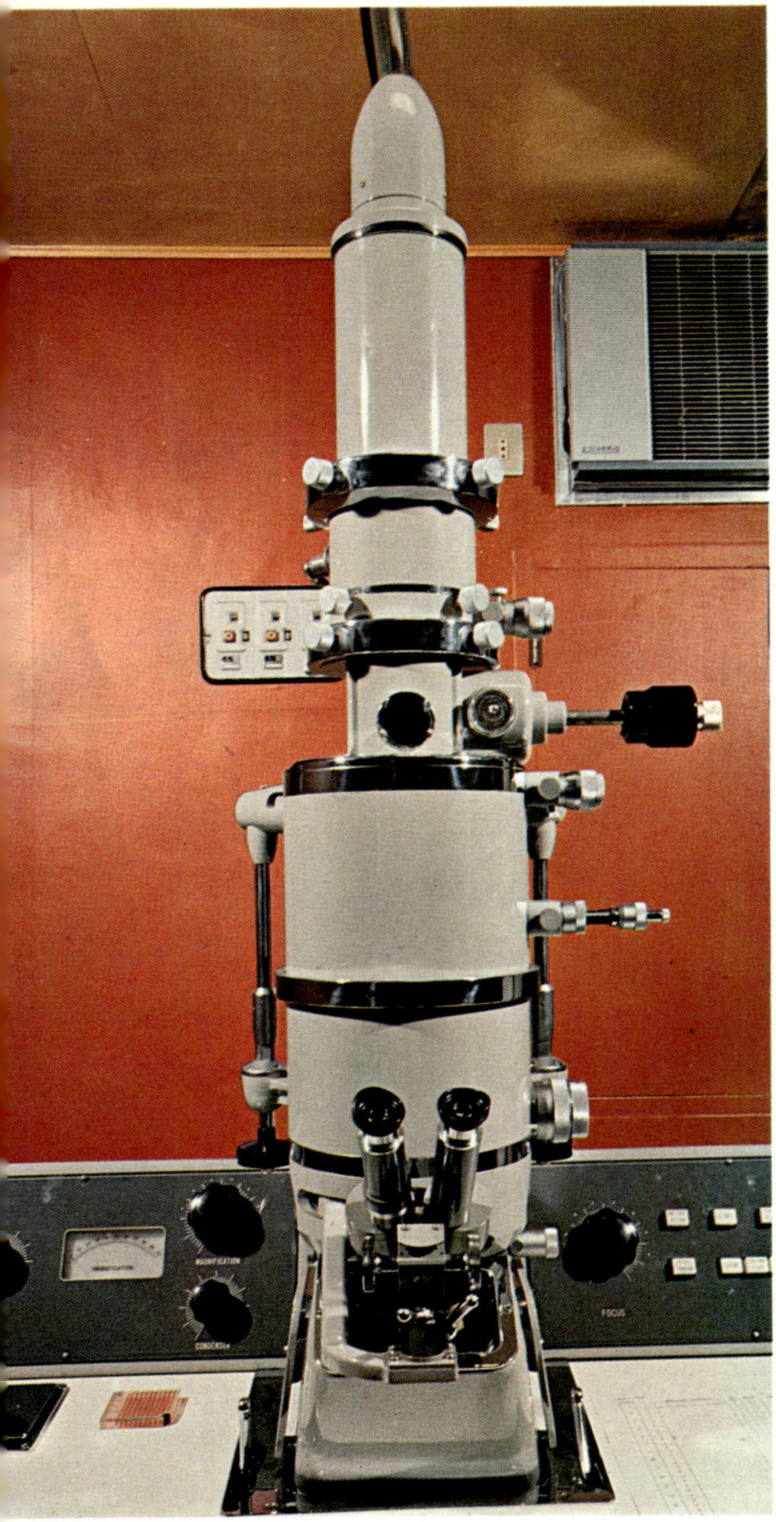

Jenner's work, of course, was the pioneer achievement in the former of these, while Pasteur had fought anthrax and rabies in the same way and Koch's tuberculin produced an active immune response. In the field of passive immunity, Behring and Kitasato's work was followed by treatments against plague and also the development of diagnostic tests for such conditions as diphtheria (the Schick test, 1913).

We have seen how the nineteenth century and the first years of the twentieth provided several of the means of achieving victory in the fight against infection, through the sciences of bacteriology, which characterized more and more organisms responsible for individual diseases, and immunology, which showed how the host responded to pathogens and enabled therapy to be devised to make best use of this response. It is now known that phagocytosis is the principal defence mechanism against bacteria, and so when the blood is deficient in normal white cells (as in some diseases of the bone marrow) the body falls prey to infections of all kinds. Phagocytosis probably removes the bacteria that have been made ineffective by antibodies, which are not often directly lethal. Other components in the serum necessary for the function of antibodies are 'complement', which has already been mentioned,

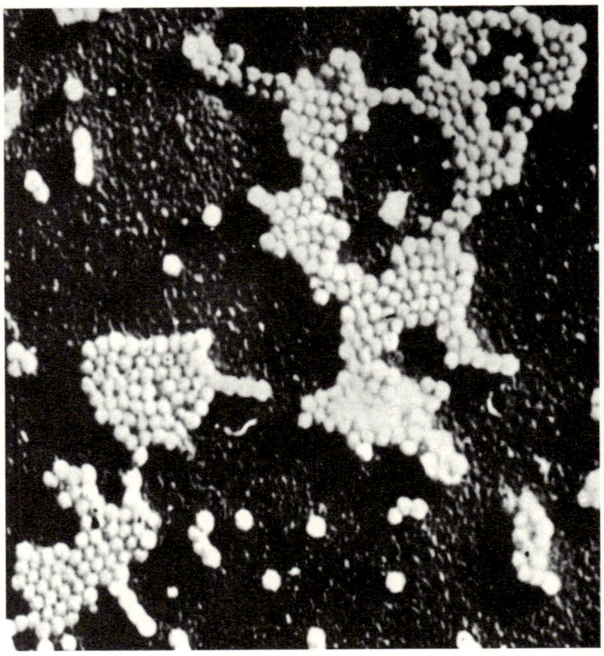

which spread throughout almost the entire world, killing some twnty-one million people. The first great medical victory against viruses was the production of an effective vaccine against poliomyelitis by Salk in 1954. This was followed by the Sabin vaccine, based on attenuated virus, which is taken orally. Both these vaccines act by stimulating the body's own defences to produce antibodies.

Electron microscope.

Poliomyelitis virus. *Electron microscope photograph.*

and 'opsonin', a group of substances discovered by Sir Almroth Edward Wright (1861–1947) which are probably antibodies that facilitate phagocytosis.

The serum of a healthy adult will contain very many different antibodies, each specific for a single disease: thus the antibodies of diphtheria will not give protection against tetanus. Antibodies are all proteins of the gamma-globulin group; all have a molecular weight of 160,000 to 1,000,000 and are identical chemically, so the differences which confer disease-specificity are very small. They are all produced by cells in the bone marrow and lymph nodes. The Australian Sir Frank Macfarlane Burnett (*b.* 1899) has remarked on the paradox that the self-same cells in the body which destroy worn-out cells (like red blood cells) without the production of antibodies also get rid of foreign organisms with antibody production. This tolerance to one's own proteins is a learned reaction, acquired in the foetus before birth; injection of an antigen into a foetus in utero produces a lifelong tolerance to the antigen. Conversely, it is today believed that in certain diseases previously of unknown aetiology, the body loses its tolerance to a particular tissue, which is therefore damaged by immune processes. Among such 'auto-immune' conditions are Hashimoto's disease of the thyroid (named after the Japanese pathologist who first described it in 1912) and pernicious anaemia, in which the stomach lining is damaged, thereby impairing the absorption of vitamin B_{12}.

Today immunology has a bearing on still other aspects of medicine, including cancer treatment and spare-part surgery (because grafted donor tissues and organs tend to be rejected by the immune responses of the healthy body–this problem is discussed further on page 289).

Two further fields of achievement against infections have been the recognition of the role of insects in the transmission of disease and the development of virology.

Sir Patrick Manson (1844–1922), the 'father of modern tropical medicine', brought the existence of insect vectors (transmitters) to the attention of the medical world with a paper in 1877 in the *Medical Report of the Imperial Maritime Customs, China* in which he showed that a minute parasitic worm found in the human bloodstream–the cause of elephantiasis–was transmitted to man by the mosquito *Culex fatigans,* in which it developed. The principle of insect transmission of disease, suggested long before in Susruta's writings, was soon applied to the investigation of other disorders. In 1882 Carlos Juan Finlay (1833–1915) reported evidence of the part played by the mosquito *Aëdes aegypti* in the spread of yellow fever in Cuba, and this was proved by Walter Reed and others in 1900. The causative agent of malaria, a protozoal plasmodium, was first seen by Charles Louis Alphonse Laveran (1845–1922) of Algiers in 1880, and in 1898 Sir Ronald Ross (1857–1932) found the parasite in the stomach of the Anopheles mosquito after it had fed on the blood of malarial patients, thus proving that the insect was responsible for the transmission of the disease. This knowledge was at once applied to the prevention of the disease; Ross won a Nobel prize in 1902 and Laveran in 1907.

A new type of micro-organism began to be recognized in the first decades of the present century–Rickettsia, which are intermediate between bacteria and viruses in their size and characteristics. Charles Nicolle (1866–1936) showed in 1910 that the agent of infection of typhus fever was the body louse. It has already been noted how this terrible epidemic disease was given one of its first accurate descriptions by Fracastoro, the author of *Syphilis,* who at the same time enunciated the modern doctrine of the specific characters and infectious nature of fevers. The organism responsible for typhus remained unidentified for over 350 years. In 1909 Howard Ricketts (1871–1910) demonstrated the cause of a related disease, Rocky Mountain spotted fever, by examining the blood from infected patients. He died of typhus in the following year. In 1916 Henrique da Rocha-Lima (1879–1945) at last identified the agent responsible for typhus, which he named *Rickettsia prowazeki,* after Ricketts and another victim Prowazek.

The term virus for centuries signified a poison produced by living beings and causing infectious disease. Viruses have been identified in the last forty years in large numbers in a way comparable to bacteriological discoveries of the end of the nineteenth century. This recent success is the result of special laboratory methods and particularly the use of the electron microscope–which makes visible minute particles beyond the resolving power of the ordinary instrument–stimulated by a number of terrible twentieth-century epidemics.

The most memorable of these was the great

Perhaps the greatest landmark in the development of modern drugs was the discovery of penicillin by Alexander Fleming. In 1928, while studying a culture of staphylococci, Fleming noticed that a fungus which had contaminated the specimen caused the bacteria around it to disappear – the mould seemed to be destroying the staphylococci. This phenomenon was further investigated by Florey and Chain, who finally isolated penicillin in 1940. Soon, when its remarkable therapeutic properties became known, the drug was produced in the United States in huge quantities. In time, as drug-resistant bacteria evolved, there were developed numerous other antibiotics, as they are called, such as streptomycin and aureomycin.

Culture of Penicillium mould.

influenza pandemic of 1918 to 1919, which spread throughout Europe, Russia, Canada, South America, New Zealand, Australia, Africa, India, China and Japan, an estimated twenty-one million people dying of the disease (two million in Europe alone). The first wave, in June and July, affected many, but the ones to die were generally the old and those already ill. In October and November there were many more deaths from pneumonia, while in the following February a severe recurrence killed many more. The virus, which like all others passes through the finest filter (in contrast to bacteria), was transmitted to ferrets by Smith, Andrewes and Laidlaw in 1933, and cultured on developing eggs by Burnet two years later. This was virus A, which was found in London; a second virus, influenza B, was isolated in 1940 by Francis in New York.

Encephalitis lethargica or 'sleepy sickness' accompanied influenza, appearing in 1917 and continuing until 1926, when it virtually disappeared. It produced drowsiness, fits and coma, and if the patient recovered, a common sequel was a form of Parkinson's disease. Another virus disease of the nervous system is poliomyelitis. This was first described at the end of the eighteenth century, but its epidemic and infective nature was not recognized until the work of Medin (1890) and Wickman (1907). In 1909 Simon Flexner (1863–1946) and Paul A. Lewis (1879–1929) succeeded in producing paralysis in monkeys with virus derived from infected nasal secretion. Later the properties of the virus were fully established and several different varieties emerged; and in 1954 Jonas Salk introduced his vaccine, made from killed virus grown on monkey kidney cells and given by injection. More recently the oral Sabin vaccine, based on attenuated virus, has come into general use. These vaccines provide real protection; it should be remembered that viruses – from that of the common cold to smallpox – are unaffected by antibiotics and virtually the sole defence against them is a good level of antibodies.

The treatment of bacterial diseases with drugs began, as has been noted, with Ehrlich's salvarsan. Such early agents were toxic and not very effective, however, and it was not until 1935, with the introduction of Prontosil by Gerhard Domagk (1895–1964), that the era of modern chemotherapy could be said to have begun. Prontosil contained sulphanilamide, which had been synthesized as long before as 1908, and after Domagk several investigators worked out that the sulphonamide group in the compound was the effective part. In 1938 a new drug, sulphapyridine (M and B 693), was first used in the treatment of pneumonia, and since then this and many other sulphonamides have become an important and permanent part of the pharmacopoeia.

That many bacteria and fungi in the soil survive in the face of great competition for foodstuffs is a remarkable fact, and is due to their production of substances which spread into the surrounding soil and kill, or inhibit the growth of other species. This is the phenomenon of antibiosis and these substances are antibiotics. It was recognized for some time before Fleming's discovery of penicillin, for the physicist John Tyndall (1820–1893) observed in 1876 the selective bacteria-inhibiting action of Penicillium mould, while Pasteur and Joubert showed in the next year that air-borne organisms inhibited anthrax.

Sir Alexander Fleming (1881–1955) made his first contribution to microbiology when he discovered lysozyme, which could dissolve living bacteria, in tears and egg white. His historic chance observation was made in 1928, when he noticed that contamination of a culture of staphylococci on an agar plate with the fungus *Penicillium notatum* caused colonies around the mould to disappear. Fleming continued his work at St Mary's Hospital, Paddington, London, for a while and published his observations in 1929. Investigation of the problem was pursued at Oxford by Sir Howard Florey and Ernst Chain, and penicillin was isolated in 1940. Within a few years it was being produced in America from cultures in vats of thousands of gallons of nutrient solution, and its use in the war greatly reduced Allied casualties. The emergence of drug-resistant bacterial strains was noted first with sulphonamides and then with penicillin; the discovery of other antibiotics, like streptomycin (introduced in 1944 by Schatz, Bugie and Waksman), chloramphenicol (Smadel and Jackson, 1947) and aureomycin (Duggar and others, 1948), as well as the synthesis of new variants of penicillin, has partly overcome this problem, and today effective drugs are available for the treatment of nearly all bacterial diseases.

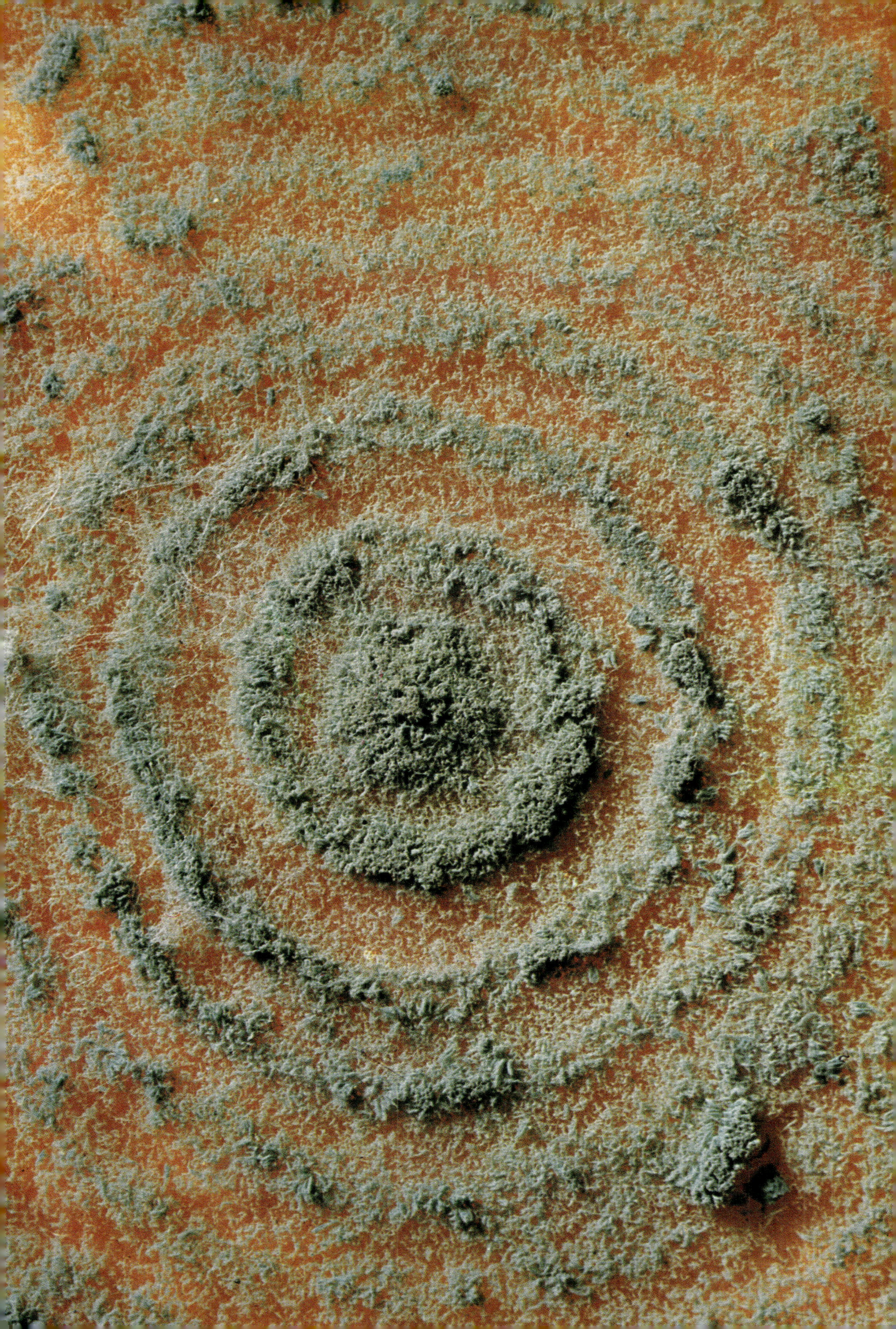

X-rays and radiotherapy

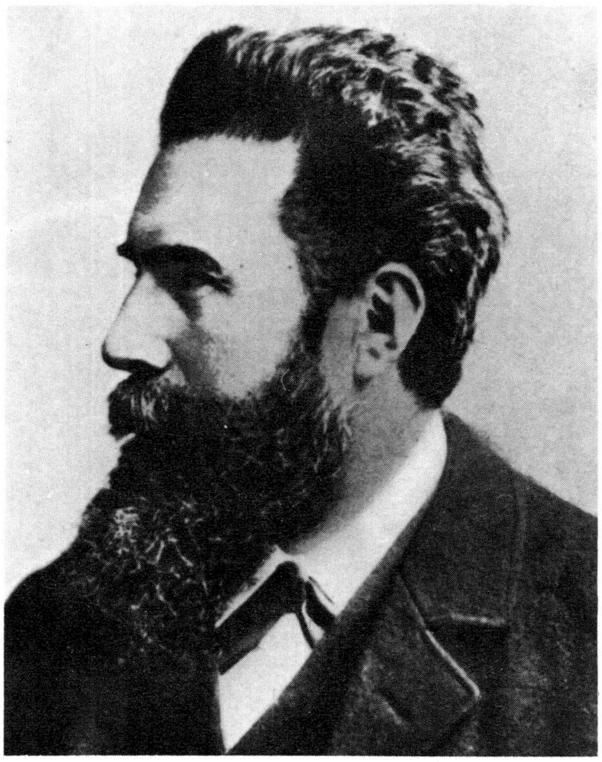

Scientific research has made contributions of inestimable value to the progress of medicine through pharmacology, immunology, endocrinology and chemotherapy. Of equal importance in general terms, but of paramount value in medical and surgical practice, is radiology. Of all the means of diagnosing the site and nature of physical diseases, X-rays are the most important because they enable the anatomy of the internal organs and tissues of the body to be seen and pathological changes to be revealed.

Wilhelm Konrad Roentgen (1845–1923) began studying the electrical phenomena described by Crookes and Hertz when he was professor of physics at the university of Würzburg. His experiments involved the passage of electricity through vacuum tubes; his momentous discovery occurred on the evening of 8 November, 1895, when he noted that, while passing current through such a tube, a sheet of cardboard coated with barium platinocyanide was shining brightly in his unlit laboratory. The physicist found that this fluorescence was a result of radiation coming from the tube. He called the radiation X-rays, because of the unknown nature of the phenomenon; he soon found that the X-rays

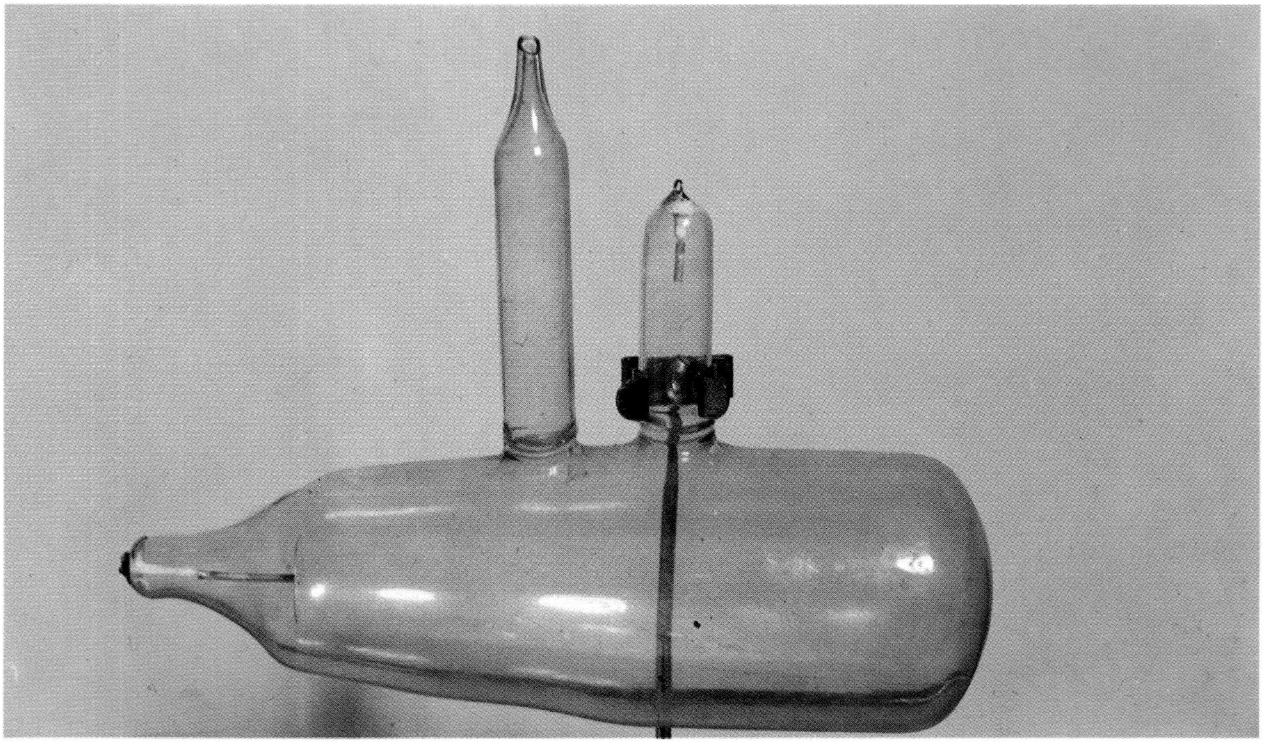

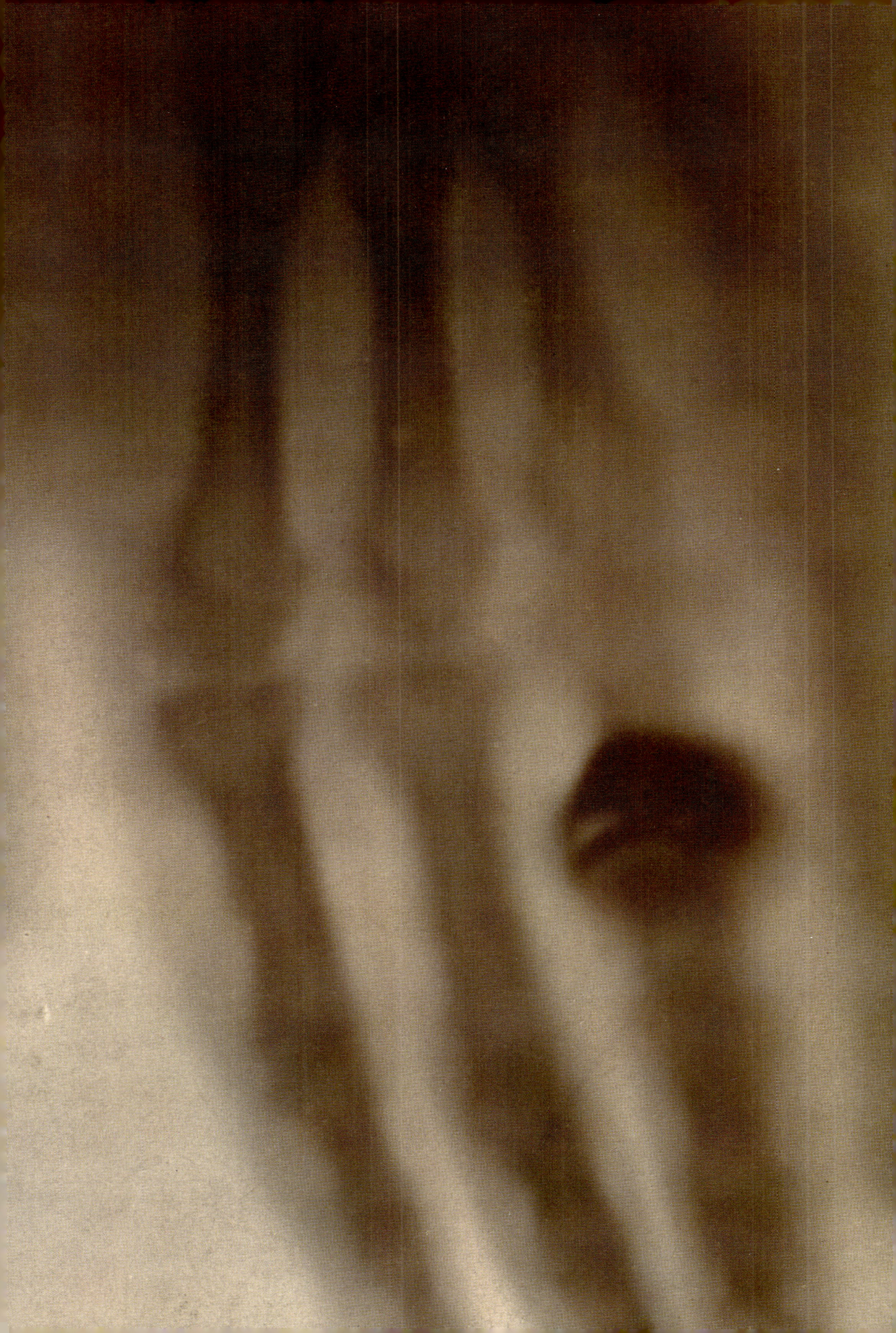

Previous pages:
Wilhelm Konrad Roentgen.

One of the first X-ray tubes. *Science Museum, London.*

First radiograph by Roentgen (22.12.1895), of his wife's hand. *Institute of Physics, University of Wurzburg.*

These pages:
Radiography room at the St Louis hospital, Paris, at the turn of the century.

Radiology apparatus built by Drault in 1896 on the orders of Antoine Béclère.

had the property of penetrating dense bodies opaque to light waves and giving an image on a photographic plate as well as on a fluorescent screen.

Thus he put solid objects between the Crookes tube and a wooden box in which he had placed a plate, and discovered that an impression could be recorded on the plate, on which showed the form of each object. In another experiment, the physicist used his own hand: the bones were clearly shown on the plate, while the soft tissues were scarcely noticeable, as can be seen in his early photograph of his wife's hand, with a ring on the fourth finger. On 28 December, 1895, Roentgen reported his sensational findings in his *Preliminary Communication to the President of the Physical-Medical Society of Würzburg,* fully aware of the implications of these mysterious rays for diagnosis, and within a few weeks his discovery had been greeted all over the world as one of the most important in medical history.

X-rays were used immediately in hospitals to diagnose fractures, bone diseases and foreign bodies. The first apparatus was primitive and emitted weak radiation; to obtain a radiograph it was necessary to allow an exposure time of nearly thirty minutes. It was soon noticed that X-rays caused unpleasant and slowly healing skin burns. The necessity of reducing the exposure time was at once recognized, and in 1913 this was achieved with the introduction of the heated cathode which emitted a greater quantity of electrons of higher energy than a cold cathode. During the First World War, ample use was found for the improved equipment, which required an exposure of a few seconds, in locating bullets and shell fragments.

Improvement had continued and today X-ray films require only two-hundredths of a second exposure and give pictures of higher definition. Technical advances involve filters, diaphragms and more efficient fluorescent materials, on the one hand, and new investigative methods on the other.

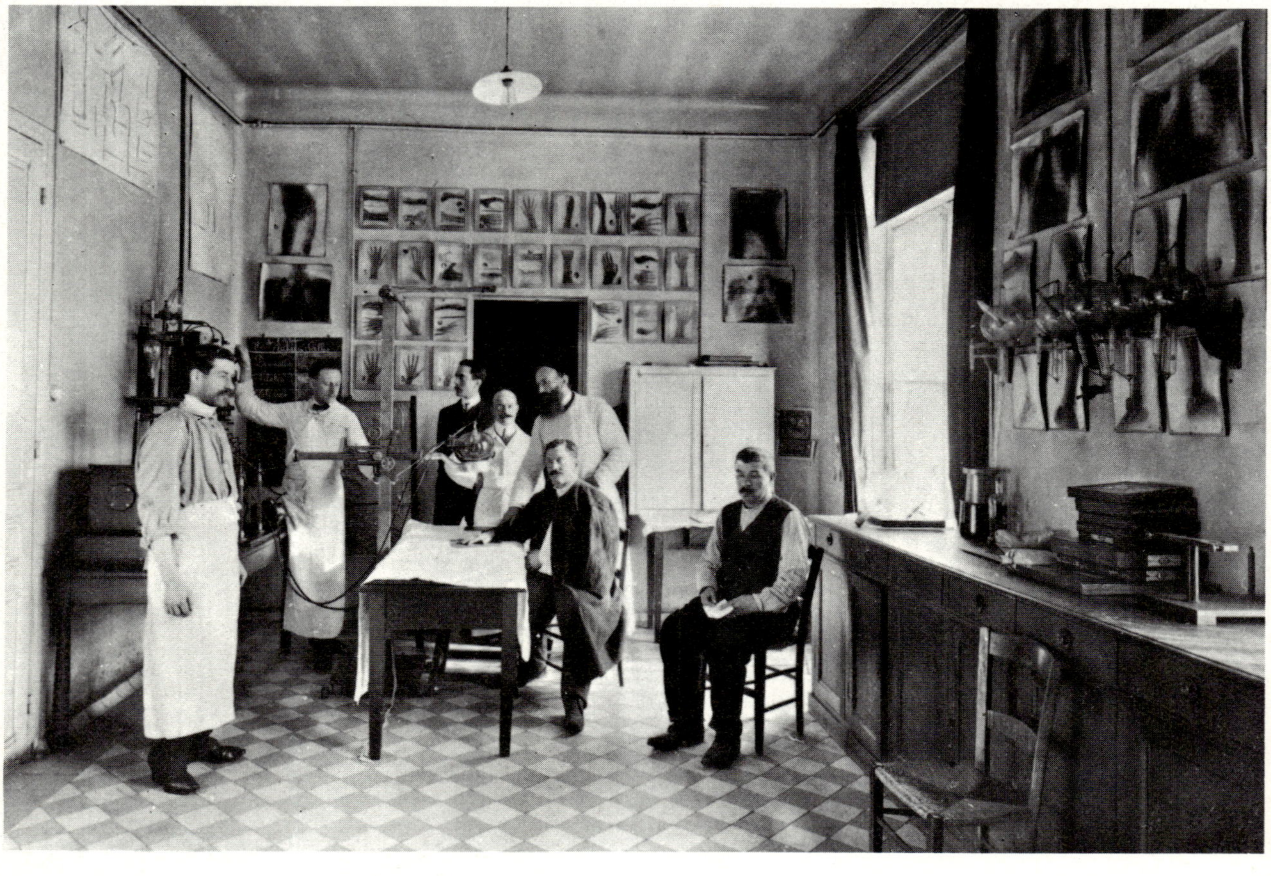

It was a chance discovery by a German physicist that gave modern medicine one of its most powerful tools – X-rays. While studying certain electrical phenomena, which involved passing electricity through a vacuum tube, Wilhelm Roentgen noticed a fluorescence which he realized was produced by radiation coming from the tube. He found that this radiation could penetrate bodies opaque to light waves and produce an image on a photographic plate as well as on a fluorescent screen. He made many X-ray plates, including one of his wife's hand, in which the bones and a ring could be clearly seen, with the soft tissues visible only as a shadow. Very soon, X-ray equipment was installed in many hospitals for the diagnosis of fractures and bone disease and the detection of foreign bodies.

W. B. Cannon (1871–1945), while a medical student, introduced the use of bismuth – which is radio-opaque – for visualizing the intestines and stomach of animals. Contrast radiography has developed from this, and now barium sulphate taken by mouth is used to outline the gastro-intestinal tract, while iodinated substances can be injected into veins to show the kidneys and into arteries to show the circulation in any part of the body, including the brain. The various body cavities can also be outlined by the injection of air. Tomography enables a plane section of any organ to be visualized.

The hands and exposed parts of the first radiologists suffered chronic and painful rashes and burns; many of these pioneers, ignorant of the powerful biological effect of X-rays, in fact died of skin cancer and leukaemia. Doctors began to use the new rays to treat skin diseases shortly after they were discovered, and then to treat skin cancer, and a few years later, when their powerful actions on germinal or rapidly dividing cells were known, to treat a wide range of malignant diseases. With lead shields and accurate dosimetry, radiotherapy became practical, although deep-seated lesions could not be dealt with satisfactorily at first because of the poor penetration of the rays and severe skin effects.

Natural radioactivity was discovered in uranium salts by the great French physicist Henri Becquerel, Nobel prize-winner for 1903. Becquerel found that a photographic plate was blackened by the invisible rays emitted by uranium salts even when wrapped in a layer of black paper and of silver. In 1898 Pierre Curie and his assistant, later his wife, Maria Sklodovska, isolated polonium and discovered radium. Pierre purposely produced a burn on his arm with radium, which was soon found to be destructive to animal tissues and effective in the treatment of tumours. The Curies were awarded a Nobel prize in 1904. Like Roentgen, prize-winner in 1901, they refused to patent their discovery. When her husband died in 1906, Marie Curie succeeded to his chair of physics at the Sorbonne and in 1910 she achieved the isolation of metallic radium.

The major problem of radiotherapy was to reach the tumour with radiation strong enough to attack or even destroy it, while damaging the normal cells as little as possible. As we have noted, the first X-rays from low-voltage apparatus had limited therapeutic value because of skin damage. The first machine capable of emitting radiation which could reach comparatively deep-seated tumours, such as those of the breast, was of 250,000 volts. Before the Second World War more powerful and bulkier machines were built, including some with voltages in the millions; in use these proved to be disappointing. After the war, radiotherapy entered a new phase thanks to electronic technology and isotope chemistry.

The development of the therapeutic uses of radium paralleled that of X-rays, whose effects on tissues are similar. In the form of radioactive needles and seeds, implanted into malignant tissue, it has found an important place in the treatment especially of tumours of the cervix, bladder and tongue.

Since the discovery in 1931 of artificial radioactivity by Irene Curie and her husband Frédéric

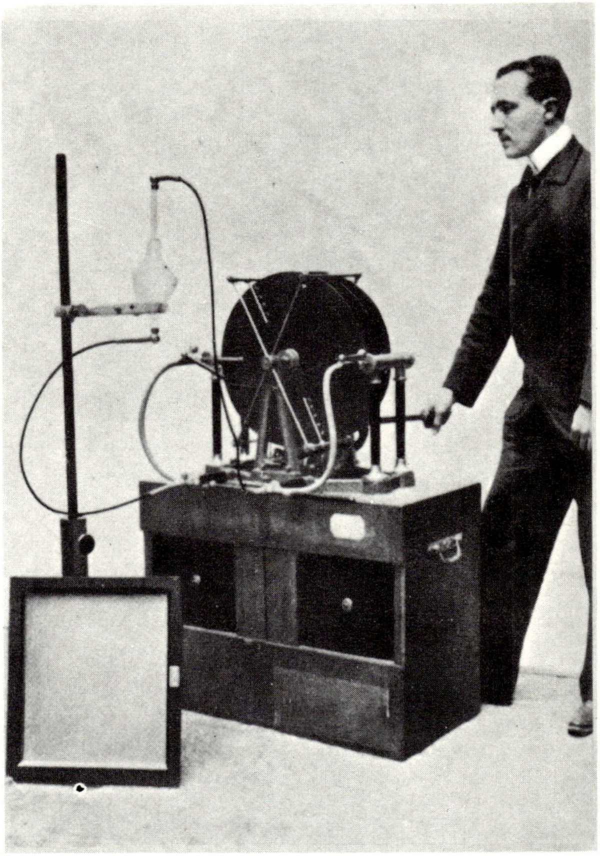

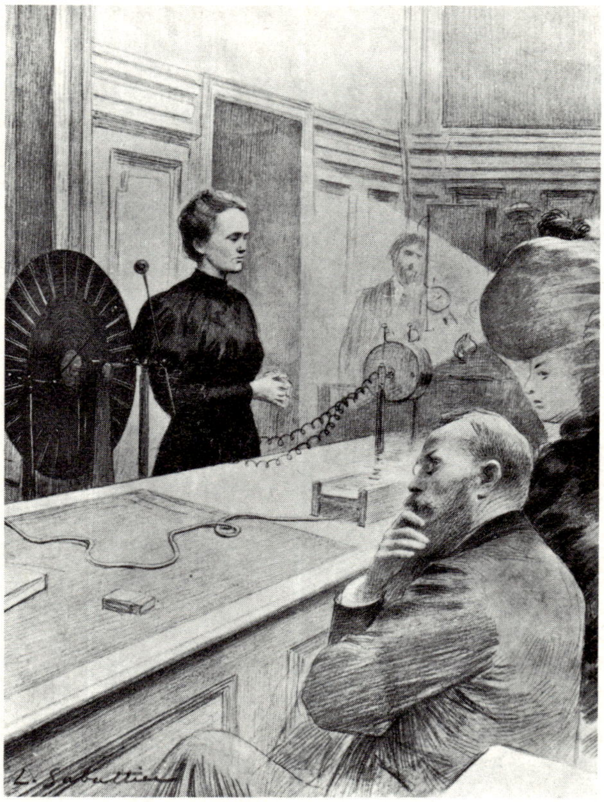

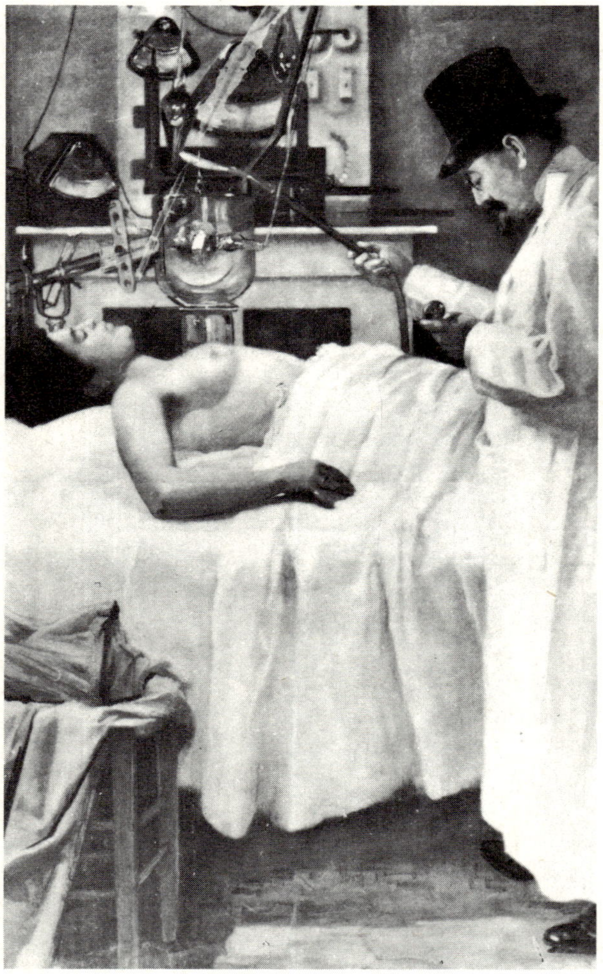

It was soon noticed that X-rays caused unpleasant and slow-healing skin burns, and the need for shorter exposure times was recognized. This was achieved in 1913, with the introduction of the heated cathode, which emitted a greater quantity of electrons than Roentgen's original cold cathode. At the same time, it was seen that the damaging effect of the radiation could have positive applications: soon X-rays were

Joliot, radioactive isotopes have found innumerable uses in medical research, diagnosis and treatment.

From the chemical viewpoint, radioactive isotopes are indistinguishable from stable isotopes of the same atomic number, but they differ in their emission of alpha and beta particles (helium nuclei and electrons) and gamma rays (X-rays). Their presence is thus detectable with appropriate apparatus, and they can take part in the body in the same processes as their stable counterparts.

The use of minute quantities of isotopes as tracers to outline metabolic pathways in the body began with the work of G von Hevesy, and has led to the concept of 'the dynamic state of body constituents' (whereby all the molecules of the tissues are in a constant state of flux) as well as detailed knowledge of the metabolism of fats, carbohydrates, proteins and electrolytes. Substances such as iron, hormones or drugs can be 'labelled' and their fate followed through the body. Information about the growth and multiplication of cells can be obtained by the use of nucleic acid precursors containing radioactive hydrogen or carbon.

In diagnosis, isotopes are used to measure abnormal activity of various parts of the body. Radioactive iodine is taken up by the thyroid, and after a patient has drunk a small quantity of this substance the gland can be scanned for uptake. Other radioactive substances are concentrated in tumours, and this fact is of particular value in the localization of brain tumours. Red blood cells can be tagged and their life span in the body calculated in some cases of anaemia. Abnormal kidney blood flow can be investigated by the excretion of a labelled compound. These and many other uses indicate the importance of isotopes as diagnostic tools.

From the point of view of therapy, the chief use of an isotope is that of iodine in cases where the thyroid gland is overactive. Here a much larger quantity is used than in diagnosis; the isotope accumulates in the thyroid and the rays it emits damage the hormone-producing cells. As has been mentioned, isotopes have supplanted high-voltage X-rays: telecobalt therapy utilizes the emission from an unstable form of cobalt to irradiate deep tumours intensely for a short period. This technique has the advantage of reducing radiation damage to neighbouring tissues.

being used with some success in treating skin cancer.

Natural radioactivity was found in uranium salts by Becquerel and later radium was discovered by the Curies. The use of radium and later of artificial radioisotopes extended the scope of radiotherapy, especially in the treatment of deep-seated tumours. The isotopes are also used as 'labels' on substances being investigated in the body.

Marie Curie inaugurating her course on radioactivity at the Sorbonne, Paris.
Early attempt to treat cancer with X-rays, by Dr Chicolot. *Painted by the doctor in 1908.*
Measuring radio-iodine in a patient's thyroid gland using a Geiger counter.

Following pages:
Artificial valves in the heart. (The X-ray photograph also shows part of the vertebral column, the ribs and the shadow of the breasts.)

Another therapeutic use of cell-damaging ionizing radiation is in suppressing the immune mechanisms of the body and so enabling grafts of foreign tissue to be accepted. As explained previously, antibody production will cause rejection of tissue from any other individual (except an identical twin) and irradiation of the whole body combined with cortisone and other drugs which counter the immune response, is at present essential to the success of spare-part surgery.

The cornea has been grafted from one person to another with good results on innumerable occasions. The operation was first performed by E. von Hippel (1867–1939) in 1888 and brought into general use through the work of the American R. Castroviejo and the Russian V. P. Filatov. The cornea has no blood vessels and so immune mechanisms hardly come into action. With organs such as the kidney, liver and heart, where transplantation is technically possible, there is a very different state of affairs.

The American Nobel prize-winner Alexis Carrel (1873–1944) began kidney transplantation in 1902 and reported his results in 1908. He grafted kidneys from one cat to another; most of his animals died rapidly but one survived for two months. Following this pioneering achievement, years of experimental study culminated in the first human graft in 1950 by R. H. Lawler. Since then, improved techniques, tissue typing and immunosuppressive drugs have allowed successful transplants from corpses and unrelated donors.

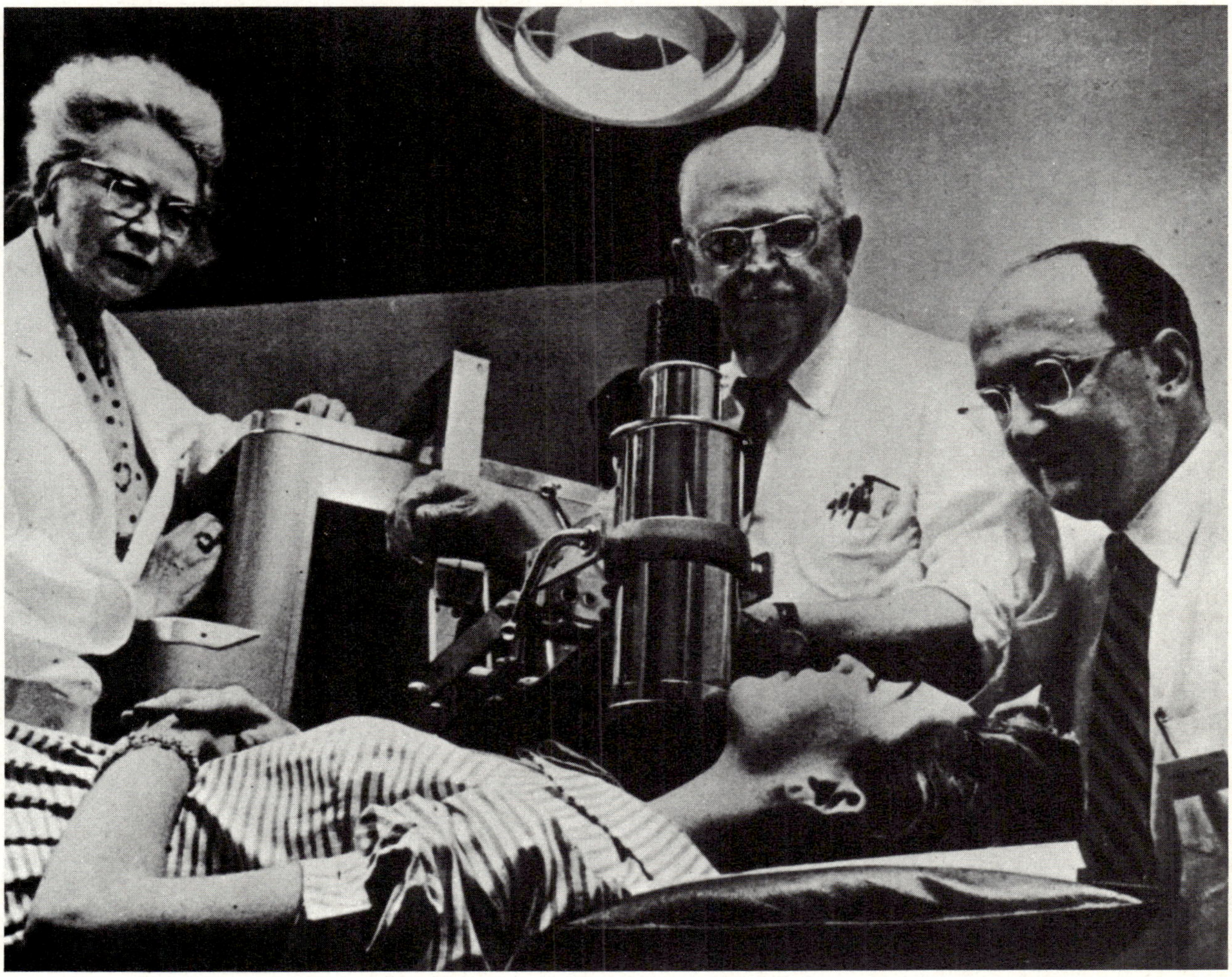

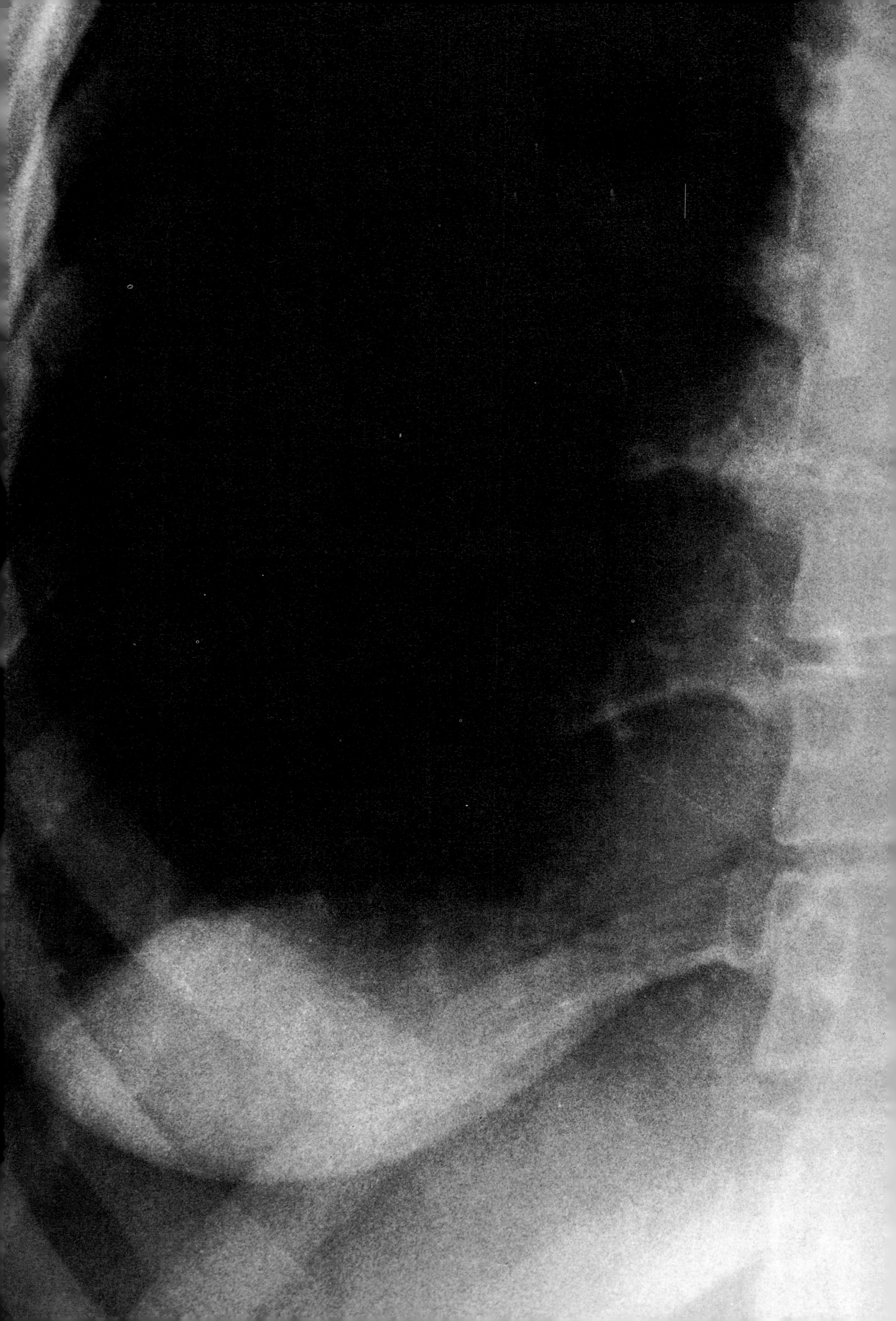

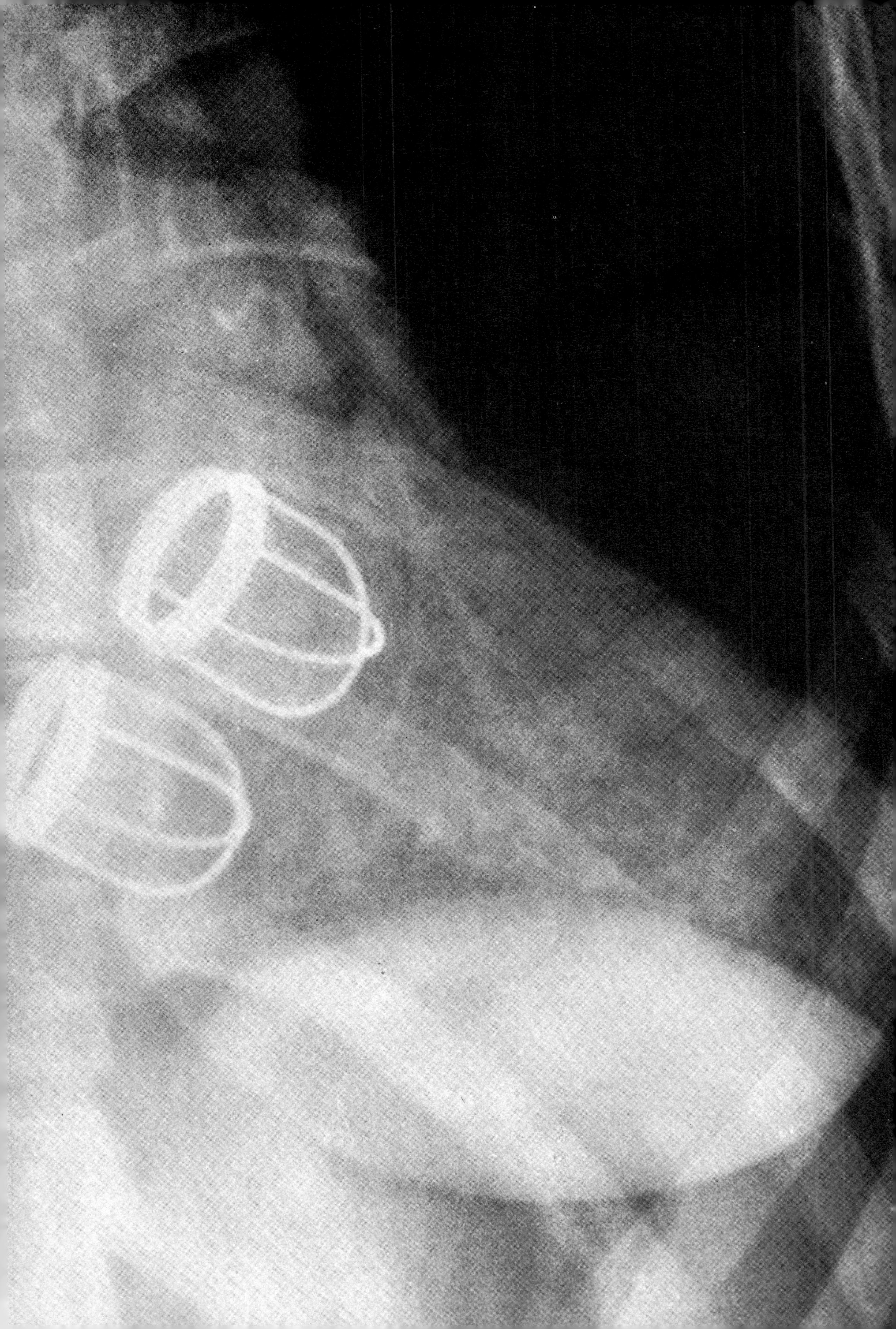

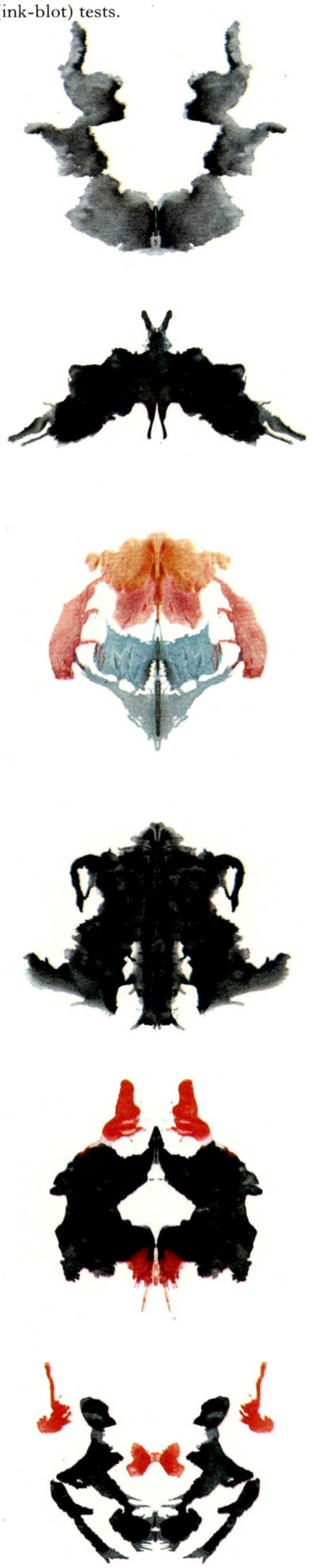

Rorschach (ink-blot) tests.

Nervous and mental diseases

What we know to be mental illness belonged, for early man, to the sphere of the supernatural. The earliest psychiatry was conceived in terms of spirit possession and the driving out of demons, and the most ancient psychotherapeutic procedures involved charms and amulets which incorporated magical powers of sacred animals and embodied health-giving properties. Amulets protected from evil not only individuals but also whole communities, and some, now with special religious significance such as phylacteries and scapulars, survive to the present day. However, through the centuries the vehicles of faith and magic in healing gradually changed from material to ritual, from precious objects to secret words and formulae and mystical numbers, while the civilized world endowed its religions with therapeutic powers.

Faith-healing, stimulated by the spread of Christianity, involved a simplification of primitive magical treatment; as faith alone was sufficient to produce a cure, the various symbolic vehicles of healing could be cut out. This did not occur all at once, and for many centuries pagan wizardry and medical folklore were linked in healing with spiritual abstraction. The church attempted to substitute exorcisms for magical formulae and herbal preparations, but the leeches, or lay wizard-doctors, remained popular, especially in Britain. A collection of their writings from before the Norman Conquest includes a psychiatric prescription: 'When a devil possesses the man or controls him from within with disease; a spew drink or emetic, lupin, bishopwort, henbane, corpleek: pound these together, add ale for a liquid, let it stand for a night, add fifty bibcorns of cathartic grains and holy water – to be drunk out of a church bell.'

Leechdom gradually built up an enormous collection of remedies, perpetuated by oral tradition and slowly becoming mingled with fragments of astrology, prayer and mumbo-jumbo. Some of it persists in the form of household cures, but as a therapeutic corpus it ceased to exist when the Church proclaimed that it alone had the power to work miraculous cures through the exorcism of demons. Nevertheless, in such treatments as 'cramp-rings' for epilepsy, made from coins offered on Good Friday and blessed by prayer and sacred inscriptions, the new religion showed its indebtedness to the old learning.

The study of the phenomena of mental illness at

For primitive man, mental disease and physical disease were one. Both were due to the possession of the victim by evil spirits, so that treatment was directed towards ridding him of his demon. The earliest psychiatry thus involved magic and ritual, embodied to some extent in amulets and material charms. For a long period after the rise of Christianity, spiritual treatment, or faith-healing, and the charm-laden medicine of folklore coexisted and were used alike to help the mentally ill. But as the church became more powerful and authoritarian, unorthodoxy was suppressed and folk remedies were stigmatized as witchcraft, as indeed were manifestations of psychiatric illness. It was only with the Renaissance, and the victory of knowledge over superstition, that a more rational attitude was entertained.

a rational and scientific level began with Hippocrates, who, in asserting that all disease resulted from natural causes, remarked that the 'sacred' disease epilepsy was no more divine in origin than any other, and to regard it as such was merely ignorance. The influence of Hippocrates was felt centuries later in Rome, when a humanist movement developed at the end of the pre-Christian era. The writings of Celsus are especially important in this context and *De re medica* includes a chapter on mental disorders with systematic clinical observation and therapy; treatments of many disorders are admirable in their directness and practicality, but by advocating the use of starvation, beating and chains for the violent or excited patient Celsus merely expresses his frustrations (shared with psychiatrists in the next eighteen centuries).

After the fall of the Roman Empire and the passage of medical learning into the Islamic-Jewish schools, rational psychiatry stood still as magic played a prominent part in treatment, while in western Europe healing by faith lay in the hands of the Church and through it the King and the monasteries.

With the development of closely knit urban communities, the persistence of superstition and the spread of epidemics, some of which were entirely hysterical and most aggravated by hysteria, mental illness became a mass problem; while previously it was possible to desert the sick individual, leaving the ill to their own resources, to wander or to rot, now whole populations were affected and the inability of the Church to control the situation resulted in the persecution of anti-authoritarian or nonconformist elements in the society. Thus there arose in the Middle Ages the science of witchcraft, a discipline which attempted to explain in terms of demon-possession what at large the Church could not control and in individual terms criminality, psychoses, dementia, impotence and hysteria. Since mental illnesses became recognized as manifestations of Satan, the persecution of witches by the organized Church drew attention away from the empirical study of psychiatric disturbances. This began again only with the Renaissance, when the spread of anatomical and physiological knowledge strengthened medicine and enabled such men as Johann Weyer (1515–1576) to expose the fallacies of demonology and the Malleus Maleficarum. Weyer stressed that cases should be regarded as individuals and suggested rational treatment to follow a diagnosis made after careful observation.

Neurology, the branch of medicine which deals with functions and disturbances of the brain, spinal cord and nerves, took a step forward with the Renaissance, but the ideas of the previous millennium were replaced relatively slowly. Galen recognized that motion and sensation, the two basic qualities of animal life, were related to the nervous system, and he distinguished motor from sensory nerves and ascribed to the brain the controlling influence over these functions. As has been noted, his writings show some remarkable neurological observations, but his concept of the transformation of vital spirit into animal spirit in the rete mirabilis, unsupported in man by anatomical evidence, was upheld into the sixteenth century and led even Vesalius into error. In the seventeenth and early eighteenth centuries, however, Willis and Morgagni added greatly to the knowledge of the workings of the brain, but at the same time the problem of the mind-brain relationship remained obscure and there was little rationalization of psychiatric treatment. Thus Willis, remembered today for his work on the cerebral circulation and for his recognition of the brain as the seat of the will as well as the mind, was nevertheless a demonologist and advocated forcible methods for dealing with the mentally ill.

The humanist ideas of the second half of the eighteenth century and the rebirth of the concept of citizenship altered the philosophy of disease treatment, hospital care and the rights of the mentally sick, while new analytical trains of thought bore neurology along novel paths. An important name is that of William Cullen (1710–1790), the spiritual head of the sect of 'neuropathologists' and a great influence for many years. By asserting that 'life, so far as it is corporeal, consists in the excitement of the nervous system and especially of the brain, which unites the different parts, and forms them into a whole', he paved the way for modern neurophysiology and the work of Pavlov and Sherrington.

At this time doctors began systematically to differentiate and classify psychiatric diseases in the manner customary for physical complaints. This led to a nosology, the means of a more precise diagnosis, without which all treatment would be empirical. Violent methods gave way to therapy designed for helpless patients in need of care, and

An early voice on the side of reason was that of Johann Weyer, who condemned witch-hunting and who regarded the mentally sick in the way that any doctor should regard any patient. The first attempts to classify psychiatric disease were made in the eighteenth century, and at the same time restraint, starvation, close confinement and other violent methods began to be supplanted by more humane treatment. Among the names remembered for their liberal achievements are William Tuke and Philippe Pinel. The first, a Quaker, founded in 1794 a retreat in York, while the latter, physician at the Bicêtre and Salpêtrière in Paris, humanized the treatments of patients under his care.

Knowledge of the workings of the physical nervous system, as distinct from the mind, advanced rapidly

this change of attitude on the part of physicians and society accompanied the transformation of 'madhouses' into 'asylums', well-regulated hospitals where the insane might be nursed rather than filthy prisons where they could be left to die. This movement began in Italy with Vincenzo Chiarugi in 1774 and in England it was initiated by William Tuke, a Quaker tea merchant who founded a retreat at York in 1794. In France, Philippe Pinel was the first to apply to the insane the humanitarian principles of the revolutionaries. Appointed physician to the asylum at Bicêtre in 1793, he proceeded to release his fettered charges and showed, with his superior practical sense, that insane people, like any sick human beings rather than beasts, could be treated by physicians without loss of dignity. He stated that moral persuasion was better than intimidation and force, and that strong personality on the part of the physician was the greatest factor in success. He put great store in good administration, and having reformed the Bicêtre he moved to the Salpêtrière where by careful observation and note-taking he gradually built up a method of clinical psychiatry.

In the early nineteenth century psychiatry and neurology were developing in a number of other ways. Mesmerism, despite being surrounded at first by spectacular showmanship, was to provide a powerful psychotherapeutic tool. Phrenology, whereby moral and intellectual qualities were supposedly ascertainable from a study of the external configuration of the skull, was initiated by Franz Joseph Gall (1758–1828) and elaborated to extreme length by his followers; its value is in allowing for the first time that different regions of the brain might serve specific purposes, and from

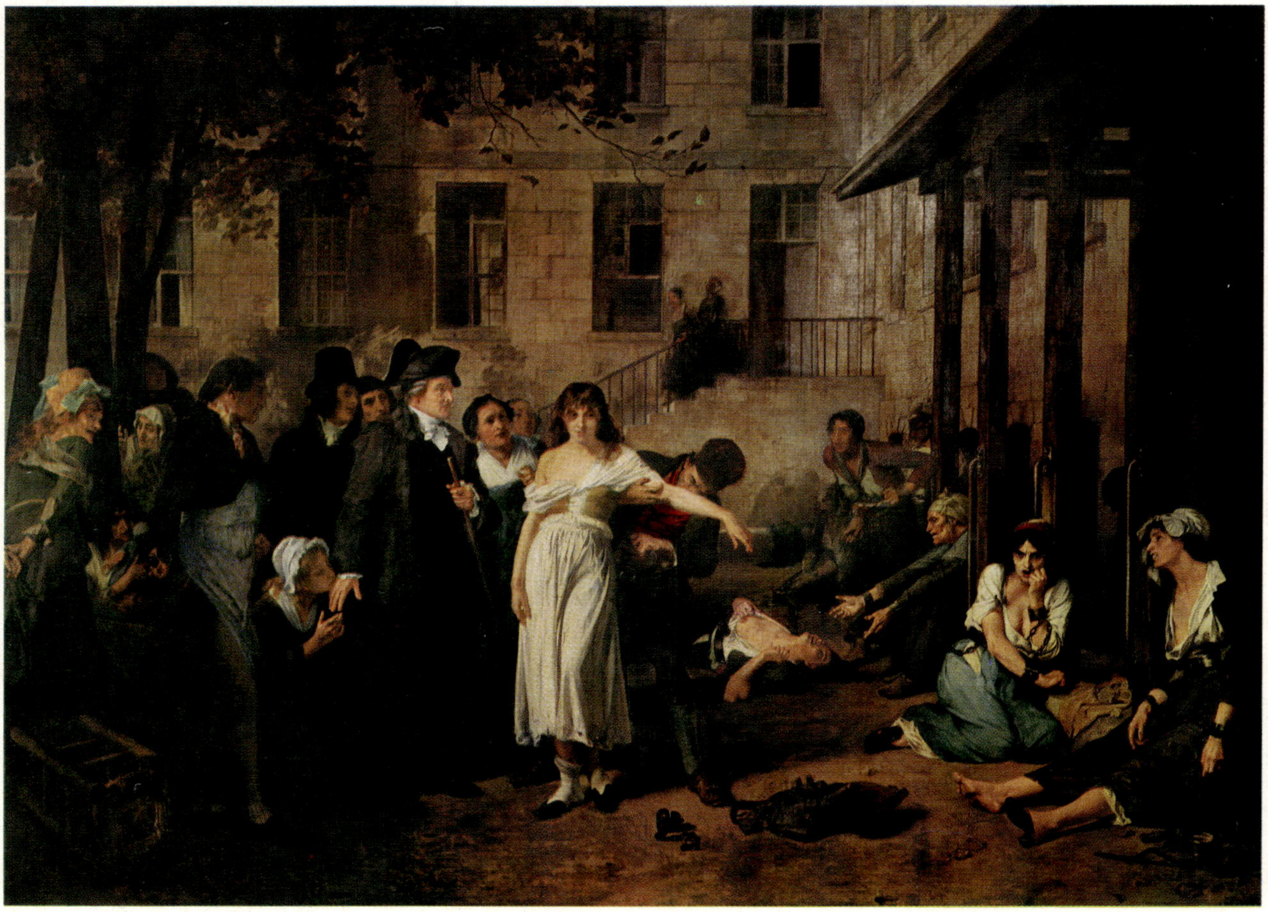

throughout the nineteenth century. Particularly in England and France neurophysiological mechanisms were elucidated, while clinical neurology developed as a study in its own right. The greatest French neurologist was Jean-Martin Charcot, who voiced some of the fundamental concepts of brain physiology and disease, while in England John Hughlings Jackson described the basic features of nervous action.

Philippe Pinel visiting mental patients at the Salpêtrière, Paris, 1795.

Drawings by Paul Richter showing phases of hysteria. *From Etudes cliniques sur la grande hysterie ou histero-epilepsie by Richter, Paris, 1881.*

it developed the seminal concept of cerebral localization. Before long, the great physiologist Marie Jean Pierre Flourens (1794–1867), an opponent of Gall, sited sensation and will in the cerebrum and showed that the cerebellum was responsible for co-ordination of movement and the medulla for respiration. Clinical observation continued to improve, and clear pictures of disease entities emerged; a classic is the 1817 essay of the Hoxton general practitioner and freethinker James Parkinson (1755–1824) on 'shaking palsy' (Parkinson's disease).

Experimental results continued to clarify neurophysiology. Charles Bell (1774–1842) and François Magendie (1783–1855) showed that the anterior and posterior roots of the nerves coming from the spinal cord were functionally distinct, and were concerned respectively with sensibility and movement, and Marshall Hall (1790–1857) expounded the idea of the reflex arc.

The advance of knowledge in this field in the mid-nineteenth century accompanied improved diagnosis, for in no other branch of medicine as in neurology can a disease state be related to a disturbance in part of the nervous system. Brown-Séquard threw light on the sensory and motor functions of the spinal cord, Claude Bernard on the sympathetic nerves, and Paul Broca (1824–1880) on the association of speech disturbance (aphasia) with damage to a small part of the left cerebral hemisphere. The synthesis was achieved by Jean-Martin Charcot (1825–1893), under whom the Salpêtrière in Paris became the centre of neurology. Charcot's reputation and genius lay in his universal approach, for he was the first to use regional criteria (acknowledging the concept that different parts of the nervous system have different functions) and pathological criteria (following Laënnec) in diagnosis. He described exactly such conditions as tabes dorsalis, motor neurone disease and multiple sclerosis, and he produced a masterly account of hysteria and hypnotic states, distinguished from organic disturbances by careful evaluation of symptoms and physical signs. It is said that Charcot's assistants used sometimes to coach their patients to produce 'hysterical' signs under the eyes of the master, but his work has no less value on this account, for by defining hysteria and hypnosis, which the Salpêtrière school thought to be identical, he transformed these subjects from a spectacle into a science.

In the 1880s the Nancy school under Hippolyte Bernheim (1840–1919) argued against Charcot's thesis that a hysterical disposition occurred only in certain patients, and showed that hypnotism was but an intensification of normal suggestion. This idea was widely adopted in the closing years of the century, and hypnotism came to be used in the treatment of neuroses and alcoholism. Dominated by Charcot and Bernheim, French psychiatry continued to concern itself mainly with neuroses, and this emphasis was of great importance as it led to the discovery of psychoanalysis. Here the name of Pierre Janet (1859–1947) should be mentioned; he formulated a concept of mental automatism in hysteria and recognized hysterical dissociation and the existence of unconscious factors.

Meanwhile, in Germany the study of cellular

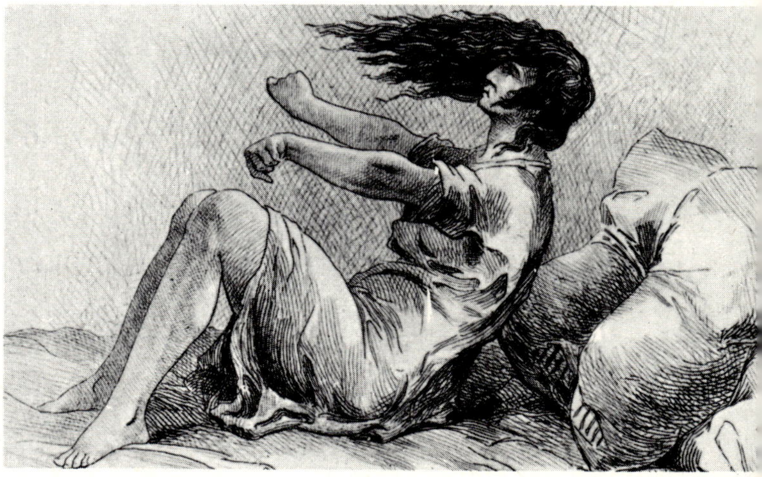

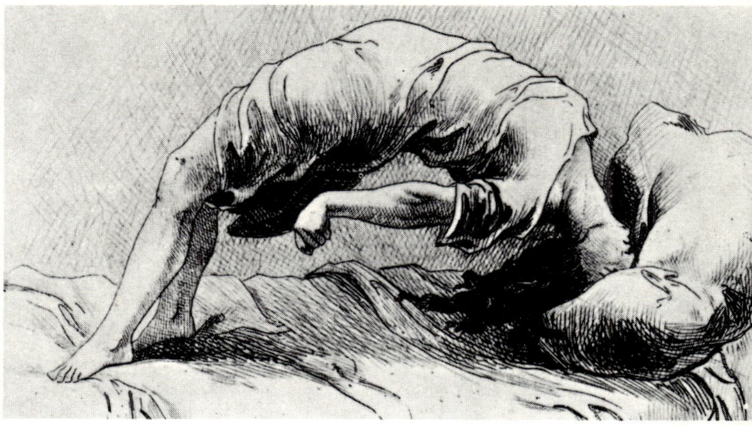

In Germany, neurological and psychiatric illnesses were closely studied in the nineteenth century. But the approach was self-limiting in that it described and pigeon-holed diseases, but ignored the causes. French psychiatrists were more dynamic. Some concerned themselves with hypnosis and the study of hysteria, and it was thus that Sigmund Freud was introduced to psychiatry. After a grounding in the neurological sciences in Vienna, Freud went to Paris to work with Charcot at the Salpêtrière in 1885. Then he began his studies in hysteria, and after returning to Vienna he extended his psychoanalytical researches to the entire field of neuroses. Freud's ideas on the sexual origin of neurosis shocked his contemporaries and continue to upset many people even today. In fact, much of Freud's work has been

pathology led to the adoption of an organic approach to mental diseases and a lessening of interest in metaphysical problems. This approach was of value in the elucidation of the various types of psychosis due to organic disease, but proved constricting, as when Theodor Meynert (1833–1892) classified all mental illness on an anatomical basis. Thorough clinical observation enabled Emil Kraepelin (1856–1926) to clarify other psychoses, such as dementia praecox (renamed schizophrenia by Bleuler), and manic-depressive states, but in general German psychiatry in the late nineteenth century tended to be too dogmatic, and progress came to a standstill.

Sigmund Freud (1856–1939) threw light on the unconscious factors adumbrated by Janet. He first studied neuroanatomy and neuropathology in Vienna and in 1885 went to the Salpêtrière. Modern psychoanalytic methods can be said to have been initiated by Freud in the following year, when he returned to Vienna after working with Charcot on hypnosis as a treatment for 'hysterical' patients. He found that this method was not always effective since only some of his patients could be hypnotized, and even those that could be were not often helped. Together with Josef Breuer (1842–1925), he evolved a method whereby patients could be induced to discuss their emotional problems not by hypnosis but by the process of free association, whereby 'powerful emotional drives swept the uncontrolled thoughts in the direction of psychic conflict'.

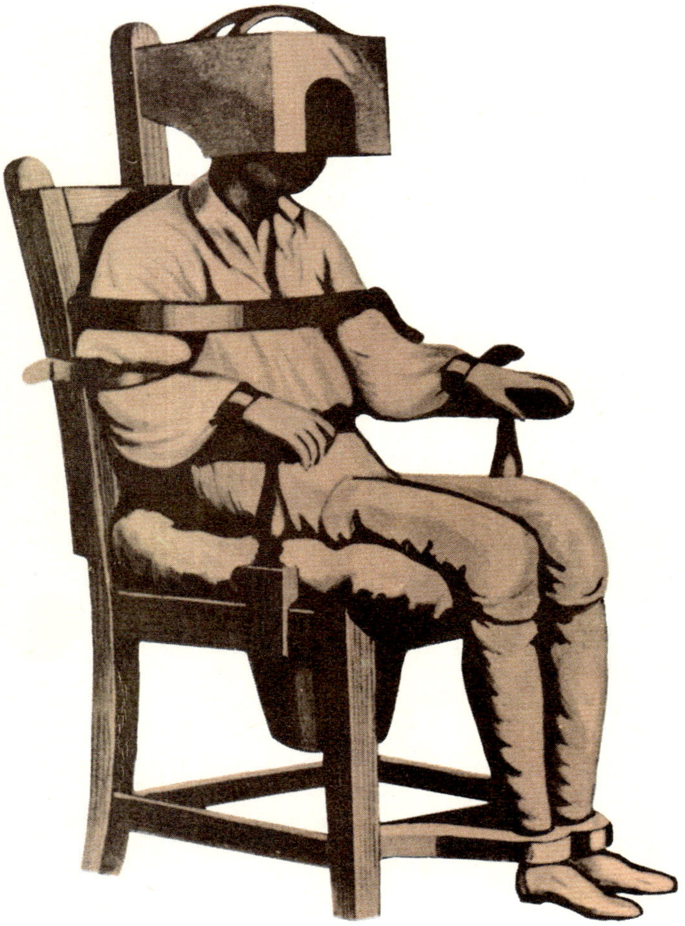

From his observations of patients under these conditions Freud found that forgotten or painful memories could often be related to traumatic sexual experiences in childhood; he concluded that hysteria resulted from childhood seduction and obsessional neurosis from guilt of active participation in such an event. He then elaborated his hypothesis of unconscious motivation, repression and resistance (whereby an experience becomes and is maintained unconscious) and the causation of neurosis. This resulted from repression of painful memories that were 'incompatible with the other dominant tendencies of the personality'.

However it was not long before Freud discovered that childhood seduction could only occasionally be implicated. Slips of the tongue and dreams were unconsciously motivated in many cases, and other processes might be at work. Freud thus elaborated the concepts of infantile sexuality and the Oedipus complex to explain imagined seduction by the parent of the opposite sex. Briefly, the infant in growing up was thought to go through three phases in which the main desires were satisfied by the mouth, the anus and the genitalia. Pre-genital sexuality ended at the age of three, but conflicts sooner or later might cause fixation at a regression to an earlier phase. At three, boys wanted the attention of their mother and resented their father—the Oedipus complex. Girls would later develop an Electra complex whereby they would desire their father and reject their mother, and these complexes were regarded as the source of anxiety, whereby libido was dammed up and not directed into the proper channels of adult sexuality and mature behaviour.

modified by later knowledge, but the fundamental validity of many of his concepts is generally recognized today. Freud revolutionized our approach to mental illness: at a time when society was just beginning to emerge from attitudes which today seem barbaric, he taught that the springs of many mental conditions should be sought in the experiences and problems of the patient.

Rush's tranquilizing chair. *From James Thacher's American Medical Biography, Boston, 1828.*

Sigmund Freud.

About this time Freud classified mental functions into conscious, preconscious and unconscious (the last being actively repressed and not able voluntarily to be recognized), and later he developed his theories of the ego (the conscious being), the superego (parental and social 'conscience') and the id (the source of mental energy, desires and libido). The id is the only mind of the newborn child and gradually becomes overshadowed by the ego and the superego; its aims remain, however, and repression, inhibition and sublimation of these leads respectively to neurosis, sexual deviation and artistic creativity.

Freud's final contribution was to attribute the origin of all anxiety to separation from the mother, which resulted in unknown internal danger. His various followers have changed his basic theories in a number of ways and have all underplayed the sexual theme on which he put so much emphasis. Carl Gustav Jung (1875–1961) introduced the idea of archetypes and the collective unconscious, a repository of experiences belonging to the race, and the concept of intraversion and extraversion. Alfred Adler (1870–1937) suggested that the inferiority complex was the most important driving factor in the armoury of the libido. Otto Rank (1884–1939), taking the childhood theme to extremes, postulated that anxiety began in the womb at the time of birth, when the child is subjected to a temporary asphyxia.

From the second half of the nineteenth century neurology was advanced on the one hand by anatomy and microscopy, especially in Germany, and on the other by physiological discoveries. Histological methods revealed the fine structure of the nervous system; Louis Ranvier (1835–1922) showed the minute architecture of peripheral nerves, Wladimir Betz (1834–1894) the giant motor cells in the cerebral cortex and Willy Kühne (1837–1900) the end-plates of motor nerves in muscle. At the same time morbid anatomy gave precise pathological meaning to a variety of nervous diseases. On the neurophysiological front advantage was taken of graphic methods of recording and electrical apparatus to study nervous tissues. The electrical excitability of nerve and muscle had long been known; Gustav Fritsch (1838–1897) and Eduard Hitzig (1838–1907) were the first to show (in 1870) that excitation of particular areas of the cerebral cortex could produce contraction of localized groups of muscles. Many other investigators developed knowledge of cerebral localization, vital to diagnosis and treatment, and with the discovery by Caton of Birmingham of the intrinsic electrical activity of the brain, the development of the electroencephalograph (EEG) was foreshadowed.

Neurophysiology in England was crowned at the end of the century by the work of Charles Sherrington (1861–1952), who developed the views of Bell and Magendie on spinal activity and in *The integrative action of the nervous system* produced the classic work on the nature of reflexes, one which is the foundation of modern ideas of the functioning of the brain and spinal cord. Meanwhile clinical neurologists in France and Germany widened the

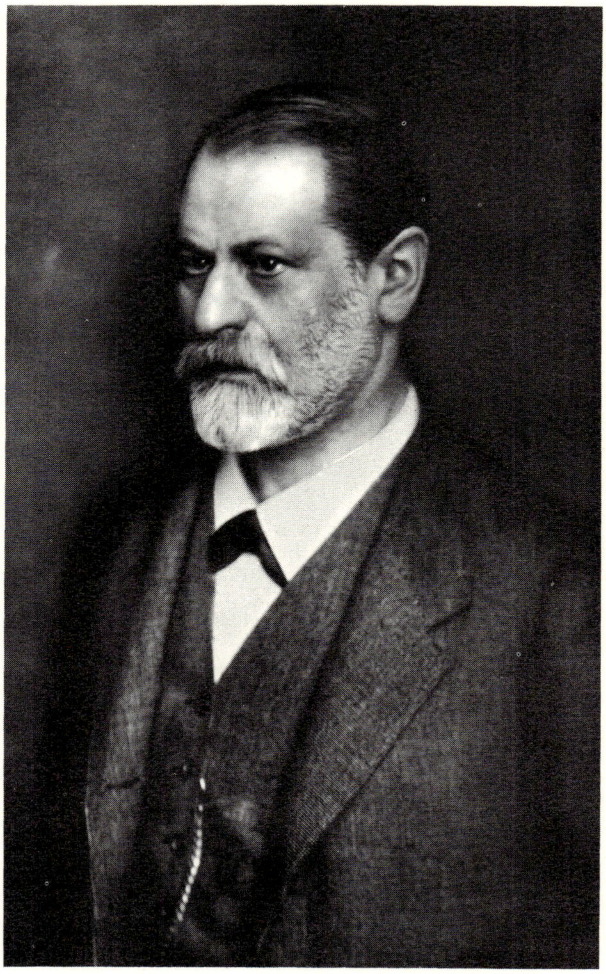

Since the latter part of the nineteenth century, knowledge of the structure, function and pathology of the nervous system has advanced on several fronts. In Germany, much work was done on the anatomy and microscopic anatomy, while in England the great neurophysiologist Sherrington produced his classic account of the nature of the reflexes. This work was complemented by that of the Russian Pavlov, who introduced the concept of conditioned reflexes. In many countries, clinicians began to describe many nervous, as distinct from mental, diseases. The greatest figure in this field was Hughlings Jackson, who really founded modern neurology with his studies of epilepsy and paralysis.

Jackson's emphasis on accurate systematic observation of signs and symptoms paved the way for the

frontiers of knowledge by describing many hitherto unrecognized forms of nervous disease, many still known by the name of their discoverer. It was in England, however, that modern neurology began with the work of the Yorkshireman John Hughlings Jackson (1835–1911), who, influenced by Brown-Séquard, came to the National Hospital for the Paralysed and Epileptic in London soon after its foundation in 1860. He defined the nervous system as an organ arranged and working at different levels of evolution, and he distinguished between 'discharging' and 'destroying' lesions, the effect of the former being the epileptic fit and that of the latter paralysis. In both cases one part of the body (hand, face or foot) might be principally affected, and Jackson described the convulsion as 'the mobile counterpart' of the stroke. He stated that

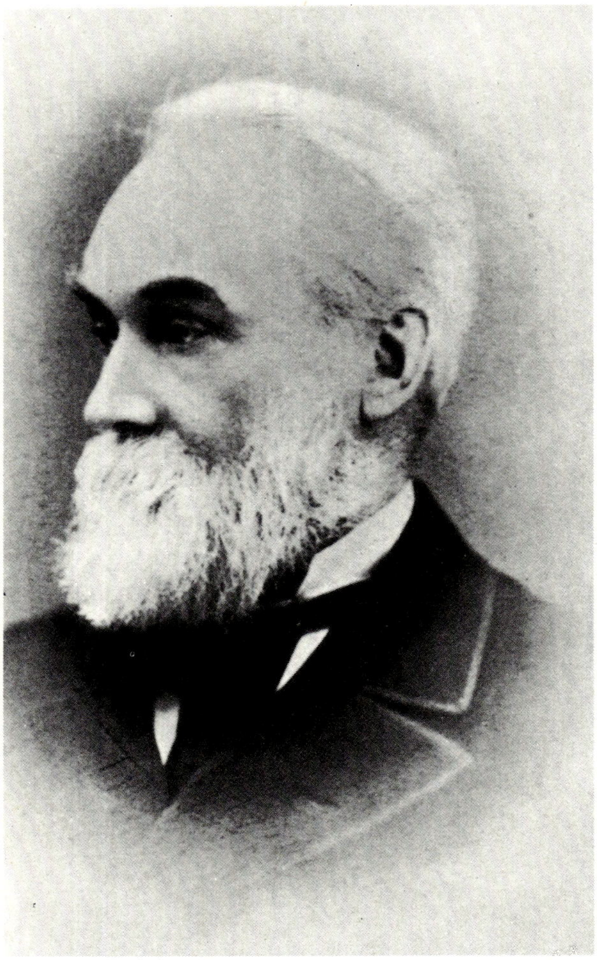

dissolution of nervous function always progressed from the most voluntary, most specialized and most differentiated, to the most automatic, least specialized and least differentiated–paralysis, aphasia and dementia all obeyed this law.

Lord Brain (1895–1967) remarked that 'the discoverer of a substantial thing, such as a bacillus, an extract or a disease, achieves more certain immortality than one who discovers a principle, for permanently valid principles soon become part of current thought and in time appear so obvious as to have needed no discovery.' Jackson was the formulator of principles, and his name is deeply embedded in the vocabulary of nervous diseases. He enunciated the general rule that 'epilepsy is the name for occasional sudden, excessive, rapid and local discharge of the grey matter (of the brain)' and it is after him that a particular type of fit, the Jacksonian attack, is called. He wrote about a patient suffering from such attacks:

'A man, forty-eight years of age, was admitted for convulsive attacks, which he described very minutely. They were, by his description, like that on which the following observation was made. One day when waiting his turn to be seen by the physician, his right hand began to twitch, the thumb and index fingers taking the lead. The fingers were soon partially flexed in a curve. . . . Next the whole arm twitched, but it did not rise; the exact sequence of involvement of its several parts was not ascertained, as the man was dressed. In about two minutes from the first, the right side of the face began to twitch, but before movement of it was discernible the patient said he felt 'it' in his face. The right eye was closed, the right cheek was drawn up, and both jaws came together. The mouth was drawn to the right. . . . The right ocular aperture was a little closer than the other, but both were narrowed. Both sides of the forehead were wrinkled upwards. There was no deviation of the head nor of the eyes; the leg was not affected and the patient could talk in any part of the fit. He begged me to let the porter take hold of his hand–to unclench it–as the porter could manage it better. The fit ceased very suddenly. After the attack the arm, which was weak before the fit, was completely paralysed, quite limp, and fell forward when he stooped, and it had not recovered completely when he left the hospital fourteen days later.'

Jackson and his associates in London developed

pinpointing of tumours for surgery. Today, other aids are available to the neurosurgeon, allowing precise and effective operation with minimal damage. The other great advance, which like neurosurgery belongs entirely to this century, is in the use of drugs in the treatment of certain neurological and psychiatric diseases. The management of schizophrenia and depression has been revolutionized by new drugs.

systematic neurology. Sir William Gowers (1845–1915), like Jackson, interested himself in epilepsy and produced a masterly book on this subject. It was at the National Hospital that a tumour of the nervous system was for the first time pinpointed in diagnosis and successfully removed.

In the twentieth century neurology and psychiatry have gained, like all branches of medicine, from developments in new methods of research and discoveries in different fields, which tend to fertilize each other. Thus biochemistry has revealed not only the existence and identity of chemical transmitters in the nervous system but also provides tests for the diagnosis of many diseases and has given a possible clue to the nature of schizophrenia. Advances in pharmacology have on the one hand given the scientist tools to investigate nervous functions and on the other hand effective treatment for such conditions as epilepsy, Parkinsonism and myasthenia gravis, while psychiatry has been revolutionized in the past decade by psychotropic drugs (like the phenothiazines and monoamine oxidase inhibitors) which have powerful effects on mental disturbances while leaving awareness and intelligence unimpaired. Anatomists have demonstrated the fine structure of the brain. Overshadowing everyone else's work in this field is that of the great Spaniard Santiago Ramon y Cajal (1852–1934), who developed the use of specialized staining methods. The electron microscope is now revealing new facts. Radiology and isotope chemistry enable the neurologist to confirm his diagnosis by outlining the cerebral blood vessels (arteriography) and ventricles (pneumoencephalography and ventriculography) and scanning the brain for an area of radioactivity indicating isotope uptake by a tumour.

Neurosurgery has benefited particularly from advances in anaesthesia. Here the name of Harvey Cushing (1864–1939) should be recorded. This pioneer extended the scope of the field beyond brain tumours, which he was the first to classify in a systematic and comprehensive manner according to prognostic and clinical criteria. Thanks to Cushing, neurosurgery now provides treatment for brain and spinal tumours, head injury, hydrocephalus and some cases of epilepsy and intractable pain, and more recently developments in neuroanatomy and

John Hughlings Jackson

Pavlov operating.

Operation by Herbert Olivecrona, the Swedish neurosurgeon (b 1891).

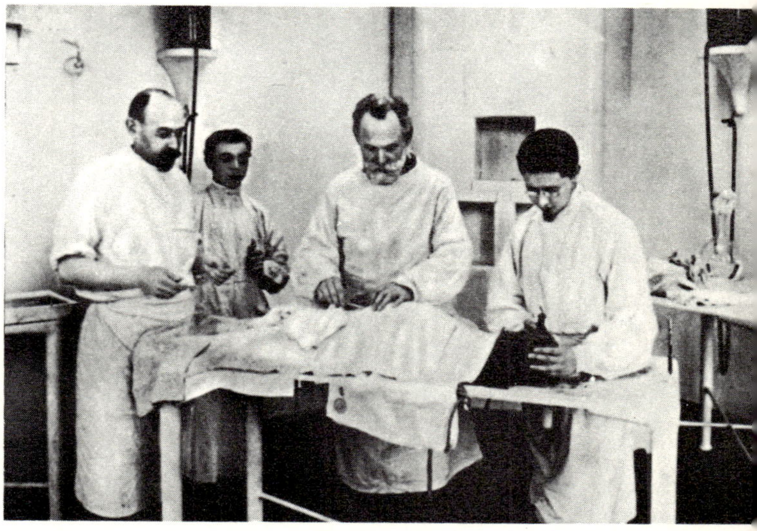

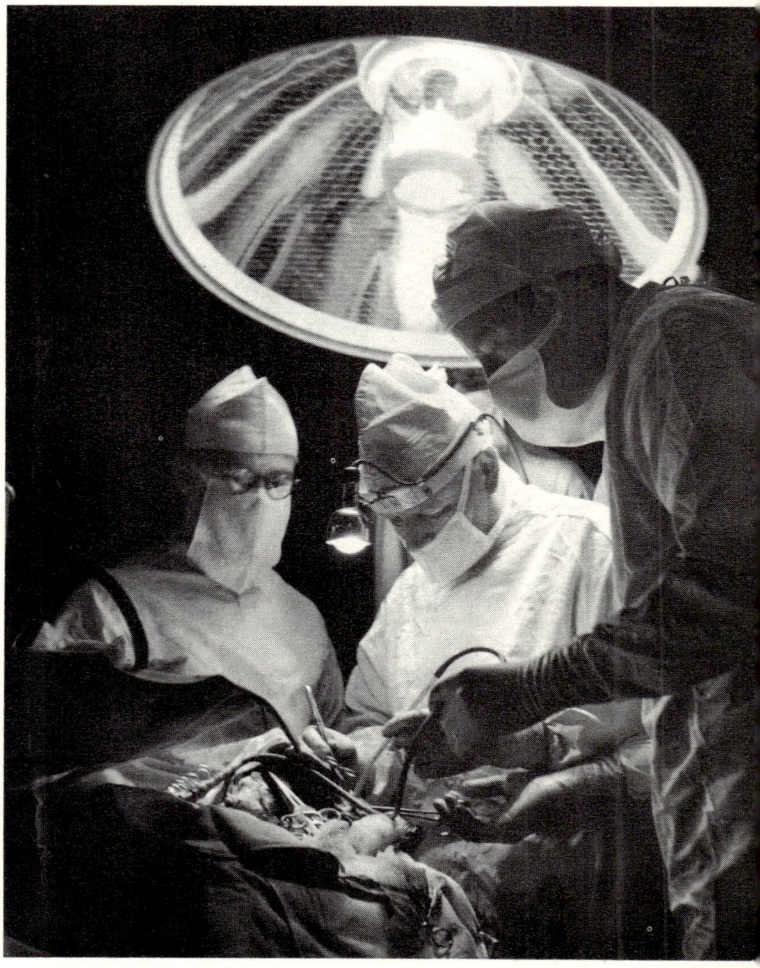

Among the modern investigational tools in nervous and psychiatric disease is the electroencephalograph, developed by H. Berger in 1929. This machine amplifies and records on paper the minute changes of electrical potential in the brain, about 1/20,000 volt, which are associated with nerve-cell activity. Some brain diseases produce characteristic alterations in the EEG record, which is thus valuable in diagnosis. Neurological disorders are also investigated at the cellular level, using both light and electron microscopy, in the attempt to relate clinical signs with changes observable in the nervous tissues. These studies play an important part in the understanding of nervous activity.

Part of an electroencephalograph tracing

Purkinje nerve cells of the human cerebellum.

physiology have enabled a successful surgical attack to be made on Parkinson's disease. The surgeon may also come to the aid of the psychiatrist, by carrying out leucotomy (cutting the connexions between the frontal lobes and other parts of the brain) on severely crippled mental patients. The operation, originated by Egas Moniz (1874–1955), damages the personality and has fallen into disrepute, but is still sometimes of use.

The physiology of the nervous system is now well understood at the cellular level. Exploration of the nature of the nerve impulse began with the work of Keith Lucas (1879–1916) and continued with Lord Adrian (*b.* 1889) and others, using valve amplifiers and cathode ray tubes, and micromethods have enabled electrical recordings to be made from individual nerve fibres and brain cells. Information continues to be gained about the activity of the brain as a whole. Sherrington apart, the most important name in this field is that of Ivan Petrovich Pavlov (1849–1936), much of whose

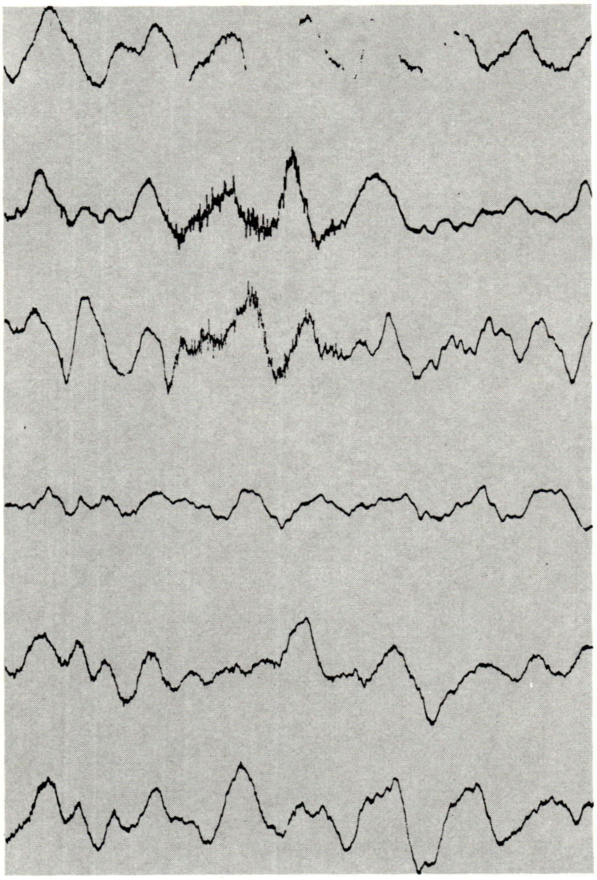

work on conditioned reflexes was carried out in the latter part of the last century. He showed that frequent repetition of specific stimuli could produce reflexes bearing no direct relationship to the stimulus; thus bell-ringing, after having been sufficiently associated with the exhibition of food, could produce in dogs a flow of gastric juice even in the absence of food. Pavlov contrasted ordinary reflexes, which were momentary and transitory, with conditioned reflexes, which became gradually reinforced to become chronic manifestations. From his physiological findings he turned to psychiatry; having produced artificial neuroses in dogs by presenting two similar conditioning stimuli, he postulated that hysteria was the result of conflicting, overwhelmingly strong or weak repetitive stimuli impinging on the balanced mechanism of conditioning. Animals could be reconditioned back to normal, which suggested a therapy for neurotic patients. This turned out not to be very effective in the long run, but Pavlovian theory has been vindicated in human physiology, and at the present time, when doubt is being cast on fine cerebral localization of function, a holistic approach to the workings of the nervous system is of great value.

In contrast to neurology, where knowledge accrues little by little, psychiatry, having been overwhelmed by two revolutions—the psychoanalytical and pharmacological—in the present century, is today in a state of flux. As ever, there are two fundamental approaches to diagnosis and therapy, the psychological and the organic, but if there is a present-day trend it is to attempt to link these and to correlate in treatment psychoanalysis, modern drugs and assessment of the mentally sick individual in the background of his own environment. However, the problems to be resolved by modern psychiatry are not just those of the overtly ill mental patient. Psychosomatic diseases, physical states brought on by emotional conflict or stress, are being recognized more and more. Besides, human existence must be seen in a psychological perspective, and psychiatric ideas thus impinge on all aspects of everyday life. For this reason the branches of child psychology and industrial psychology have developed and psychiatric social help is available to the community: contemporary psychiatry entails not only the modernization of mental hospitals and hospital treatment but the evolution of altogether new and different systems of care.

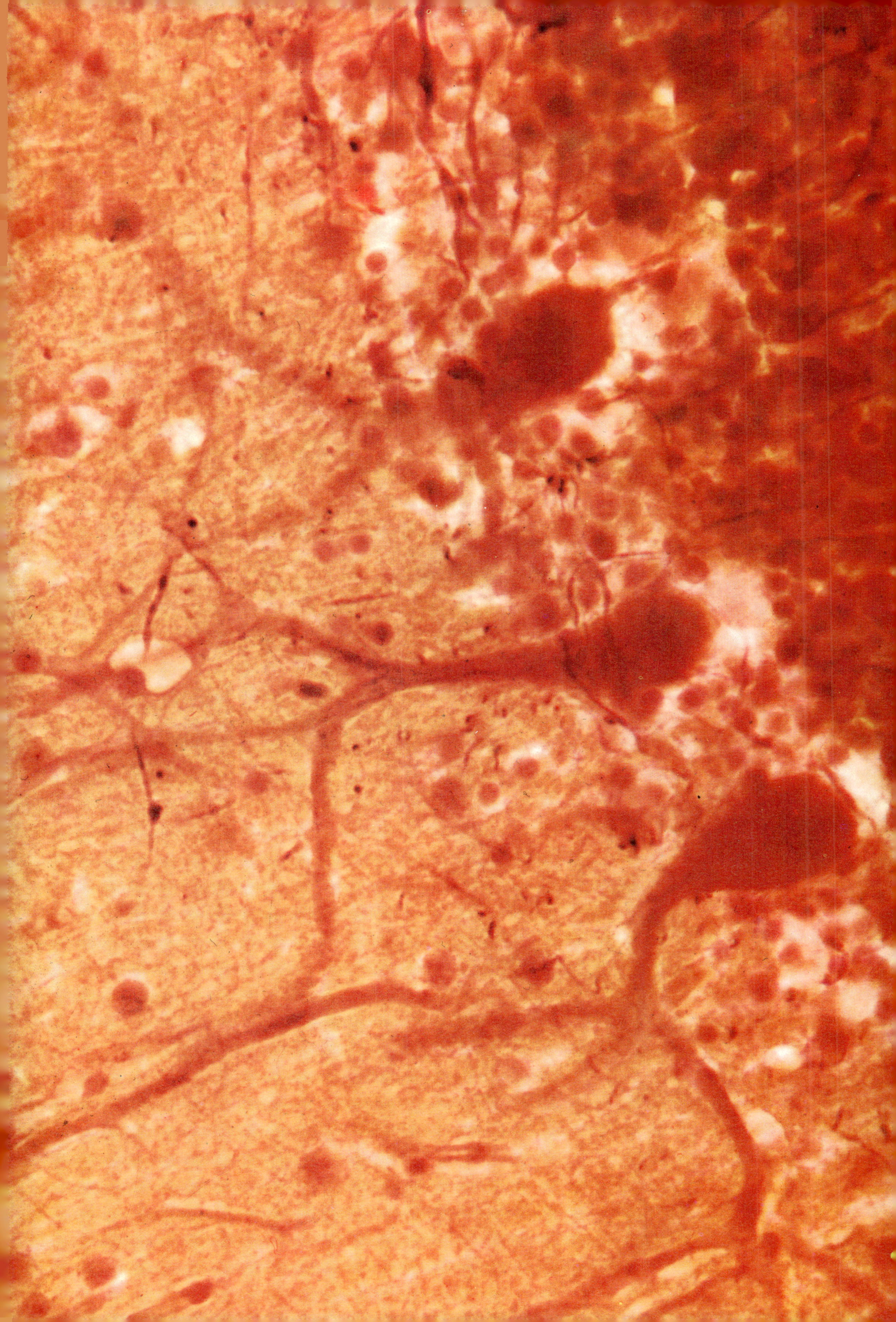

From earliest times, societies have recognized a need to protect the health of their citizens: a healthy society is obviously stronger than one riddled with disease. The health laws of the ancient Israelites protected them through their most difficult times. The Romans made the next great step in this field, but it was the plagues of the Middle Ages and after that really awoke societies to the necessity for organized medical services, along with control of living and working conditions. The nineteenth century saw the beginning of real involvement by states in such areas as housing, education and health insurance, all of which form an essential background to modern medical practice.

Maternity clinic. *Painting by Ben Shahn, 1940. Downtown Gallery, New York.*

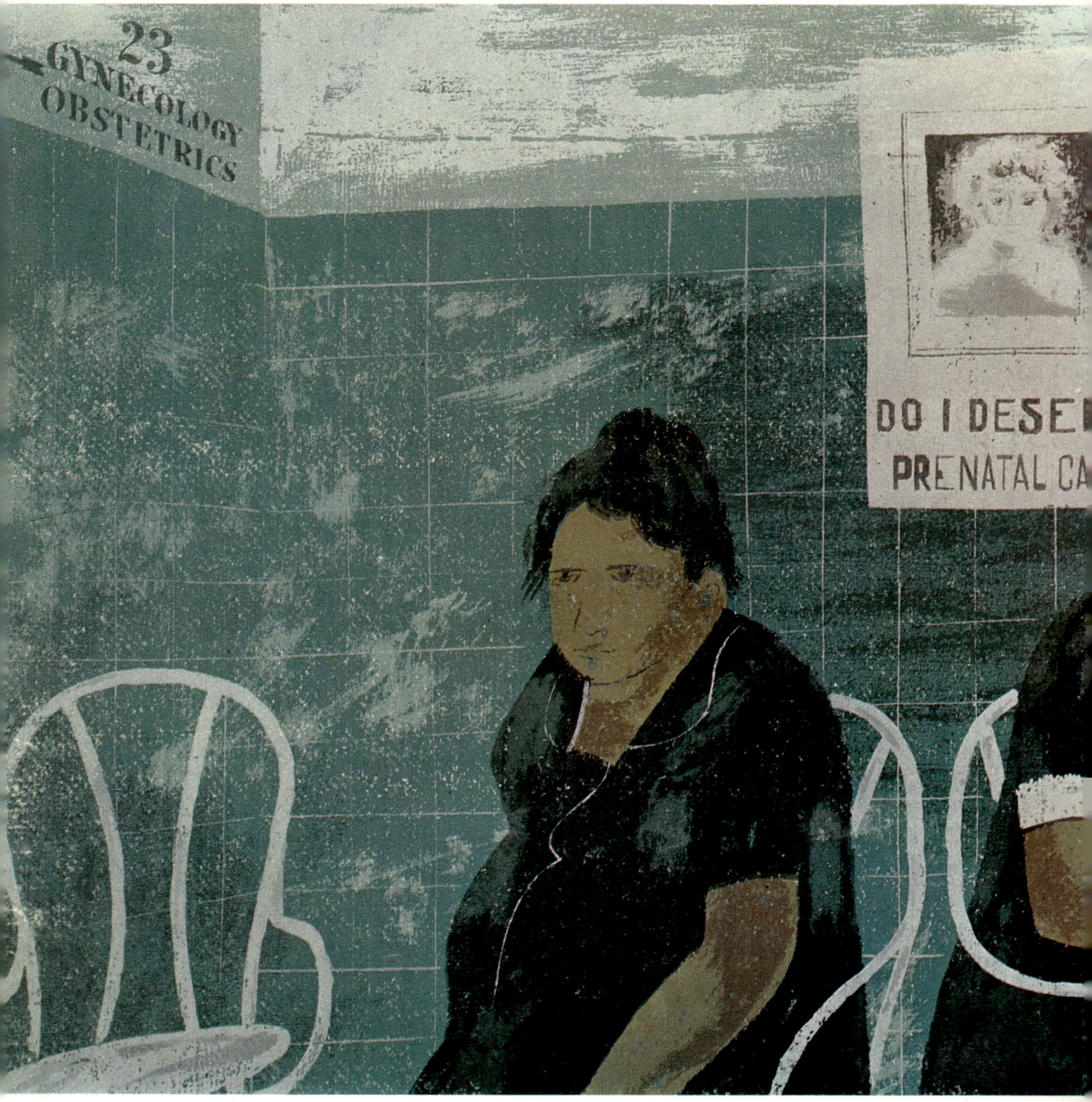

Medicine in modern society

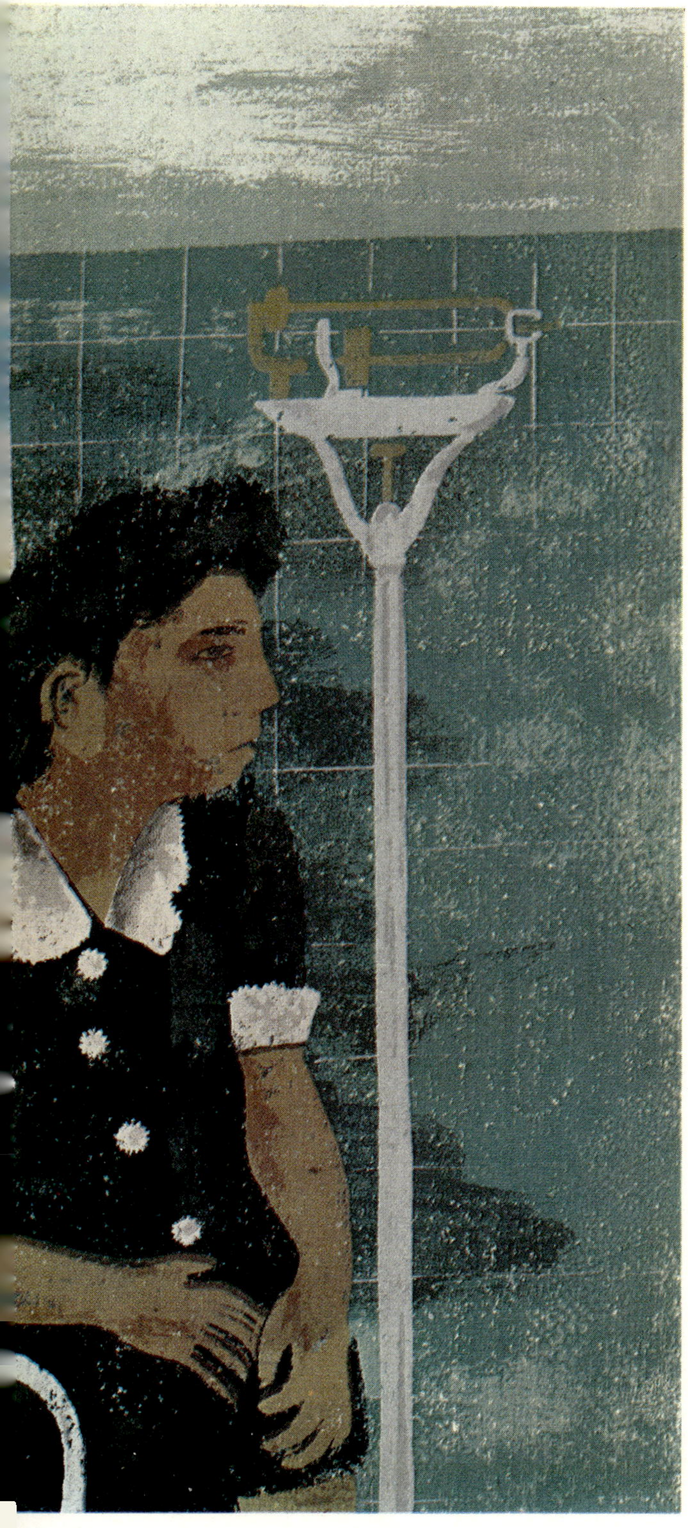

Many of the landmarks of public health through the ages have already been noted in this book, from the hygienic legislation of the Jews and the sewer system of ancient Rome to the foundation of industrial medicine by Ramazzini and the reform of hospitals by Florence Nightingale and Lord Lister. The early achievements in this field were of no use against such lethal epidemics as the Black Death; and in the Middle Ages and afterwards, with the flourishing growth of crowded, walled cities, the lowering of standards of personal and communal hygiene resulted in every possible infectious disease being widespread.

One of the greatest problems in these cities was the disposal of solid excreta. As late as the eighteenth century faeces and urine were thrown into the streets, and in London, at the sites of such now salubrious places as Belgrave Square, Hyde Park Gardens and University College, the excreta were collected and dumped in refuse piles. An answer to this problem had been provided two hundred years earlier by Sir John Harington (1561–1612), with his invention of the water-closet, in which for the first time the disposal of faeces and urine was controlled by mechanical means. His discovery was recorded in his *New discourse of a stale subject, called the Metamorphosis of Ajax* (1596), the classical allusion being a pun on 'a jakes' (the old word for privy); and it prepared the way for the public health era. Unfortunately refuse was flushed into cesspools whose contents soaked into the earth, thus polluting wells, or were drained into rivers; in London, the Thames and Serpentine became no better than open sewers.

The Industrial Revolution produced hundreds of thousands of jerry-built hovels in which disease was favoured by lack of ventilation and light, in addition to overcrowding. The importance of fresh air under such conditions was realized early. Stephen Hales (1677–1761), the parson of Teddington who measured everything he could lay his hands on, thereby becoming one of the great names of plant and animal physiology, devised in 1743 a ventilator by means of which fresh air could get into prisons, the holds of ships, mines and other confined spaces. This invention was at once widely used, producing improvement of health and living conditions. William Wells (1757–1817), physician to St Thomas' Hospital, followed it up with a study of humidity, which he recognized as important in

Medical science today makes possible treatments that even at the beginning of our century would have seemed nothing short of miraculous. Physicians are armed not only with the knowledge of disease that is the fruit of study in every corner of the world, they also have truly effective therapies for the great majority of known diseases. Powerful and specific drugs, accurate and safe surgery, and hospitals equipped with an enormous armoury of diagnostic and therapeutic equipment exist to back up the work of every doctor–at least in principle. In fact, the great problem of modern medicine is beginning to be seen as the organization of its services to make all this available to every man, woman and child who needs treatment. Even the most wealthy modern state cannot realistically provide all the resources, of money

relation to comfort and health in enclosed surroundings.

The repeal of the evil window tax in 1803 helped a little with light and ventilation, but in smoky industrial towns there was little enough light, and this, combined with the poverty of the urban diet in comparison with that of the peasants of agricultural England, resulted in rickets, 'the English disease'. People were still unaware that there were such things as deficiency diseases, although scurvy was successfully treated with citrus fruit in 1747 by James Lind (1716–1794), this replacement of vitamin C being later paralleled by the use in rickets of cod liver oil and light, and Sir Edward Mellanby's recognition that this disease could be corrected by adequate amounts of vitamin D in the diet. Certainly in the nineteenth century the food intake of the poor consisted mainly of the cheap energy-providing carbohydrate foods, deficient in vitamins and essential minerals: the per capita consumption of refined sugar rose from a few pounds a year at the start of the century to a hundredweight at the end.

The new era really began with the work of Sir Edwin Chadwick, through whose efforts the Public Health Act of 1848 was passed. Determined to improve the lot of the working classes in the large towns, he prepared a report on their sanitary conditions and showed why mortality was greatest in the slums; his findings revealed such a distressing picture that they were received by Parliament 'with astonishment, dismay, horror and even incredulity'. The Act of 1848 put into practice for the first time the principle that a state was responsible for the health of its people.

One of Chadwick's innovations was the use of glazed earthenware pipes for sewage, which greatly reduced the possibility of contamination of drinking water. At the same time it was decided that shallow wells should be abolished and main water supply introduced. This was partly thanks to the detective work of the anaesthetist John Snow, who collected data on a number of outbreaks of cholera and showed the disease to be water-borne.

The cholera pandemics began in the early 1830s and produced great apprehension as well as a good deal of thorough epidemiological investigation. The official report on the first outbreak in Paris in 1832 began 'When a deadly scourge, such as famine, pestilence, or an epidemic strikes a great city, the first feeling that it arouses is terror. Everyone has but one thought, one object: to escape the evil. Those whose position or wealth allows it flee in all haste; those–and they are in the majority–for whom flight is impossible, forced to remain, give way to fatal despondency, already considering themselves doomed to an early death, living in continual terror, more afflicted by the real misfortunes which they bring upon themselves than by the scourge which they dread but which may not assail them.' One particularly severe outbreak occurred in Soho, London, in 1854, with 14,000 cases and 618 deaths; Snow suggested that an invisible living agent was responsible and traced the infection to a well in Broad (now Broadwick) Street, which was contaminated from a leaking cesspool.

It will have been gathered that during the second half of the nineteenth century the efforts of the state were directed at improvement of the physical environment rather than at implementing the recent advances in medicine at the individual level. That preventive medicine alone was not enough in reducing disease in the poor was revealed forcibly at the end of the century, when the alarming discovery was made that half of the army recruits for service in South Africa were physically unfit. It became increasingly recognized that poverty and everything that went with it predisposed strongly to disease. The state awoke to this dangerous situation in time for the Great War, introducing school meals, the School Medical Service (1907) and the National Insurance Act of 1911. The last of these provided free medical services for a large part of the working population, and was modelled on a system that had been working effectively in Germany for many years. It marked the beginnings of state medicine and presaged the five acts of 1944-1948 which provided a comprehensive system of social security for everyone in Great Britain.

In fact there had been some sort of community medical care in England for 400 years before the National Health Service Act of 1946. In the sixteenth century doctors were employed at Newcastle and Barnstaple and paid out of the poor rates, while the Poor Law of Elizabeth I (1601) required the 'necessary relief of the lame, old, blind, and such other among them being poor and not able to work' *and of manpower, required to fulfill this dream.*

However, in almost all of the world's developed countries, there exist insurance schemes or free or subsidised health services for all. Britain pioneered this with the foundation of the National Health Service in 1948. In Russia and the other communist countries, too, the health of citizens is the responsibility of the state.

Women's clinic in the USSR.

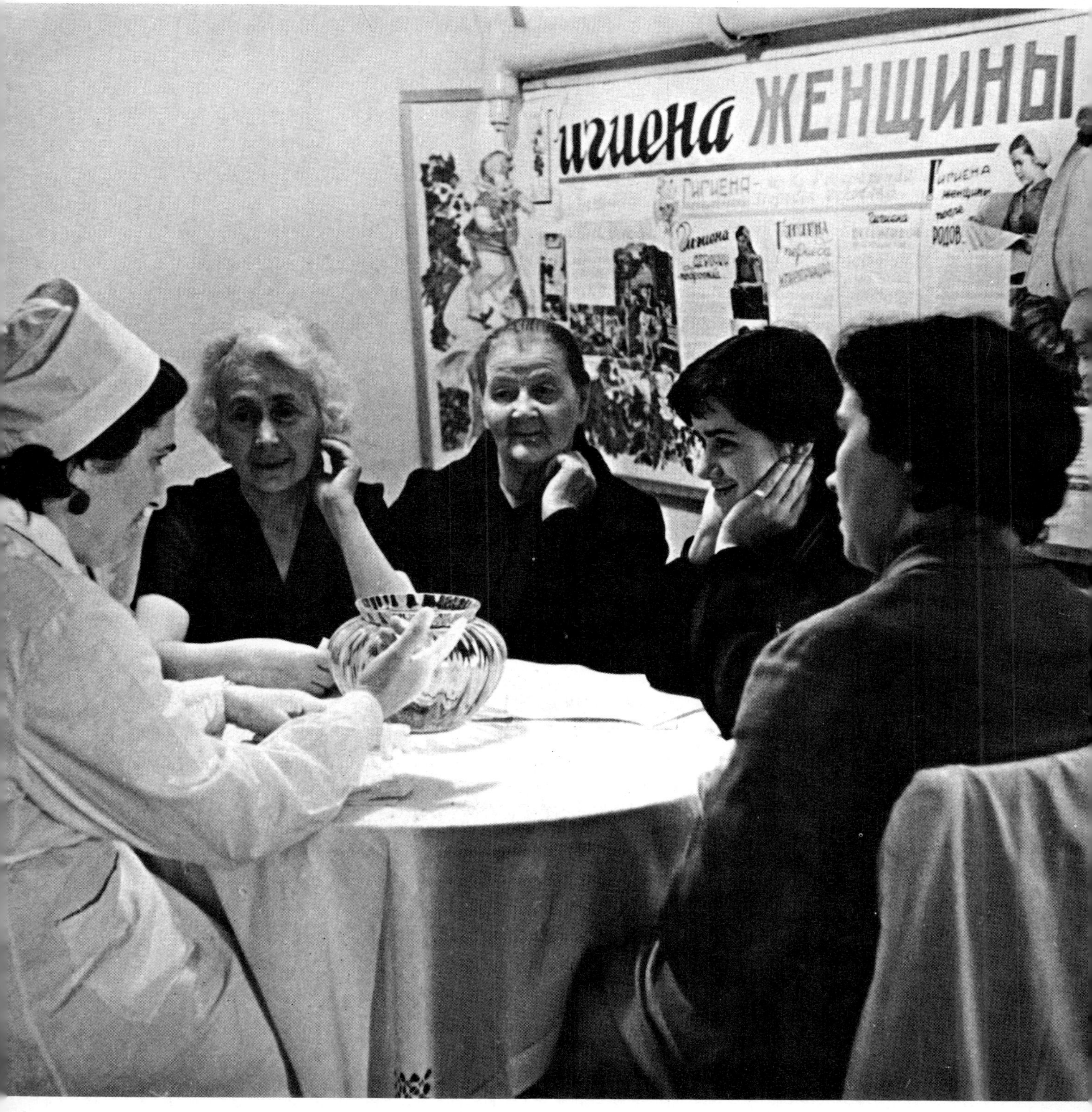

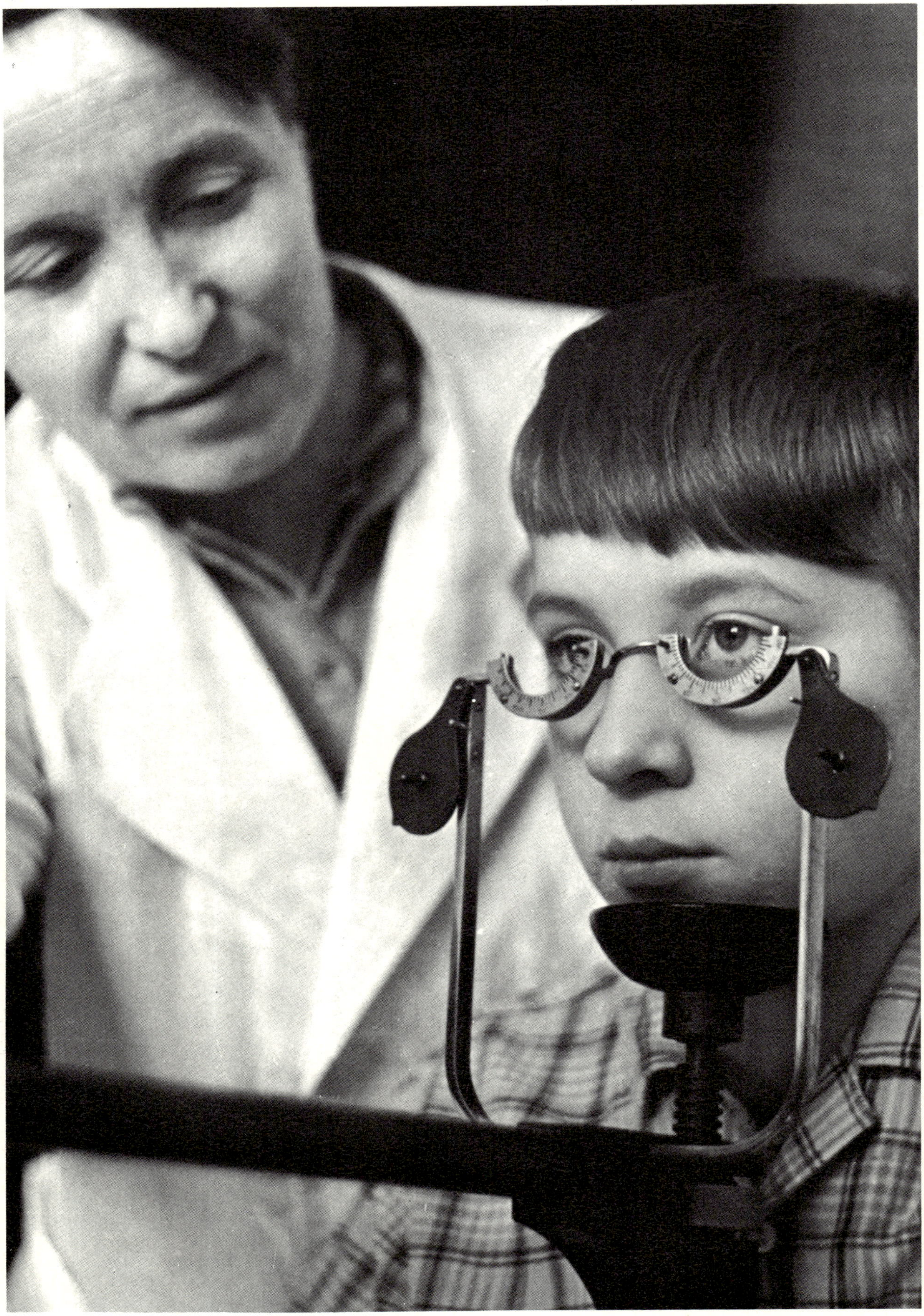

Among the earliest state health regulations in Britain and many other countries were those protecting children. Until the mid-nineteenth century, children had no special protection and many worked long hours in appalling conditions. Today, it is one of the basic principles of most societies that children should not work, and should be provided with free education, as well as complete medical protection. They are vaccinated against several diseases as babies, and are carefully observed throughout their early years. As a result, many diseases have practically disappeared.

Testing a child's eyesight in the USSR.

Vaccinating a child against German measles in the United States.

Tuberculosis prevention in the USSR.

–thus providing medical care in theory, at least.

The epidemics that harassed the population through the seventeenth century led to the foundation of almshouses and also public dispensaries, which were provided in towns by the physicians to supply cheap medicines for the poor sick. Nevertheless the physicians, governed by their Royal College, remained aloof, charged high fees and took no part in the care of the less wealthy; the poor obtained their remedies from the apothecaries, who, while not allowed to charge for giving advice, nevertheless gradually assumed the role of general practitioners. By the end of the eighteenth century the apothecary was 'the physician to the poor at all times and to the rich whenever the disease is without danger'. Although well-educated and often with polished manners, he was still looked down on by the privileged classes.

Jenner was a surgeon-apothecary: after he had become famous, efforts were made to admit him to the Royal College of Physicians. This entailed his passing an examination in Latin. There was no way round this; and Jenner refused, for he was by nature modest and not an Establishment figure. It was not until 1858, with the passing of the Medical Act, that the apothecaries became fully respectable and gained recognition as professional men. By then, twenty-four years after the New Poor Law, which enabled local boards of guardians to appoint district medical officers and pay them for their services, there were four thousand state-salaried practitioners treating four million patients annually. It is interesting also that there was then, as now, much argument over such topics as salaried service and free choice of doctor.

The American writer Emerson considered that 'the health standard of a nation is a fair gauge of its intelligence, and its degree of social development'. Although only the development of the health services in Britain has been described, a number of general points are illustrated. Thus no country can reach a high health standard purely through knowledge of the cause and cure of disease; there must in addition be a social structure within which the appropriate measures for the cure of disease can be taken even in the absence of epidemics, and in peacetime. The application of such measures seems always to have lagged behind their theoretical justification, and it is to be hoped for the future that the under-developed countries acquire efficient local self-government to enable prejudices to be removed and preventive medicine to be carried out while making the best use of available resources.

In the meanwhile, in emergent states Western

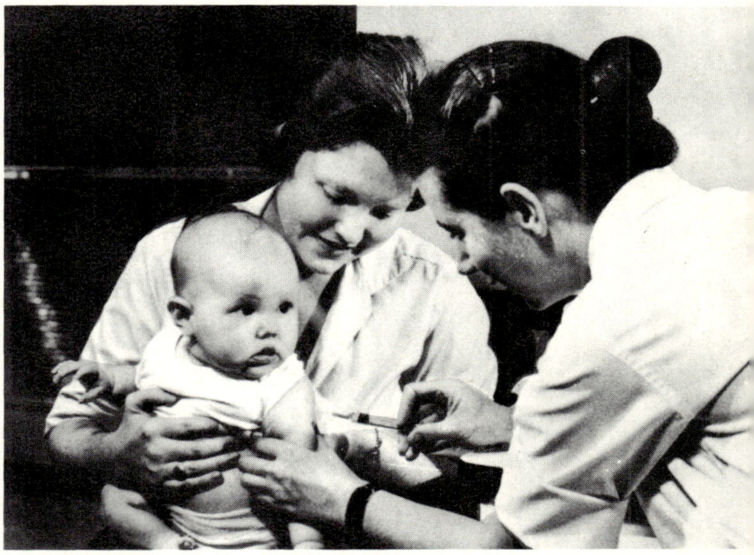

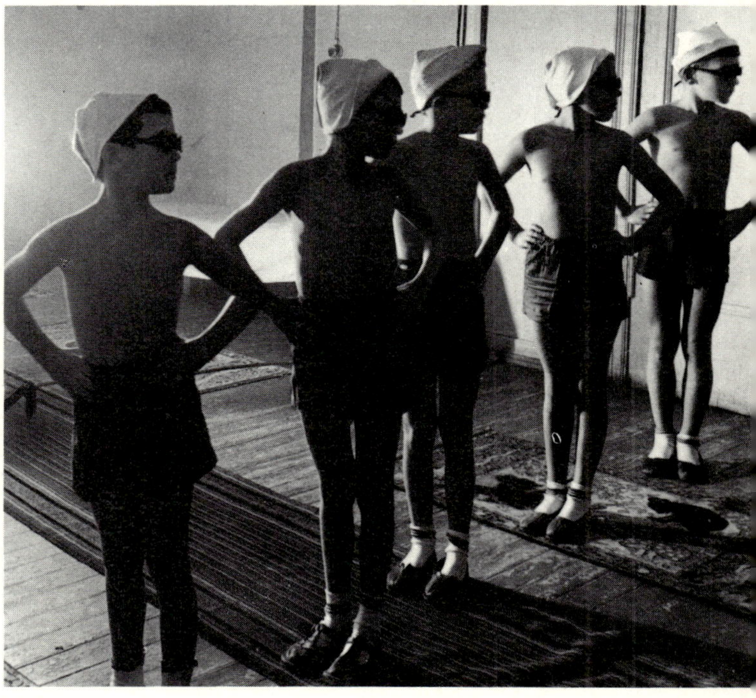

In the modern world, doctors find themselves facing many new problems which have nothing to do with infections and so on, but which are the direct product of our rapidly evolving way of life. Man is reaching out into entirely new spheres, including space travel, where his previous experience is only of limited value. But the many strains and stresses of modern urban society are almost as unknown a factor as space or supersonic flight : psychiatric diseases present modern medicine with its most intractable problems. At the same time, as drugs and surgery and special nursing successfully prolong healthy and normal life, the problems of the aged become more important. Similarly, medicine can now keep alive many people with serious disabilities who would otherwise not have survived : the welfare and occupation of these patients

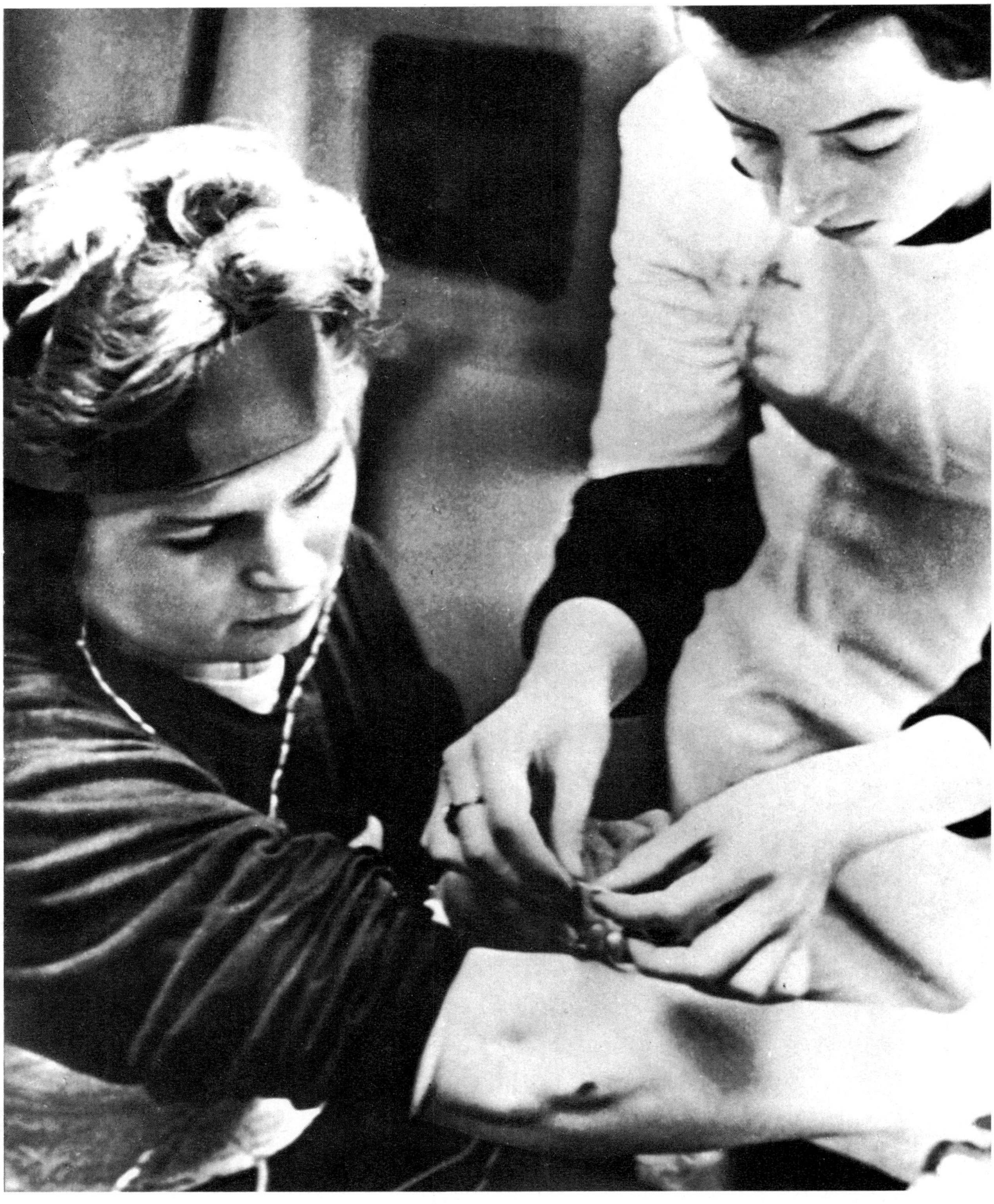

is another task to tax the resources not only of medicine, but of society as a whole. But the greatest single problem facing man and medicine today is that of the underdeveloped countries, where hundreds of thousands of people die of undernourishment and of diseases for which there has long been a cure. The provision of health services on a world-wide scale is the responsibility of the World Health Organization.

medicine is faced with great practical problems. Villagers, with their own idea of government and its punitive powers and indifference to people in remote communities, may well regard the health educator with suspicion. He, in turn, may be totally ignorant of their traditional system of medicine and find himself competing ineffectually with it.

We have now come full circle and once again we look at primitive medicine, this time from the viewpoint of world health. The work of social anthropologists is especially valuable in throwing light on the basic elements of traditional medicine. The physician in the under-developed community may or may not understand such factors as local methods of prophylaxis and treatment, the importance of the supernatural, the part played by the native healers, and the involvement of a whole family in the illness of an individual. Certainly he will recognize the importance of achieving liaison with the traditional practitioner. A French doctor in Equatorial Africa has written of his success in getting local medicine men to travel with him in his car, dressed in white coats, and to make contact with villagers, while another doctor, in Togoland, held conferences with herbalists and diviners, and found that many people, having been given advice and magical therapy, were told to go to the new hospital for further investigation and treatment.

Health education and medical aid is now being provided on an enormous scale by the World Health Organization, a specialized agency of the United Nations. This organization has 129 member countries and regional offices in Brazzaville, New Delhi, Manila, Alexandria, Copenhagen and Washington and acts, under the terms of its constitution, 'as the directing and coordinating authority on international health work.' Among the many projects that it sponsors, it helps to provide governments with the technical information required to protect and promote the health of their peoples, to demonstrate effective methods of disease control, to supply better trained doctors and nurses and to strengthen existing national health services, to establish international standards for drugs, and to stimulate and coordinate medical research.

Valentina Terezkhova undergoing a medical check-up before her space flight.

Medical check-up for the aged in the United States: a volunteer having the air-capacity of his lungs measured.

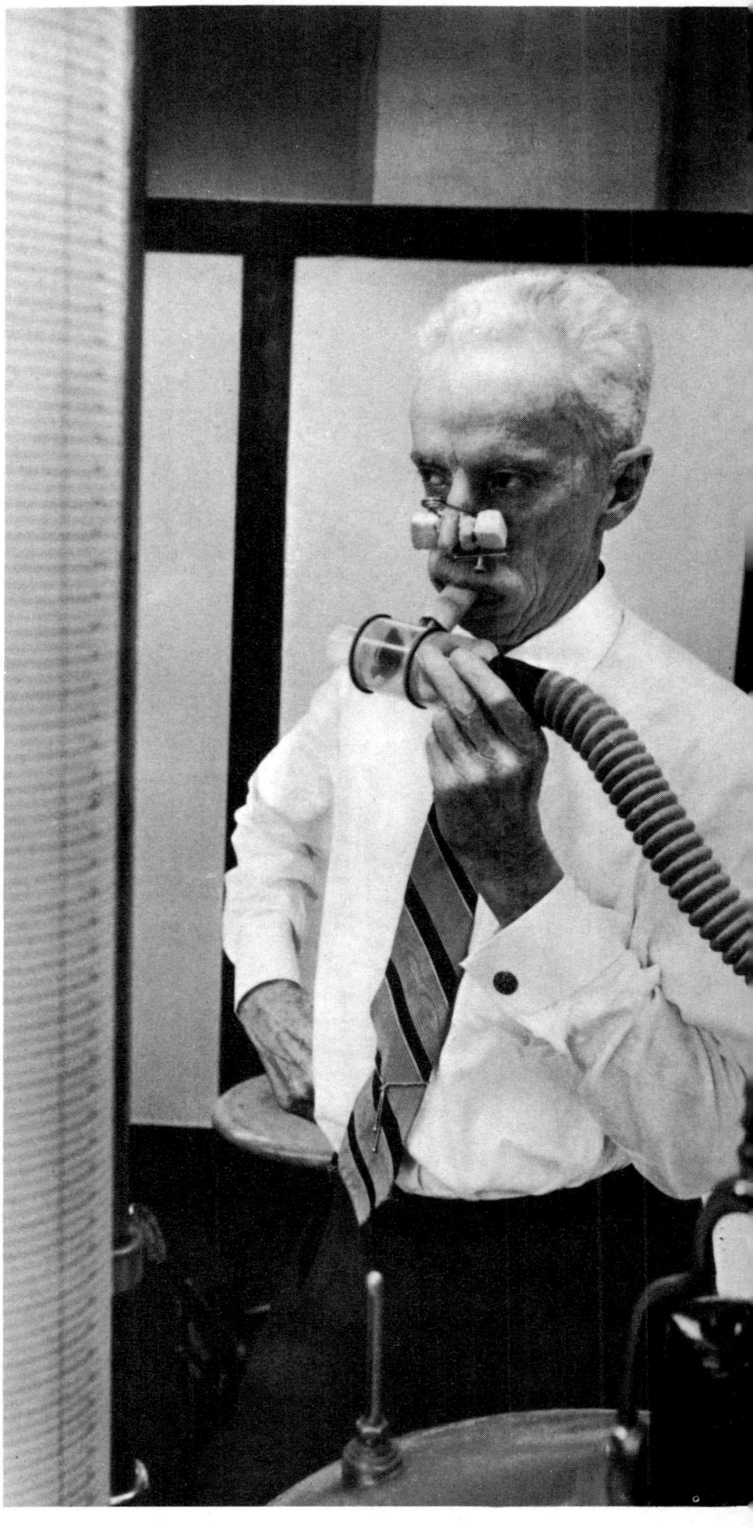

The Constitution of the WHO was signed on 22 July 1946 by the representatives of sixty-one states and came into force on 7 April 1948. In the twenty years of its existence the organization has carried out massive campaigns in developing countries to eradicate malaria and control tuberculosis, venereal diseases, water-borne infestations and a wide range of communicable diseases. It has worked to improve nutrition, child health and mental welfare. Not only the underprivileged nations but also the Western states have benefited from its pharmacological and cancer programmes.

We conclude this chapter with the principles enunciated in the Constitution of the WHO—principles which embody the highest ideals of medicine today:

Health is a state of complete physical, mental and social well-being and not merely the absence of disease or infirmity.

The enjoyment of the highest attainable standard of health is one of the fundamental rights of every human being without distinction of race, religion, political belief, economic or social condition.

The health of all peoples is fundamental to the attainment of peace and security and is dependent upon the fullest co-operation of individuals and states.

The achievement of any state in the promotion and protection of health is of value to all.

Unequal development in different countries in the

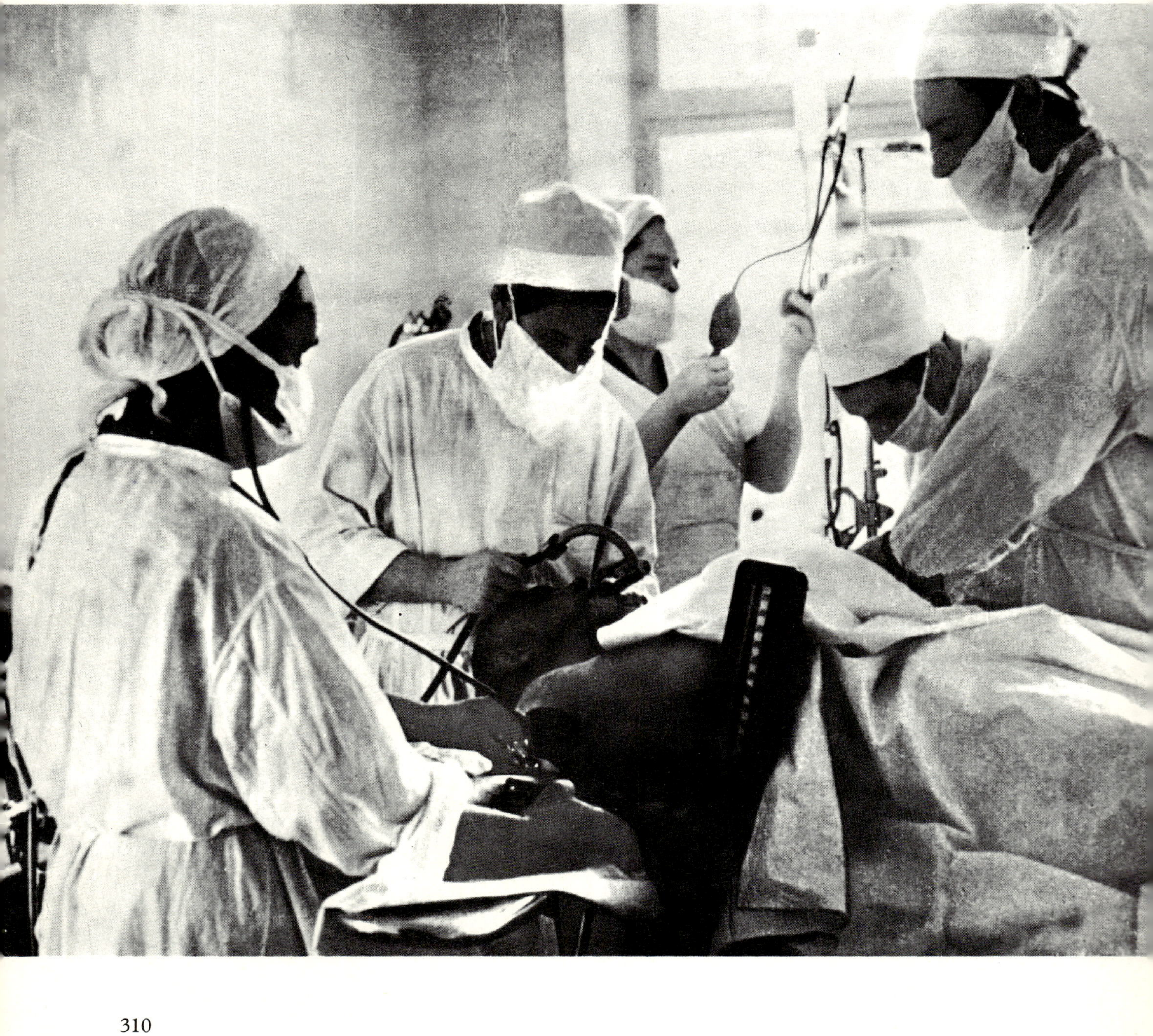

promotion of health and control of disease, especially communicable disease, is a common danger.

Healthy development of the child is of basic importance; the ability to live harmoniously in a changing total environment is essential to such development.

The extension to all peoples of the benefits of medical, psychological and related knowledge is essential to the fullest attainment of health.

Informed opinion and active co-operation on the part of the public are of the utmost importance in the improvement of the health of the people.

Governments have a responsibility for the health of their peoples which can be fulfilled only by the provision of adequate health and social measures.

These pages:
Revival of a man declared to be clinically 'dead', at a medical centre in Moscow.

Operation performed with the use of a microscope, in Hospital 67, Moscow.

Following pages:
Surgical operation on the heart by Professor Dogliotti, using cardiac bypass.

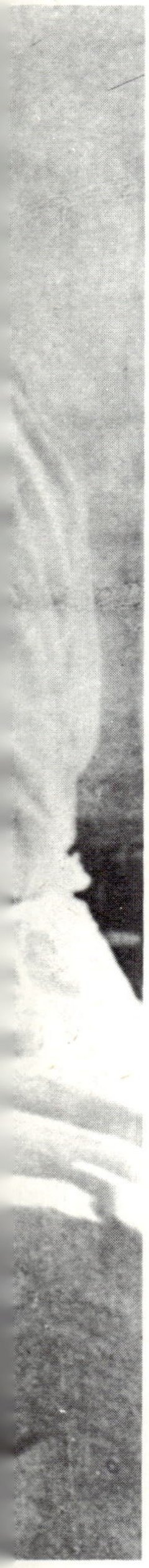

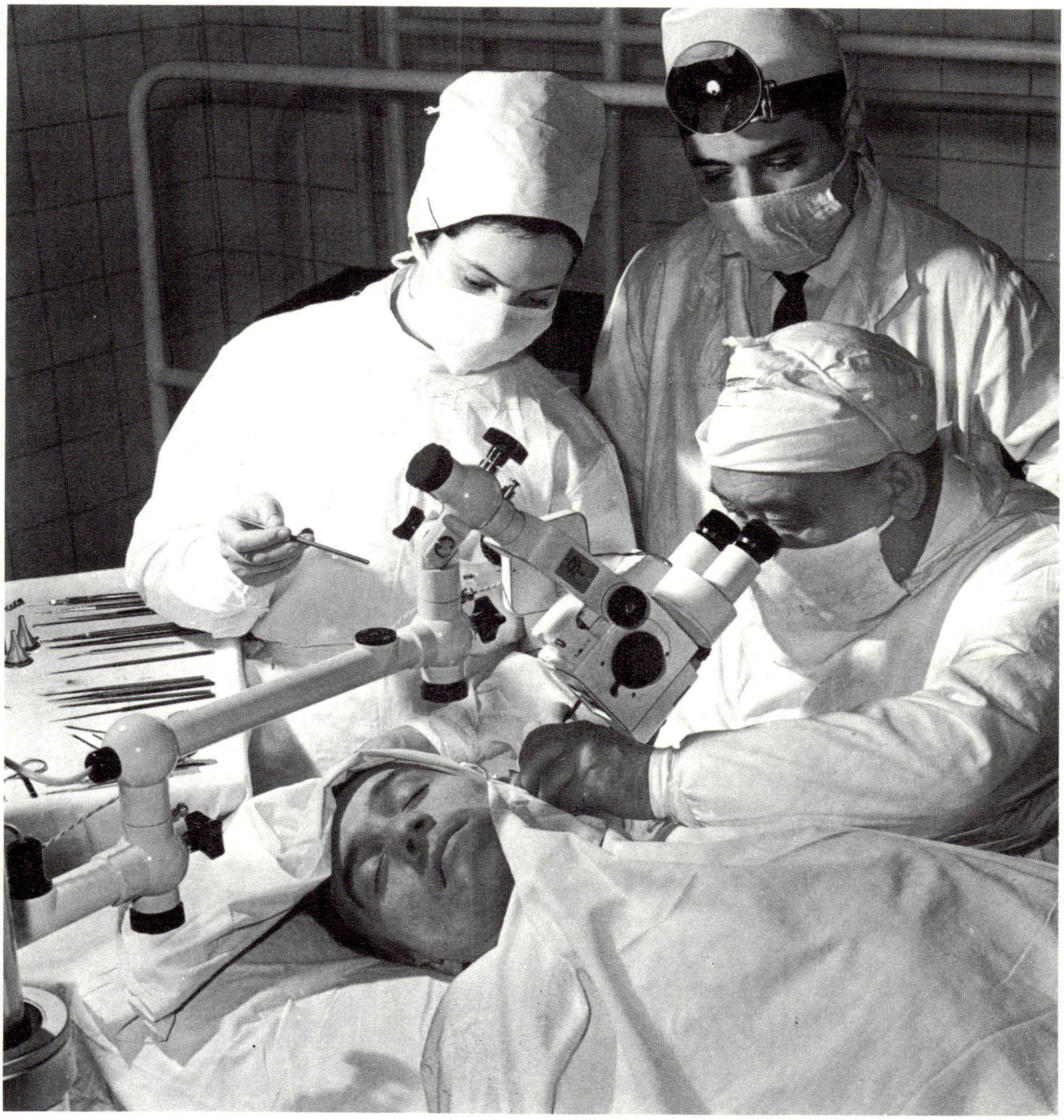

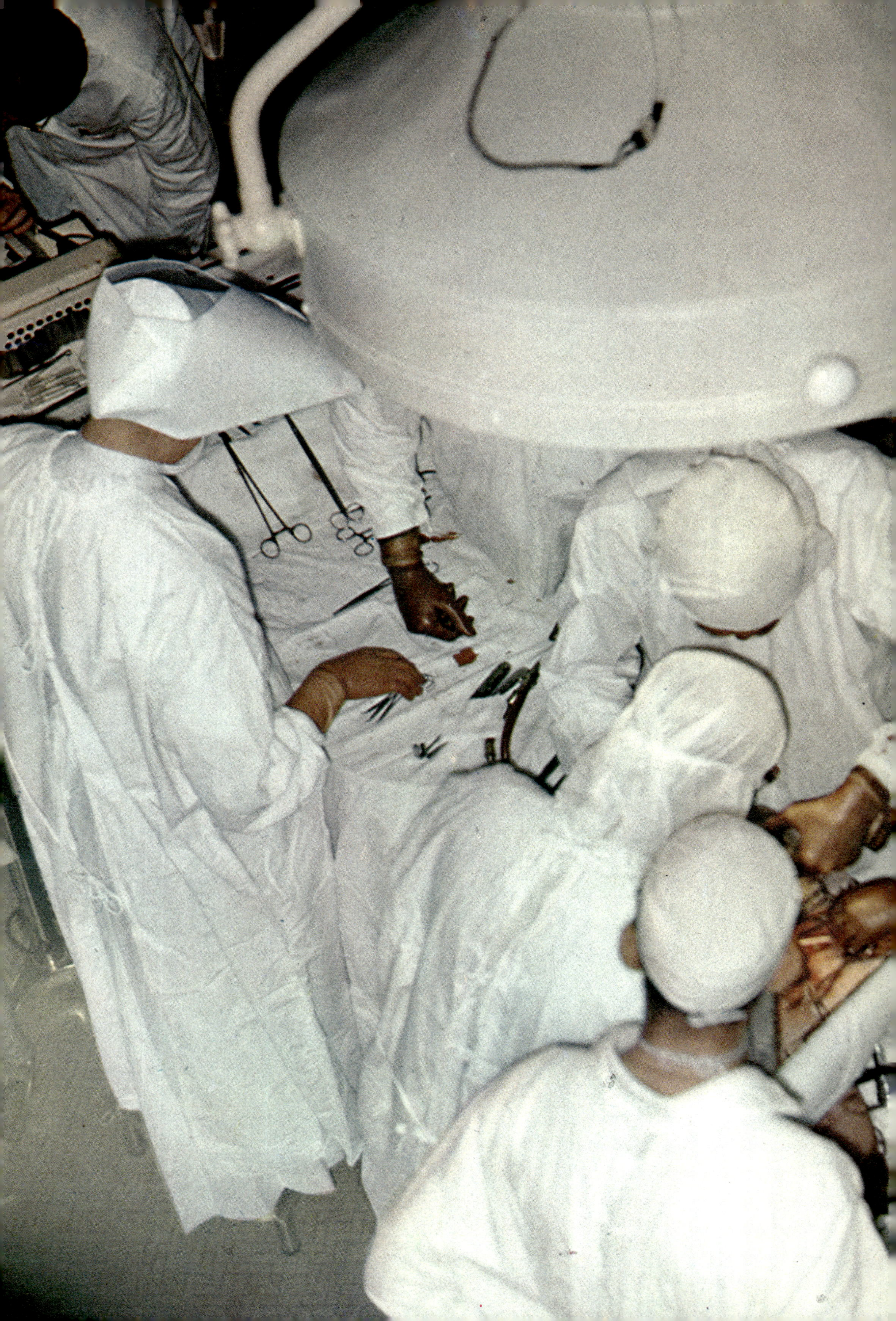

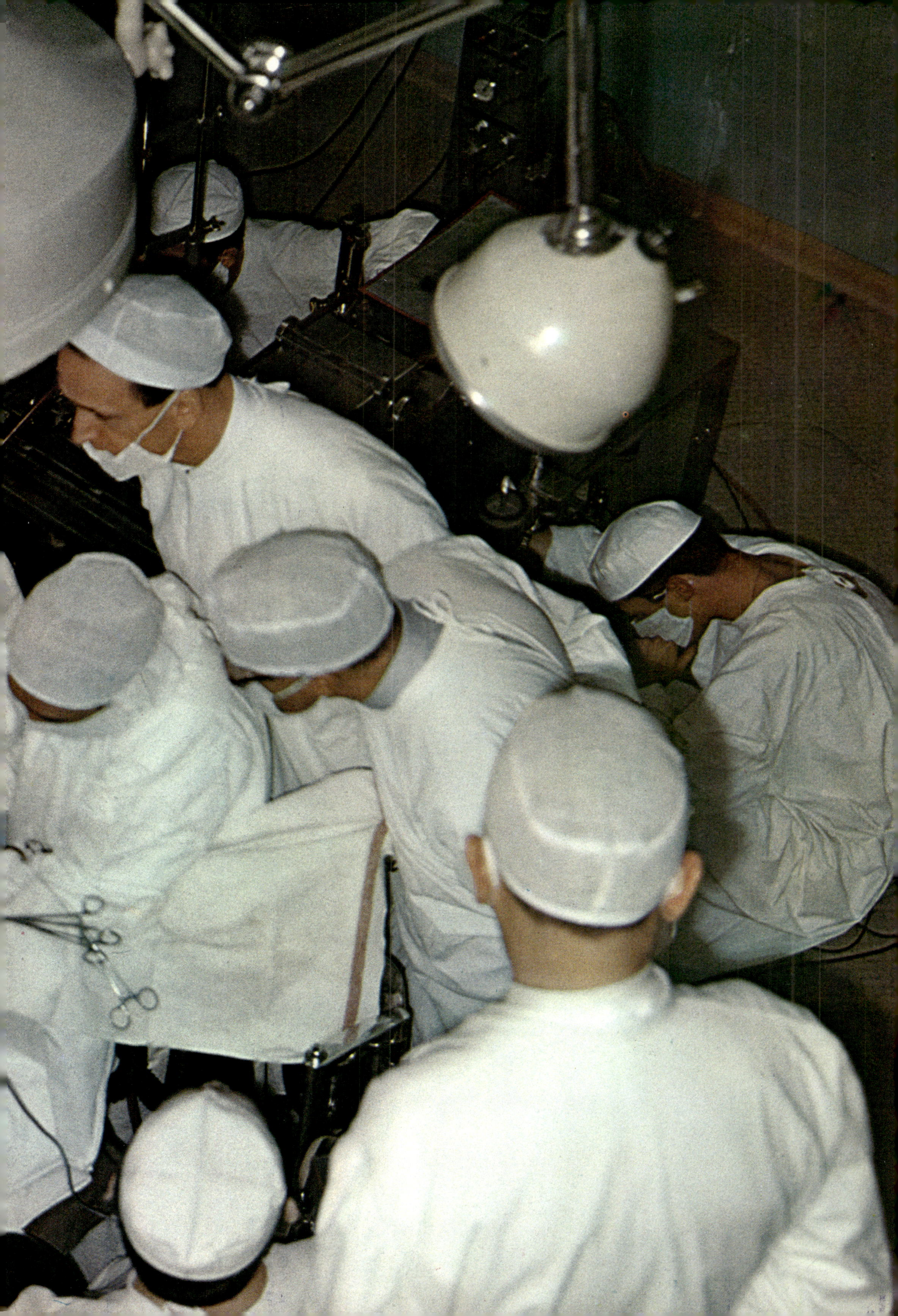

Medicine past and future

What is the value of medical history at the present time? What is the usefulness of a knowledge of medicine of the past to people of today? Before answering these questions it must be said that medical history remains largely separated from medical practice: medical historians are more often historians than practising doctors, and the training of most medical students, in Europe and America, generally ignores all but the most superficial excursions into the subject. Too often the new doctor leaves medical school in total ignorance of the evolution of his art and science, contemptuous of the mistakes of earlier generations of physicians and surgeons and at the same time half-blinded to new developments in medicine. To laymen, medical history must often seem of even less relevance to the present or the future.

Yet the inescapable truth–and the value of medical history is to remind one of it–is that today's medicine is something that has been built up over the centuries, succeeding eras seeing more or less important additions to the corpus of medical knowledge and practice. The significance of many past discoveries to the present time has been pointed out in this book. The humane and yet reserved doctor is the descendent on one hand of Hippocrates and Sydenham, and on the other, of the Aesculapian priests. His ability to diagnose disease starts with his taking a history from the patient: this is something that again stems from the ancients, from Hippocrates and Galen, and it is something which has nothing to do with scientific method. His clinical diagnostic methods, however, do belong to the age of science, and are the development of systems worked out in the eighteenth and nineteenth centuries by such people as Auenbrugger, Laënnec, and the Parisian and Queen Square neurologists. Already in the mid-twentieth century many of these procedures have become old-fashioned and supplanted by more modern techniques. Thus a very elaborate examination of the chest by the traditional practice of 'inspection, palpation, percussion and auscultation' is no longer needed, and the old methods are partly bypassed, because an equivalent or even a greater amount of information about the state of the lungs can be obtained very simply by X-raying the patient. New methods of pathological and chemical diagnosis have evolved, more rationally and less empirically based than the mediaeval practice of

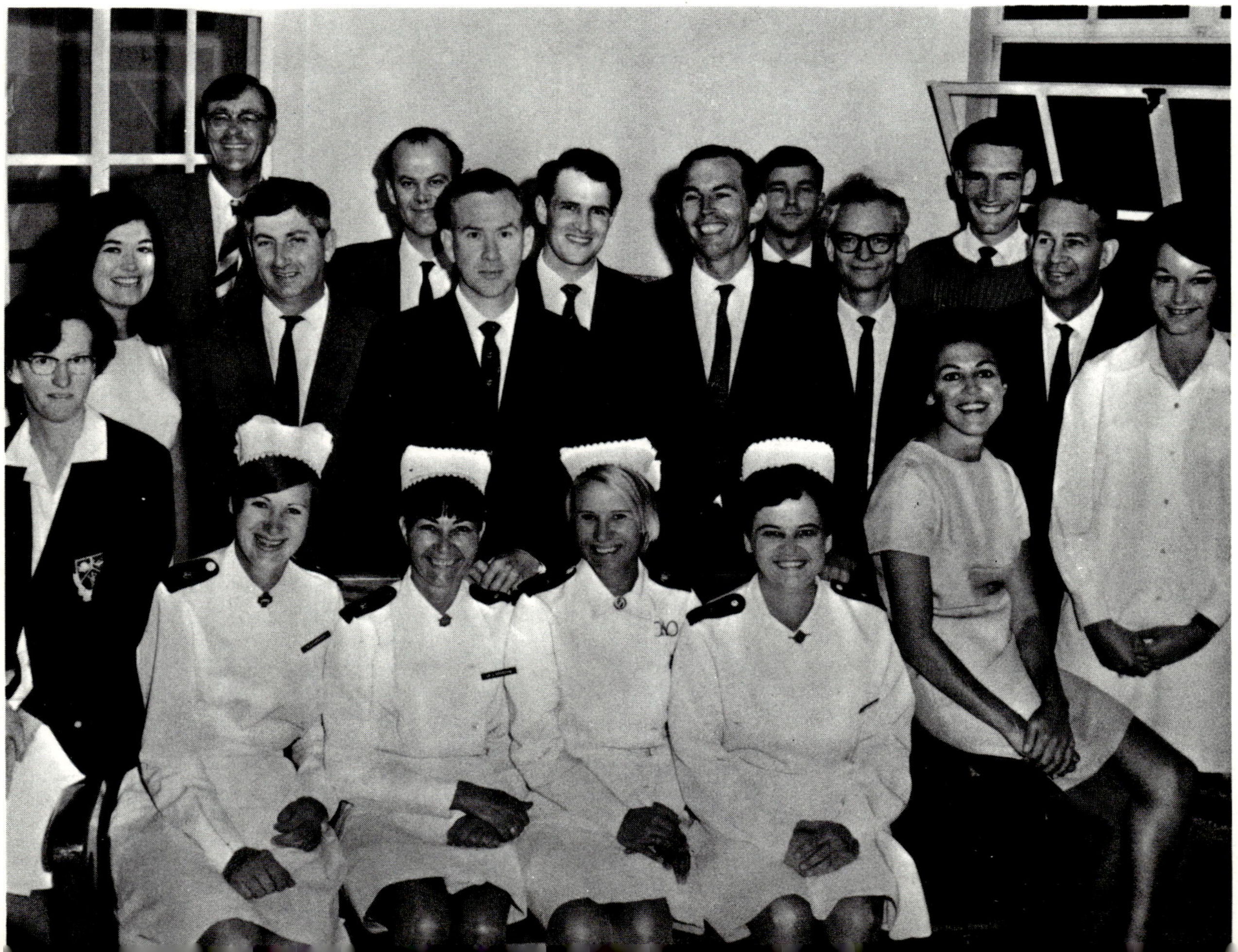

Dr. Christian Barnard (standing fourth from right) and his team at the Groote Schuur Hospital, Cape Town, who performed the first successful human heart transplant.

Great Britain. An artificial kidney machine designed for operation by the patient in his home.

urinoscopy but occupying nevertheless an equivalent position in medical science. In due course the innovations of today will be themselves largely succeeded, a number surviving as valuable incorporations into the evolving mass of medicine.

More than ever before in the past the doctor finds himself faced by problems of life and death. So many new life-saving remedies are available that these problems loom larger than ever. Now it seems possible that life can be prolonged well beyond normal not only by drugs but by the replacement of diseased organs by healthy ones. Kidney transplantation is well past the experimental stage. Heart transplantation is established, in technique at least, and when the difficulties imposed by the body's immune response have been overcome, this and liver replacement may be invaluable life-savers for a number of patients. The doctor, then, has to decide when to treat and when not to. The solution to this problem lies partly within history, and is a traditional one–the doctor's function through the ages has been to relieve suffering and to preserve lives. But today, with the advance of medicine, certain questions arise with increasing urgency. For example, is the prolongation of a useless or unhappy existence part of a doctor's duty? Many a difficult medical decision may depend upon the answer to this question, and such decisions will become more and more common as medicine continues to advance. In many hospitals from time to time patients with severe brain damage are kept 'alive' for long periods on machines which provide artificial respiration. But when the experience of the doctor tells him that there is no real hope of recovery, the question becomes inevitable–when should the machine be turned off?

Another lesson for today provided by medical history is that old remedies should not be discarded just because they are old, because this does not necessarily make them worthless. Drugs and methods of therapy come into use for a while and then fall out of fashion, sometimes to be revived years, decades or even centuries later. Ephedrine and acupuncture, two modern treatments, are part of ancient Chinese therapy. Colectomy, a modern operation for ulcerative colitis, was advocated (for different purposes) by the Victorian surgeon Arbuthnot Lane. What so often happens is that advance in the knowledge of the usefulness or otherwise of a remedy occurs not so much from research into the remedy as from a general advance of knowledge of medicine or the condition that is being treated. Thus a constant revision of ideas of therapy is necessary in the context of medicine as a whole.

Recent words of Kenneth Keele provide the conclusion to this book:

'In the past the connection between medicine and its history has often been tenuous. This is partly a result of its excessive localization into nations and continents. Times are changing. We can now reach any part of the globe in a matter of hours and make contact with medicine at all stages of its historical evolution. This is a condition of the present–and the future. More and more, therefore, will it become necessary to have some comprehension of the history of medicine as exemplified in all the countries of the world.'

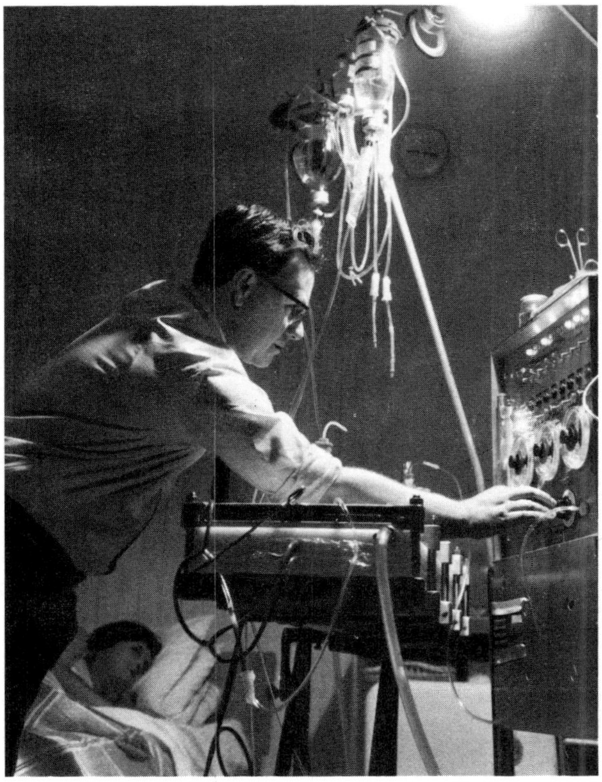

Picture Acknowledgments

The publishers wish to thank the following individuals and organisations for the use of their photographs in this book.
(The numbers refer to the page, the letters to the position on the page, reading across then down):
Alinari: 50/51, 56/57, 98; AME Archive: 12, 17a, 22a, 23, 25a, 28b, 31, 51a, 52a, 73, 109b, 124, 146, 178a, 194b, 222, 224, 240b, 261ab, 279, 280a, 284a, 287; Arborio Mella: 3, 6, 22/23, 24, 27c, 32b, 33ab, 42c, 48, 49, 50ab, 51b, 55, 59b, 62/63, 65, 66/67, 68/69, 70, 72, 75, 77, 78bc, 82b, 83, 85, 86, 87, 88, 89b, 90, 93, 105, 113, 116/117, 121, 122, 123b, 125, 130, 131b, 132a, 136, 140ab, 152, 157a, 158, 159, 166, 168ab, 169, 179, 180, 182b, 190ac, 192ab, 193abc, 196, 196/197, 198a-g, 201, 203ab, 210, 217, 225, 228b, 246/247, 247b, 258, 263, 270, 275, 278c, 285, 292, 294, 295, 297; Basle University Library: 164ab, 165; Berlin Museum of Ethnology: 14; Bertarelli Collection: 94ab, 95, 96/97, 99, 226, 233b, 242, 247a, 248, 252/253, 261c; Bettmann Archive: 216a, 244ab, 260b, 296; Bevilacqua: 16c, 27b, 27d, 29, 37, 52b, 53, 153, 195, 199, 204, 205, 223b, 228a, 230, 232, 271ab, 278b, 283, 284b, 301; Bibliothèque Nationale: 38, 39a, 40, 41, 42ab, 44, 45, 103, 106/107, 112, 114, 115a, 118ab, 119, 173, 174, 187a; Bodleian Library, Oxford: 9, 32a, 126, 127; British Museum: 20/21; W. Bruggmann: 19; Bulloz: 214; CEAM Archive: 25b, 26, 59a, 60, 61, 89a, 143ab, 161, 194a, 197ab, 207, 208, 236/237, 239, 249, 251, 266, 269bc; Centre de Photographie Médicale de l'Assistance Publique, Paris: 190b, 235, 256ab, 257, 259ab, 264a, 274, 286, 288b; Cinecolorfoto: 13ab; Elettra Cliché: 28a, 84, 92, 120b, 151, 188/189, 214/215, 220/221, 227, 265, 273; Fotofast: 36, 115b, 128/129, 134, 135, 150b, 156, 157b, 162, 163, 178b, 181, 182a, 184ab, 185, 187b, 213, 229; Fototeca EST: 109a, 120cd, 240a, 250b, 269a; Gernsheim Collection: 264b; Giraudon: 132b, 133; André Held: 100/101; Hans Hinz: 170/171; Hodder and Stoughton Ltd: 298; Kodansha Ltd: 17b, 30/31, 108; University of Leipzig: 27a; Louvre Museum: 242/243; Mansell: 238; MAS: 131c; Mercurio: 110/111, 144, 148/149, 167, 223a, 255, 277; National Hospital, London: 300; National Portrait Gallery: 200a; Novosti Agency: 299a, 305, 306, 307b, 308, 310, 311; Professor Olivecrona: 299b; Civic Museum, Padua: 131d; Paris Match: 200b; Pasotti: 14/15; Patellani: 290/291; Marcella Pedone: 79, 262ab; Photo B.N.: 288a; PIME: 47; Rassegna Medica Lepetit, Milan: 123ac; Reitberg Museum, von der Heydt Collection: 18b; Oscar Savio: 43ab, 76/77, 78a; Scala: 81, 104, 138/139, 147, 148, 150a, 154, 155, 175, 176/177, 191, 218/219, 302/303; Stickelmann: 160; Syndication International: 315; United Press International: 314; USIS: 280b, 289, 307a, 309; National Library, Vienna: 39b, 183a, 186ab, 216/217, 218; The Wellcome Trustees: 35, 172, 250a, 298; Institute of Culture, Worms: 186c.
We would also like to thank the British Medical Journal for permission to use the quotation from an article by K. D. Keele published 19th November, 1966.

INDEX